There is no question that this book will make a significant contribution to the field of psychological testing and assessment in South Africa. Such a book is long overdue and it should serve the field of psychology well into the future. I suspect that this will become a classic text in the field and will be used as a reference for graduate students and psychologists for many years to come.

Juvia P. Heuchert, Professor of Psychology, Allegheny College

Psychological Assessment in South Africa provides a good balance between conceptual and applied dimensions in psychological assessment, with specific emphasis on core considerations and principles derived from and applicable to the multicultural and multilingual context of South Africa. By virtue of their scope, foci, scholarly merit and contextual relevance, the themes addressed will appeal to a wide range of readers, including but not limited to students, academics and practitioners. The utility, cultural sensitivity and relevance of the assessment tools and techniques is central to the theory and practice of psychological assessment and this book offers a significant contribution to the extension and the advancement of knowledge in this domain.

Associate Professor Maria Damianova, Monash South Africa, a campus of Monash University Australia; Counselling and Educational Psychologist

Psychological Assessment IN SOUTH AFRICA

Research and Applications

Edited by Sumaya Laher and Kate Cockcroft

WITS UNIVERSITY PRESS

Wits University Press
1 Jan Smuts Avenue
Johannesburg
South Africa
www.witspress.co.za

First published 2013

ISBN 978-1-86814-578-2 (print)
ISBN 978-1-86814-579-9 (digital)

Edited by Karen Press
Cover design by Fly Creative
Layout and design by Baseline Publishing Services
Printed and bound by Paarl Media

Contents

Section Two: Personality and projective tests: conceptual and practical applications

Tables and figures

Acknowledgements

We would like to thank the following individuals and committees from the University of the Witwatersrand: the Dean of the Faculty of Humanities, Professor Tawana Kupe, the Assistant Dean of the Faculty of Humanities Research Committee, Professor Mark Leon, the Head of the School of Human and Community Development, Professor Maria Marchetti-Mercer, as well as the University of the Witwatersrand's Research Office, for their generous contributions towards the publication of this book. Professor Norman Duncan is also acknowledged for the significant role he played in ensuring the publication of this book.

We are also greatly indebted to many people who selflessly agreed to review a chapter, purely as an exercise in academic citizenship and as a contribution to a high standard of academic knowledge. We have listed their names below:

Dr Daleen Alexander (University of the Witwatersrand)
Dr Zaytoon Amod (University of the Witwatersrand)
Dr Maurice Aronstam (University of Pretoria)
Dr Katherine Bain (University of the Witwatersrand)
Dr Ronel Blom (Umalusi)
Dr Olaniyi Bojuwoye (University of the Western Cape)
Dr Marita Brink (Private Practitioner)
Dr Michelle Buchler (Centre for Education Policy Development)
Dr Nicolaas Claassen (Private Practitioner)
Dr Nicoleen Coetzee
Mr Patrick Connolly (Private Practitioner)
Dr Maria Damianova (Monash, South Africa)
Professor Marie de Beer (University of South Africa)
Dr Karina de Bruin (University of Johannesburg)
Dr Fiona Donald (University of the Witwatersrand)
Ms Renate Gericke (University of the Witwatersrand)
Dr Charmaine Gordon (Private Practitioner)
Ms Tanya Graham (University of the Witwatersrand)
Dr Kirston Greenop (Mindset South Africa)
Dr Salome Human Vogel (University of Pretoria)
Ms Celeste Joyce (Private Practitioner)
Mr Jan Knoetze (Rhodes University)
Professor Hennie Kriek (University of South Africa)
Dr Stacey Leibowitz-Levy (Private Practitioner)
Professor Marilyn Lucas (University of the Witwatersrand)
Ms Susan Malcolm-Smith (University of Cape Town)
Dr Macalane Malindi (North-West University)
Professor David Maree (University of Pretoria)
Professor Karen Milner (University of the Witwatersrand)
Professor Mokgadi Moletsane (University of the Western Cape)
Ms Sharon Moonsamy (University of the Witwatersrand)
Dr Reagan Murphy (Cork University, Ireland)

Professor Drienie Naude (North-West University)
Ms Ruby Patel (Rhodes University)
Mr Jarrod Payne (Millward Brown)
Dr Esther Price (University of the Witwatersrand)
Dr Cas Prinsloo (Human Sciences Research Council)
Mr Gregg Quy (TNS Research Surveys)
Ms Ilse Ruane (University of Pretoria)
Ms Alida Sandison (Nelson Mandela Metropolitan University)
Dr Vanessa Scherman (University of Pretoria)
Ms Enid Schutte (University of the Witwatersrand)
Mr Joseph Seabi (University of the Witwatersrand)
Dr Lee Senior (Private Practitioner)
Mr Ian Siemers (University of the Witwatersrand)
Professor Marius Stander (North-West University)
Dr Inette Taylor (Private Practitioner)
Dr Nicola Taylor (University of Johannesburg / Jopie van Rooyen & Partners)
Mr Tesfay Teferi (University of Eritrea)
Professor Andrew Thatcher (University of the Witwatersrand)
Professor Linda Theron (North-West University)
Mrs Nanette Tredoux (Psytech South Africa)
Professor Oliver Turnbull (University of Bangor, Wales)
Dr Rene van Eeden (University of South Africa)
Dr Clifford van Ommen (Massey University, New Zealand)
Ms Liesl Vogt (Private Practitioner)
Dr Jacki Watts (Private Practitioner)
Mrs H Williams (North-West University)

Acronyms and abbreviations

15FQ	Fifteen Factor Questionnaire
15FQ+	Fifteen Factor Questionnaire Plus
16PF	Sixteen Personality Factor Questionnaire
16PF5	Sixteen Personality Factor Questionnaire Fifth Edition
16PF-SA92	Sixteen Personality Factor Questionnaire – South African 1992 version
ABE	Adult Basic Education
ABET	Adult Basic Education and Training
ABLSA	Augmented Baltimore Longitudinal Study of Aging
ACL	Adjective Construct Checklist
ADHD	Attention Deficit/Hyperactivity Disorder
AIDS	Acquired Immunodeficiency Syndrome
ANA	Annual National Assessments
ANCOVA	Analysis of Covariance
ANOVA	Analysis of Variance
APA	American Psychological Association
APIL	(Conceptual) Ability, Processing of Information, and Learning
ARICD	Association for Research in Infant and Child Development
ART	antiretroviral treatment
ASB	Aptitude Test for School Beginners
ASCT	Attachment Story Completion Task
BAI	Beck Anxiety Inventory
BB-CAB	Broad Band Competency Assessment Battery
BDI-II	Beck Depression Inventory-II
BEE	black economic empowerment
BHS	Beck Hopelessness Scale
BITE	Bulimia Investigatory Test Edinburgh
BTI	Basic Traits Inventory
BULIT	Bulimia Test
CAS	Cognitive Assessment System
CAT	Computerised Adaptive Testing (chapter 10)
CAT	Children's Apperception Test (chapters 24, 25)
CAT	computer-administered testing system (chapter 29)
CAT-S	Beginners Children Apperception Test – Supplement
CDQ	Career Development Questionnaire
CFI	comparative fit index
CFT	Concept Formation Test
CHC	Cattell-Horn-Carroll
cm	centimetre
COL	Curve of Learning
COPE	Coping Orientations to Problems Experienced
CORE-OM	Clinical Outcomes in Routine Evaluation – Outcome Measure
CPAI	Chinese Personality Assessment Inventory
CPAI-2	Cross-Cultural Personality Assessment Inventory – 2

CPP	Cognitive Process Profile
CTT	classical test theory
DA	dynamic assessment
DAM	Draw-A-Man Test
DAP	Draw-A-Person Test
DAP: IQ	Draw-A-Person Intellectual Ability Test for Children, Adolescents and Adults
DAP-SPED	Draw-A-Person Screening Procedure for Emotional Disturbance
DAT	Differential Aptitude Test
DET	Department of Education and Training
DIF	differential item functioning
DSM	*Diagnostic and Statistical Manual of Mental Disorders*
EAC	experimental astronomy curriculum
EAT	Eating Attitudes Test
ECD	Early Child Development
EDI	Early Development Instrument
EDI	Eating Disorders Inventory (chapter 22)
EFA	Education For All
EI	emotional intelligence (chapter 16)
EQ	emotional intelligence (chapter 17)
FAS	Foetal Alcohol Syndrome
FCI	Fluid-Crystallised Index
FDGRS	Family Drawing Global Rating Scale
FET	Further Education and Training
FFM	Five-Factor Model
FSIQ	Full Scale Intelligence Quotient
g	the general intelligence factor / general intelligence
GAB	General Adaptability Battery
GDM	Group Dynamic Modification
GMDS	Griffiths Mental Development Scales
GMDS-ER	Griffiths Mental Development Scales – Extended Revised
GQ	General Quotient
GSAT-CAT	General Scholastic Aptitude Test (adaptive version)
GTISA	Group Test for Indian South Africans
HFD	Human Figure Drawing
HFDT	Human Figure Drawing Test
HIV	Human Immunodeficiency Virus
HOR	House of Representatives
HPCSA	Health Professions Council of South Africa
HR	Human Resources
HSRC	Human Sciences Research Council
HTP	House-Tree-Person Test
IAC	Initial Assessment Consultation
ICC	item characteristic curve
ICD	*International Classification of Mental and Behavioural Disorders*

ICG	Inventory of Complicated Grief
IE	Instrumental Enrichment
ImPACT	Immediate Postconcussion Assessment and Cognitive Testing
IPAT	Institute for Personality and Ability Testing
IPER	Institute for Psychological and Edumetric Research
IQ	intelligence quotient
IRT	item response theory
ISB	Incomplete Sentence Blank
ITC	International Test Commission
JPA	*Journal of Psychology in Africa*
JSAIS	Junior South African Individual Scales
K-ABC	Kaufman Assessment Battery for Children
KABC-II	Kaufman Assessment Battery for Children – Second Edition
KDS	Kinetic Drawing System
KFD	Kinetic Family Drawing
KR-20	Kuder-Richardson Formula 20
KSD	Kinetic School Drawing
KTT	Knowledge Transfer Test
LCI	Locus of Control Inventory
LPAD	Learning Potential Assessment Device
LPCAT	Learning Potential Computerised Adaptive Test
LRI	Life Roles Inventory
LSAS	large-scale assessment studies
MACI	Millon Adolescent Clinical Inventory
MAPI	Millon Adolescent Personality Inventory
MBA	Master of Business Administration
MBMD	Millon Behavioural Medicine Diagnostic
MBTI	Myers-Briggs Type Indicator
MCCI	Millon College Counselling Inventory
MCI	Mild Cognitive Impairment
MCMI-III	Millon Clinical Multiaxial Inventory – III
MIPS-Revised	Millon Index of Personality Styles – Revised
MLE	mediated learning experience
MMPI	Minnesota Multiphasic Personality Inventory
M-PACI	Millon Pre-Adolescent Clinical Inventory
MPC	Mental Processing Composite
MPI	Mental Processing Index
MSCI	My System of Career Influences
MTBI	mild traumatic brain injury
NARA	Neale Analysis of Reading Ability – Revised
NEO-FFI	Neuroticism–Extraversion–Openness Five-Factor Inventory
NEO-PI-R	Revised NEO Personality Inventory
NIPR	National Institute for Personnel Research
NQF	National Qualifications Framework
NSAGT	New South African Group Test
NSAIS	New South African Individual Scale

OPPro	Occupational Personality Profile
OPQ	Occupational Personality Questionnaire
PACL	Personality Adjective Check List
PAI	People Assessment in Industry
PASS	Planning, Attention, Simultaneous and Successive
PDS	Post-traumatic Diagnostic Scale
PIB	Potential Index Battery
PINS	*Psychology in Society*
PIQ	Performance Intelligence Quotient
POI	Perceptual Organisation Index
PPA	Personal Profile Assessment
PPG	Paper-and-Pencil-Games
PRI	Perceptual Reasoning Index
PSI	Processing Speed Index (chapters 2, 3)
PSI	person separation index (chapter 16)
PTCI	Post-traumatic Cognitions Inventory
PTSD	post-traumatic stress disorder
RAPM	Raven's Advanced Progressive Matrices
RCPM	Raven's Coloured Progressive Matrices
RCS	Rorschach Comprehensive System
RISB	Rotter Incomplete Sentence Test
RMSEA	root mean square error of approximation
ROI	return on investment
RPL	Recognition of Prior Learning
RSPM	Raven's Standard Progressive Matrices
SACMEQ	Southern African Consortium for Monitoring Education Quality
SACNA	South African Clinical Neuropsychological Association
SAJBM	*South African Journal of Business Management*
SAJHRM	*South African Journal of Human Resource Management*
SAJIP	*South African Journal of Industrial Psychology*
SAJP	*South African Journal of Psychology*
SANDF	South African National Defence Force
SAPI	South African Personality Inventory
SAT	Senior Aptitude Test
SAWAIS	South African Wechsler Adult Intelligence Scale
SCARED	Screen for Child Anxiety and Related Emotional Disorders
SCL-90	Symptom Checklist-90
SCOR-R	Social Cognition and Object Relations Scale – Revised
SDS	Self-Directed Search
SEE	standard error/s of estimate
SEM	standard error/s of measurement
SEM	structural equation modelling (chapter 20)
SHL	Saville and Holdsworth Limited

SIOPSA	Society for Industrial and Organisational Psychology of South Africa
SSAIS	Senior South African Individual Scales
SSAIS-R	Senior South African Individual Scales – Revised
STF	Systems Theory Framework
TAT	Thematic Apperception Test
TRAM	Transfer, Automatisation and Memory
UK	United Kingdom
US	United States
USA	United States of America
VCI	Verbal Comprehension Index
VIQ	Verbal Intelligence Quotient
VS	Values Scale
WAIS	Wechsler Adult Intelligence Scales
WAIS-III	Wechsler Adult Intelligence Scale – Third Edition
WAIS-IV	Wechsler Adult Intelligence Scale – Fourth Edition
WAIS-R	Wechsler Adult Intelligence Scale revised version
WDRB	Woodcock Diagnostic Reading Battery
WISC	Wechsler Intelligence Scale for Children
WISC-III	Wechsler Intelligence Scale for Children – Third Edition
WISC-IV	Wechsler Intelligence Scale for Children – Revised Fourth Edition
WISC-R	Wechsler Intelligence Scale for Children – Revised
WJ-III	Woodcock Johnson Tests of Achievement – Third Edition
WJ-R	Woodcock Johnson Tests of Achievement – Revised
WMI	Working Memory Index
XBAI	isiXhosa translations of the Beck Anxiety Inventory
XBDI-II	isiXhosa translations of the Beck Depression Inventory-II
XBHS	isiXhosa translations of the Beck Hopelessness Scale
ZAD	zone of actual development
ZPD	zone of proximal development

1 Contextualising psychological assessment in South Africa

S. Laher and K. Cockcroft

Psychological assessment in South Africa is a controversial topic primarily, but not exclusively, because of its links to South Africa's troubled past. The history of South Africa is a chequered one, characterised by ethnic and racial interaction, integration and conflict (Heuchert, Parker, Stumpf & Myburgh, 2000). The tribal groups that occupied the country prior to the arrival of white settlers in 1650 followed patterns of merging and splitting that were similar to those in most other parts of the world. Some groups were formed voluntarily and others by conquest and subjugation. In 1652, the ancestors of present-day Afrikaans-speaking South Africans arrived. They were originally mainly of Dutch ancestry, and later also of German and French ancestry. Slaves from the former Dutch colonies in the East (mainly the territories now forming part of Malaysia) were also brought to the Cape at this time. In 1834 all slaves were emancipated. Around the same time a common language developed amongst the groups in the Cape consisting of a mixture of words from the Malay, Khoisan, Portuguese, French and Bantu languages, but with Dutch as a base. Towards the late 19th century this language was recognised as Afrikaans. Although the former slaves spoke the same language (Afrikaans) as the white settlers, after 1948 they were separated into two groups based on skin colour – namely, white Afrikaners and coloured Afrikaners. The other main white group in South Africa consisted of English-speaking South Africans who arrived in the early 1800s with the aim of 'settling the frontier' (Heuchert et al., 2000, p.113).

In the 1860s, British settlers recruited indentured labourers from India primarily to man the sugar, tea and coffee plantations in the Natal region. These labourers were promised good wages and the right to settle as free men after five years. The failure to implement the freedom policies for Indians led to Gandhi forming the Natal Indian Congress, the first mass political organisation in South Africa. At the same time, members of the Indian merchant class also came to South Africa and were instrumental in setting up trade in the then Transvaal region of the country. Even though this merchant class had more freedom than the indentured Indian labourers and Malay former slaves, they were still regarded as an inferior group by the white population. Together with the indigenous South African tribes, coloureds and Indians were classed as a 'black' group. Relationships between the white Afrikaners and white English-speaking South Africans were tense – so much so that two wars were fought between the two groups. However, they were united in their efforts to subjugate black South Africans (Heuchert et al., 2000).

In 1948 the National Party, which was the dominant political party at the time, instituted a formal system of racial segregation called apartheid. Apartheid ensured the reservation of social, economic and political privilege for white South Africans, while black South Africans (referred to as 'non-whites') were denied access to basic material resources, opportunities and freedom. This divide-and-rule tactic also created further social stratification within the black population. South African Indians, particularly the merchant classes, had a higher socio-economic status, followed by coloureds, while the section of the population most discriminated against was the indigenous African tribal groups. While opportunities and freedom for Indians and coloureds were curtailed, these groups had better access to infrastructure and basic resources such as water, electricity and housing, whereas the indigenous groups were denied even this. Indigenous African groups were encouraged or forced to accept a tribal identity by means of a series of policies that separated and removed people to rural 'homelands' such as Bophuthatswana, Venda and Transkei. Urban residents were separated by racial classification and forced to live in separate residential areas. Those urban areas set aside for indigenous Africans were very small, with little or no infrastructure, resulting in further oppression of this group of people (Heuchert et al., 2000).

The role of psychological assessment within this turbulent history was equally contentious. According to Claassen (1997), psychological testing came to South Africa through Britain, and the development of psychological tests in South Africa followed a similar pattern to that in the USA. There was a difference, however. South African tests were developed in a context of unequal distribution of resources as a result of apartheid policies. According to Nzimande (1995), assessment practices in South Africa were used to justify the exploitation of black labour and to deny black people access to education and economic resources. Sehlapelo and Terre Blanche (1996) make the similar point that tests were used in South Africa to determine who would gain access to economic and educational opportunities.

Under apartheid, job preference was given to white individuals and a job reservation policy was put in place that ensured employment for whites. Psychometric testing and psychological assessment were misused to support this policy; for example, tests that were developed and standardised on educated white South Africans were administered to illiterate, uneducated or poorly educated black South Africans, and the results were used as justification for job reservation and preference. They were also used to indicate the superiority of the white intellect over the black intellect, and thus to further justify the logic of the apartheid system. This practice resulted in a general mistrust of psychological assessment, and more specifically psychometric testing, amongst the black population in South Africa (Foxcroft & Davies, 2008; Nzimande, 1995; Sehlapelo & Terre Blanche, 1996).

It is important to note that discriminatory practices in psychological testing were not exclusively a product of the apartheid regime. As early as 1929, Fick was conducting research on black children using the Army Beta Test, which was standardised for use on white children. The black children performed noticeably more poorly on the test than the white children. Fick (1929) initially concluded that environmental and educational factors were primary factors in understanding the poor performance of black children. Ten years later, he opined that differences in nonverbal intelligence tests were more likely due to innate differences between blacks and whites (Fick, 1939). However, the Interdepartmental Committee on Native Education (1936) released a report that highlighted the irregular assessment practice of using a test normed on white people to assess black individuals.

Also prior to the advent of apartheid, the National Institute for Personnel Research (NIPR) was established under the leadership of Simon Biesheuvel. The institute focused largely on tests which could identify the occupational suitability of black individuals who had very little or no formal education. Biesheuvel (1943) argued that black individuals were not familiar with the content of items on tests or with the type of test material used, and so he introduced the concept of 'adaptability testing' (Biesheuvel, 1949) and developed the General Adaptability Battery (GAB).

While the NIPR focused on developing tests for industry, the Institute for Psychological and Edumetric Research (IPER) developed tests for the educational and clinical spheres. These two bodies dominated the field of psychological assessment from the 1950s to the late 1980s, when both divisions were incorporated into the Human Sciences Research Council (HSRC). The HSRC specialised in developing local measures. This was necessary primarily because of the sanctions imposed by other countries on South African access to their test materials. Although the work done by the HSRC is often criticised, it needs to be recognised that it was one of the most productive agencies for psychological assessment in South Africa and, in a number of ways, created the foundation on which the field stands today.

The release of Nelson Mandela in 1990 and the first democratic election in 1994 marked a turning point in South African history. The system of apartheid had failed, and a system that promoted mutual respect, democracy, freedom of expression and transparency was developed and legislated in a very progressive Constitution. Since 1994, South Africa has experienced rapid transformation in all spheres – social, political and economic. In this climate, it was vital that past inequalities be redressed and that a way forward be found that subscribed to the country's new-found democratic identity.

Psychology, particularly psychometrics and assessment, had played a controversial role in the previous political dispensation of the country and there now arose a pressing need for research and practice in the field to redress the negative effects of these practices. Around this time, the HSRC was restructured and the unit devoted to testing and assessment was repositioned. HSRC tests, as well as international tests such as the Sixteen Personality Factor Questionnaire (16PF) for which the HSRC held copyright in South Africa, were sold to private organisations such as Jopie van Rooyen and Partners, Saville and Holdsworth

Limited (SHL), Psytech and Mindmusik. These organisations took over the test distribution, adaptation and development role.

At the turn of the millennium, South African psychologists were more aware than ever of the need to create instruments or utilise pre-existing instruments in a fair and unbiased manner (Abrahams & Mauer, 1999a; 1999b; Foxcroft, Paterson, Le Roux & Herbst, 2004; Laher, 2007; 2008; 2011; Meiring, 2007; Nel, 2008; Sehlapelo & Terre Blanche, 1996; Taylor & De Bruin, 2006; Van Eeden & Mantsha, 2007). This shift in consciousness was strongly linked to legislation promulgated in Section 8 of the Employment Equity Act No. 55 of 1998 which stipulated that '[p]sychological testing and other similar assessments are prohibited unless the test or assessment being used (a) has been scientifically shown to be valid and reliable; (b) can be applied fairly to all employees; and (c) is not biased against any employee or group'. Unlike other countries where issues of bias and fairness are addressed by the codes of conduct of professional organisations of psychologists, in South Africa the importance of fair and unbiased testing and assessment was incorporated into national law (Van de Vijver & Rothmann, 2004).

The value of psychological testing remains a contested one in South Africa (Foxcroft, 2011). Its critics see it as being of limited value for culturally diverse populations (Foxcroft, 1997; Nzimande, 1995; Sehlapelo & Terre Blanche, 1996). Others argue that, regardless of its flaws, testing remains more reliable and valid than any of the limited number of alternatives. Since testing plays a crucial role within assessment internationally, proponents suggest that the focus be on valid and reliable tests for use within multicultural and multilingual societies (Plug in Foxcroft, 1997).

South Africa is 18 years into democracy and it is essential to determine whether the field of psychological assessment has found a way to address these criticisms. Many academics and practitioners have been extremely active in the discipline of psychological assessment. However, although a substantial portion of this work has been presented at various local and international conferences, it has not always been published and is therefore not widely available. Thus, one of the aims of this book is to collate existing research on commonly used measures and assessment practices so that practitioners and researchers can make informed decisions about their usage with local populations.

Since the 1990s, there have been several excellent and useful textbooks published on psychological assessment, but these tend to be targeted at an introductory level for undergraduate students and, in some cases, for specialist student groups (see Foxcroft & Roodt, 2008; Huysamen, 1996; Kaliski, 2006; Moerdyk, 2009). There is no South African text that approaches the complex phenomenon of psychological assessment in a more in-depth, critical manner. Having taught psychological assessment as a subject at postgraduate level for a number of years, and with our collective experience in the field, we conceptualised this book as a text that would bring together the range of work on psychological assessment in South Africa currently available.

Our aim is to provide an accessible text that gives a comprehensive and critical overview of the psychological tests most commonly used in South Africa, as well as of research conducted on these instruments. Strauss, Sherman and Spreen (2006) state that a working knowledge of tests without the corresponding knowledge of the psychometric properties and the research that accompanies their use renders us inadequate as practitioners. Thus, we hope that this book will provide readers with an understanding of critical issues relevant to psychological test use in the South African context, including the strengths and weaknesses of psychological tests that have been identified based on empirical research.

Further, we felt it was valuable to present a few alternative approaches to the more traditional views of psychological assessment, some of which have a distinctly South African flavour, such as the chapter on Recognition of Prior Learning (RPL) as a way of evaluating an individual's acquired learning and skills. In addition to its local relevance, the book interrogates the current Eurocentric and Western cultural hegemonic practices that dominate the field of psychological assessment and engages in international debates in psychological theory and assessment.

In compiling this book, we examined past issues of the *South African Journal of Psychology* and the *South African Journal of Industrial Psychology*, as well as some issues of *Psychology in Society* and the *Journal of Psychology in Africa*, to establish potential assessment areas and tests currently in use in South Africa, as well as to identify key individuals working in the field. The HSRC needs survey published in 2004 (see Foxcroft et al., 2004) was also a useful source of information. In addition to this, we examined conference programmes in order to locate those who were working in the field of psychological assessment. Invitations to submit abstracts for this book were sent to all individuals identified in this way. Following this, a general call to submit abstracts for the book was sent to all heads of local psychology departments. The chapters presented in this book represent the culmination of this effort.

When authors were invited to contribute to the book, we were careful not to impose too rigid a structure on the format, rather allowing each author to find the structure that best matched their particular chapter focus. Thus, the reader will note slight variations in presentation across the chapters. Furthermore, since the book is intended to be a specialist research text, primarily for postgraduate and professional use, the chapters read more like research articles than textbook chapters. Each chapter addresses significant and sophisticated arguments, and because they are written by local experts in the field who are strong supporters of their fields or instruments, the arguments may not always be evenly balanced. Nonetheless, most chapters maintain a critical focus and the final judgement is left up to the reader.

The chapters form natural groupings into three sections. Sections One and Two focus on particular psychological instruments. The chapters in these sections each provide a brief introduction to the instrument, including its history, development and psychometric properties. This is typically followed by a detailed critical examination of the instrument in the South African context, incorporating local research. These chapters emphasise the applied, practical nature of assessment, as well as the challenges inherent in assessment within a particular area or domain. The first two sections also include more generalist chapters pertaining to particular assessment methodologies, such as projective techniques and dynamic assessment. Sections One and Two also, for the most part, address assessment from traditional perspectives. Although dynamic assessment is addressed in Section One, and many of the chapters in the first two sections identify progressive ways in which the tests can be used effectively in South Africa, these sections should be supplemented by the chapters in Section Three that offer a broader perspective. This final section is a collation of chapters that highlight issues pertinent to the domain of psychological assessment, but which could not be accommodated within the areas highlighted in the previous two sections – for example, questions of ethics and computerised testing. Many of the chapters in this section go beyond the boundaries of what is traditionally conceptualised as psychological assessment, as the reader is encouraged to think about what constitutes psychological assessment, and to consider innovative ways of addressing the challenges facing assessment practitioners in South Africa. Each of the sections of the book is outlined in detail below.

Section One: Cognitive tests: conceptual and practical applications

Cognitive tests are still largely viewed with suspicion in South Africa as a result of their past misuse to enforce and support divisive racial apartheid practices. We need to move beyond this thinking and understand how these tests can benefit society. Consequently, this section details both locally and internationally developed tests of cognitive processes, together with relevant research that has been done on these measures. The section includes discussions of the Wechsler tests, which are widely considered to be the 'gold standard' in intelligence testing (Ivnik, Smith & Cerhan, 1992). In their chapters on the Wechsler Intelligence Scale for Children – Revised Fourth Edition (WISC-IV) and the Wechsler Adult Intelligence Scale – Third Edition (WAIS-III), Shuttleworth-Edwards and colleagues stress the need for, and describe the process of, obtaining preliminary normative data on these tests for South Africans. Given the educational inequalities still pervasive in South African society, these authors highlight quality of education as an important variable along which research samples should be stratified and which should be considered when conducting and interpreting intelligence quotient (IQ) assessments.

Although the norms for local IQ tests are both outdated and inappropriate for all South Africans, we have included a discussion of these tests as they are still widely used. Consequently, the Senior South African Individual Scales – Revised (SSAIS-R) is presented in its own chapter, together with the (limited) research on its use. Theron, in her chapter on the Junior South African Individual Scales (JSAIS), provides considerable and valuable tips on using the test qualitatively to comment on various aspects of the child's readiness to cope with formal schooling. She points out how the test can be informative in providing insight regarding the child's level of resilience and coping. Read this chapter together with that of Amod and Heafield on school readiness assessment and you are likely to have a balanced view of methods used to determine readiness for school entry and to identify preschool children who may benefit from additional stimulation programmes, learning support or retention.

This section of the book demonstrates that there is a range of conceptualisations of intelligence and how it should be measured. The traditional, static approaches to intelligence presented at the outset of this section have been widely criticised as reflecting only Western, Eurocentric, middle-class values and attitudes (Nell, 1999). Against the background of increased demand for nondiscriminatory assessment procedures, both locally and internationally, dynamic assessment has been proposed as a fairer assessment methodology that views intelligence as changeable and grants the testee the opportunity to demonstrate how effectively she or he can take up instruction. The chapter by Amod and Seabi on dynamic assessment presents some of the ways in which this approach may be beneficial to South African assessment practice. De Beer takes this issue further in her chapter on the Learning Potential Computerised Adaptive Test (LPCAT), which she has developed as a formal measure of learning potential that evaluates not only an individual's present level of performance, but also their potential levels of performance if relevant learning opportunities can be provided. Similarly, the chapter by T. Taylor on the (Conceptual) Ability, Processing of Information and Learning (APIL) test and Transfer, Automatisation and Memory tests (TRAM-1 and TRAM-2) shows how these learning potential tests can be employed to assess how a person copes with novel problems under standardised conditions. Given the unequal educational and employment conditions available to many South Africans, these tests represent a much fairer approach to making occupational decisions about individuals.

In addition to dynamic assessment, criticisms of traditional intelligence tests and their theoretical bases have resulted in several additional conceptualisations of intelligence. Among them are the Planning, Attention, Simultaneous and Successive (PASS) cognitive processing model proposed by Naglieri and Das (1988). This section includes a chapter on the Cognitive Assessment System (CAS) (discussed by Amod in chapter 8) which developed from this theory. The CAS differs from traditional measures in that it was designed to evaluate the cognitive processes underlying general intellectual functioning and is purportedly less influenced by verbal abilities and acquired knowledge. As such, it is likely to be a vital tool in ensuring equitable assessment procedures.

One of the most influential and more recent models of intelligence is that of Cattell-Horn-Carroll (CHC), which emphasises several broad classes of abilities at the higher level (for example, fluid ability (*Gf*), crystallised intelligence (*Gc*), short-term memory, long-term storage and retrieval, and processing speed) as well as a number of primary factors at the lower level. The CHC framework is the preferred interpretation model to be used when assessing functioning on the Kaufman Assessment Battery for Children (K-ABC), and is discussed by Greenop, Rice and De Sousa in chapter 7. Like the CAS, the K-ABC was designed to measure how children receive and process information, and to outline their cognitive strengths and weaknesses, and thus represents a deviation from the traditional IQ approach.

The reader may notice that this section does not include any chapter specifically addressing the assessment of nonverbal intelligence. It is important to acknowledge the value of such measures, particularly in cross-cultural contexts, where language may be a barrier to optimal cognitive performance. Considerable research has been conducted using the Raven's Progressive Matrices in South Africa (see Cockcroft and Israel, 2011 for a brief review). These are useful for individuals whose test performance may be confounded by language, hearing or motor impairments, or educational disadvantage. While not culture-free, they are more culture-fair than traditional IQ tests.

It would have been remiss not to include discussion of some measures of developmental assessment in this section. The chapter by Jacklin and Cockcroft on the Griffiths Mental Development Scales (GMDS), one of the most popular developmental tests used locally, is a valuable compendium of the local, and often unpublished, research done on these scales. Of the 135 million infants born throughout the world each year, more than 90 per cent live in low-income or developing countries such as South Africa. Despite this, only a small percentage of published research addresses children who come from such backgrounds (Tomlinson, 2003). It is therefore important that such research becomes available through publication. This will ensure that the different circumstances of infants and young children be carefully considered as part of psychological assessments, since social factors, notably maternal education level, are among the strongest predictors of poor developmental outcome in infants (Brooks-Gunn, 1990).

Finally, the assessment of brain-behaviour relationships draws primarily on cognitive measures, and so this section concludes with a chapter on neuropsychological assessment. Neuropsychological assessment is at last coming into its own in South Africa, with the opening of the registration category and the promulgation of a scope of practice for neuropsychologists. The chapter by Lucas outlines the current status of neuropsychological assessment in South Africa, as well as the major challenges facing this field of assessment. The latter include the complexity and diversity of the country's population, varying levels and qualities of education, socio-economic status discrepancies and rapid acculturation. The chapter presents some of the local research that has been done to address these challenges.

Section Two: Personality and projective tests: conceptual and practical applications

Aside from cognitive tests, personality tests make up the next broad domain within the field of psychological assessment. Personality is a multifaceted construct and its definition varies depending on the epistemological framework that one subscribes to. An examination of textbooks on personality theory and general introductory psychology texts reveals that most theories of personality fall into one of eight theoretical categories – namely, the psychodynamic, lifespan, cognitive, social learning, humanistic/existential, behaviourist, biological/behavioural genetics, or dispositional/trait theoretical approach (see Ellis, Abrams & Abrams, 2009;

Friedman & Schustack, 2009; Larsen & Buss, 2008; Meyer, Moore & Viljoen, 2003; Naidoo, Townsend & Carolissen, 2008; Ryckman, 2008; Schultz & Schultz, 2009; Weiten, 2009). However, when it comes to the assessment of personality, instruments generally fall into one of two categories: either the objective, self-report personality inventories, which have their roots in the dispositional and, to a lesser extent, humanistic approaches, or the projective inventories, which originated primarily within the psychodynamic tradition. Section Two includes chapters on the objective and projective measures. The arguments that projective tests do not solely measure personality and are capable of assessing broader domains of the self and identity are noted. However, these tests do fit in well with the rubric and arguments presented in other chapters in this section. As in Section One, the chapters included in this section do not focus solely on the instruments.

Chapters on the objective personality tests are presented first. These chapters cover the 16PF, the Myers-Briggs Type Indicator (MBTI), the Fifteen Factor Questionnaire Plus (15FQ+), the NEO Personality Inventory (Revised) (NEO-PI-R), the Occupational Personality Profile (OPPro), the Occupational Personality Questionnaire (OPQ), the Basic Traits Inventory (BTI) and the Millon family of instruments, particularly the Millon Clinical Multiaxial Inventory – III (MCMI-III). It is evident from these chapters that aside from the BTI, there are no emic self-report personality questionnaires in South Africa. However, each of these chapters provides information on the particular test's applicability in South Africa. Van Eeden, Taylor and Prinsloo, for example, discuss the adaptation of the 16PF, particularly the Sixteen Personality Factor Questionnaire – South African 1992 version (16PF-SA92), from its entry and early adaptations to date with the 16PF5, in chapter 14. Laher discusses the NEO-PI-R in chapter 18, and uses contemporary research to demonstrate the limited utility of the inventory in South Africa.

The inclusion of these chapters is useful, not only in terms of the description and research provided for each instrument, but also because of the various challenges identified for personality testing in South Africa. All of the chapters make reference to test adaptation within the South African context. They also highlight issues of language proficiency, response bias and social desirability, amongst others. Tredoux provides the necessary background to, as well as current findings on, the 15FQ+ in chapter 15. This chapter is particularly useful in terms of its frank consideration of issues of language proficiency. Taylor and De Bruin's chapter on the BTI (chapter 16) makes reference to research conducted on response bias.

Personality traits are different to personality types, where a personality type is defined as a 'unique constellation of traits and states that is similar in pattern to one identified category of personality within a taxonomy of personalities' (Cohen & Swerdlik, 2004, p.126). A personality trait is also different to personality states, which are generally emotional reactions that vary from one situation to another (Kaplan & Saccuzzo, 2008). The chapter by Knott, Taylor, Oosthuizen and Bhabha on the MBTI (chapter 17) provides research on the use of a type inventory in South Africa and in so doing critically examines the strengths and limitations of this inventory in South Africa.

Chapters 19 and 20 on the OPPro and the OPQ provide information and research on tests used primarily in organisational settings. The inclusion of these two chapters also highlights the tension between tests used in research and those used in practice, in terms of subscription to theoretical positions. With the 16PF, the MBTI, the NEO-PI-R and the Millon instruments, for example, the epistemological underpinnings are clear. However, with both the OPQ and the OPPro, the research presented is testament to their utility, but their theoretical underpinnings are not clear. This leads to a broader debate around the validity and utility of such instruments. It is hoped that this book will allow the reader access to all the necessary information to make an informed judgement on these issues.

Patel and Laher present a chapter on the Millon family of instruments (chapter 21). The chapter provides a brief introduction to the instruments and then focuses on the MCMI-III. Aside from the information presented on the MCMI-III, the chapter also highlights interesting debates that transcend the boundaries of psychological assessment and link to the cognate fields of psychopathology and clinical psychology. The cross-cultural debates around mental illness are briefly addressed, thereby providing the reader with a stimulating opportunity to view assessment within the context of the broader debates taking place in the field of psychology.

These issues are addressed further in the chapters by Edwards and Young (chapters 22 and 23), who discuss the principles of psychological assessment as they apply to clinical and counselling settings. In chapter 22 they show how, in a multicultural society such as South Africa, the principles of assessment should be flexibly adapted to working with clients from different backgrounds and in different settings. Following on from this, in chapter 23 the same authors present a chapter on assessment and monitoring of symptoms in the treatment of psychological problems. They discuss the particular difficulties inherent in using self-report scales in cultural contexts different from those in which they were developed and validated. The authors recommend that practitioners first evaluate such scales within carefully conducted systematic case studies, as outlined in the chapter. Where such an evaluation provides evidence for the clinical utility of a scale, the scale can then be used to serve many valuable functions which include highlighting symptoms relevant for diagnosis, case formulation and treatment planning, as well as providing practitioners with continuous feedback about the effectiveness of their intervention strategies, thereby allowing for therapeutic adjustments that ultimately benefit the client.

As mentioned in the introduction to this section, projective tests are a special kind of personality test. They are based on the assumption that, when presented with ambiguous or unstructured stimuli, people tend to project onto these stimuli their own needs, experiences and unique ways of interacting with the world (Lezak, Howieson & Loring, 2004). As such, they provide the practitioner with a glimpse into the client's inner world that would be difficult to obtain by other methods. The general chapter on projective techniques by Bain, Amod and Gericke (chapter 24) shows how projective responses tend to differ depending on gender and cultural group, among other factors. These findings are extended in the final three chapters in Section Two (chapters 25, 26 and 27), which focus on specific projective tests – namely, the Thematic Apperception Test, the Draw-A-Person Test and the Rorschach Inkblot Test.

From Sections One and Two it is evident that psychological assessment in South Africa is still dominated by formal testing in both research and practice, but that those working in the field have been quite innovative in researching and adapting tests to our specific needs. The manner in which the authors of Sections One and Two engage with assessment issues in their field indicates their awareness of the benefits and limitations of relying solely on psychological testing to make informed decisions about individuals. Furthermore, these chapters highlight the need for alternative forms of psychological assessment in South Africa. This need is explicitly addressed in the chapters in Section Three, which reflect some of the future trends (both actual and suggested) in psychological assessment in South Africa.

Section Three: Assessment approaches and methodologies

Again and again in the chapters in Sections One and Two, the caution is raised about the need to use Western-developed (etic) tests in a manner that is sensitive to contextual and cultural differences. Many invaluable suggestions are made by the authors in Section Three about how test results can be interpreted in fair and ethical ways that are culturally appropriate. It is thus appropriate to commence the section with Coetzee's chapter, 'Ethical perspectives in assessment' (chapter 28). This chapter identifies key ethical considerations for research and practice in psychological assessment, and puts forward the valuable argument for the development of an 'ethical consciousness' (Bricklin, 2001, p.202).

Chapter 29 by Tredoux provides an excellent introduction to the field of computerised testing in South Africa, and presents contemporary debates in the area. In chapter 30, Shuttleworth-Edwards and colleagues show specifically how some of this methodology can be used for medical management in the sports concussion arena, using the Immediate Postconcussion Assessment and Cognitive Testing (ImPACT) approach. The authors show how this computerised neurocognitive approach has potential for wide application beyond the sports concussion field.

This section also presents some of the conceptual approaches that have much potential for addressing the diverse needs of the range of groups that we assess in South Africa. In chapter 31, Amod discusses the Initial Assessment Consultation (IAC) approach, a shared problem-solving approach to child assessment, focusing on collaboration with parents, caregivers and significant others such as teachers, with the aim of facilitating learning and empowering clients and their families.

Chapter 34 by Osman on RPL may at first glance appear out of place in a book on psychological assessment, as RPL's application has generally been focused on higher education practice. However, in this chapter the application of RPL is extended to the psychological assessment domain, as it is proposed as a complementary procedure that can give insight into an individual's acquired knowledge and experience.

It is quite evident that thus far the book has presented no chapter on vocational or organisational assessment. As indicated earlier, there are some very good local texts that provide these. De Bruin and De Bruin (2008) provide a very useful chapter on vocational assessment, while Moerdyk's (2009) book provides a useful introduction to psychological assessment in the organisational context. In Section Three, we have included two chapters that attempt to take these issues further.

Watson and McMahon present a chapter on vocational assessment (chapter 32). They briefly discuss the traditional approaches to vocational assessment and identify the limitations inherent within these. This provides the basis for the introduction of more qualitative approaches to career assessment and counselling. The main tenets of this more narrative approach are introduced, and the My System of Career Influences (MSCI) technique is presented by way of example. Chapter 33 by Milner, Donald and Thatcher provides an interesting perspective on psychological assessment in the workplace by linking it to issues of transformation. The authors draw on organisational justice theory to address concerns regarding psychological assessment and organisational transformation.

In keeping with the theme of exploring the broader domain of psychological assessment, chapter 35 by Kanjee presents some large-scale assessment studies conducted in South Africa. This chapter highlights the fact that assessment extends beyond the traditional individual and group settings. It also proposes that if psychological assessment is to be transformed, large-scale studies are a necessity. As the psychological assessment fraternity, we need to think more creatively about ways to achieve this.

In the concluding chapter 36, we consider the information presented in this book and attempt to amalgamate it into suggested directions for psychological assessment practitioners in South Africa to take. It is hoped that this collaborative volume will provide the reader with a solid understanding of the challenges and opportunities facing psychological assessment in South Africa, as well as an awareness of the considerable research that has already been undertaken in this regard.

References

Abrahams, F. & Mauer, K. F. (1999a). The comparability of the constructs of the 16PF in the South African context. *Journal of Industrial Psychology, 25(1)*, 53–59.

Abrahams, F. & Mauer, K. F. (1999b). Qualitative and statistical impacts of home language on responses to the items of the Sixteen Personality Factor Questionnaire (16PF) in South Africa. *South African Journal of Psychology, 29*, 76–86.

Biesheuvel, S. (1943). *African Intelligence*. Johannesburg: South African Institute of Race Relations.

Biesheuvel, S. (1949). Recent advances in personnel research in South Africa. *Journal of the South African Institute of Personnel Management, 4*, 6–19.

Bricklin, P. (2001). Being ethical: More than obeying the law and avoiding harm. *Journal of Personality Assessment, 77(2)*, 195–202.

Brooks-Gunn, J. (1990). Identifying the vulnerable young children. In D. E. Rogers & E. Ginsberg (Eds), *Improving the Life Chances of Children at Risk* (pp. 104–117). New York, NY: Plenum Press.

Claassen, N. C. W. (1997). Cultural differences, politics and test bias in South Africa. *European Review of Applied Psychology, 47(4)*, 297–307.

Cockcroft, K. & Israel, N. (2011). The Raven's Advanced Progressive Matrices: A comparison of relationships with verbal ability tests. *South African Journal of Psychology, 41(3)*, 363–372.

Cohen, R. J. & Swerdlik, M. E. (2004). *Psychological Testing and Assessment* (6th edition). Boston, MA: McGraw-Hill.

De Bruin, G. P. & De Bruin, K. (2008). Career counselling assessment. In C. Foxcroft & G. Roodt (Eds), *An Introduction to Psychological Assessment in the South African Context* (2nd edition, pp. 248–262). Cape Town: Oxford University Press.

Ellis, A., Abrams, M. & Abrams, L. D. (2009). *Personality Theories: Critical Perspectives.* Thousand Oaks, CA: Sage Publications.

Fick, M. L. (1929). South African intelligence tests: Comparisons of various racial groups. *Social and Industrial Review, 8*, 701–705, 791–794.

Fick, M. L. (1939). *The Educability of the South African Native.* Pretoria: South African Council for Educational and Social Research.

Foxcroft, C. D. (1997). Psychological testing in South Africa: Perspectives regarding ethical and fair practices. *European Journal of Psychological Assessment, 13(3)*, 229–235.

Foxcroft, C. (2011). Some issues in assessment in a developing world context: An African perspective. Paper presented at the Association for the Study of Evaluation and Assessment in Southern Africa International Conference, Towards Valid Assessment: Efficiency, Relevance and Social Consequence. North West University, Vanderbijlpark, July 11–13.

Foxcroft, C. & Davies, C. (2008). Historical perspectives on psychometric testing in South Africa. In C. van Ommen & D. Painter (Eds), *Interiors: A History of Psychology in South Africa* (pp. 152–182). Pretoria: Unisa Press.

Foxcroft, C., Paterson, H., Le Roux, N. & Herbst, D. (2004). *Psychological Assessment in South Africa: A Needs Analysis. The Test Use Patterns and Needs of Psychological Assessment Practitioners.* Pretoria: Human Sciences Research Council.

Foxcroft, C. & Roodt, G. (2008). *An Introduction to Psychological Assessment in the South African Context* (3rd edition). Cape Town: Oxford University Press.

Friedman, H. S. & Schustack, M. W. (2009). *Personality: Classic Theories and Modern Research* (4th edition). Boston, MA: Pearson.

Heuchert, J. W. P., Parker, W. D., Stumpf, H. & Myburgh, C. P. H. (2000). The Five-Factor Model of personality in South African college students. *American Behavioral Scientist, 44(1)*, 112–125.

Huysamen, G. K. (1996). *Psychological Measurement: An Introduction with Psychological Examples.* Pretoria: Van Schaik.

Interdepartmental Committee on Native Education (1936). *Report of the Interdepartmental Committee on Native Education, 1935–36 (UG 29-36).* Pretoria: Interdepartmental Committee on Native Education.

Ivnik, R., Smith, G. E. & Cerhan, J. H. (1992). Understanding the diagnostic capabilities of cognitive tests. *Clinical Neuropsychologist, 15(1)*, 114–124.

Kaliski, S. (2006). *Psycholegal Assessment in South Africa.* Cape Town: Oxford University Press.

Kaplan, R. M. & Saccuzzo, D. P. (2008). *Psychological Testing: Principles, Applications and Issues.* Pacific Grove, CA: Brooks/Cole.

Laher, S. (2007). Personality reconceptualised: A Millonian approach? *South African Journal of Psychology, 37*, 82–95.

Laher, S. (2008). Structural equivalence and the NEO-PI-R: Implications for the applicability of the Five Factor Model of personality in an African context. *South African Journal of Industrial Psychology, 34(1)*, 76–80.

Laher, S. (2011). The applicability of the NEO-PI-R and the CPAI-2 in the South African context. Unpublished PhD dissertation. University of the Witwatersrand, Johannesburg.

Larsen, R. J. & Buss, D. M. (2008). *Personality Psychology: Domains About Human Nature.* Boston, MA: McGraw-Hill.

Lezak, M. D., Howieson, D. B. & Loring, D. W. (2004). *Neuropsychological Assessment* (4th edition). New York, NY: Oxford University Press.

Meiring, D. (2007). *Bias and Equivalence of Psychological Measures in South Africa.* Ridderkerk: Labyrint Publication.

Meyer, W., Moore, C. & Viljoen, H. (2003). *Personology: From Individual to Ecosystem.* Sandton, Johannesburg: Heinemann.

Moerdyk, A. (2009). *The Principles and Practice of Psychological Assessment.* Pretoria: Van Schaik.

Naglieri, J. A. & Das, J. P. (1988). Planning-Arousal Simultaneous-Successive (PASS): A model for assessment. *Journal of School Psychology, 26,* 35–48.

Naidoo, P., Townsend, L. & Carolissen, R. (2008). Mainstream theories and non-mainstream approaches to personality. In L. Swartz, C. de la Rey, N. Duncan & L. Townsend (Eds), *Psychology: An Introduction* (2nd edition, pp. 117–139). Cape Town: Oxford University Press.

Nel, J. A. (2008). Uncovering personality dimensions in eleven different language groups in South Africa: An exploratory study. Unpublished PhD dissertation. University of the North-West, Potchefstroom.

Nell, V. (1999). Standardising the WAIS-III and the WMS-III for South Africa: Legislative, psychometric, and policy issues. *South African Journal of Psychology, 29(3),* 128–137.

Nzimande, B. (1995). To test or not to test? Paper presented at the Congress on Psychometrics for Psychologists and Personnel Practitioners. Council for Scientific and Industrial Research, Pretoria, June 13–14.

Ryckman, R. (2008). *Theories of Personality.* Belmont, CA: Thomson Wadsworth.

Schultz, P. & Schultz, S. E. (2009). *Theories of Personality* (9th edition). Belmont, CA: Thomson Wadsworth.

Sehlapelo, M. & Terre Blanche, M. (1996). Psychometric testing in South Africa: Views from above and below. *Psychology in Society, 21,* 49–59.

Strauss, E., Sherman, E. M. S. & Spreen, O. (2006). *A Compendium of Neuropsychological Tests* (3rd edition). Oxford: Oxford University Press.

Taylor, N. & De Bruin, G. P. (2006). *Basic Traits Inventory: Technical Manual.* Johannesburg: Jopie van Rooyen & Partners.

Tomlinson, M. (2003). Culture and infancy: A critical examination. *South African Journal of Child and Adolescent Mental Health, 15(1),* 45–48.

Van de Vijver, F. J. R. & Rothmann, S. (2004). Assessment in multicultural groups: The South African case. *South African Journal of Industrial Psychology, 30(4),* 1–7.

Van Eeden, R. & Mantsha, T. R. (2007). Theoretical and methodological considerations in the translation of the 16PF5 into an African language. *South African Journal of Psychology, 37(1),* 62–81.

Weiten, W. (2009). *Psychology: Themes and Variations.* Belmont, CA: Brooks/Cole.

Section One

Cognitive tests: conceptual and practical applications

2 WAIS-III test performance in the South African context: extension of a prior cross-cultural normative database

A. B. Shuttleworth-Edwards, E. K. Gaylard and S. E. Radloff

The focus of this chapter is on the Wechsler Adult Intelligence Scale – Third Edition (WAIS-III) and its application within the South African context.[1] While there is now a fourth edition of the Wechsler Adult Intelligence Scale, WAIS-IV (Wechsler, 2008), the only cross-cultural research within the South African context to date is in respect of the WAIS-III, the normative implications of which continue to have crucial relevance for practitioners wishing to employ a WAIS in this country.

Importantly, two distinct categories of norms have been delineated in the psychometric assessment literature: (i) population-based norms (*standardisation data*) representative of the general population that are typically derived on large samples and presented in association with a newly developed test; and (ii) norms that closely approximate the subgroup to which an individual belongs (*within-group norms*), such as form the basis of the leading normative guidebooks in clinical neuropsychology (Mitrushina, Boone, Razani & D'Elia, 2005; Strauss, Sherman & Spreen, 2006).

The objective of standardisation data is to allow for the location of an individual's ability relative to the general population, for purposes such as institutional placement. In contrast, the purpose of within-group norms is to allow for comparisons of an individual's level of performance with the subgroup that best approximates his or her unique demographic characteristics for *diagnostic* purposes, and is the impetus behind the data for presentation in this chapter.

Within-group norms with fine levels of stratification are regularly reported descriptively in terms of means and standard deviations, and may be based on small sample numbers (for example, n < 10, and in some instances the sample numbers may be as low as n = 1 or 2). Nevertheless, such normative indicators are considered less prone to the false diagnostic conclusions that may accrue via comparisons with population-based standardisation data that are not demographically applicable in a particular case (Lezak, Howieson & Loring, 2004; Mitrushina et al., 2005; Strauss et al., 2006).

The history of the Wechsler Adult Intelligence Scales

Historically, the various WAIS in current usage have their origins in the release of the Wechsler-Bellevue Intelligence Scale Forms I and II in 1939 and 1944, respectively (Wechsler, 1939; 1944). Over the years, the adult Wechsler tests in their various refined and updated versions, currently covering the age range from 16 to 89 years, have accumulated a wealth of endorsement through clinical and research experience. Consequently, despite a number of alternative intelligence tests of an exemplary nature being devised, the Wechsler tests remain the gold standard for the individual measurement of intelligence worldwide within clinical psychology, clinical neuropsychology, forensic and correctional services, and postgraduate university training, and for the evaluation of general cognitive ability (Flanagan & Kaufman, 2009; Lichtenberger & Kaufman, 2009).

The original Wechsler-Bellevue Forms 1 and 2 (Wechsler 1939; 1944) were replaced in 1955 by the WAIS, and in 1981 the test was submitted in a revised version (WAIS-R) (Wechsler, 1955; 1981). The WAIS-III appeared in 1997 (Wechsler, 1997), and very recently a fourth edition, WAIS-IV, has been released (Wechsler, 2008). Wechsler's original adult intelligence quotient (IQ) tests, up to and including the WAIS-R, took the same basic form of a Verbal IQ comprising six subtests, and a Performance IQ calculated from five subtests, together making up the Full Scale IQ (FSIQ). The WAIS-III departed from this format somewhat by offering four separate entities of a Verbal Comprehension Index (VCI), a Perceptual Organisation Index (POI), a Working Memory Index (WMI) and a Processing Speed Index (PSI), in addition to allowing for the calculation of the Verbal, Performance and FSIQ scores (Wechsler, 1997). Finally, the format of the newly published WAIS-IV (Wechsler, 2008) mirrors the format of the fourth edition of the Wechsler Intelligence Scale for Children (WISC-IV) (Wechsler, 2004). The four Index scores devised for the WAIS-III have been retained, although the Perceptual Organisation Index has been renamed the Perceptual Reasoning Index (PRI), and a number of changes have been introduced around the subtest structure with a view to improving measures of working memory and processing speed. Furthermore the test format has made the dramatic shift of dropping the Verbal and Performance IQ scores, such that only an FSIQ is now available.

The history of the Wechsler Adult Intelligence Scales in South Africa

Within South Africa, the Wechsler-Bellevue Intelligence Scale was adapted and normed for white Afrikaans-speaking and white English-speaking South Africans from 1954 to 1969, and was renamed the South African Wechsler Adult Intelligence Scale (SAWAIS) (1969). Until recently, the SAWAIS was used extensively in South Africa across all race groups, and is probably still in use by some, despite criticism of its outdated questions and standardisation data (Nell, 1994; Shuttleworth-Jordan, 1995). The development of a more up-to-date standardisation of a suitable intelligence test for use within South Africa was clearly necessary. Accordingly, following the demise of the apartheid regime, the Human Sciences Research Council (HSRC) decided to norm the most recent version of the WAIS in the form of the WAIS-III (Claassen, Krynauw, Paterson & Mathe, 2001). Following extensive consultation with local experts in the assessment field, the data collection for the standardisation took place over a two-year period from 1997 to 1998, on an English-only administration of the WAIS-III in respect of four race groups (black, coloured, Indian and white). Participants in the age range 16–69 were the target group, and totalled 900 individuals who spoke English at home most of the time. A subset of 664 individuals in the age range 16–55 was investigated for differences in performance between four race groups (black, coloured, Indian and white). A few minor modifications were made to content items to make the test more culturally relevant (for example, the term 'dollar' was replaced with 'rand'), but no substantial alterations were made. The resultant South African WAIS-III manual (Claassen et al., 2001) provides raw score conversion tables reflecting the *combined* (that is, aggregated) outcome of all four race groups across nine age groups within the age span 16–69 years.

However, the investigation into WAIS-III race differences for the 16–55-year-old subset within the HSRC standardisation sample revealed substantial differences in performance on a continuum from highest to lowest scores for the white, Indian, coloured and black groupings (mean FSIQs of 108.34, 99.98, 101.02 and 92.51, respectively) (Claassen et al., 2001, p.59). The researchers considered these differences to be 'a reflection of the outcomes of quality of education experienced' (p.62), a factor that was not controlled for in the sampling procedure. Consequently, the decision to aggregate the data from all four race groups, although perhaps more palatable politically, raises concern about the utility of this standardisation for valid clinical use, in that data are too lenient for the typical white South African testee, and too stringent for the typical black South African testee. In that the mean scores for the Indian and coloured subgroups fell between the two extremes of the white and black groups, the standardisation has optimal relevance for valid neurodiagnostic interpretation in respect of these two median groups.

Accordingly, it is apparent that there are significant problems in the application of the Wechsler tests to different race groups, as has been comprehensively reviewed elsewhere (Shuttleworth-Edwards, Kemp, Rust, Muirhead, Hartman & Radloff, 2004), not due to the influence of race itself, but due to the influence on cognitive test performance of differential socio-cultural variables that may or may not happen to be associated with a particular race. There is an accumulating body of US and South African cross-cultural research that has called upon the variable of quality of education in particular as crucial in explaining lowered cognitive test performance for particular groups, in spite of matching for educational level (Manly, 2005; Manly, Byrd, Touradji, Sanchez & Stern, 2004; Manly, Jacobs, Touradji, Small & Stern, 2002; Shuttleworth-Edwards et al., 2004; Shuttleworth-Jordan, 1996). Importantly, inferior performance in association with relatively disadvantaged education compared with advantaged education is observed to occur not only on verbal tasks, but also on so-called culture-fair performance tasks.

Reasons offered for this phenomenon are that those who are exposed to relatively advantaged Western schooling systems are more likely to acquire problem-solving strategies for learning rather than placing high value on pure rote learning, as well as to absorb (rather than specifically learn) a superior degree of test-taking familiarity and sophistication (Grieve & Viljoen, 2000; Nell, 1999).

The problem of test-taking differences, therefore, is not solved merely through stratification by race, in that the *acculturation* process (that is, the rapid shift among non-Westernised individuals from rural to Westernised urban conditions) will result in *heterogeneity* of psychometric test performance *within* race groups in association with variations in quality of education (Manly, 2005; Shuttleworth-Edwards et al., 2004). More specifically, the concept of acculturation carries with it the implication that the more an individual acquires the skills and exposure to a Western middle-class context, the more his or her IQ score will increase (Ogden & McFarlane-Nathan, 1997). Van de Vijver and Phalet (2004) use an analogy of a continuum of acculturation, ranging from no adjustment and marginalisation to complete adjustment or assimilation to the other culture.

In South Africa especially, the potential for dramatic heterogeneity *within* the previously disadvantaged race groups applies, in that under the apartheid regime vastly discrepant educational facilities were made available for white individuals compared with other-than-white individuals from the time that the South African government began passing legislation to ensure variations in quality of education according to race (Claassen et al., 2001). The traditionally black South African schools were undersupplied with basic resources such as books and desks, and teachers were required to teach large classes. There was a long history of nomenclature provided for 'black' education departments during the course of the apartheid era, a review of which is beyond the scope of the present chapter. Throughout this period the majority of black South Africans were educated in schools of inferior quality, with restricted curricula. In the years leading up to democratisation the Department of Education and Training (DET) was responsible for curricula in all government schools for 'Africans'. These DET schools, which were attended by the vast majority of the school-going population, received only 5–25 per cent of the financial resources that were expended on white Afrikaans and white English first-language pupils. These latter groups were educated in elite private or 'Model C' government schools (modelled on the British public school system) that were of a comparatively far superior quality (Kallaway, 1984).

From 1991, Model C schools became multiracial and restrictions that had applied to the former DET schools were dismantled. However, the problem of poor resources remains for most of these beleaguered schools, with the conditions in some township schools having worsened, especially in the relatively impoverished Eastern Cape (Cooper, 2004; Cull, 2001; Matomela, 2008a; 2008b; Van der Berg, 2004). What has changed since the dismantling of apartheid is that there have been widely differing schooling opportunities for increasing numbers of other-than-white individuals who have been in a position to access the well-resourced, traditionally white advantaged schools, and consequently the quality of education attained by South African individuals (that is, their positioning on the acculturation continuum) may vary substantially both across and within ethnic groups, with differential effects on psychometric test performance. Nell (1999), taking account of this phenomenon, predicted that the representativeness of the HSRC WAIS-III standardisation of Claassen et al. (2001) would be flawed due to vastly different types of educational exposure amongst black individuals in South Africa as a legacy of the apartheid structure, a factor (as indicated above) that had not been taken into account in the sampling procedure. The failure to stratify for quality of education in respect of the South African WAIS-III standardisation, therefore, provided the impetus for further, more strictly stratified cross-cultural research on the WAIS-III within the South African context that would take race into account in association with both level and quality of education.

South African cross-cultural research

An extensive literature search indicates that there appears to be no other published cross-cultural research in respect of the WAIS-III to date worldwide, besides the South African research of Shuttleworth-Edwards et al. (2004) (hereafter Study 1) discussed below. In a follow-up study (hereafter Study 2), the research was refined, and the results of that study are presented in this chapter. For descriptive purposes (as per Strauss et al., 2006), the closely interrelated terms 'race' and 'ethnicity' are used here to differentiate the more genetic aspects of racial identity (race) from those socio-cultural aspects that happen to be associated with a particular race such as tribe, home language and geographical affiliation (ethnicity).

Study 1: The work of Shuttleworth-Edwards et al. (2004)

In response to the limitations of the South African WAIS-III standardisation in regard to the lack of control for quality of education, an investigation was conducted into an English administration of the WAIS-III test (Shuttleworth-Edwards et al., 2004), on a sample of white South African English and black southern African participants in the age range 19–30 who spoke English as their home language, and/or were working or studying in the medium of English in the Eastern Cape (that is, they were considered to be fluent in English). A further language check was put in place via the testers' observations of English fluency during the administration of the test, on the basis of which it was not considered necessary to exclude any of the participants.

The above language fluency criteria for Study 1 are in keeping with those of the HSRC's Claassen et al. (2001) standardisation, in that a requirement for their chief norm group was that all participants had English as their home language. However, on this basis the HSRC group was unable to find sufficient numbers to fill their sampling grid for black participants with lower levels of education than Grade 12, and therefore additional black participants were included in the sample who had met a set criterion on an English language test. Importantly, Claassen et al. made a comparison of WAIS-III data for a selection of black participants in their study depending on whether they (i) reported English as their *home* language, (ii) reported English as the language they used at *work* most of the time, or (iii) passed the inclusion criterion on the basis of the English *language test.* The results indicated that the 'work' and 'language test' groups did not differ significantly from each other, demonstrating a performance of around 90 for each one of the four Index scores. The Claassen et al. 'home' language group revealed performance of around five to ten IQ points higher than this for the four Index scores, a finding that was attributed to that group's relatively higher educational level compared with the other two groups. Accordingly, it was considered that the mode of control for basic proficiency in English employed for Study 1 was adequate and broadly equivalent to that of the Claassen et al. study (that is, participants being asked whether they used English at home and/or at work and/or for their studies most of the time).

The sample was further stratified according to sex (female versus male), ethnicity (black southern African versus white South African English), level of education (Grade 12 versus Graduate) and quality of education (advantaged versus disadvantaged). Disadvantaged education was operationalised as those participants who had been exposed to schooling at institutions formerly under the control of the DET (hereafter Ex-DET/township schooling); advantaged education was operationalised as those participants who had been exposed to the formerly white *English-medium* private or Model C schooling (hereafter Private/Model C schooling).

The results of this Shuttleworth-Edwards et al. (2004) research indicated that scores for the black southern African and white South African English groups with advantaged education were comparable with the US standardisation, whereas scores for black African participants with disadvantaged education were significantly lower than this. The outcome gave credence to the warning of Nell (1999) that the HSRC standardisation was potentially problematic in failing to control for quality of education in the standardisation. There was, however, a limitation of the Shuttleworth-Edwards et al. study (Study 1) in terms of homogeneity of ethnic affiliation amongst the black participants. At the time that the research was conducted (1998–1999), it was difficult to find black Xhosa participants in the Eastern Cape with more than four years of consecutive privileged (Private/Model C) education, largely due to the fact that South Africa had become a democracy only four to five years before the research began.[2] Consequently, it was necessary to include other-than-Xhosa black African participants in the privileged educational category, with resultant inconsistency in the number of Xhosa individuals across groups, and particularly reduced numbers of Xhosa participants in the educationally advantaged Graduate subgroup. Both the disadvantaged and advantaged Grade 12 black groups consisted of 90 per cent Xhosa participants. Similarly, the disadvantaged Graduate black group consisted of 100 per cent Xhosa participants. However, the advantaged Graduate black group comprised only 20 per cent Xhosa participants; the rest of the group was made up of 60 per cent Shona and 20 per cent Tswana first-language Zimbabweans, respectively.

On analysis, this mixed southern African black Private/Model C Graduate group in Study 1 is less than ideal, not only in terms of its ethnic heterogeneity, but also because it happened to represent a particularly superior group educationally, in that 80 per cent of the group had experienced advantaged education during primary and high schooling that was commensurate with white schooling. The six Shona-affiliated participants in this group had received particularly advantaged education in Zimbabwe, which in the 1980s and early 1990s was recognised for its high quality of education, and 80 per cent of the group were postgraduate students at one of the relatively elite formerly white English-medium South African universities. This provided further impetus to conduct additional research, with a view to refining the cross-cultural data obtained in the Shuttleworth-Edwards et al. (2004) study.

Study 2: An extension of Shuttleworth-Edwards et al. (2004)

The aim of Study 2 was to refine the data obtained by Shuttleworth-Edwards et al. (2004) in a cross-cultural investigation on the WAIS-III (English administration) stratified for both level and quality of education, by recruiting additional young adult Xhosa participants in order to create a sample in which there were equal numbers of exclusively Xhosa participants with South African education in all the subgroups.

Method used in the study

Sampling procedure: The sampling method employed for Study 2 was essentially the same as that used for the Shuttleworth-Edwards et al. (2004) study (Study 1), with the exception of recruiting black subgroups that were exclusively of Xhosa ethnic origin, rather than having groups that included some black participants who were not of Xhosa ethnic origin. The terminology for level of education was changed to permit greater specificity in terms of years of education completed, from 'Grade 12' to '12+ Education', and from 'Graduate' to '15+ Education'. Similarly, the term 'DET' schooling applied in the earlier research was changed to 'Ex-DET' schooling, thereby reflecting the discontinuation of DET schooling since the dismantling of the apartheid system.

A sampling matrix was devised in order to stratify for relevant variables, including sex (male versus female), ethnicity (black South African Xhosa versus white South African English), level of education (12+ Education versus 15+ Education), and quality of education (disadvantaged Ex-DET/township schooling versus advantaged English-medium Private/Model C schooling). The participants in the original study (Study 1) formed the basis of the sample for the new study (Study 2). However, all non-Xhosa participants from Study 1 were excluded (n = 14), and for the purposes of the new study, 16 participants of Xhosa affiliation were added to the sampling matrix in order to replace these exclusions and achieve balanced subgroup numbers, as follows: Ex-DET 12+ Education group (n = 2 additions), Ex-DET 15+ Education group (n = 2 additions), Private/Model C 12+ Education group (n = 3 additions), Private/Model C 15+ Education group (n = 9 additions). The final sample (age range 19–31 years) had the following mean age and sex distributions: 12+ Education Ex-DET, mean age = 24.7, n = 11 (5F; 6M); 12+ Education Private/Model C, Mean age = 21.75, n = 12 (6F; 6M); 15+ Education Ex-DET, mean age = 27.83, n = 12 (5F; 7M); 15+ Education Private/

Model C, mean age = 25.09, n = 11 (5F; 6M). As in the previous study, Ex-DET-educated participants tended to be slightly older than those educated in Private/Model C systems, but the age difference was not considered to be of relevance, as it remained well within the decade bracket normally used for stratification purposes (Lezak et al., 2004). Furthermore, there are minimal differences in the conversion of raw to scaled scores between the ages 18–19, 20–24, 25–29 and 30–34 (Wechsler, 1997). Commensurate with this, a correlation analysis revealed weak and negative correlations for age in relation to Subtest scores ($-0.004 < r < -0.348$), Index scores ($-0.058 > r > -0.307$) and IQ scores ($-0.138 > r > -0.312$).

As with Study 1, for inclusion in Study 2 all participants were required to have English as their home language and/or to be either studying or working in the medium of English (that is, they were considered to be fluent in English). Also, as with the original study, a language check was put in place via the testers' observations of English fluency during the administration of the test, on the basis of which it was not considered necessary to exclude any of the participants. Initially for Study 2, attempts were made to recruit participants from the Eastern Cape. However, in order to meet the target numbers for the sample groups, it was necessary to include Xhosa participants who were born and schooled in the Eastern Cape but were living in Cape Town or Gauteng. As in Study 1, in order to obtain a nonclinical sample potential participants were excluded from Study 2 if they reported a history of head injury, cerebral disease, learning disability, substance abuse or mental illness.

Quality of education: In accordance with the sampling procedure used in Study 1, to qualify for the Ex-DET group in Study 2 participants had to have attended a former DET school throughout high school, which invariably meant that they had also experienced former DET primary schooling. To qualify for the Private/Model C group, participants had to have attended four or more years of Private/Model C schooling. Thus, a participant could have a disadvantaged (Ex-DET) primary school education and an advantaged high school education (Private/Model C) and be included in the Private/Model C category. An Analysis of Variance (ANOVA) comparing participants with Model C schooling to those with private schooling on the Subtest, Index and IQ scores revealed no significant differences ($p > 0.05$ in all instances), and warrants the use of Private/Model C as one category. The 12+ Education group comprised participants with Grade 12 and possibly one or two years of tertiary education; the 15+ Education group comprised participants with three or more years of successfully completed tertiary education, resulting in the completion of a degree or a diploma. The newly constituted pure Xhosa Private/Model C 15+ Education subgroup consisted of seven university graduates, all from previously advantaged English-medium universities, and four technikon (university of technology) graduates with a diploma. An ANOVA comparing the technikon and university graduates revealed no significant difference between the two groups for any of the Subtest, Index or IQ scores ($p > 0.05$, in all instances), and warrants inclusion of those with at least a three-year degree or diploma in the same category.

Overall, however, the newly constituted Xhosa Private/Model C 15+ Education group in Study 2 had less tertiary education than the original Mixed

African Private/Model C 15+ Education group of Study 1, in that only 54.44 per cent of the Xhosa group had completed postgraduate studies, compared with 80 per cent of the Mixed African group. Furthermore, only 27.27 per cent of the Xhosa group had attended advantaged primary school compared with 80 per cent of the Mixed African group. Thus, the Xhosa Private/Model C 15+ Education participants in Study 2 differed from the Mixed African Private/Model C 15+ Education participants in Study 1, both in having received a lower level of tertiary education and in having had less advantageous primary-level schooling.

In summary, with reference to the three black subgroups, it can be seen that they had been exposed to varying levels of quality of education which can be conceptualised along Van de Vijver and Phalet's (2004) continuum: the Xhosa Ex-DET participants had experienced disadvantaged primary and high schooling, the Xhosa Private/Model C 15+ Education group had generally experienced disadvantaged primary schooling and advantaged high schooling, and the Mixed African 15+ Education group from the previous research had experienced high-quality education throughout primary and high school that was commensurate with the white English Private/Model C 15+ Education group.

Data collection and data analysis

In accordance with the protocol of the previous research, participation in the study was voluntary. Each participant who met the requirements of the sampling matrix completed a biographical questionnaire and the WAIS-III, administered in English by a trainee clinical psychologist. Tests were scored and converted into Scaled, Index and IQ scores according to the WAIS-III manual (Wechsler, 1997). Responses to the Verbal subtests were scored by the researcher and an independent clinician blind to the aims of the study, who also checked the accuracy of the Scaled, Index and IQ scores.

T-test comparisons were run comparing the data for each black Mixed African subgroup from the original research to those for each newly configured black Xhosa subgroup. There were no significant differences for any of the Subtest, Index and IQ comparisons between groups, with the exception of the 15+ Education Mixed African Private/Model C group from the original research and the equivalent newly formed Xhosa group, where the Mixed African group revealed significantly superior scores to the Xhosa group for the WMI, the PSI and Performance IQ (PIQ) ($p = 0.025$, $p = 0.035$ and $p = 0.044$, respectively).

For the purposes of descriptive comparison and clinical practice, normative tables were drawn up separately for 12+ Education subgroups (see Table 2.1) and 15+ Education subgroups (see Table 2.2), incorporating all the data for the newly constituted pure Xhosa groups, as well as data from the original research for the 12+ Education and the 15+ Education white English subgroups, as well as the 15+ Education Mixed African Private/Model C group. The 15+ Education Mixed African Private/Model C group was the only data set for black participants included in the normative tables from the original research, as it was the only subgroup to reveal significant differences from its equivalent newly constituted pure Xhosa subgroup.

Table 2.1 WAIS-III data for 12+ years education, stratified for race/ethnicity and quality of education (N = 37)*

Race/ethnicity Quality of education Test	Black South African Xhosa Ex-DET (n = 11) Mean (SD)	Black South African Xhosa Private/Model C (n = 12) Mean (SD)	White South African English Private/Model C (n = 14) Mean (SD)
*Subtest scores***			
Picture Completion	6.82 (2.60)	9.42 (2.84)	12.21 (3.26)
Vocabulary	4.82 (1.47)	8.67 (3.08)	10.57 (2.68)
Digit Symbol	6.18 (2.09)	10.42 (3.23)	11.50 (1.87)
Similarities	6.64 (1.50)	9.92 (2.87)	11.00 (2.88)
Block Design	6.55 (2.30)	8.33 (2.42)	11.14 (2.91)
Arithmetic	7.18 (2.04)	8.67 (3.58)	10.00 (2.91)
Matrix Reasoning	7.55 (3.05)	10.83 (3.79)	12.43 (2.79)
Digit Span	6.82 (2.52)	9.42 (2.68)	10.86 (3.63)
Information	6.55 (2.58)	9.00 (2.13)	10.29 (2.27)
Picture Arrangement	5.00 (2.37)	8.33 (2.06)	10.57 (2.28)
Comprehension	7.00 (2.79)	11.33 (2.96)	10.50 (2.18)
Symbol Search	5.82 (2.56)	7.92 (2.35)	10.07 (2.70)
L-N Sequencing	8.00 (3.55)	10.92 (2.61)	11.14 (2.93)
Object Assembly	5.55 (2.11)	6.92 (3.29)	9.79 (3.02)
Index scores			
VCI	77.73 (9.10)	95.33 (12.53)	103.14 (11.36)
POI	81.55 (10.27)	96.92 (15.68)	111.86 (15.36)
WMI	83.27 (14.43)	97.58 (15.76)	103.86 (16.17)
PSI	78.55 (9.91)	95.33 (13.49)	104.29 (11.97)
IQ scores			
VIQ	79.00 (7.25)	96.67 (12.92)	102.71 (10.96)
PIQ	77.00 (9.21)	96.25 (15.69)	110.50 (13.46)
FSIQ	76.55 (8.29)	96.42 (13.68)	106.57 (12.15)

Notes: * For comparative purposes this *12+ years of education* table is in respect of Study 2 normative data derived for the two newly constituted pure black South African Xhosa subgroups (columns 1 and 2), and Study 1 original normative data for the white South African English subgroup (column 3). ** L-N Sequencing = Letter-Number Sequencing; VCI = Verbal Comprehension Index; POI = Perceptual Organisation Index; WMI = Working Memory Index; PSI = Processing Speed Index; VIQ = Verbal IQ; PIQ = Performance IQ; FSIQ = Full Scale IQ.

Table 2.2 WAIS-III data for 15+ years education, stratified for race/ethnicity and quality of education (N = 47)*

Race/ethnicity Quality of education Test	Black South African Xhosa Ex-DET (n = 12) Mean (SD)	Black South African Xhosa Private/Model C (n = 11) Mean (SD)	Black African Mixed Private/Model C (n = 10) Mean (SD)	White South African English Private/Model C (n = 14) Mean (SD)
*Subtest scores***				
Picture Completion	8.83 (3.19)	10.64 (2.62)	11.20 (2.30)	13.00 (2.72)
Vocabulary	10.08 (3.26)	13.27 (1.79)	13.10 (1.66)	15.43 (2.14)
Digit Symbol	8.58 (2.35)	9.00 (3.52)	10.90 (2.73)	12.43 (1.91)
Similarities	10.83 (2.86)	13.55 (2.16)	12.60 (2.32)	13.57 (2.31)
Block Design	8.08 (3.18)	8.36 (2.34)	9.60 (1.78)	11.64 (2.50)
Arithmetic	8.58 (2.94)	8.18 (2.09)	11.70 (2.98)	13.50 (1.91)
Matrix Reasoning	9.42 (2.71)	10.00 (3.07)	12.40 (3.41)	13.36 (3.03)
Digit Span	9.58 (1.88)	9.73 (2.72)	11.40 (2.99)	12.86 (2.74)
Information	10.08 (2.15)	12.00 (2.37)	13.10 (1.66)	13.86 (1.51)
Picture Arrangement	6.42 (1.78)	8.82 (3.03)	12.00 (3.62)	11.43 (2.53)
Comprehension	11.08 (1.98)	13.82 (1.66)	13.90 (2.42)	13.93 (1.82)
Symbol Search	7.42 (2.15)	7.73 (2.41)	10.40 (2.01)	11.78 (2.33)
L-N Sequencing	10.17 (2.37)	11.18 (3.09)	12.10 (2.51)	13.57 (2.24)
Object Assembly	6.00 (2.17)	5.82 (2.09)	8.30 (1.57)	9.86 (2.69)
Index scores				
VCI	101.75 (13.35)	116.36 (10.74)	116.00 (8.78)	124.29 (8.41)
POI	92.42 (14.93)	97.45 (11.74)	105.90 (10.87)	116.29 (10.60)
WMI	96.25 (9.69)	97.82 (10.86)	109.70 (11.46)	119.79 (11.23)
PSI	88.92 (10.00)	91.09 (13.39)	103.30 (11.07)	111.64 (11.07)
IQ scores				
VIQ	99.58 (8.93)	110.36 (9.10)	116.10 (7.50)	124.93 (8.20)
PIQ	88.42 (12.32)	95.55 (14.10)	107.80 (11.82)	116.14 (9.78)
FSIQ	94.50 (10.65)	104.36 (11.30)	113.40 (9.03)	123.00 (8.44)

Notes: * For comparative purposes this *15+ years of education* table is in respect of Study 2 normative data derived for the two newly constituted pure black South African Xhosa subgroups (columns 1 and 2), and Study 1 original normative data for the black African mixed and white South African English subgroups (columns 3 and 4, respectively). ** L-N Seq. = Letter-Number Sequencing; VCI = Verbal Comprehension Index; POI = Perceptual Organisation Index; WMI = Working Memory Index; PSI = Processing Speed Index; VIQ = Verbal IQ; PIQ = Performance IQ; FSIQ = Full Scale IQ.

The tables were structured to reflect the subgroups in order from least to most exposure to advantaged education, reading from the left to the right side of the tables as follows:

- Table 2.1: 12+ Education Xhosa Ex-DET group (*disadvantaged Ex-DET education during both primary and high school*), 12+ Education Xhosa Private/Model C group (*mainly disadvantaged Ex-DET primary school education but advantaged Private/Model C high schooling*), 12+ Education white English Private/Model C group from the original study (*advantaged Private/Model C education throughout primary and high school*);
- Table 2.2: 15+ Education Xhosa Ex-DET group (*disadvantaged Ex-DET education throughout both primary and high school*), 15+ Education Xhosa Private/Model C group (*mainly disadvantaged primary schooling but advantaged Private/Model C high schooling*), 15+ Education Mixed African Private/Model C group from the original study (*mainly advantaged primary schooling and advantaged high schooling*), 15+ Education white English Private/Model C group from the original study (*advantaged Private/Model C education throughout primary and high school*).

Results and discussion

Perusal of Tables 2.1 and 2.2 from left to right, each arranged in ascending order of quality of education per subgroup, reveals how performance of the 12+ and 15+ Education groups on Subtest, Index and IQ scores increases in close association with the rising levels of quality of education. This finding in respect of more carefully refined ethnic groups, taken together with detailed attention to nuances of quality of education, continues to be in accordance with earlier research that demonstrated superior cognitive test performance in association with superior quality of education and vice versa (for example, Manly et al., 2002; 2004; Shuttleworth-Edwards et al., 2004), and provides an excellent demonstration of Van de Vijver and Phalet's (2004) description of acculturation as being on a continuum.

In Table 2.1, it is of note that the FSIQ score of 96.42 for the 12+ Education Xhosa Private/Model C group is a relatively close equivalent of the FSIQ of 92.51 reported for the black group within the South African WAIS-III standardisation of Claassen et al. (2001), a score that is only 10 points lower than the FSIQ of 106.57 obtained in respect of the advantaged 12+ Education white English Private/Model C group, such that these scores all fall in the average range. However, there is a significant lowering of the Grade 12+ Education Xhosa Ex-DET group in relation to the Grade 12+ Xhosa Private/Model C group of 20 points, with the disadvantaged Ex-DET group scoring in the borderline range (FSIQ = 76.55). These divergent findings *within* the black Xhosa group in the present study suggest that the Claassen et al. (2001) sampling was for a relatively advantaged group of black participants, and that the standardisation is not suitable for use with Xhosa individuals from educationally disadvantaged backgrounds. The consequence of not taking this factor into account when using the South African WAIS-III standardisation manual is that erroneous conclusions are likely to be drawn in respect of scholastic and occupational placements, as well as compensation claims.

Perusal of specific subtest differences across both the 12+ and 15+ Education groups reveals that Object Assembly is the subtest that is most consistently significantly lower for the black Xhosa groups, including those with advantaged education, with scores all falling in the extremely low range (5.55 up to at best 6.92), followed closely by Symbol Search (5.82 to 7.92), Picture Arrangement (5.00 to 8.82), and Block Design (6.55 to 8.36). This aspect of the outcome lends substantial support to the observation from cross-cultural researchers that performance skills *in addition* to verbal skills are vulnerable to socio-cultural effects, and indeed cannot be seen to be culture-fair (Ardila, 1995; Manly et al., 2004; Ostrosky-Solis, Ramirez & Ardila, 2004; Rosselli & Ardila, 2003). In contrast, the most culture-fair task overall across both the 12+ and 15+ Education Xhosa groups appeared to be Letter-Number Sequencing, where there were no extremely low scores in evidence for any of the groups, including those with disadvantaged education, and all scores fell within the low average to high average range (8.00 to 11.18). The finding of relatively robust performance for Letter-Number Sequencing, despite educational disadvantage, is in keeping with the research of Engel, Santos and Gathercole (2008) which demonstrated that tests of working memory involving well-learned basic material such as numbers and letters, as distinct from higher-level numerical concepts and reasoning such as are called upon in the Arithmetic subtest, are relatively free of socio-economic influences. Overall the specific subtest results support the notion that reasoning ability and exposure to visuoperceptual construction tasks are functions affected by deficiencies in educational input, whereas verbal attention and concentration skills are less affected and/or preferentially promoted, as might be expected in an approach to education that focuses on rote learning rather than problem-solving (see earlier discussion concerning approaches to learning in disadvantaged educational settings, citing Grieve & Viljoen, 2000; Nell, 1999).

Conclusion

In summary, the newly presented research in respect of two *levels* of education (12+ and 15+ years of education), as reflected in Tables 2.1 and 2.2 respectively, has demonstrated the effect of quality of education across fine gradations of different degrees of disadvantaged and advantaged education at primary and high school levels. Accordingly it is clear that refinement of the Shuttleworth-Edwards et al. (2004) data was warranted, in that a less pure group in respect of ethnic (Xhosa) affiliation in that study happened also to be associated with a higher level of quality of education, a factor that in turn produced the expected advantageous effect on WAIS-III test performance. Overall, the normative data presented serve to emphasise the marked disparities in the South African educational system as a legacy of the apartheid system, and accordingly, as warned by Nell (1999), it is essential to make the *within* race group distinction for scientifically meaningful psychometric test indications, between those educated in the well-resourced English-medium Private/Model C schools and those educated in the impoverished Ex-DET/township schools. On the basis of this research it is evident that lowering associated with disadvantaged education amounts to as much as 20 IQ points, and renders the Claassen et al. (2001) South African WAIS-III standardisation problematic when making interpretations in respect of that population group.

While accepting the practical implications of the data is in order, it is important to be cautious about making assumptions concerning causality on the basis of these data, in that superior quality of education cannot be denoted as the sole cause of the raised WAIS-III scores amongst the Xhosa advantaged Private/Model C groups, compared with the Xhosa disadvantaged Ex-DET/township groups. Other closely interrelated factors are likely to be contributing to the picture, in that individuals with higher intellectual capacity in the first instance would be more likely to access advantaged educational opportunities, due to inherent ability and/or due to the fact that their parents have higher intellectual capacity, a higher level of education, and associated improved financial means. However, the purpose of this research was not to establish causation, nor was it to develop standardisation data for the general South African population. Rather, the objective was to provide demographically relevant *within group* normative indications on IQ test performance for a young adult South African group of black Xhosa and white English affiliation, further stratified for level and quality of education, to facilitate diagnostic accuracy for neurodiagnostic and psycho-legal purposes, and to make reality-based educational and occupational placements.

Clearly, a limitation of the research was that the sampling pool comprised small numbers. However, as indicated above, the use of small sample numbers in respect of well-stratified sample groupings is considered preferable to data with large sample numbers without adequate stratification (Mitrushina et al., 2005; Strauss et al., 2006). The present study was well controlled for all the crucial variables of age, level and quality of education, in addition to race and ethnic origin. Similarly, it is considered that there was adequate control for language usage in that all participants drawn into the sample were required to be speaking English at home, at work, or in their study situations most of the time, these being selection criteria that were demonstrated by Claassen et al. (2001) to be as discriminating of basic language proficiency for sampling purposes as a language test. Despite the small subgroup numbers, the data appear robust in that they are entirely commensurate with the differential performance expected in association with both level and quality of education.

Additional research is needed to explore effects for other South African language groups, and individuals with lower levels of education, as well as older and younger age groups. The cross-cultural outcome demonstrated here in respect of the WAIS-III will have broad application for the interpretation of test performance on the WAIS-IV, given the current absence of any other available research of this kind on either of these tests. However, to achieve greater specificity further research in this area should advisedly employ the improved later edition of the test.

Notes

1 Acknowledgements are due to the National Research Foundation and the Rhodes University Joint Research Council for funding utilised for the purposes of the first author's cross-cultural research.

2 The term 'Xhosa' is used to denote the amaXhosa people whose first language is isiXhosa.

References

Ardila, A. (1995). Directions of research in cross-cultural neuropsychology. *Journal of Clinical and Experimental Neuropsychology, 17,* 143–150.

Claassen, N. C. W., Krynauw, A. H., Paterson, H. & Mathe, M. (2001). *A Standardisation of the WAIS-III for English-speaking South Africans.* Pretoria: Human Sciences Research Council.

Cooper, B. (2004). 'Burn-out' threat saps teacher's morale. Unions cite assessment system, workloads for discontent. *The Herald,* Port Elizabeth, July 7.

Cull, P. (2001). EC Matric results show west-east split. Results mirror the spending patterns of the apartheid era. *The Herald,* Port Elizabeth, December 31.

Engel, P. M., Santos, F. H. & Gathercole, S. E. (2008). Are working memory measures free of socioeconomic influence? *Journal of Speech, Language and Hearing Research, 51(6),* 1580–1587.

Flanagan, D. P. & Kaufman, A. S. (2009). *Essentials of WISC-IV Assessment* (2nd edition). Hoboken, NJ: John Wiley & Sons.

Grieve, K. W. & Viljoen, S. (2000). An exploratory study of the use of the Austin maze in South Africa. *South African Journal of Psychology, 30,* 14–18.

Kallaway, P. (1984). *Apartheid and Education: The Education of Black South Africans.* Johannesburg: Ravan Press.

Lezak, M. D., Howieson, D. B. & Loring, D. W. (2004). *Neuropsychological Assessment* (4th edition). New York, NY: Oxford University Press.

Lichtenberger, E. O. & Kaufman, A. S. (Eds) (2009). *Essentials of WAIS-IV Assessment.* Hoboken, NJ: John Wiley & Sons.

Manly, J. J. (2005). Advantages and disadvantages of separate norms for African Americans. *The Clinical Neuropsychologist, 19,* 270–275.

Manly, J., Byrd, D., Touradji, P., Sanchez, D. & Stern, Y. (2004). Literacy and cognitive change among ethically diverse elders. *International Journal of Psychology, 39,* 47–60.

Manly, J., Jacobs, D., Touradji, P., Small, S. & Stern, Y. (2002). Reading level attenuates differences in neuropsychological test performance between African-American and white elders. *Journal of the International Neuropsychological Society, 8,* 341–348.

Matomela, D. (2008a). Eastern Cape schools far from ready for 2008. *The Herald,* Port Elizabeth, January 14.

Matomela, D. (2008b). New year, same old story. *The Herald,* Port Elizabeth, January 17.

Mitrushina, M., Boone, K. B., Razani, J. & D'Elia, L. F. (2005). *Handbook of Normative Data for Neuropsychological Assessment* (2nd edition). New York, NY: Oxford University Press.

Nell, V. (1994). Interpretation and misinterpretation of the South African Wechsler-Bellevue Adult Intelligence Scale: A history and a prospectus. *South African Journal of Psychology, 24(2),* 100–109.

Nell, V. (1999). Standardising the WAIS-III and the WMS-III for South Africa: Legislative, psychometric, and policy issues. *South African Journal of Psychology, 29(3),* 128–137.

Ogden, J. A. & McFarlane-Nathan, G. (1997). Cultural bias in the neuropsychological assessment of young Maori men. *New Zealand Journal of Psychology, 26*, 2–12.

Ostrosky-Solis, F., Ramirez, M. & Ardila, A. (2004). Effects of culture and education on neuropsychological testing: A preliminary study with indigenous and nonindigenous population. *Applied Neuropsychology, 11*, 186–193.

Rosselli, M. & Ardila, A. (2003). The impact of culture and education on non-verbal neuropsychological measurements: A critical review. *Brain and Cognition, 52*, 326–333.

Shuttleworth-Edwards, A. B., Kemp, R. D., Rust, A. L., Muirhead, J. G. L., Hartman, N. P. & Radloff, S. E. (2004). Cross-cultural effects on IQ test performance: A review and preliminary indications on WAIS-III test performance in South Africa. *Journal of Clinical and Experimental Neuropsychology, 26(7)*, 903–920.

Shuttleworth-Jordan, A. B. (1995). Against mutton masquerading as lamb: Additional commentary on the interpretation and misinterpretation of the SA-WAIS. *South African Journal of Psychology, 25*, 244–246.

Shuttleworth-Jordan, A. B. (1996). On not reinventing the wheel: A clinical perspective on culturally relevant test usage in South Africa. *South African Journal of Psychology, 26(2)*, 96–102.

South African Wechsler Adult Intelligence Scale (SAWAIS) Manual (1969). Johannesburg: National Institute for Personnel Research, Human Sciences Research Council.

Strauss, E., Sherman, E. M. S. & Spreen, O. (2006). *A Compendium of Neuropsychological Tests: Administration, Norms and Commentary* (3rd edition). New York, NY: Oxford University Press.

Van der Berg, S. (2004). Throwing money at education problem isn't enough. *Sunday Times*, July 4.

Van de Vijver, F. J. R. & Phalet, K. (2004). Assessment in multicultural groups: The role of acculturation. *Applied Psychology: An International Review, 53*, 215–236.

Wechsler, D. (1939). *The Measurement of Adult Intelligence*. Baltimore, MD: Williams & Wilkins.

Wechsler, D. (1944). *The Measurement of Adult Intelligence* (3rd edition). Baltimore, MD: Williams & Wilkins.

Wechsler, D. (1955). *The Wechsler Adult Intelligence Scale: Manual*. New York, NY: Psychological Corporation.

Wechsler, D. (1981). *The Wechsler Adult Intelligence Scale – Revised (WAIS-R): Manual*. New York, NY: Psychological Corporation.

Wechsler, D. (1997). *The Wechsler Adult Intelligence Scale – Third Edition (WAIS-III): Manual*. San Antonio, TX: Psychological Corporation.

Wechsler, D. (2004). *WISC-IV (UK): Wechsler Intelligence Scale for Children – Fourth UK Edition*. London: Harcourt Assessment.

Wechsler, D. (2008). *Wechsler Adult Intelligence Test – Fourth Edition (WAIS-IV): Manual*. Austin, TX: Pearson.

3 WISC-IV test performance in the South African context: a collation of cross-cultural norms

A. B. Shuttleworth-Edwards, A. S. van der Merwe, P. van Tonder and S. E. Radloff

The Wechsler Intelligence Scales have led the way in assessment of intelligence for almost seven decades, since the release of the original Wechsler-Bellevue Intelligence Scale in 1939 (Saklofske, Weiss, Beal & Coalson, 2003). Despite exemplary characteristics of other new and revised versions of intelligence tests, the Wechsler tests remain, and in the foreseeable future are likely to remain, the most widely used standardised measures for individual testing of children and adults worldwide, covering the age range from 2.5 to 89 years (Flanagan & Kaufman, 2009). The intermediate age ranges are catered for by the Wechsler Intelligence Scale for Children (WISC) which, when first released in 1949, marked the division of the Wechsler Intelligence Scales into separate tests for children and adults (Saklofske et al., 2003).

The WISC has gone through two previous revisions (WISC-R, 1974; WISC-III, 1991) prior to the most recently released version of the WISC-IV (Wechsler, 2003; 2004) that is intended for use with children aged 6 years to 16 years 11 months. The current version of the test was revised to keep up with changes in norms as population scores become inflated over time (known as the Flynn effect), as well as to ensure that test items remain current and unbiased (Prifitera, Weiss, Saklofske & Rolfhus, 2005). It also encompasses a fundamental theoretical shift, as it was designed with current trends in factor analysis theories in mind and thereby is considered to have introduced stronger psychometric properties (Baron, 2005). The test remains a good measure of *g* (the general intelligence factor) and consistently measures the same constructs across age groups 6 to 16 (Keith, Fine, Taub, Reynolds & Kranzler, 2006). The results of the US standardisation confirmed that the WISC-IV achieved high levels of reliability, with test-retest reliability being at least .76, but mostly in the .80s, and with subtest scores being less stable compared to Index scores and the Full Scale Intelligence Quotient (FSIQ); convergent validity with preceding editions of the Wechsler tests, including the WISC-III, yielded correlations from at least .73, but mostly in the high .70s and high .80s (Wechsler, 2003).

Based on new neurological models of cognitive function, the WISC-IV's main departure from the traditional Wechsler model is that it improves on the test's ability to evaluate perceptual reasoning, working memory and processing speed (Wechsler, 2003). This has been achieved by making changes to some subtests and/or incorporating new subtests, and by the creation of four domain Index scores including the Verbal Comprehension Index (VCI), the Perceptual Reasoning Index (PRI), the Working Memory Index (WMI) and the Processing Speed Index (PSI). The VCI was designed to replace the Verbal IQ (VIQ) and measures verbal knowledge, reasoning and conceptualisation, and the PRI was designed to replace the Performance IQ (PIQ) and measures interpretation, reasoning and organisation of visually presented nonverbal information; the WMI measures attention, concentration and working memory for verbal material, and the PSI measures speed of mental and graphomotor processing (Strauss, Sherman & Spreen, 2006). The test still allows for the calculation of a FSIQ derived from the four domain Index scores, thus representing a general composite score for the entire scale.

Specifically, in order to calculate the four composite Index scores and forming the basis of the FSIQ, the WISC-IV consists of a core battery of ten subtests, including Vocabulary, Similarities and Comprehension, which contribute to the VCI score; Block Design, Picture Concepts and Matrix Reasoning, which contribute to the PRI score; Digit Span and Letter-Number Sequencing, which contribute to the WMI score; and Coding and Symbol Search, which contribute to the PSI score. In addition there are five supplementary subtests, including Picture Completion, Cancellation, Information, Arithmetic and Word Reasoning. It is possible to replace one or more of the subtests from the core battery with one of the supplementary subtests within the same functional modality, thereby enhancing the test's flexibility.

WISC-IV standardisation and demographic indications

The WISC-IV has been standardised on a USA population of 2 200 children equally distributed for males and females, and an ethnic stratification that matches the 2000 USA census data closely (that is, white majority and other-than-white minority). In addition the test has been adapted and standardised for use in Canada, the UK, France and Belgium, the Netherlands, Germany, Austria and Switzerland, Sweden, Lithuania, Slovenia, Greece, Japan, South Korea and Taiwan (Van de Vijver, Mylonas, Pavlopoulos & Georgas, 2003). For the UK standardisation (used for the purposes of the present research), minor changes to content items were carried out in order to make the test more culture-specific, rather than a comprehensive rewriting of the test being undertaken (Wechsler, 2004). Comparisons between the US WISC-IV subtest raw scores and those derived from the WISC-IV (UK) version across each age group demonstrated close correspondence between the two sets of data. In the case of the UK standardisation, stratification for race/ethnic group was based on the UK 2001 census data, resulting in a sample that was made up of a majority of white individuals, including 87.6 per cent white and 12.4 per cent relatively evenly distributed black, Asian and other (Chinese and mixed) individuals (Wechsler, 2004).

Various demographic influences have been investigated in respect of the US standardisation sample of the WISC-IV, including the effects of sex and race. No differences were found for sex, with the exception of a small superior performance for boys over girls on the PSI of approximately five points (as reviewed in Strauss et al., 2006), thereby obviating the need for sex-specific normative data. However, substantial differences were found to be present for race. Specifically, persistent group differences between African-Americans, Hispanics and whites in the WISC-IV standardisation sample have been demonstrated, with white children achieving higher IQ scores than their African-American and Hispanic peers of 11.5 and 10 points, respectively (Prifitera et al., 2005; Sattler & Dumont cited in Strauss et al., 2006). The differences observed between these groups on individual Index scores varied, but PSI and WMI scores showed the least variation between groups. Differences between ethnic groups tended to increase with age, and Strauss et al. (2006) attribute this to the negative environmental influences which have a cumulative effect on development of cognitive abilities, especially in groups consisting of largely disadvantaged individuals.

Additional cross-cultural research in respect of any of the WISC tests is sparse, and only two studies were identified in respect of black African-American individuals. Kusch, Watkins, Ward, Ward, Canivez & Worrell (2001) demonstrate that factor loadings revealed anomalies for a referred black sample, and Brown (1998) reports that African-American children in her study performed 20 points below the mean of 100 for the WISC-III composite scores. Specifically with reference to the African continent, the only published cross-cultural research to date on the WISC in any of its forms appears to be that by Zindi (1994), who demonstrated a 25 point IQ differential on the WISC-R between black Zimbabwean children and white British children matched for social class, and he showed almost the same magnitude of difference on the Raven's. Evidence for test differences such as this between ethnic groups raises concerns about the use of the WISC-IV in the multicultural South African situation. While there has been an attempt to standardise the Wechsler Adult Intelligence Scale – Third Edition (WAIS-III) for a South African population (Claassen, Krynauw, Paterson & Mathe, 2001), to date there has been no attempt at South African standardisation of any of the Wechsler intelligence tests for children, including the WISC-IV.

The intricacies that are involved in cross-cultural test influences generally, in addition to those that pertain specifically to the South African context, warrant further elaboration.

Cross-cultural test issues

Two sets of issues relating to cross-cultural test influences are discussed here: issues pertaining to race and culture, and those involving education.

Race and culture

The influence of 'culture' and attitudes towards testing, which is a function of learning and experience acquired through social interaction, should be taken into account when assessing all individuals (Lezak, Howieson & Loring, 2004; Mitrushina, Boone, Razani & D'Elia, 2005). It is now commonly accepted in the cross-cultural literature that focusing on ethnicity/race differences alone may lead to faulty claims with regard to test performance, as cultural influences such as acculturation to the predominant culture amongst others, including literacy levels and English fluency, quality of education and socio-economic status, may better serve as an explanation for variance in test scores (Ardila, 1996; Harris & Llorente, 2005; Manly, Byrd, Touradji & Stern, 2004; Manly, Jacobs, Touradji, Small & Stern, 2002; Shuttleworth-Edwards, Kemp, Rust, Muirhead, Hartman & Radloff, 2004). In the South African context, due to the legacy of apartheid, test users need to acknowledge that race is a particularly potent mediator of the quality of education, economic opportunities, urbanisation and socio-economic status of many South Africans, and as such cultural issues are likely to impact on test performance (Nell, 1999). Stead (2002), like other researchers (for example, Van de Vijver & Rothmann, 2004), has highlighted two possible approaches that can be followed to address this problem.

Firstly, Stead cites researchers such as Sehlapelo and Terre Blanche who argue that non-indigenous (for example, US and European) tests should not be used in South Africa because of the questionable validity of test scores among black South Africans. This line of argument calls for the development of tests specific to the South African context, in that tests that have been developed elsewhere are inherently problematic for use in this country. Secondly, Stead draws attention to the contrasting argument of researcher Shuttleworth-Jordan (1996), who proposes that rather than 'reinventing the wheel', minor content modification and standardisation of existing tests is sufficient to allow for their use with a substantial proportion of previously disadvantaged black South Africans. This argument is based on the fact that many black South Africans have experienced an acculturation process, including moving from rural to urbanised conditions, and in the process have had the opportunity to access Westernised education and develop literacy in English. Accordingly, Shuttleworth-Jordan (1996) strongly advocates norming of commonly employed, internationally based cognitive tests for use in the South African context, rather than producing newly devised tests without the benefit of a long history of test refinement through clinical and research practices.

Commensurate with the latter position, it was decided by the Human Sciences Research Council (HSRC) to norm the most recent Wechsler test in current international use at that time, that is the WAIS-III, in its *English administration*, rather than devising a new South African-specific IQ test for use in the newly democratised South Africa (Claassen et al., 2001). The standardisation was achieved in respect of a young adult population only (age range 19–30). Notably, the Claassen et al. HSRC standardisation of the WAIS-III has been heavily criticised as being flawed due to the lack of control for quality of education *within* the other-than-white populations in the norm sample (Nell, 1999; Shuttleworth-Edwards et al., 2004). This is a factor that is of particular pertinence for cross-cultural researchers in both the adult and child populations, and demands further exploration.

Education, including quality of education

As is commonly documented, level of education is a highly significant variable of neuropsychological test performance, and specifically educational attainment correlates significantly with scores on intelligence tests (Ardila, 1996). However, researchers have shown that scores on intelligence tests are positively correlated not only with level of education (grades achieved), but also with performance on reading comprehension and mathematical knowledge, that is, with subjects closely linked to curriculum content (Brody, 1997; Byrd, Jacobs, Hilton, Stern & Manly, 2005). Byrd et al. (2005) conclude that while educational level has been documented to be a strong predictor of performance on intelligence tests, reading level and literacy are more accurate reflections of academic achievement than years of education. Further research reveals lowered cognitive test performance amongst elderly African-Americans from the south and north of the USA that is attributed to the factor of quality of education, in that some individuals were more likely to have had lower quality of education because of segregated schooling (Manly et al., 2004). In a key article included in a special edition of *The Clinical Neuropsychologist* on African-American normative data, Manly cautions that separation of test battery norms purely in terms of ethnicity is not scientifically meaningful due to the 'tremendous [within-group] heterogeneity in cultural, educational, linguistic and environmental exposure' (Manly, 2005, p.274). Manly's observation has particular relevance in light of disparate educational opportunities historically within South Africa, and current developments in association with 20 years of democratisation.

It is clearly apparent that South Africa's racialised past has left a legacy of educational inequality that sets ethnic groups apart. A negative effect on educational achievement is most clearly evidenced for the underprivileged black group (Fleisch, 2007). Prior to the desegregation of South African schools in 1991, white learners, as well as a minority of learners from other race groups who had the financial means, attended privately funded independent schools (hereafter termed private schools) or government-funded Model C schools run by various provincial departments of education. These children enjoyed access to more than 75 per cent of available resources (Broom, 2004; Claassen et al., 2001). Private and former Model C schools remain well resourced, and children educated in these schools achieve academic competency, perform in the upper range and comprise the majority of university entrants and graduates (Fleisch, 2007). Conversely, black learners attended schools run by the Department of Education and Training (DET) and coloured learners attended schools run by the House of Representatives (HOR), the coloured House of Parliament. These children attended vastly under-resourced schools and were mostly taught by underqualified teachers, and currently the vast majority of black and coloured South African children (those from working-class and poor families) are still attending former DET or HOR schools (hereafter termed township schools), making up approximately 80 per cent of all learners in South Africa (Broom, 2004; Claassen et al., 2001; Fleisch, 2007).

Although township schools are generally referred to as 'previously disadvantaged', many continue to be relatively ill-resourced or have resources that may be underutilised (Matomela, 2008a; 2008b). These schools often lack basic supplies, books or even desks. They also receive only basic government funding; there is absenteeism from the classroom (of teachers and learners); ineffective teaching methods are used; there are higher teacher–learner ratios in township schools; and teachers are often underqualified, have weak subject knowledge and do not cope with changing demands of the curriculum. Moreover, the township teachers are often not fully proficient in the English language, although tuition is normally expected to occur in English in these schools from Grade 3 (Fleisch, 2007). All these factors, therefore, contribute to a poorer quality of education in township schools (Cooper, 2004; Fleisch, 2007; Nell, 1999). In short, the inequality in the South African education system continues, especially in the relatively poor Eastern Cape Province (Cull, 2001; Matomela, 2008a; 2008b).

In the apartheid era, the educational divide between private and Model C schooling and township schooling was almost exclusively manifested along racial lines. Since democratisation, however, this is no longer the case, in that increasing numbers of black and coloured children attend the traditionally white English-medium private and former Model C schools, thereby being exposed to relatively better-resourced and advantaged educational settings. This, in turn, is likely to impact on IQ test performance differentially *within* these ethnic groups. Therefore, as indicated above, failure to take the within-groups variable of quality of education into account has resulted in heavy criticism being levelled at the Claassen et al. (2001) WAIS-III standardisation attempt. Specifically in order to redress the shortfall in this regard, Shuttleworth-Edwards et al. (2004) set about generating preliminary normative indications for the WAIS-III (English administration), in respect of a predominantly South African sample that was stratified for white English first-language and black African first-language individuals who were either working or studying in the medium of English, and that in turn was stratified for both level (Grade 12 and graduate) *and* quality of education (advantaged private/ former Model C schooling versus disadvantaged township schooling).

The results of this study revealed significant effects for both level and quality of education in the direction of poorer performance for Grade 12s versus Graduate groups across both black African and white English first-language groups, and for disadvantaged schooling in relation to advantaged schooling *within* the black African first-language group of around 25 IQ points. It was deemed imperative, therefore, given the absence of any further available cross-cultural research on the WISC series of tests, to extend the Shuttleworth-Edwards et al. (2004) WAIS–III investigation downwards with a cross-cultural investigation into WISC-IV test performance in respect of a South African child population that was similarly stratified for both race and quality of education.

The WISC-IV norming study

An investigation into WISC-IV performance was conducted by the present researchers, using the WISC-IV (UK) version of the test (Wechsler, 2004) that is virtually identical to the WISC-IV (US) version of the test (Wechsler, 2003), with the objective of producing comparative normative indications for the ten core subtest scores, four Index scores and the FSIQ score that could be utilised in typical clinical situations as they currently apply in the South African context. Importantly, this type of *within-group* normative study, which is finely stratified for demographic characteristics such as race and language, needs to be differentiated from a test standardisation that pertains more broadly to the general population (Strauss et al., 2006). Typically, the within-group normative study is in respect of relatively small subgroup samples when compared with the typically large standardisation sample, and subgroup normative data are frequently presented in the descriptive form of means and standard deviations (Mitrushina et al., 2005; Strauss et al., 2006).

Procedure and sample distribution

Building on the research of Shuttleworth-Edwards et al. (2004), preliminary normative data were collected for a Grade 7 South African child sample stratified for race and language (white English, black Xhosa, white Afrikaans, coloured Afrikaans) and quality of education (advantaged private/former Model C schooling versus disadvantaged township schooling). In order to ensure a nonclinical sample, the following exclusion criteria applied: repeated grade at any stage; presence of a learning disability; history of medical, psychiatric or neurological disorder. The final combined sample (N = 69) was made up of Grade 7 participants with an age range of 12 to 13 years, as summarised in Table 3.1.

Table 3.1 Grade 7 samples, stratified for ethnicity,* language,** quality of education*** and sex

Ethnic group	First language	Education	Sex		Sample (N = 69)
			M	F	
White	English	Private/Model C	n = 6	n = 6	n = 12
Black	Xhosa	Private/Model C	n = 6	n = 6	n = 12
Black	Xhosa	DET Township	n = 6	n = 6	n = 12
White	Afrikaans	Model C	n = 6	n = 6	n = 12
Coloured	Afrikaans	Model C	n = 6	n = 3	n = 9
Coloured	Afrikaans	HOR Township	n = 6	n = 6	n = 12

Notes: *White, black, coloured; **English, Xhosa, Afrikaans; ***Advantaged, disadvantaged.

Level of education

To ensure an equal performance distribution, the researchers consulted with the schools to verify learners' marks for Grade 6 and Grade 7. This was done as the objective was to test a cross-section of children across all performance levels, so that the sample would be representative of normally performing children within a specific targeted school situation. This was not possible within the coloured Afrikaans advantaged schooling group, however, as this group did not typically perform well academically, and learners in this group tended to be in the bottom performance range within their class.

School sampling

The white English and black Xhosa Grade 7 learners were sampled from schools in Grahamstown (Eastern Cape, South Africa), with a balanced distribution for attendance at either a private or former Model C school. The white Afrikaans and coloured Afrikaans Grade 7 learners included white Afrikaans and coloured advantaged learners attending former Model C schools only, due to the lack of availability of private Afrikaans-medium schools in the area where the study was taking place. To complete the sample, Afrikaans learners with advantaged education were drawn from Port Elizabeth and Cape Town, as well as from Grahamstown.

Age and sex

Participants were all between the ages of 12.01 and 13.11 years (mean = 13.04, SD = 0.34). Age differences between the comparative groups were not statistically significant ($p > 0.05$ in all instances). A target total of n = 12 participants with equal sex distribution was met for all groups, with the exception of the coloured Afrikaans advantaged group that yielded a total of n = 9 participants, with an unequal sex distribution of males (n = 6) and females (n = 3).

Data collection

The data were collected by intern clinical/counselling psychologists assisted by psychology honours students trained in the administration of the test. Whereas the WAIS-III norming initiatives in South Africa of Claassen et al. (2001) and Shuttleworth-Edwards et al. (2004) employed an English-only administration of the test, this route was not deemed appropriate for children at Grade 7 level, as in a clinical setting it is considered appropriate to conduct testing in a child's language of tuition. Accordingly, white English and black Xhosa advantaged learners who were from English-medium schools were given the standardised English administration, as it was assumed that they had received good-quality English language tuition. A Xhosa-speaking intern clinical psychologist was used as a translator for testing black Xhosa disadvantaged learners, who were given test instructions in English followed by a spontaneous Xhosa translation of the instruction, as this practice mirrored mixed Xhosa/English language use in these classrooms. Afrikaans participants who were from Afrikaans-medium schools were tested in Afrikaans by testers proficient in spoken Afrikaans, on the basis of an Afrikaans translation of the test devised by a bilingual postgraduate student specifically for the purposes of the research. It was acknowledged that this approach deviated from the ideal of using formally translated and standardised tests. However, the *modus operandi* was typical of the current mode of test application in clinical settings (given the absence of standardised translations), and the research aim was to provide preliminary normative indications to facilitate clinical practice, rather than a large-scale standardisation of the test.

Results and discussion

From the normative table (Table 3.2) it is clear that WISC-IV performance revealed a clear continuum of a downward trend in association with lower quality of education. In other words, the overall trend was that groups with advantaged

Table 3.2 WISC-IV performance of English, Xhosa and Afrikaans Grade 7 learners, stratified for advantaged versus disadvantaged education (N = 69)

	Advantaged				Disadvantaged	
Index or subtest	**Group 1 White English adv. (n = 12)**	**Group 2 White Afrikaans adv. (n = 12)**	**Group 3 Black Xhosa adv. (n = 12)**	**Group 4 Coloured Afrikaans adv. (n = 9)**	**Group 5 Black Xhosa disad. (n = 12)**	**Group 6 Coloured Afrikaans disad. (n = 12)**
VCI	**M = 120.92 (SD = 14.76)**	**M = 92.58 (SD = 12.40)**	**M = 101.30 (SD = 10.12)**	**M = 85.00 (SD = 6.08)**	**M = 80.42 (SD = 13.59)**	**M = 65.08 (SD = 11.25)**
Similarities	M = 14.08 (SD = 2.35)	M = 8.92 (SD = 3.03)	M = 12.33 (SD = 2.35)	M = 7.44 (SD = 1.59)	M = 6.42 (SD = 3.50)	M = 4.33 (SD = 3.20)
Vocabulary	M = 13.75 (SD = 2.49)	M = 8.42 (SD = 2.39)	M = 9.08 (SD = 2.07)	M = 6.78 (SD = 1.92)	M = 7.08 (SD = 3.61)	M = 3.17 (SD = 1.19)
Comprehension	M = 12.92 (SD = 3.26)	M = 8.75 (SD = 2.26)	M = 9.58 (SD = 2.43)	M = 7.89 (SD = 1.27)	M = 6.50 (SD = 2.68)	M = 4.58 (SD = 2.07)
PRI	**M = 111.67 (SD = 18.10)**	**M = 97.50 (SD = 16.83)**	**M = 92.75 (SD = 7.57)**	**M = 90.67 (SD = 10.09)**	**M = 80.83 (SD = 11.21)**	**M = 73.83 (SD = 12.04)**
Block Design	M = 11.83 (SD = 2.66)	M = 10.17 (SD = 4.28)	M = 8.33 (SD = 1.92)	M = 7.11 (SD = 2.09)	M = 6.42 **(SD = 1.93)**	M = 4.92 (SD = 2.02)
Picture Concepts	M = 11.67 (SD = 2.43)	M = 9.67 (SD = 2.84)	M = 10.00 (SD = 2.34)	M = 10.00 (SD = 3.00)	M = 7.67 (SD = 2.64)	M = 6.92 (SD = 2.84)
Matrix Reasoning	M = 10.75 (SD = 3.28)	M = 8.92 (SD = 2.54)	M = 8.08 (SD = 2.02)	M = 8.33 (SD = 1.73)	M = 6.58 (SD = 1.93)	M = 5.33 (SD = 2.35)
WMI	**M = 101.25 (SD = 13.37)**	**M = 97.00 (SD = 12.13)**	**M = 100.08 (SD = 10.08)**	**M = 85.67 (SD = 12.45)**	**M = 86.50 (SD = 12.99)**	**M = 71.00 (SD = 11.78)**
Digit Span	M = 11.42 (SD = 3.61)	M = 8.83 (SD = 2.95)	M = 10.42 (SD = 2.23)	M = 6.78 (SD = 2.28)	M = 7.25 (SD = 2.42)	M = 6.00 (SD = 2.17)
Letter-Number Sequencing	M = 9.25 (SD = 2.90)	M = 10.33 (SD = 2.02)	M = 9.83 (SD = 2.17)	M = 8.33 (SD = 3.20)	M = 8.17 (SD = 3.27)	M = 4.00 (SD = 3.02)
PSI	**M = 96.17 (SD = 14.89)**	**M = 96.17 (SD = 15.09)**	**M = 84.50 (SD = 12.30)**	**M = 84.33 (SD = 6.12)**	**M = 79.83 (SD = 16.28)**	**M = 75.33 (SD = 11.24)**
Coding	M = 8.00 (SD = 2.66)	M = 8.33 (SD = 2.77)	M = 7.08 (SD = 2.64)	M = 6.00 (SD = 1.23)	M = 5.83 (SD = 2.73)	M = 6.00 (SD = 1.95)
Symbol Search	M = 10.75 (SD = 2.56)	M = 10.25 (SD = 2.77)	M = 7.33 (SD = 2.61)	M = 8.56 (SD = 1.59)	M = 6.92 (SD = 3.48)	M = 5.00 (SD = 2.63)
FSIQ	**M = 112.83 (SD = 13.17)**	**M = 94.42 (SD = 13.25)**	**M = 93.92 (SD = 5.85)**	**M = 82.67 (SD = 7.43)**	**M = 77.08 (SD = 13.79)**	**M = 64.25 (SD = 9.73)**

Notes: VCI = Verbal Comprehension Index; PRI = Perceptual Reasoning Index; WMI = Working Memory Index; PSI = Processing Speed Index; FSIQ = Full Scale IQ; M = mean; SD = standard deviation.

schooling performed better than those with disadvantaged schooling. The historically advantaged white English group obtained the highest mean scores across all four indices, as well as on the FSIQ. This group also obtained the highest mean scores on 8 out of 10 of the core subtests. When the advantaged groups were ranked according to their performance on the WISC-IV, the white English advantaged participants performed best. Next best were white Afrikaans advantaged and black Xhosa advantaged participants, with lower mean scores compared to the white English advantaged group but with largely corresponding scores when compared to each other. The coloured Afrikaans advantaged participants achieved the poorest performance in the advantaged grouping.

A further downward trend was observed between advantaged and disadvantaged groups. Within the disadvantaged grouping, black Xhosa disadvantaged participants performed somewhat better than their coloured Afrikaans disadvantaged counterparts, who obtained the weakest mean scores on all four indices and on the FSIQ, as well as the lowest mean scores on 9 out of 10 of the core subtests, with the exception of the Coding subtest for which they were marginally better than the black Xhosa disadvantaged group and the same as the coloured Afrikaans advantaged group.

Importantly, the downward trend of IQ test performance in association with quality of education was true for all Index scores in both the verbal and non-verbal modalities. However, the overall lowering for disadvantaged education was much higher for the VCI (a massive 55 points overall), and somewhat less for the other three Index scores in descending order of PRI (40 points), WMI (30 points) and PSI (20 points). Lowering in nonverbal areas is consistent with the observation of cross-cultural researchers such as Nell (1999), who emphasise the effect of differential test-taking attitudes and test-wiseness on all cognitive test performance, not just on acquired verbal function. The relative preservation of the WMI and PSI demonstrated on the present research (compared with the VCI and PRI) is consistent with indications on the WISC-IV cross-cultural research of Sattler & Dumont (cited in Strauss et al., 2006), and Prifitera et al. (2005) referred to earlier, in respect of Hispanic and African-American children.

Across all indices and the FSIQ, mean scores of the South African Grade 7 white English advantaged group were equivalent to, or somewhat higher than, mean scores of the US/UK standardisation samples. The generally higher mean scores for the white English advantaged group can be accounted for in that the South African sample was specifically stratified for ethnicity/first language, level of education and quality of education, which is not the general practice when tests are standardised. Further, the higher mean scores for the Grade 7 white English advantaged sample compared with the white Afrikaans advantaged sample may be accounted for by the facts that (i) a proportion of the white English advantaged participants received private schooling whereas the Afrikaans sample was purely made up of non-private, Model C learners; and (ii) the WISC-IV was administered in Afrikaans to white Afrikaans-speaking learners, and it is possible that the translation of the test may have impacted negatively on the outcome for this group on verbal items in particular.

Similar sampling and administrative explanations may apply to the finding of lower scores for the coloured advantaged group compared with the black advantaged group, in that (i) the black group was drawn from both private *and* Model C schooling (whereas the Afrikaans sample was purely made up of non-private Model C learners); and (ii) the black group would have had the advantage of receiving test instructions in English in the standardised form (in contrast to getting the test instructions in the Afrikaans form, as per the administration mode that was applied with the Afrikaans learners). Additional sampling effects that may have contributed generally to the relatively depressed performance for the Afrikaans advantaged group are that the coloured Afrikaans advantaged population tended to be amongst the lower achievers in the bottom half of the class, and furthermore this was the only unbalanced group in respect of sex (three female compared with six male participants).

It is of particular note that, while the performances of the advantaged groups in respect of the FSIQ ranged from high to low average along the continuum, the performances of the disadvantaged groups were in the borderline and extremely low (mild mental retardation) ranges for the black Xhosa disadvantaged and coloured Afrikaans disadvantaged groups respectively (see Table 3.2, Groups 5 and 6). As all participants in the study were representative of a nonclinical population, and were judged to be of average academic standard and had never failed a grade before, the findings are cause for concern. The important implication arising from these norms is that when practitioners apply the WISC-IV US or UK norms to individuals who are currently attending relatively disadvantaged schools, or who have a substantive background of exposure to such poorer quality of education, they need to exercise caution to avoid potential misdiagnosis.

For instance, children with disadvantaged educational exposure may be mistakenly classified as mentally handicapped or intellectually compromised, with the implication of the need for placement in special educational streams or special needs schools, when this is not actually applicable. Such erroneous placement would in turn cause further disadvantage in terms of educational exposure, by virtue of the child having been removed from the challenge of mainstream education, and would in addition be harmful to self-esteem as a consequence of the child's perception of him- or herself as being intellectually subnormal. In addition, treatment or compensation for the presence and extent of damage following brain trauma will be extremely difficult to evaluate with any accuracy if the specific effect of disadvantaged education is unknown. Lowered scores may result in an overestimate of the extent of damage, and thereby contribute to a falsely applied sick image, or unwarranted financial compensation. Conversely, for those with relatively advantaged education, if interpretations of test data are applied with the expectation of significantly lowered scores on the basis of race alone when this is not applicable, the presence of clinically significant lowering due to brain dysfunction may be overlooked. Such misdiagnosis could preclude a child from receiving appropriate medical interventions which might even be life-saving, or could preclude the child from special educational support when it is indicated, and/or could deprive the child of deserved financial compensation.

Conclusion

The WISC-IV is the most recent advance in the Wechsler series of intelligence scales for children covering the age range 6 years to 16 years 11 months (Wechsler, 2003), with stronger psychometric properties than earlier versions of the test (Baron, 2005; Prifitera et al., 2005). However, it has never been standardised for a South African population, nor have any South African standardisations been undertaken for preceding versions of the test.

This chapter has presented the results of preliminary norms established for a Grade 7, largely Eastern Cape population in the age range 12 to 13 years across participants stratified for race, language, and disadvantaged versus advantaged education. The resultant norms are thus very specific to the demographic features of the groups investigated, as well as being regionally specific. Therefore caution should be exercised when applying the norms to individuals from other regions of South Africa, or to individuals from other ethnic/language groups such as other than Xhosa-speaking black African language groups. Nevertheless, the outcome reveals substantive lowering in association with disadvantaged education across all race groups of as much as 20 to 30 IQ points, replicating the earlier South African WAIS-III study of Shuttleworth-Edwards et al. (2004), and earlier research in relation to the WISC-R and WISC-III of Zindi (1994) and Brown (1998), respectively. In accordance with the observations of Nell (1999) and Manly (2005) noted above, the research confirms in robust fashion that ethnicity in itself is not a meaningful norming category. Significant heterogeneity *within* ethnic groups, particularly in terms of quality of education, should therefore be accounted for in test interpretation with multicultural and multilingual populations. It is essential that appropriate cross-cultural norms such as those explicated here are used in clinical practice to ensure that misdiagnosis is avoided.

Although sample numbers were relatively small within the Shuttleworth-Edwards et al. (2004) study (n = 10 to 12 participants per subgroup), data that are well stratified for the pertinent variables of age, level of education, ethnicity and/or quality of education are considered to have more validity than poorly stratified data on large sample numbers (Lezak et al., 2004; Mitrushina et al., 2005; Strauss et al., 2006). Accordingly, the research is published in a leading international journal of clinical neuropsychology, and cited in a number of seminal neuropsychology assessment texts (for example, Grant & Adams, 2009; Strauss et al., 2006). A current literature search failed to reveal any further cross-cultural reports since the Shuttleworth-Edwards et al. (2004) study in respect of any of the adult and child Wechsler Intelligence Scales, including the WAIS-R, WAIS-III, WAIS-IV, WISC-R and WISC-IV, such that the indications from this 2004 South African study on the WAIS-III have remained the most pertinent to date, with a glaring gap in cross-cultural information in respect of the child versions of this series of intelligence scales.

The data in this chapter in respect of the WISC-IV, while also in respect of small sample numbers, similarly gain validity in that the sample is well stratified for the relevant socio-cultural variables. Further, clear replication of the adult findings in this child-oriented research, of a downward continuum of IQ

Pattern Completion, Missing Parts and Form Board subtests of the Performance scale, enabling the measurement of both power and speed. The core subtests form the basis for the Full Scale IQ (FSIQ) and are used to derive the Verbal and Nonverbal IQs. The Memory for Digits and Coding subtests are additional subtests, to be used if further diagnostic information is required, and are not included in the composite scales. The reason for this is that their low factor analytic loadings suggest that they make a small contribution to general intelligence and they do not load clearly on the verbal or nonverbal factor.

Thurstone's method was used to arrange the items within the subtests. Homogenous items that measured the same ability were added, in ascending order of difficulty, to each subtest (Van Eeden, 1997b).

Table 4.1 Description of subtests of the SSAIS-R and what they measure

Subtest	Description and rationale
	Verbal scale
Vocabulary	Five cards with four pictures per card. The testee must indicate the picture that is most relevant to a given word. There are 10 words for each card, with a total of 50 words. It measures receptive language skills, the ability to understand single words out of context, long-term memory, concept formation and verbal learning ability.
Comprehension	Fifteen questions about conventional social situations and everyday practices. It assesses social reasoning skills, long-term memory, logical reasoning and general knowledge.
Similarities	Fifteen pairs of concepts where the testee must determine the degree of similarity between each pair. It measures the quality of verbal reasoning (abstract, functional, concrete), verbal concept formation, long-term memory, ability to form associations, classification and deduction of rules.
Number Problems	Twenty arithmetical problems, of which 11 are presented only verbally and the remaining 9 are also presented on cards. It evaluates numerical reasoning, logical thinking, long-term and working memory and attention.
Story Memory	A short story containing 43 facts, which is read to the testee. It assesses short-term memory skills for contextualised auditory information, verbal learning and attention.
	Nonverbal scale
Pattern Completion	Nineteen partially completed patterns which the testee must complete using a pencil. Three sections of each pattern are complete, requiring the testee to deduce the rule for completion of the fourth segment. This is a nonverbal measure of logical thinking, visual perception, concept formation and attention.
Block Designs	Fifteen items which require the re-creation of a model (either concrete or on cards) using between four and nine plastic cubes. It evaluates nonverbal problem-solving, visual-spatial analysis and synthesis, perceptual organisation, visual-motor coordination and attention.

continued →

Subtest	Description and rationale
Missing Parts	Twenty pictures, each with an essential part missing, which the testee must identify, verbally or nonverbally. It measures contact with reality, ability to distinguish between essential and non-essential visual information, visual perception, long-term visual memory and the ability to understand the whole in relation to its parts.
Form Board	A board containing six coloured shapes which the testee must re-create using three to four loose parts. It assesses visual perception, visual concept formation, visual-spatial analysis and synthesis and visual motor coordination.
Additional subtests	
Memory for Digits	A series of digits are read out by the examiner and the testee must repeat them in the same sequence for the Forwards section and in reverse sequence for the Backwards section. It determines the testee's working memory, auditory sequencing and auditory attention.
Coding	Digits from one to nine, each with an accompanying symbol, are provided in a key at the top of the page. The testee must complete the accompanying symbol for a random array of 91 digits within 120 minutes. This measures visual-associative learning, psychomotor speed, visual-motor integration and coordination, as well as attention.

The time required to administer the SSAIS-R is approximately 90 minutes, and it has instructions and scoring in both English and Afrikaans. There is no evidence that the English and Afrikaans versions of the SSAIS-R are equivalent. Despite this, separate norms are only provided for each language for the Vocabulary subtest. In terms of scoring the test, subtest standard scores range from 0 to 20 and it is possible that the test may not be sufficiently sensitive for very low-functioning children. Tables are provided to convert raw scores to scaled scores, which have a mean of 10 and a standard deviation of 3. Confidence intervals based on standard errors of estimate (SEE) and true scores are provided in the manual for each age range for both the environmentally disadvantaged (that is, English- and Afrikaans-speaking coloured and Indian children from socio-economically deprived backgrounds) and non-disadvantaged (that is, English and Afrikaans first-language white children from advantaged backgrounds) normative samples. The SEE gives an indication of the probable limits of a child's true test score (IQ in this case). A confidence interval of 2 SEE should provide a sufficient range within which a true score is likely to fall (Van Eeden, 1997b).

Information necessary for calculating the significance and frequency of discrepancies for an individual's subtest profile are provided in the *Background and Standardisation* manual (Van Eeden, 1997b). It is important to note that the nonverbal subtests for children aged 12 years and older are less suitable for profile analysis in the case of more intelligent learners (two standard deviations or more above the mean for 12- and 13-year-olds, and one standard deviation above the mean for 14–16-year-olds) (Van Eeden, 1997b). In these cases statistically significant deviations do not necessarily point to a weakness in the learner's profile, as the scores may still fall well within (or above) the average range of functioning. Although significant differences should be investigated further, in these cases it is important to base hypotheses on additional information and not just on a single score.

The statistical significance of Verbal versus Nonverbal scale differences is provided in the *Background and Standardisation* manual (Van Eeden, 1997b). Differences between the Verbal and Nonverbal scales should be interpreted with caution, as they may in certain instances be statistically significant, but may not have practical significance. Thus, a difference between the Verbal and Nonverbal scales may be calculated as statistically significant, when in practice such differences occur relatively frequently in the general population and are consequently not practically significant. It is also important to remember that the FSIQ score cannot be interpreted meaningfully if there is a significant difference between the VIQ and the PIQ. Tables for prorating are not provided, which is appropriate, since prorating introduces unknown measurement error and violates standard administration procedures.

Demographic variables

A limited set of demographic influences has been examined in respect of the SSAIS-R – namely, home language and gender. According to Van Eeden (1997b), there was a significant difference in performance on both the Verbal and Nonverbal scales of the SSAIS-R between English- and Afrikaans-speaking children ($p < .05$), in favour of the former group. Claassen (1987) cites the higher socio-economic status of the English-speaking learners as a possible reason for this difference.

In terms of gender effects, there was no significant difference between boys and girls in their performance on any of the composite scales of the SSAIS-R, despite the popular belief that girls are more verbally orientated, while boys are regarded as more mathematically and spatially adept. There is, however, some empirical support for such beliefs. For example, Bee and Boyd (2004) found that American primary school boys scored significantly higher on numerical reasoning tasks than matched girls, whereas the girls scored significantly higher on verbally related tasks. That such differences did not emerge on the SSAIS-R is advantageous, as it eliminates the need for gender-specific normative data.

While comparisons between the environmentally disadvantaged and non-disadvantaged groups are noticeably absent, the means and standard deviations are provided for each group so that these comparisons can be made. When calculated, there were significant differences across all age groups and subtests ($p < .0001$) in favour of the non-disadvantaged group, which increased with age. Strauss, Sherman and Spreen (2006) attribute such increases to the fact that adverse environmental influences exert a cumulative effect on cognitive abilities, and these increases may be more evident within disadvantaged groups.

No data are provided in respect of parental education, although this would be expected to influence performance on the SSAIS-R, since parents who have a tertiary education are likely to enter professional occupations, and subsequently to belong to middle-to-high socio-economic groups. This in turn influences access to financial resources, diet, health care, quality of education, exposure to books and technology, parent-to-child ratio, parental knowledge of child development and familiarity with Western cultural mores, which are all likely to have an effect on child development and psychological functioning (Brislin, 1990; Flynn & Weiss, 2007; Nell, 1997; Owen, 1991). While no local data exist to support this, the mean FSIQ of children of US parents who had completed college was found to be 22 points higher than that of children whose parents had less than nine years of education (Sattler & Dumont, 2004).

Normative data

When the SSAIS was revised in 1985, a proportionally stratified sample of 500 learners (100 per age group, for ages 7, 9, 12, 14 and 16 years) was drawn from each of the legacy education departments (i.e. the Houses of Delegates (Indians), Representatives (coloureds) and Assembly (whites); black Africans had no parliamentary representation and were thus not included in the standardisation sample), using a method of controlled selection. Stratification variables included province, medium of instruction and area. Items were eliminated which favoured one or more race groups over the others. For inclusion, an item had to discriminate between learners within the different age groups and the distribution of difficulty values had to be as wide as possible. Items were then arranged in ascending order of difficulty in each subtest (Van Eeden, 1997b).

The original test norms were based on a sample of 2 000 children, with 200 at each year from ages 7 years to 16 years 11 months. The children were drawn from white, Indian and coloured racial groups, and spoke either Afrikaans or English as their home language. Because of their low representation, children attending private and special needs schools were not included. Norms were stratified again according to province, medium of instruction and area (Van Eeden, 1997b).

Since the SSAIS-R content is based on Western cultural knowledge, environmentally disadvantaged children would be handicapped in terms of knowledge of and familiarity with the cultural content of the test. A positive correlation was found between socio-economic status, particularly socio-economic deprivation, and performance on the SSAIS-R (Van Eeden, 1997b). Consequently, a separate sample of 4 767 coloured and Indian children was also drawn up. Thus, the norms in Part III: Tables of Norms represent norms for English and Afrikaans first-language children who can be considered non-environmentally disadvantaged. A second set of norms exists for the proportional or environmentally disadvantaged sample, in an appendix to the manual.

Two additional studies explored the validity of the SSAIS-R with 14- and 15-year-old high school learners who had an African language as their mother tongue and were attending private schools (Van Eeden, 1993), and 14- and 15-year-old learners attending Model C schools who had an African language as their mother tongue (Van Eeden, 1997a). These studies were motivated by the growing need to use the SSAIS-R with children who did not have English as their mother tongue and because 'differences in the quality of education cause substantial variations of proficiency in English among children of the same age' (Van Eeden, 1993, p.1).

In terms of the first study, the sample comprised 105 learners who were attending private schools in Johannesburg and Pretoria. Of this group, 35 children had English as their home language and 70 spoke an African language at home. The former group formed a comparison group for the latter group. They were all said to be reasonably proficient in English, as determined by performance on a Scholastic Achievement Test in English. When their performances were compared, the English first-language group showed significantly higher levels of performance. The performance of the children who spoke an African language at home was comparable to that of the non-environmentally disadvantaged group. The relatively small sample size may have influenced these results. It was concluded from the study that the norms for the proportional (environmentally disadvantaged) norm group should be used if a child is not tested in his or her mother tongue. Further, the SSAIS-R was shown to be reasonably reliable for use with children who did not speak English at home, but who had some proficiency in English. However, it was advised that confidence intervals based on the standard errors of measurement (SEM) be used to indicate the possible range of a child's true score.

The second study, which explored the validity of the SSAIS-R for 14- and 15-year-old learners at Model C schools who had an African language as their mother tongue, was published in 1997 (Van Eeden, 1997a). This employed a similar methodology and sample sizes to the 1993 study and reached the same conclusions as the 1993 study had done.

It is no longer valid to compare South African children along language (or ethnic) lines in order to determine performance. It is now apparent that quality of schooling plays a critical role in determining the outcome of IQ testing (Shuttleworth-Edwards, Kemp, Rust, Muirhead, Hartman & Radloff, 2004). In South Africa, schools are still living with the legacy of apartheid and although they are now racially desegregated, there are still marked inequalities between independent (privately funded) schools, former Model C government schools and schools located within townships and rural areas. The former two types of schools are far better resourced than the latter, in which learning is hampered by poorly trained teachers, high teacher–learner ratios and lack of educational resources, to name but a few of the problems these schools experience (Fleisch, 2007). Shuttleworth-Edwards et al. (2004) note this issue, and in the preliminary normative data that they have collected for white English first-language and black African first-language South Africans on the Wechsler Intelligence Scale for Children (Fourth Edition) (WISC-IV), they have stratified their sample for quality of education (advantaged versus disadvantaged).

Psychometric properties

In order to determine scaled and standard scores from the standardisation data, raw scores from the normative sample were normalised for each age group. Scaled scores were then derived from these distributions. This resulted in 16 six-month age bands, with scaled scores ranging from 1 to 19 for each age group. Composite Verbal and Nonverbal, as well as Full Scale scores, can also be derived, which are based on sums of scaled scores.

Internal reliability and standard error of measurement

Within the non-environmentally disadvantaged group, internal consistency reliability coefficients using the Kuder-Richardson Formula 8 for subtests 1 to 10 and the Kuder-Richardson Formula 12 for subtest 11 range from 0.59 (Missing Parts, ages 13 and 14 years) to 0.91 (Block Designs, 8-, 10- and 12-year-olds) for the subtest scores. The reliability coefficients for the composite scales were calculated using Mosier's formula and range from 0.86 (Nonverbal scale, 12-year-olds) to 0.95 (Full Scale, 9-, 10-, 11-, 13- and 15-year-olds). It is important to consider the reliability coefficients and the SEM when interpreting subtest and composite scale scores. The average SEM across age for the FSIQ is 3.51 IQ points; others range from .83 to 1.90 scaled score units (subtests) and from 3.29 to 5.43 IQ points (composite scores). The *Background and Standardisation* manual (Van Eeden, 1997a) provides more detail on this, and on SEM by age.

Content validity

The development of the SSAIS-R, as well as its predecessors, the SSAIS and NSAIS (which both had good content validity), was based on the Wechsler model of intelligence. The process of development included bias analyses on the standardisation sample results. Quality assurance procedures were carried out by employing psychologists and counselling psychology students from the University of Stellenbosch for administration and scoring, and researchers from the Human Sciences Research Council (HSRC) for data entry and analysis. It should be noted that the standardisation version of the test included more items than the final published version; a maximum of 20 per cent of a subtest was dropped following standardisation (Van Eeden, 1997b).

Construct validity

Overall, the Verbal subtests are significantly intercorrelated at $p < .01$ or $.05$, supporting the construct validity of this scale. The Nonverbal subtests are similarly intercorrelated. The correlations are in no instance so high that a particular subtest does not also have specific variance. (If the specific variance exceeds the error variance and can account for a minimum of 25 per cent of the variance, a test has adequate variance). In particular, Form Board, Memory for Digits and Coding have considerable specific variance. On the other hand, the Comprehension and Similarities subtests do not have adequate variance, and nor does the Block Designs subtest for learners between the ages of 13 and 15 years. The Comprehension and Similarities probably measure a composite verbal reasoning factor, while Block Designs is likely to measure a composite nonverbal reasoning factor for the mentioned age groups, rather than other specific abilities. Although the Missing Parts subtest has adequate specific variance for certain age groups (8-, 10-, 12-, 13-, 14- and 16-year-olds), it is smaller than the error variance, particularly in the non-environmentally disadvantaged sample. Thus, the specificity of a subtest for a particular age group needs to be taken into account when interpreting scaled score deviations from the learner's scaled score averages (Van Eeden, 1997b).

Factor analysis was also used to examine the intercorrelations between the subtests and to obtain more information about the structure of underlying abilities on the SSAIS-R. The results, which are presented in detail in the *Background and Standardisation* manual, indicate which subtests share variance and thus measure the same construct. The first unrotated factor of a principal components analysis was, with two exceptions, .30 or greater for all age groups, supporting the construct validity of the subtests as measures of intelligence. However, it is preferable that loadings of .50 or higher be used for including subtests to evaluate general intelligence. Neither Story Memory (for ages 11, 13, 15 and 16 years) nor Missing Parts (for ages 7, 11, 13 and 15 years) meets this criterion. In most cases, Form Board, Memory for Digits and Coding do not satisfy this criterion for the non-environmentally disadvantaged sample (Van Eeden, 1997b), suggesting that they do not load on a common 'intelligence' construct.

Exploratory factor analysis, using a three-factor structure, based on the expectation of verbal, nonverbal and freedom from distractibility factors, was initially used, but the factor loadings could not be meaningfully interpreted and a two-factor structure was thus specified. This represented a verbal and a nonverbal factor. The correlations between the two rotated factors indicate a single, higher-order factor (*g*). However, the rotated factors also have specific variance. Thus, there is confirmation of the theoretical structure of the SSAIS-R: namely, that the subtests measure a general intelligence factor as well as verbal and nonverbal intelligence. Four of the five Verbal scale tests load on the verbal factor – namely, Vocabulary, Comprehension, Similarities and Story Memory. The fifth subtest, Number Problems, loads on both the verbal and nonverbal factors and is likely to also measure freedom from distractibility as it taps working memory. All of the Performance scale subtests load on the nonverbal factor – namely, Pattern Completion, Block Designs, Missing Parts and Form Board, although Form Board shares a low correlation with the other subtests, has low communalities and a relatively low loading on *g* and thus also measures more specific abilities (Van Eeden, 1997b).

Memory for Digits and Coding both showed low loadings on *g* and thus make a very small contribution to general intelligence. In addition, they do not load clearly on a verbal or nonverbal factor. Consequently, they are not included in the calculation of the FSIQ. Despite the fact that a freedom from distractibility factor could not be extracted, information on this ability can be obtained from the latter subtests, particularly the Digit Span subtest, as well as Number Problems (Van Eeden, 1997b).

There are no reported studies that determine the factor structure of the SSAIS-R in clinical populations.

Correlations with other intelligence tests

The Verbal, Nonverbal and Full Scale scores of the SSAIS-R correlated significantly ($p < .01$) with the New South African Group Test (NSAGT) and the Group Test for Indian South Africans (GTISA) for both the non-environmentally disadvantaged and the disadvantaged norm groups (Van Eeden, 1997b). This suggests that the SSAIS-R was measuring the same construct as these group measures of cognitive ability.

While many published studies use the SSAIS-R to gauge South African children's intellectual abilities as part of a larger investigation, very few have examined its psychometric properties. Cockcroft and Blackburn (2008) investigated how effectively the subtests of the SSAIS-R were able to predict reading ability, as assessed by performance on the Neale Analysis of Reading Ability – Revised (NARA) (Neale, 1989). The findings were consistent with literature that had identified a correlation between the Vocabulary subtest of the Wechsler Intelligence Scale for Children – Revised (WISC-R) and reading ability generally (Muter, Hulme, Snowling & Stevenson, 2004). Cockcroft and Blackburn also found gender differences in this regard, with the ability to reason abstractly, deduce rules and form associations appearing to be particularly important for boys' reading comprehension. Auditory memory for text appeared to impact on girls' reading, but not boys', while visual sequencing abilities did not appear to be as important as the aforementioned skills for reading in the early stages of development (the children in the study were in Grade 2).

Concurrent validity

When the SSAIS-R was normed, teachers were asked to rate each child on a five-point scale which assessed their language skills and general intellectual ability. This was used as the criterion for determining whether the SSAIS-R was able to differentiate between children of differing intellectual abilities. There was no separation by age. The correlations between this criterion and the composite and scaled scores on the SSAIS-R were, with a few exceptions, significant ($p < .01$), indicating that the SSAIS-R has the ability to differentiate between children in terms of their intellectual ability (Van Eeden, 1997b).

Predictive validity

The main role of children's intelligence tests has been to identify students at risk of academic failure. The early diagnosis of potential school failure can alert teachers and parents to the need for preventative intervention, tailored to the strengths and weaknesses revealed by an intelligence test. However, the capacity of derivatives of the original Wechsler tests, such as the SSAIS-R, to predict academic achievement (and especially academic failure) has been the subject of some controversy (De Bruin, De Bruin, Dercksen & Cilliers-Hartslief, 2005; Van Eeden & Visser, 1992). The extent to which a Full Scale intelligence test score is a useful predictor of academic success depends partly on the age of the person being tested. For example, Jensen (1980) reviewed the voluminous literature and found that the typical range of correlations between intelligence test scores and school grades in the USA was 0.6 to 0.7 for the elementary grades, 0.5 to 0.6 for high school, 0.4 to 0.5 for college and 0.3 to 0.4 for graduate school, while Kaufman (1990) cites an overall correlation of 0.5 between intelligence test scores and school performance for US children. The predictive validity of the SSAIS-R for school achievement is similar, with correlations ranging between 0.24 and 0.51 (for the NonVerbal scale) and between 0.20 and 0.63 (for the Verbal scale) depending on the grade and subject (Van Eeden, 1997b). The Verbal scale of the SSAIS-R similarly appears to be slightly more strongly correlated with academic success than the NonVerbal scale (Van Eeden, 1997b). This is probably a result of the highly verbal nature of much of the school curriculum. When the predictive validity of the SSAIS-R was calculated, in some instances the numbers within a grade were small (less than 100), which is problematic and may have resulted in non-significant or low correlations. Since the South African school curriculum has changed considerably since the 1990s, these statistics are no longer valid.

Conclusion

Although psychometrically sound, the SSAIS-R is based on a dated theoretical model, with newer IQ tests (for example, WISC-IV) subscribing to the more recent Cattell-Horn-Carroll (CHC) framework (Flanagan, McGrew & Ortiz, 2000), which is more comprehensive. This framework is a synthesis of the factor analytic work of Carroll (1993; 1997) and Horn and Noll (1997) and emphasises several broad classes of abilities at the higher level (for example, fluid ability (*Gf*), crystallised intelligence (*Gc*), short-term memory, long-term storage and retrieval, processing speed) and a number of primary factors at the lower level (for example, quantitative reasoning, spelling ability, free recall, simple reaction time). However, the IQ tests based on the latter theory have been criticised for the fact that there are as yet relatively few studies of the validity of CHC theory with regard to diagnosis and intervention in clinical populations, while considerable empirical data exist on the clinical validity and diagnostic utility of the Wechsler scales. The demographics of South African children and the educational curriculum have changed so substantially since the original development of the SSAIS-R that restandardisation and renorming of the test are critically overdue.

A further issue in IQ test use is the finding that the developed world has demonstrated substantial IQ gains in the 20th century (see Flynn & Weiss, 2007) and these increases are also being evidenced in less developed parts of the world, such as Kenya (Daley, Whaley, Sigman, Espinosa & Neumann, 2003). It is consequently not unreasonable to assume that South African children may demonstrate similar increases in IQ. These gains illustrate what is happening in educational settings and suggest that certain of children's cognitive skills are being enhanced over time. Gains have been particularly prominent on those WISC subtests that assess processing speed and abstract classification, skills which appear to have developed because of their social and educational significance. This finding, known as the Flynn effect, indicates that intelligence is dynamic, and further corroborates the need to redevelop and renorm tests of intelligence on a regular basis (Flynn & Weiss, 2007).

While Shuttleworth-Jordan (1996) has proposed that the South African psychometric community focus on norming commonly employed cognitive tests for use in the South African context, rather than 'reinventing the wheel' with the development of new tests, she qualifies this statement by adding that the focus be on *internationally based* intellectual tests. This proposal is already being acted upon with Shuttleworth-Edwards et al.'s investigations into the WISC-IV, reported on in chapter 3 of this volume.

References

Bee, H. & Boyd, D. (2004). *The Developing Child*. Boston, MA: Pearson.

Brislin, R. W. (1990). *Applied Cross-cultural Psychology*. New York, NY: Sage Publications.

Carroll, J. B. (1993). *Human Cognitive Abilities: A Survey of Factor Analytic Studies*. New York, NY: Cambridge University Press.

Carroll, J. B. (1997). The three-stratum theory of cognitive abilities. In D. P. Flanagan, J. L. Genshaft & P. L. Harrison (Eds), *Contemporary Intellectual Assessment: Theories, Tests and Issues* (pp. 122–130). New York, NY: The Guilford Press.

Claassen, N. C. W. (1987). *Manual for the General Aptitude Test: Intermediate Level*. Pretoria: Human Sciences Research Council.

Cockcroft, K. & Blackburn, M. (2008). The relationship between Senior South African Individual Scale – Revised (SSAIS-R) subtests and reading ability. *South African Journal of Psychology, 38(2)*, 377–389.

Daley, T. C., Whaley, S. E., Sigman, M. D., Espinosa, M. P. & Neumann, C. (2003). IQ on the rise: The Flynn effect in rural Kenyan children. *Psychological Science, 14*, 214–219.

De Bruin, K., De Bruin, G. P, Dercksen, S. & Cilliers-Hartslief, M. (2005). Predictive validity of general intelligence and Big Five measures for adult basic education and training outcomes. *South African Journal of Psychology, 35(1)*, 46–57.

Flanagan, D. P., McGrew, K. S. & Ortiz, S. O. (2000). *The Wechsler Intelligence Scales and Gf-Gc Theory: A Contemporary Approach to Interpretation*. Boston, MA: Allyn & Bacon.

Fleisch, B. (2007). *Primary Education in Crisis: Why South African Schoolchildren Underperform in Reading and Mathematics*. Cape Town: Juta.

Flynn, J. R. & Weiss, L. G. (2007). American IQ gains from 1932 to 2002: The WISC subtests and educational progress. *International Journal of Testing, 7(2)*, 209–224.

Horn, J. L. & Noll, J. (1997). Human cognitive abilities: Gf-Gc theory. In D. P. Flanagan, J. L. Genshaft & P. L. Harrison (Eds), *Contemporary Intellectual Assessment: Theories, Tests and Issues* (pp. 53–91). New York, NY: The Guilford Press.

Jensen, A. R. (1980). *Bias in Mental Testing*. London & New York, NY: Methuen & Free Press.

Kaufman, A. S. (1990). *Assessment of Adolescent and Adult Intelligence*. Boston, MA: Allyn & Bacon.

Muter, V., Hulme, C., Snowling, M. J. & Stevenson, J. (2004). Phonemes, rimes, vocabulary and grammatical skills as foundations of early reading development: Evidence from a longitudinal study. *Developmental Psychology, 40*, 665–681.

Neale, M. D. (1989). *Neale Analysis of Reading Ability*. Berkshire: NFER-Nelson Publishing Co.

Nell, V. (1997). Science and politics meet at last: The insurance industry and neuropsychological norms. *South African Journal of Psychology, 27*, 43–49.

Owen, K. (1991). Test bias: The validity of the Junior Aptitude Tests for various population groups in South Africa regarding constructs measured. *South African Journal of Psychology, 21(2)*, 113–118.

Sattler, J. M. & Dumont, R. (2004). *Assessment of Children: WISC-IV and WPPSI-III Supplement*. San Diego, CA: Jerome M. Sattler.

Shuttleworth-Edwards, A. B., Kemp, R. D., Rust, A. L., Muirhead, J. G. L., Hartman, N. L. & Radloff, S. E. (2004). Cross-cultural effects on IQ test performance: A review and preliminary normative indications on WAIS-III test performance. *Journal of Clinical and Experimental Neuropsychology, 26(7)*, 903–920.

Shuttleworth-Jordan, A. B. (1996). On not reinventing the wheel: A clinical perspective on culturally relevant test usage in South Africa. *South African Journal of Psychology, 26(2)*, 96–102.

Strauss, E., Sherman, E. M. S. & Spreen, O. (2006). *A Compendium of Neuropsychological Tests: Administration, Norms and Commentary* (3rd edition). New York, NY: Oxford University Press.

Van Eeden, R. (1993). *The Validity of the Senior South African Individual Scale – Revised (SSAIS-R) for Children Whose Mother Tongue is an African Language: Private Schools*. Pretoria: Human Sciences Research Council.

Van Eeden R. (1997a). *Manual for the Senior South African Individual Scale – Revised (SSAIS-R): Background and Standardisation*. Pretoria: Human Sciences Research Council.

Van Eeden, R. (1997b). *The Validity of the Senior South African Individual Scale – Revised (SSAIS-R) for Children Whose Mother Tongue is an African Language: Model C Schools*. Pretoria: Human Sciences Research Council.

Van Eeden, R. & Visser, D. (1992). The validity of the Senior South African Individual Scale – Revised (SSAIS-R) for different population groups. *South African Journal of Psychology, 22(3)*, 163–171.

5 Assessing school readiness using the Junior South African Individual Scales: a pathway to resilience

L. C. Theron

School readiness is a crucial construct in the life of a child: being ready to learn and to interact meaningfully with a group of peers and teachers is predictive of later achievement, resilience and well-being (Duncan et al., 2007; Edwards, Baxter, Smart, Sarson & Hayes, 2009). By assessing how ready a child is to make the transition to a formal school environment, and how ready the child is to learn formally, it becomes possible to identify children who are at risk of poorer outcomes (Roodt, Stroud, Foxcroft & Elkonin, 2009). Identification of risk is not done to label children, but rather to extend a helping hand to children who have not yet developed the necessary foundational cognitive, perceptual, physical, social and emotional skills to cope with the multiple demands of formal schooling. This helping hand comes in the form of recommendations for timely, suitable interventions that can potentially enable children to navigate pathways towards resilience.

Drawing on ten years of professional experience as a practising educational psychologist, I will comment in this chapter on how school readiness can be assessed using the Junior South African Individual Scales (JSAIS). Following a brief introduction to the JSAIS, I will draw the reader's attention to the limitations of the JSAIS as a school readiness measure and suggest ways in which psychometrists and psychologists can compensate for this. I will provide pointers to using the JSAIS diagnostically with regard to social and emotional readiness for school, concentration difficulties, language barriers and physical difficulties. I will also emphasise that interpretation of JSAIS results should be nuanced by cognisance of the realities of our multicultural and violent South African context. In essence, this chapter will aim to encourage interns and practitioners not to limit the JSAIS to use as a measure of intelligence, but to use it as a tool to comment qualitatively (rather than just quantitatively) on children's readiness for formal learning.

Defining school readiness

Simply put, school readiness is concerned with how prepared, or ready, a child is to profit from schooling (Reber & Reber, 2001). Despite the apparent simplicity of the aforementioned statement, school readiness is a widely debated term and one that often causes parents and preschool teachers, not to mention children themselves, some distress. Although school readiness is anticipated to occur around the age of six, its meaning involves more than arrival at a chronological age (De Witt, 2009).

In North America, school readiness is typically understood to encompass physical health and adequate motor development, social and emotional maturity, positive attitudes to learning, language development, and cognition and general knowledge (Dockett & Perry, 2009). Similarly, in South Africa school readiness is understood to denote emotional, intellectual, social and physical readiness as well as school maturity (De Witt, 2009). As such, school readiness signifies preparedness and capacity to cope with the multiple and complex challenges commensurate with formal schooling. Clearly then, it is more than a given age or mere cognitive readiness.

Given the complexity of what is implied by school readiness, suggestions that school readiness assessments not be limited to a one-off, single-context appraisal and that they be multidimensional (Panter & Bracken, 2009) begin to make good sense. Nevertheless, the reality (also for South African children) is that such assessments would probably be logistically and financially prohibitive (Panter & Bracken, 2009). The question then arises of how psychometrists and psychologists might best use available measures to comment meaningfully on school readiness. I turn now to a brief overview of the JSAIS in a bid to answer this question.

The JSAIS as a school readiness assessment tool

At the outset of any presentation of the JSAIS, it is important to acknowledge the widespread understanding that it (like other measures of cognitive functioning) has limited value. The JSAIS has not been standardised for all cultural groups making up the population of South African children: it was developed for use with white English- and Afrikaans-speaking children (Madge, 1981) and later standardised for use with Indian (Landman, 1988) and coloured children (Robinson, 1989). Furthermore, it does not provide a picture of the child as a total little person (Roodt et al., 2009). Nevertheless, despite these shortcomings, it can provide useful diagnostic information (Van Eeden & De Beer, 2009) and commentary on a child's readiness for formal schooling (Robinson & Hanekom, 1991), especially when used perceptively and critically.

The JSAIS aims to measure the intellectual skills cardinal to a child's progress in Grade 1, or a child's cognitive ability between the ages of 3 years and 7 years 11 months (Madge, 1981). Although the full battery comprises 22 tests, only 12 core tests are used to compile a child's cognitive profile. These 12 tests form the Global intelligence quotient (IQ) scale (see Table 5.1) and are variably grouped to provide a Verbal, Performance, Numerical and Memory scale. These scales form the focus of this chapter, primarily because Robinson and Hanekom (1991) have confirmed their validity for assessing school readiness close to actual school entry.

Table 5.1 Summary of global intelligence quotient scale

Test description*	Rationale
Verbal scale**	
Vocabulary This test consists of 28 cards (bound into a picture booklet), each depicting four pictures. The practitioner says a word and the child points to the picture matching the word.	It measures the child's ability to recognise, comprehend and interpret everyday language out of context. Because an auditory stimulus (a spoken word) is paired with a visual stimulus (four pictures from which the child must choose), integration of visual and verbal stimuli is required.
Ready Knowledge There are 28 brief questions which the practitioner potentially asks the six-year-old child.	It measures social reasoning skills and general knowledge (i.e. long-term memory). A child's competence in this test reflects the extent to which the child has been exposed to factual knowledge, preschool stimulation and cultural influences (Brink, 1998).
Story Memory The practitioner reads a brief story and asks the child to retell the story.	It measures short-term memory skills for narrative, or meaningfully related, auditory information when recall is unaided by specific questions.
Picture Riddles The test consists of 15 cards (bound into a picture booklet), each depicting four pictures. The practitioner verbalises the riddle and the child points to the picture matching the answer.	It measures independent reasoning skills when comprehension is dependent on relatively complex language, concrete practical judgement and understanding of rhyming words. Because an auditory stimulus (spoken riddle) is paired with a visual stimulus (four pictures from which the child must choose), integration of visual and verbal stimuli is required.
Word Association The test consists of 15 statements which the child completes.	It measures the ability to reason relationally, categorically and logically in terms of purely verbal stimuli.
Performance scale	
Form Board The test consists of 11 tasks which the child must complete (build) in a limited period of time.	It measures form discrimination and manipulation. It also allows insight into trial-and-error visual reasoning, spatial orientation and perceptual constancy.
Block Designs The test consists of 14 tasks which the child must complete (build) in a limited period of time.	It measures visual-spatial reasoning. It also allows insight into how patterns are analysed and synthesised, visual-motor coordination and speed.

Test description*	Rationale
Performance scale	
Absurdities A: missing parts The test consists of 20 cards (bound into a picture booklet). The child identifies what is missing in each picture.	It measures form discrimination and the ability to recognise essential details within a larger whole.
Absurdities B: absurd situations The test consists of 17 cards (bound into a picture booklet). The child identifies what is odd/inappropriate in each picture.	It measures visual reasoning and recognition of a visual portrayal of something absurd/inappropriate.
Form Discrimination The test consists of 32 cards (bound into a picture booklet), each depicting four figures. The child identifies which figure is different from the rest.	It measures visual form discrimination. It also provides insight into spatial orientation, visual reasoning and perceptual constancy.
Numerical scale	
Number and Quantity Concepts The test consists of 23 cards (bound into a picture booklet) containing a visual stimulus paired to a simple arithmetic question asked by the practitioner, and 15 simple, spoken-word sums (not paired with visual stimuli).	It measures basic numeracy skills and how well/accurately the child can apply these to solving simple arithmetic problems (when paired with visual stimuli and when presented as a purely auditory word sum).
Memory for Digits The test consists of six (increasingly long) auditory numerical sequences (two to seven digits) that the child must repeat; and four (increasingly long) auditory numerical sequences (two to five digits) that the child must reverse.	It measures short-term memory for auditory sequences (or non-narrative information).
Memory scale	
Story Memory As above. **Absurdities A: missing parts** As above. **Memory for Digits** As above.	As above.

Sources: Brink (1998); Madge (1981).

Notes: *All descriptions of tests in this table pertain to six-year-old children. Test descriptions for younger children can be found in the JSAIS manual (Madge, 1981). All tests, except Story Memory, are subject to discontinuation rules; details of these rules can also be found in the JSAIS manual. ** The JSAIS manual (Madge, 1981) contains guidelines on how to compute the Verbal, Performance, Memory, Numerical and Global scales, all of which form part of the gestalt of school readiness but are not enough (by themselves) to confirm school readiness.

While the JSAIS-derived scales referred to above will enable a practitioner to comment to some extent on a child's verbal, number, auditory-perceptual, visual-spatial and visual-motor abilities – all cardinal to intellectual readiness for school – they do not provide standardised scores for *emotional, social and physical readiness* or for *school maturity*. To provide meaningful commentary on these crucial facets of school readiness, the practitioner essentially needs to behave like a skilled qualitative researcher and make detailed, informed observations of the child being assessed.

In Table 5.2 I suggest *test-specific* opportunities for observation that are embedded in the JSAIS process. These suggestions are drawn from my experiences of assessing preschoolers between 2000 and 2010, including weekly assessment of the school readiness of preschool boys from multiple cultures in a private, English-medium boys' school. This rich experience has taught me to use the JSAIS as a springboard for observations that comment on comprehensive school readiness.

Table 5.2 Test-specific opportunities for school readiness observations

Verbal scale	Useful observations
Vocabulary	• Does the child echo every word? What might this suggest about **auditory processing**? • Must words be repeated? What might this suggest about **hearing**? What might this suggest about **familiarity with the language of testing**? What might this suggest about **concentration skills**? • Does the child dither/withdraw when uncertain? What might this suggest about **confidence levels** and/or **anxiety**? • Are many/most words unfamiliar to the child? What might this suggest about **familiarity with the language of testing**? What might this suggest about **language stimulation**? • Is the child curious about words that he/she does not know? What might this suggest about **attitude to learning**? Might a lack of obvious curiosity be related to **cultural mores**?
Ready Knowledge	• Must questions be repeated? What might this suggest about **hearing** or about **processing**? What might this suggest about **concentration skills**? • How does the child phrase answers? For example, a six-year-old child's answer to me about why we cannot touch the sun was '*Our hands not big*'. If single words, or poorly constructed phrases (as in the example given) or clumsy syntax, are predominantly used, what might this suggest about **expressive language skills**? • Does the child make many articulation errors whilst answering? What might this suggest about **expressive language skills**? • Does the child provide convoluted answers where a simple sentence might have sufficed? What might this suggest about **expressive language skills**? • How does the child's answer match the question? For example, a six-year-old boy's answer to 'Name two things that are seen in the sky and nowhere else' (Question 10) was '*Because you are in the cloud*'. What might this suggest about **receptive language skills** and/or **auditory processing**?

Verbal scale	Useful observations
Ready Knowledge	• Does the child **perseverate** or **stick to a previous theme**? For example, do answers to subsequent questions retain an earlier question's focus (in my experience, the answer to Question 12 often reflects perseveration around animals (see answer to Question 11). A more extreme example relates to a six-year-old who answered '*You have eyeballs to see with*' in response to Question 7. Then he answered '*Eyeballs ... they help you to see ... and you see out of the window ... and you look at all the people*' in response to Question 10. Later, in response to Question 14, he answered: '*Because it's your eyeballs.*' What might this suggest about **concentration skills** or about capacity to **shift mental set / mental flexibility**? • Do the questions spark stories? For example, in response to the question about what a chemist does (Question 17), a boy eagerly told me in great detail about his brother who had gone to a chemist and what had transpired there. What might this suggest about his levels of **distractibility** and **concentration skills**? • Can the child generally not answer questions relating to time concepts (see Questions 12, 18, 19, 20, 21, 22, 27)? What might this suggest about the development of **time concepts**? • Does the child hear 'mat' for 'gnat' (see Question 24)? What might this suggest about **auditory discrimination**? • Does the child have accurate answers to factual questions (see, for example, Questions 11, 16, 17, 23, 24, 25)? If not, might this be related to how well the child has been **stimulated**? Might this be related to the child's **socio-economic background**? Might this be related to the child's **culture**? Might this be related to **long-term memory**?
Story Memory	• Does the child refuse this task / panic? What might this suggest about **confidence levels** and/or **shyness** and/or **anxiety**? • How does the child narrate the story? In well-constructed sentences or clumsy phrases? With multiple articulation errors? With convoluted descriptions for simple concepts (e.g. '*There were two little rat-type animals*' for mice)? With incorrect plurals (e.g. '*sheeps*', '*mouses*') or incorrect conjugation of the past tense (e.g. '*they goed to frogs*')? What might any of the aforementioned suggest about **expressive language skills** and **language development**? • Does the child narrate the story chronologically? Does the child remember the gist but not the detail? Are the details altered (e.g. tea becomes '*coffee*', twinkle becomes '*star*')? What might this suggest about **listening skills**? • Does the child recall only the first or last third of the story? What might this suggest about **concentration skills**? • Does the child confabulate? This may demonstrate the point at which focus and/or memory declined. What might this say about **concentration skills**? What might this say about **imagination** and **fantasy**? • Does the child appear to pay attention during the reading of the story? Does the apparent concentration match what is recalled? If not, what might this suggest about **distractibility**?

continued →

Verbal scale	Useful observations
Story Memory	• If the child is unable to recall the story or is adamant that he/she remembers nothing, what response would you get if you asked simple questions (such as 'Who is the story about?' / 'Where did they go?' etc.)? Clearly you would not use these responses to score the Story Memory test, but what **diagnostic information** might be revealed? If the child copes with these questions, what might this suggest about the **need for support** or capacity for **aided recall versus unaided recall?***
Picture Riddles	• Does the child struggle with longer riddles, or does the answer reflect comprehension of only one part of the riddle? What might this suggest about **auditory processing**? What might this suggest about **concentration**? • Do the pictures spark stories? For example, some six-year-olds have launched into stories about their pets in response to Question 18 or about their toys in response to Question 14. What might this suggest about **distractibility**? • Does the child cope well with all riddles, except those including abstract language (see Questions 20–23)? What might this suggest about the child's **exposure to complex language / language stimulation**?
Word Association	• Does the child echo every statement? What might this suggest about **auditory processing**? • Does the child take a long time to answer? What might this suggest about **expressive language**? • How does the child process auditory detail? For example, what do answers like '*Dogs have hair and birds have wings*' or '*The sea is wet and the desert is hot*' or '*Stones are hard and wool is sheep*' suggest about **processing skills** and **attention to detail**? • How do the aforementioned differ from answers like '*Sugar is sweet and vinegar is yuck!*' or '*Dogs bark and lions ROARRRRRRR* [sound emulated]'? What does a response like this suggest about **maturity**? • Does the child often decline to answer, or answer '*not*' or '*I don't know*'? What might this suggest about **familiarity with the language of testing / language stimulation**?
Performance scale	**Useful observations**
Form Board	• Does the child work slowly? What might this suggest about **visual-motor readiness** for school? What might this suggest about **work tempo**? • Can the child discriminate between the colours and the shapes of the form-board pieces? What might this suggest about **conceptual stimulation**? What might this suggest about exposure to these concepts – are colourful shapes, or pictures of these, readily accessible in this child's **milieu**? What might this suggest about capacity to **see** colour and possible **visual barriers to learning**? • Does the child demonstrate poor trial-and-error skills? What might this suggest about the child's capacity to **problem-solve**? • Does the child play with the shapes? What might this suggest about readiness to **work formally**?

Performance scale	Useful observations
Form Board	• Do the shapes spark comment? For example, children have sometimes commented that parts of the circle look like '*a slice of pizza*'. Do these comments reflect **creativity**, or do they interfere with task completion, and what might this then suggest about a **mature work ethic**? • Does the child quit when tasks within this test are challenging? What might this say about **emotional readiness** to learn? What might this suggest about **perseverance** and **task completion**? • Does the child become visibly frustrated and/or angry when tasks within this test are challenging? Very occasionally, children I have assessed have slammed the form board or swept the pieces off the table when they have found this to be a challenging task. What might that say about **frustration tolerance** and **emotional/social readiness to learn**?
Block Designs	• The questions pertaining to Form Board can usually be asked of Block Designs, too. In addition: • Does the child fail to notice the colour of the blocks or the directionality of the design? What might this suggest about **attention to detail**? • Can the child only build designs that were first modelled by the practitioner? Can the child work independently from the model? How frequently does the child refer to the model? Does the child try to build the design directly on top of the model card? What might this imply about the child's capacity for **independent analysis and synthesis**? • Does the child rotate the model? What might this convey about **visual-perceptual skills**? • Does the child ignore the pattern card and build something else? What might this suggest about **age-appropriate work ethic**? About **cooperation**? About **ability to follow instructions**?
Absurdities A: missing parts	• Does the child miss finer detail? For example, in my experience children who are less focused on detail miss the finger (Card 12), the second hand (Card 14), the light (Card 15), the eyebrow (Card 19) and the peg (Card 20), but cope well with the remaining cards. What might this suggest about **attention to detail**? • Does the child provide answers that suggest unfamiliarity with the object in the picture? For example, some six-year-old boys suggest that the watch (Card 14) is missing the '*stopwatch button*'. When I meet their parents for feedback, their fathers are often wearing sports-watches without second hands. What might children's answers suggest about their **milieu** and what they have been exposed to? • Does the child perseverate – for example, provide the same answer to Questions 14 and 18? What might this suggest about **concentration skills**?

continued →

Performance scale	Useful observations
Absurdities B: absurd situations	• Does the child provide a moral or gender stereotypical answer in response to what is odd about the picture? For example, children sometimes point to the boy blowing out the candle in Card 14 and comment that '*He's being naughty because it's wrong to blow out candles*' or to the person in Card 13 and comment that he should not have '*girl's lips*'. What might answers like this suggest about the **socialisation of the child** and **how might this impact on learning**? • Does the child struggle with items that require understanding of directionality (see Cards 12, 14, 15)? What might this suggest about **spatial orientation**? • How possible is it that the absurdities presented are beyond the lived experiences of the child? For example, is it possible that the child being assessed does not typically eat with a knife and fork and so the situation depicted in Card 9 makes little sense? Or is it possible that the child being assessed has never seen a fruit tree and has no concept of how fruit grows, and so the situation depicted in Card 11 makes little sense? What might children's answers suggest about their **milieu** and what they have been exposed to?
Form Discrimination	• Does the child approach this task meticulously, or are answers provided haphazardly and impulsively? As this is typically the last test in the JSAIS-12, what might this suggest about ability to sustain a **mature work ethic** and about **concentration skills**? • Does the child comment on the patterns being in colour (or later, not)? What might this suggest about **attention to detail** and/or **distractibility**?
Numerical scale	**Useful observations**
Number and Quantity Concepts	• Must questions be repeated? What might this suggest about **hearing** or about **processing**? What might this suggest about **concentration skills**? • Does the child use the visual stimuli provided, or is the approach to this task impulsive? For example, I have experienced that impulsive children guess the number of apples, rather than counting (Question 17). What might this suggest about **concentration skills** and **formal work ethic**? • Do basic mathematical concepts like more/less/most/half/etc. have meaning for the child? What might this suggest about **stimulation relating to arithmetic**? What might this suggest about **language competency**? • Does the child cope with the questions that are paired with picture cards, but not the others? What might this suggest about ability to **work less concretely**?
Memory for Digits	• How many digits can the child recall? What might this suggest about **concentration skills**? • Can the child recall digits forwards, but not backwards? What might difficulty with the latter (which implies more complex memory and attention tasks) imply about **concentration skills**?

Note: * When practitioners assist a child in this way, an attempt is made to determine how well the child performs when a barrier to competence (for example, poor, unstructured recall capacity; anxiety; shyness) is accommodated. This method is known as 'testing the limits' (Decker & McIntosh, 2010, p.289) and will provide useful recommendations for encouraging competence (or in this instance, school readiness).

By bearing in mind the questions set out in Table 5.2, the practitioner has multiple opportunities to use the JSAIS diagnostically to gain deeper understanding of the child's emotional and social readiness for school, concentration difficulties, language barriers, and motor and physical difficulties. Using this set of questions as a guide, the practitioner is also encouraged to regard the child as an ecosystemic being (Donald, Lazarus & Lolwana, 2010) and to be sensitive to social and cultural influences on school readiness.

In addition to the above, there are a number of observations not specific to any one JSAIS test which a practitioner can potentially make throughout administration of the JSAIS that encourage deeper understanding of the emotional, social and physical facets of school readiness. These are itemised in Table 5.3.

Table 5.3 JSAIS-process opportunities for school readiness observations

Social and emotional maturity
• How well does the child ~ tolerate **pressure** (for example, the pressure of a novel situation, of being assessed, of growing tired as the assessment progresses)? ~ **separate** from parent/caregiver/teacher? ~ respond when uncertain (that is, what is the child's capacity for **risk-taking**)? ~ respond to reasonable **limits**? ~ **follow instructions**? ~ make **eye contact** (given the child's culture)? ~ tolerate **waiting** (for example, for the next task to be placed on the table, for items to be packed away)? • Does the child ~ need **encouragement**? How well does the child respond to encouragement? ~ **avoid tasks** (for example, think of reasons to exit the assessment earlier, build his/her own design when a given one is challenging)? ~ **complain** that the assessment is **too long** (or ask repeatedly to return to class)? ~ complain of **tummy aches** or of tiredness? ~ engage in **comfort behaviours**? ~ **help** spontaneously (for example, with packing away of blocks)? ~ display **curiosity**? ~ **self-correct** (for example, when an impulsive, incorrect answer is provided)? ~ **concentrate** for the duration of one test? ~ **tell stories** unrelated and/or related to the task at hand? If so, what is the quality of such completed tasks? ~ work without **chatting** / **humming** / **making sounds**? If not, what is the quality of completed tasks? ~ comment on **background noise**? If so, how does this affect task completion? ~ comment frequently on objects in the room / **ask multiple questions** about the room in which the assessment is taking place? If so, how does this affect task completion? ~ repeatedly **tap** or **thump** the answer in tests requiring answers to be pointed out? • How ~ **cooperative** is the child? ~ **tenacious** is the child? ~ **mature** is the child's **speech**? Is there evidence of '**baby talk**'?

continued →

Social and emotional maturity

- ~ **competitive** is the child? Is there a need to know about how others have done in comparison?
- ~ **approval-seeking** is the child?
- ~ **critical/realistic** is the child of his/her own efforts?
- ~ **assertive** is the child? Can he/she acknowledge difficulty / not knowing an answer?
- ~ **autonomous** is the child's functioning during completion of the JSAIS?

Physical readiness*

- How often does the child
  - ~ blink / rub his or her eyes / complain that he or she cannot see / hold material close to his or her eyes?
  - ~ speak overly loudly / ask for questions to be repeated or comment that he or she did not hear / focus on practitioner's lips / provide answers that do not match questions?
- What is the child's body posture like? How often does the child slouch / support chin or head / lie on the table / squirm or fidget?
- How
  - ~ thin is the child? Is the child's physique similar to that of a healthy six-year-old?
  - ~ easily does the child tire during the assessment?
  - ~ energetic is the child?
  - ~ coordinated is the child? How deftly does the child manipulate form-board pieces / blocks? Does the child knock objects (like blocks) off the table?

Source: Adapted from Brink (1998).

Note: * An astute practitioner needs to be constantly looking for signs of physical barriers to learning. Knowledge of typical symptoms of visual and auditory barriers (see, for example, Donald et al., 2010) is crucial, but so is sensitivity to poor body posture, extreme restlessness and inability to remain seated, all of which might denote poor muscle tone. If a child with poor muscle tone is not assisted, work tempo and attention span will probably suffer, along with optimal learning. Furthermore, practitioners need to include copying activities to comment on fine motor skills (see Conclusion).

With reference to Tables 5.2 and 5.3, it is vital to emphasise that observations need to be triangulated. Rigorous qualitative researchers strive to gather evidence which has replicability, because such evidence can be trusted. The same applies to observations made during a school readiness assessment: one instance of perseveration does not suggest an attention deficit; one instance of quitting does not suggest poor emotional readiness; one instance of brief playfulness does not suggest an immature work ethic.

Contextual considerations

As noted above, the JSAIS was originally developed for use with white South African children. Post-1994, many English-medium schools reflect the rich multicultural reality of South Africa. In my experience, many black children grow up speaking English and attend suburban English-medium schools, particularly when their parents are professionally qualified. Likewise, I have observed that white children whose home language is not English, and Chinese children, attend these schools too. How does one assess their school readiness? Should a practitioner refrain from using the JSAIS, even when these children have attended similar English-medium preschools and attend the same preparatory school? It is beyond the scope of this chapter to attempt an answer, but it is important to emphasise that caution is called for when using the JSAIS with children other than those for whom it was developed. Such caution includes reference to *diagnostic* use, and heightened awareness of test items that could discriminate against children who are not white (such as identifying 'freckles' in the Vocabulary test), or whose background is not South African (such as remembering 'in the veld' or putting flowers 'in a vase ... in the dining room' in the Story Memory test) or whose cultural practices may be different from what is typically associated with the average white South African child (see Table 5.2). In my experience, an additional contextual consideration when using the JSAIS to determine school readiness is sensitivity to the high levels of crime and loss that many South African children have experienced. Although this is not the norm, I have witnessed various JSAIS test items trigger memories of loss and/or crime. For example, in response to Question 10 (Ready Knowledge), a child answered '*My daddy*' and explained how his father now lived in the sky, following a hijacking. In response to Question 15, a different child answered that windows are made of glass because they '*don't keep baddies out*' and recounted an armed robbery in his home. Other children have answered '*dangerous*' in response to Question 10 (Word Association) and some have then narrated experiences of crime at night. A number of children have spontaneously commented on lived experiences of shootings and losses in response to Item 18 (Vocabulary). Awareness of how our South African context may lead to trauma that could tinge responses to various test items encourages more sensitive administration and interpretation of 'inaccurate' responses.

Conclusion

No school readiness test, the JSAIS included, is sufficient in and of itself. With regard to commenting meaningfully on a child's school readiness, the provision of only JSAIS-derived quantitative scales reflecting verbal, performance, memory, numerical and global intellectual functioning is relatively meaningless. When these scales are paired with sensitive, informed observations about the child's emotional, social and physical readiness and school maturity, more meaningful assessment of school readiness is possible. Ideally, further tests (such as supplementary JSAIS tests like Visual Memory for Figures or Copying, and additional measures like the Draw-A-Person-Test,[1] Wepman Auditory Discrimination test and laterality screenings (Brink, 1998)) need to be included to comment even more meaningfully on readiness to learn. In summary, then, the JSAIS has the potential to provide significant commentary on school readiness when it is used astutely as a quantitative and qualitative tool.

As noted at the outset of this chapter, school-ready children often experience greater well-being and resilience to the challenges of schooling. The onus is therefore on every practitioner who uses the JSAIS to determine school readiness to conduct a meaningful, comprehensive assessment that includes rigorous observation and qualitative comment, if the outcome is to be fair (also culturally and contextually) to the child. Finally, when the JSAIS has been used fairly and as a springboard for informed observation, the ensuing recommendations need to encourage accessible, specific and culturally appropriate interventions to hone potential for learning, ever mindful that school readiness is an early step along the complex trajectory of learning and resilience.

Note

1 Copying and drawing activities also provide opportunities to observe fine motor skills.

References

Brink, M. (1998). Clinical use of the SSAIS-R and using the JSAIS to evaluate school readiness. Unpublished workshop notes. Melville, Johannesburg.

Decker, S. L. & McIntosh, D. E. (2010). Academic achievement measures in rehabilitation. In E. Mpofu & T. Oakland (Eds), *Assessment in Rehabilitation and Health* (pp. 280–294). Upper Saddle River, NJ: Pearson Education.

De Witt, M. W. (2009). *The Young Child in Context: A Thematic Approach. Perspectives from Educational Psychology and Sociopedagogics*. Pretoria: Van Schaik.

Dockett, S. & Perry, B. (2009). Readiness for school: A relational construct. *Australasian Journal of Early Childhood, 34(1)*, 20–26.

Donald, D., Lazarus, S. & Lolwana, P. (2010). *Educational Psychology in Social Context: Ecosystemic Applications in Southern Africa* (4th edition). Cape Town: Oxford University Press.

Duncan, G. J., Dowsett, C. J., Claessens, A., Magnuson, K., Huston, A. C., Klebanov, P. & Japel, C. (2007). School readiness and later achievement. *Developmental Psychology, 43(6)*, 1428–1446. doi: 10.1037/0012-1649.436.1428.

Edwards, B., Baxter, J., Smart, D., Sarson, A. & Hayes, A. (2009). Financial disadvantage and children's school readiness. *Family Matters, 83*, 23–31.

Landman, J. (1988). *Appendix to the Manual for the Junior South African Individual Scales (JSAIS): Technical Details and Table of Norms with Regard to 6–8-year-old Indian Pupils*. Pretoria: Human Sciences Research Council.

Madge, E. M. (1981). *Manual for the Junior South African Individual Scales (JSAIS)*. Pretoria: Human Sciences Research Council.

Panter, J. E. & Bracken, B. A. (2009). Validity of the Bracken School Readiness Assessment for predicting first grade readiness. *Psychology in the Schools, 46(5)*, 397–409. doi: 10.1002/pits.20385.

Reber, A. S. & Reber, E. S. (2001). *Dictionary of Psychology*. London: Penguin Books.

Robinson, M. (1989). *Bylae tot die handleiding vir die Junior Suid-Afrikaanse Individuele Skale (JSAIS): Tegniese Besonderhede en Normtabelle vir 6–8-Jarige Leerlinge*. Pretoria: Human Sciences Research Council.

Robinson, M. & Hanekom, J. D. M. (1991). *Die JSAIS en ASB as Hulpmiddels by die Evaluering van Skoolgereedheid*. Pretoria: Human Sciences Research Council.

Roodt, G., Stroud, L., Foxcroft, C. & Elkonin, D. (2009). The use of assessment measures in various applied contexts. In C. Foxcroft & G. Roodt (Eds), *An Introduction to Psychological Assessment in the South African Context* (3rd edition, pp. 203–224). Cape Town: Oxford University Press.

Van Eeden, R. & De Beer, M. (2009). Assessment of cognitive functioning. In C. Foxcroft & G. Roodt (Eds), *An Introduction to Psychological Assessment in the South African Context* (3rd edition, pp. 128–147). Cape Town: Oxford University Press.

6 School readiness assessment in South Africa

Z. Amod and D. Heafield

Local and international research provides considerable evidence that the early years of children's lives are critical for their future development. Assessment measures can be used effectively to prevent, identify and address barriers to learning and development. Most psychology practitioners would agree that both formal and informal assessment procedures can guide parents, caregivers and educators in establishing a solid foundation for children's growth, development and potential through the provision of optimal enrichment and learning activities, as well as socio-emotional support.

The primary purpose of school readiness assessment is to predict readiness for school entry and to identify preschool children who may benefit from additional stimulation programmes, learning support or retention. Focus is placed on physical development, cognitive skills and academic readiness, as well as on the child's socio-emotional functioning. Factors considered in school readiness assessment include the child's emotional maturity, ability to follow directions, and ability to work cooperatively with peers and adult figures. In addition to early identification and support, a school readiness assessment can also serve the purpose of reassuring parents and caregivers that their child is progressing adequately. In some instances a child may be accepted a year early into school to accommodate his or her need for accelerated learning.

While school readiness assessment is an established field of practice, it has generated a great deal of controversy amongst practitioners and researchers (Carlton & Winsler, 1999; Dockett & Perry, 2009; Freeman & Brown, 2008; Goldblatt, 2004; Graue, 2006; Maxwell & Clifford, 2004). It remains a highly contentious issue in South Africa for several reasons. Concerns have been raised about the historical misuse of assessment measures, which have been seen as perpetuating exclusionary practices and an inequitable education system (Kriegler & Skuy, 1996). Some of the intellectual and school readiness assessment tools that have been locally developed have outdated norms (Foxcroft, Paterson, Le Roux & Herbst, 2004). In addition, many were not normed on a fully representative South African sample. Examples are the Junior South African Individual Scales (JSAIS) (published in 1981 and standardised for English- and Afrikaans-speaking individuals) and the Aptitude Test for School Beginners (ASB). The latter is an individually/group-administered school readiness test which was first devised in

1974 (and revised in 1994), to be used from the sixth to the eighth week of the school year. However, an advantage of this test is that it has been translated into nine official South African languages.

In response to the current limitations of locally developed tests and the absence of any new tests, a number of practitioners have relied on internationally developed tests that are not registered by the Health Professions Council of South Africa (HPCSA) (Foxcroft et al., 2004). The decision to make use of unregistered international tests presents practitioners with difficult ethical dilemmas. Concerns have been expressed by clinicians and researchers regarding the use of test instruments that are not normed for the population group for which they are used (Foxcroft et al., 2004; Foxcroft & Roodt, 2008; Nell, 2000; Venter, 2000).

As a result of apartheid, children in this country exist within extremely diverse socio-cultural and socio-economic structures. This confounding factor further complicates the issue of school readiness assessment and, in most cases, contributes significantly to developmental and emotional differences between children. The *Situational Analysis of Children in South Africa* report (The Presidency, Republic of South Africa, 2009) shows that racial inequality in children's poverty status, as well as inequalities between urban and rural areas, persists. Education White Paper 5 (Department of Education, 2001a) states that one of the goals for 2010 was to ensure that all children entering Grade 1 would have the opportunity to participate in an accredited reception-year programme. This goal has not been met, and the number of children in Early Child Development (ECD) programmes falls short of the number of children that are within the preschool age range (Department of Basic Education, 2010). Major gaps exist in relation to access and equity with regard to the provision of ECD programmes in South Africa. A staggering figure of 21 per cent of the child population is reported to have one or both parents deceased (The Presidency, Republic of South Africa, 2009). This could be related to the high incidence of HIV/AIDS in this country. In response to some of these issues, some provincial departments of education have imposed an informal moratorium on school readiness testing within South African government schools.

Considering the myriad of factors related to school readiness testing in South Africa, a child deficit model is obviously inadequate. Denying a child the right to begin school at the appropriate age based on this model, without providing a suitable alternative, could be considered both discriminatory and unfair. The objective of this chapter is to propose a more holistic and ecosystemic view of school readiness assessment, based on a critique of approaches and a discussion of developments in this field.

Approaches to school readiness assessment

Traditionally, the concept of school readiness was viewed through a rather narrow lens, resulting in an oversimplified perception of what it was and what it entailed. Consequently, the content of many school readiness tests reflected this narrow conceptualisation. Increasing evidence, however, highlights the complexity and multifaceted nature of school readiness. This in turn makes the assessment thereof anything but simple.

Past conceptualisations of school readiness tended to view the issue in one of two ways. Some theorists subscribed to the idea that readiness was a linear, maturational process. In other words, once children had reached a level of maturity that enabled them to sit still, stay focused, interact with others in socially acceptable ways and take direction from adults, they were considered to be ready to begin formal schooling (Meisels, 1998). Proponents of the maturational point of view argued that a child's developmental changes were a result of a natural biological progression rather than of learning or environmental influences. This view stemmed from the work of Arnold Gesell, a psychologist and paediatrician, who had proposed that development follows an orderly sequence and each child's distinctive genetic make-up determines his or her rate of development. It follows from this theory that a child's readiness for school is linked to his or her biological timetable (Scott-Little, Kagan & Frelow, 2006).

In contrast to the maturational view, some researchers and theorists have taken a more empirical standpoint on the concept of school readiness. This approach emphasises specific skills and knowledge that are deemed necessary to achieve success at school. According to Meisels (1998), from this perspective, being ready for school means knowing one's shapes and colours, one's address, how to spell one's name, how to count to ten and say the alphabet, and how to behave in a polite and socially acceptable manner.

The common factor underpinning both of these approaches is the focus on the individual child, and whether or not the child has reached a particular point that constitutes readiness (Dockett & Perry, 2009). In an endeavour to make decisions about whether or not children are ready for school, a plethora of mainly international school readiness and developmental tests were developed and administered to children. These included the Boehm Test of Basic Concepts, the Gesell School Readiness Test, the Brigance Inventory of Early Development and the Metropolitan School Readiness Test, many of which are still used today.

Critics draw attention to a number of problems associated with using once-off testing procedures for the purpose of evaluating a child's readiness for school. Frequently cited is the issue of validity and reliability. Freeman and Brown (2008, p.267) point out that the National Association for the Education of Young Children asserts that 'by their very nature young children are poor test takers and therefore researchers' attempts to determine an instrument's reliability and validity are fruitless'. Other problems include concerns about measuring skills in isolation, and the fact that test results often lead to inappropriate classification and mistaken placements (Carlton & Winsler, 1999; Dockett & Perry, 2009; Engel, 1991; Freeman & Brown, 2008; Meisels, 1998; Scott-Little et al., 2006). Freeman and Brown (2008) state that children's growth occurs at different rates in uneven and irregular spurts, and there is great variability among and within typically performing children. They therefore argue that tests are inadequate for measuring the complex social, emotional, cognitive and physical competencies that children need to succeed in school. These confounding variables are accentuated by the multicultural and multilingual context in which South

Africans exist. Added to this, the complexity of South African socio-political history has impacted on many spheres of life, including the current education system and the delivery of ECD programmes.

It is encouraging to note that over approximately the last two decades there has been a gradual shift in the conceptualisation of school readiness and how best to assess it. In shifting from the traditional linear and empirically (skills and knowledge) based approaches to school readiness, most psychologists now use a holistic approach which addresses the preschool child's physical, developmental, cognitive and socio-emotional functioning. A variety of tools and methods are thus used in the assessment process. In addition to conventional school readiness tests, psychologists also make use of developmental tests, intellectual assessment measures and projective tests. Developmental tests, such as the Griffiths Mental Developmental Scales (GMDS) which has been researched in South Africa and is discussed in chapter 12 of this volume, are often used to assess locomotor skills, eye-hand coordination, language ability and personal-social skills, as well as performance and practical reasoning skills. More psychologists are also making use of information processing models of cognitive functioning and are using tests such as the Kaufman Assessment Battery for Children (K-ABC) and the Cognitive Assessment System (CAS) (discussed in chapters 7 and 8). These tests are purported to be less biased in terms of cultural and language differences. Dynamic assessment measures are also being more widely used today in the assessment of learning potential (see chapter 9 for a detailed discussion).

Test results are not interpreted in isolation, but collateral information is equally important in assessing the child's readiness for school. Other sources of information that are utilised in the assessment process include preschool inventories, parent and teacher rating scales, informal observation and information obtained from parents and caregivers.

Although the concept of school readiness evaluation and the processes used to assess it continue to be viewed through a wider lens, there is still a challenge in South Africa to address the diverse needs of the population in relation to preschool assessment and to develop models of assessment that are appropriate for this context. As reflected in a South African survey, psychologists perceive an urgent need for tests that can be utilised for school readiness assessment and that would account for factors such as socio-economic status and chronological age (Foxcroft et al., 2004). The reality of the South African context is that there are groups of children from communities where parents and caregivers have access to the services of psychologists and other professionals whom they can consult with regard to their child's readiness for school, while simultaneously there are those who live in dire poverty and who are unable to afford or access these services.

In the latter cases, decisions regarding school readiness are often left to teachers and parents who may not always be fully informed about the most appropriate schooling alternatives for their children. For instance, one solution for the 'unready child' is the practice of delaying school entry. Many studies have shown that the process of delaying school entry in itself does not produce substantial benefit for the child (Carlton & Winsler, 1999; Dockett & Perry, 2009;

Engel, 1991; Maxwell & Clifford, 2004; Scott-Little et al., 2006). Carlton and Winsler (1999, p.346) argue that the practice of school readiness testing and placement 'may be creating a type of exclusionary sorting process that results in denying or delaying educational services to precisely those children who might benefit the most from such services'.

This is an important consideration in South Africa, where many children, especially those from lower socio-economic groups, either do not attend preschool because of financial constraints, or attend preschool placements that are simple day-care facilities with limited educational value. Preventing these children from accessing educational opportunities for an additional year would clearly not be in their best interest.

Another common decision amongst teachers and parents is to keep children back an additional year in preschool (Grade 0/R). Studies conducted over the past 70 years have failed to show significant benefits to students of such retention (Carlton & Winsler, 1999). In addition, if not handled sensitively, this may have detrimental effects on the child's self-esteem and attitude towards school. Some professionals argue that if the retention is handled with care and sensitivity, these children may experience the year in a positive manner, and may gain self-confidence related to enhanced scholastic performance. Unfortunately, an extra year for many children simply means more of the same, and their specific learning difficulties may not be addressed, resulting in limited progress.

Another concern related to the practice of school readiness assessments is the pressure it places on the development of preschool curriculum content. An emphasis on more academically oriented content may be the result of content from higher grades being 'pushed down' into preschool years (Scott-Little et al., 2006). Children in preschool are now expected to learn content and develop skills that were previously only expected of Grade 1 learners. Winter (2009/2010) argues that children's play is seen as less important than teaching basic reading skills to increasingly young children. She further argues that this process is creating an increasing divide between children from lower socio-economic groups and those from more affluent communities. This appears to be the case in some parts of South Africa, where significant differences in expectations exist between government and private schools. A second-language English speaker from a less enriched background may be deemed school-ready in one school and not in another.

Dynamic and creative ways need to be explored to meet the needs of preschool children so that they can cope with the demands of formal schooling and progress to reach their full potential. For instance, the establishment of an enrichment year may serve as a stepping stone to stimulate school readiness skills, and assist with adjustment to the more formally structured schooling environment.

On a global level, there appears to be a growing awareness of the need to protect children from unnecessary and inappropriate assessment and to use assessment effectively to enhance the quality of education for all children (Department of Education, 2001b; Kagan, 2003). Much of the debate about school readiness acknowledges that contextual factors play an important role in its determination. In other words, the socio-economic and cultural context in which one lives serves to define and impact upon how school readiness is perceived within families, schools and communities. Contemporary socio-cultural/social constructivist learning theory and modern transactional models of child development offer a broader view of school readiness, and may provide a new theoretical framework for understanding school readiness (Carlton & Winsler, 1999).

From a social constructivist perspective, school readiness is shaped by children's communities, families and schools. Vygotsky (1978) views learning primarily as a social process and not an isolated exploration by the child of the environment. From his viewpoint, learning precedes or leads development, and children's experiences with others and with the environment therefore propel their development forward. This is in contrast to maturational views in which development is seen as preceding learning, and the child's development therefore cannot be hastened by experience or teaching. The social constructivist view shifts the focus of assessment away from the child, and directs it to the community in which the child is living (Meisels, 1998). It therefore becomes vital to consider the context in which the child is raised and the environment in which he or she will be educated. Because different schools have different expectations of readiness, the same child with the same abilities and needs could be considered ready in one school and not in another (Maxwell & Clifford, 2004). School readiness therefore becomes a relative term. This is a relevant argument within the local context, where vast differences exist between schools as a result of the country's socio-political history.

Scott-Little et al. (2006) found that early learning standards – that is, specific skills and knowledge deemed important for children's school readiness – varied according to who was involved in the process of developing the standards, and the context in which the standards were developed. They argued that unique historical, political, institutional and policy contexts can have a significant impact on the way school readiness is conceptualised in different communities. They also found that parents and teachers had different notions about which attributes and skills were important indicators of a child's readiness for school. While parents and teachers seemed to agree that it was important for children to be healthy, socially competent and able to communicate effectively, it was found that some parents and preschool teachers accentuated academic competencies and basic knowledge more than Foundation Phase teachers did. In South Africa, school readiness assessment is in many instances perceived differently in different community settings. Entry standards and requirements in the range of schools that exist (such as private, inner-city, suburban, township, rural, informal settlement and farm schools) can differ markedly.

If parents and teachers share a common understanding and belief about the important skills and characteristics that are needed to begin formal schooling, then there will be greater congruence between the skills parents mediate to their children prior to school entry and the skills teachers look for as children enter school (Goldblatt, 2004). Goldblatt (2004) investigated South African Jewish and Muslim parents' and teachers' perceptions of school readiness, and found that the parents and teachers in her study had similar expectations regarding school readiness. However, she also noted that this study, unlike many studies conducted in the USA, was limited to middle-class socio-economic groups, thus accounting for their shared expectations.

As existing theories of school readiness have been integrated with each other, there has been a gradual emergence of a broader conceptualisation of the process. Some contemporary theorists view school readiness from an interactionist or bi-directional perspective. This approach incorporates elements of maturationist and empirical theory, and recognises the importance of the social and cultural context, following social constructivist theory. Thus, school readiness does not reside solely within the child, nor is it completely external to the child. Instead, it is an intricate tapestry of the child's own genetic make-up, skills and abilities, interwoven with the experiences and teachings received from surrounding social and cultural groups.

Considering the complexity of the concept of school readiness, the issue of assessing school readiness becomes a far more complicated matter than just determining whether children have mastered a predetermined set of skills. By redefining readiness in terms of the characteristics of the child, family, school and community, the assessment of readiness adopts a very different perspective. Freeman and Brown (2008) suggest that rather than asking, 'Is the child ready for school?', we should reframe the question by asking, 'Is the school ready for all learners?' The idea of 'ready' schools, and the assessment thereof, is an issue that has been addressed recently by a growing number of authors. Dockett and Perry (2009) argue that 'ready' schools are ones in which the necessary support structures are provided, where there is strong and effective leadership, and where an environment of mutual respect between teachers and parents is fostered. The assessment of schools could take the form of reviewing class sizes, determining the extent to which teachers have early childhood training, ensuring the implementation and development of appropriate curricula, and promoting continuity between preschools and formal schooling. This paradigm shift in school readiness assessment is consistent with the policy of inclusive education which South Africa has embraced over the last decade (Department of Education, 2001a; 2001b).

Teachers obviously form an essential ingredient in the process of assessing school readiness, and their evaluation and assessment of young learners can form a vital and useful part of this process. It is therefore essential that teachers have access to ongoing professional development and training. This has been set as a priority in South Africa (The Presidency, Republic of South Africa, 2009). Many professionals advocate that assessment should take place in the child's own natural setting, in a comfortable and nonthreatening way. In addition to this, children should be observed and assessed over an extended period, rather than on a single occasion (Carlton & Winsler, 1999; Dockett & Perry, 2009; Engel, 1991; Freeman & Brown, 2008). Teachers need to be trained to assess children's work in different contexts, using methods such as portfolio systems, observational checklists and the collection of varied examples of their work (Engel, 1991). These kinds of assessment procedures are promoted in the current South African education curriculum. Teachers should also help students to produce their best possible work by taking cognisance of their special abilities and interests. This shifts the focus away from deficits to strengths. Teachers also need to be trained to utilise a variety of approaches to teaching and learning, and to tailor their teaching and learning to suit the needs of a diverse range of children. This type of approach eliminates the need to assess children before they enter formal schooling (Carlton & Winsler, 1999). The primary purpose of assessment is therefore for instructional purposes and the development of suitable programmes, rather than for placement.

In order to enable schools and teachers to be 'ready', they need to be supported by families, communities and government. An interdisciplinary and collaborative approach is needed to address the many variables that affect children's school readiness. Dockett and Perry (2009) point out that families can provide an essential foundation in facilitating a positive start to school. Children need nurturing, encouragement and access to rich and varied learning opportunities. Families do not exist in isolation, though. The existence and accessibility of community support structures can determine the extent to which families are able to fulfil these roles (Dockett & Perry, 2009). Such support structures can make a vital contribution in South Africa, especially in addressing the needs of under-resourced and marginalised communities. Children need support to maintain optimal physical and emotional health if they are to achieve academic success (Winter, 2009/2010). Research findings from the fields of medicine, child development, cultural studies, sociology and other disciplines can provide valuable input into the development of strategies for attaining school readiness. Winter (2009/2010) stresses that in order to achieve optimal results, school readiness programmes must begin early on and continue to provide an appropriate level of support throughout childhood.

New and fundamentally different approaches to school readiness assessment are being developed and implemented in countries such as the USA, Great Britain and Australia. This is part of the major paradigm shift that is occurring in school readiness research. Dockett and Perry (2009) believe that the focus on developing community measures of readiness, rather than measures of individual children's readiness for school, is one approach that is worthy of further consideration. Examples of community measures include the Early Development Instrument (EDI), and an Australian adaptation of this model, the Australian Early Development Index. The EDI was developed at the Oxford Centre for Child Studies and assesses the whole child, by asking developmentally appropriate questions across five dimensions identified in current literature as being important. These include physical health and well-being, social competence, emotional maturity, language and cognition, and communication skills and general knowledge. The EDI is not used to diagnose individual children, but is administered for the assessment of entire classrooms, communities and school districts. It is completed halfway through the year by the child's preschool teacher. This ensures that the assessment is conducted by a professional who has had sustained contact with the child and therefore knows the child well. The results are then interpreted at a group or population level, instead of at an individual level. Because the results are based on all children in a given community, the information gathered from this type of assessment is more suitably translated into practice and policy (Guhn, Janus & Hertzman, 2007).

Such a model of assessment would need to be researched to explore its appropriateness for our local context. It may be a valuable assessment tool, given the range and diversity of schools and communities within South Africa. This type of assessment practice could help to clarify the most important needs within a given community or school, and then goals could be set to address these. In this way, the needs of many would be served, as opposed to the needs of just a few individual children. Given the financial constraints of many schools and parents, the luxury of one-on-one assessment is not an option for most parents. In addition to this, models such as the EDI incorporate multiple stakeholders and this could help to alleviate the excessive burden that is placed on teachers in this country.

The Early ON School Readiness Project is another community-based model that has emerged recently. It is based on an ecosystemic approach and requires the involvement of various stakeholders. It focuses on community awareness, parent education, professional development for childcare environments, and transition to school. The development of the model was initiated by the US government in collaboration with non-profit agencies and a university. Studies suggest that this emerging model shows promise for increasing children's developmental skills and abilities associated with school readiness (Winter, Zurcher, Hernadez & Zenong, 2007).

It is clear that a tremendous shift has taken place over the past few decades in the conceptualisation of school readiness. This, in turn, has had a significant impact on how school readiness is assessed. Nonetheless, 'readiness, it turns out, cannot be assessed easily, quickly or efficiently' (Meisels, 1998, p.21).

Research trends

In the international literature there are three main bodies of research that inform the understanding of school readiness (Rimm-Kaufman, 2004). The first consists of large-scale surveys that explore the perceptions of stakeholders, such as preschool teachers and parents, of school readiness. The second body of research focuses on definitions of school readiness by studying the relative importance of variables such as cognitive skills and chronological age. The third examines the outcomes of early educational experiences and family social processes in relation to school readiness and performance.

Examples of research conducted in the last few years include La Paro and Pianta's (2000) meta-analytic review, which indicates that preschool cognitive assessment predicts about 25 per cent of the variance in cognitive assessment in the first two years of schooling. While their findings support the importance of cognitive indicators, they also indicate that other factors account for most of the variance in early school outcomes. On the other hand, in South Africa, Van Zyl (2004) found that there was a highly significant correlation between perceptual development as part of school readiness using the ASB, and Grade 1 children's performance in literacy and numeracy. The sample in this study was 137 Afrikaans- and English-speaking children from average to above-average socio-economic backgrounds.

Winter and Kelley (2008) conducted a comprehensive analysis of several large-scale studies spanning a period of 40 years, which showed the importance of high-quality home and preschool environments for improving children's school readiness. The longitudinal studies that they reviewed indicated that children who had participated in high-quality early development programmes or learning environments were more likely to have better cognitive and language development than their peers. Positive outcomes for children from socio-economically disadvantaged backgrounds were reported, especially where programmes provided individual child-focused early intervention in conjunction with comprehensive family support services. Ramey and Ramey (2004), after reviewing evidence from randomised controlled trials, also argued in favour of the positive effect of high-quality early intervention programmes on high-risk groups of children from economically poor families This is of particular relevance to South African communities where a high level of poverty places children at risk in the formal schooling system.

Teacher professional development, behaviour and practice have been related to children's social and behaviour skills. Winter and Kelley (2008) state that there is a need for more research into the effects of early childhood programmes on these aspects of children's functioning. They also suggest that studies in third world and developing countries will expand on ways of enhancing school readiness in contexts where there is a scarcity of resources.

Conclusion

Although school readiness testing has a fairly long history in South Africa, there is a paucity of local research in this field (Goldblatt, 2004; Sundelowitz, 2001). This, together with the fact that there have been no new developments in school readiness testing for more than two decades, places practitioners at an impasse. Research and examples of best practice based on educational experience need to be documented in order to design a framework for school readiness assessment that is most suited to our unique context, and that addresses the needs of our diverse population of preschool children.

Education White Paper 6 (Department of Education, 2001b) advocates that responsibility be placed on schools, and the education system as a whole, to provide adequate support structures to accommodate a range of children and to promote optimal learning and development. This is consistent with the shift towards an interactive, bi-directional, context-appropriate concept of school readiness (Dockett & Perry, 2009; Freeman & Brown, 2008; Goldblatt, 2004; Maxwell & Clifford, 2004; Meisels, 1998; Scott-Little et al., 2006). There is a definite place for the assessment of individual learners in the interest of early identification of problems and provision of intervention and/or support, and therefore government expenditure on education should prioritise the development of early childhood programmes, the upgrading of ECD facilities and the improvement of teacher training. This will assist in addressing the current challenges faced by the education system, and provide children with better opportunities to reach their full potential.

References

Carlton, M.P. & Winsler, A. (1999). School readiness: The need for a paradigm shift. *School Psychology Review, 28(3)*, 338–353.

Department of Basic Education (2010). *2009 Country Report: South Africa*. Pretoria: Department of Basic Education.

Department of Education (2001a). *Education White Paper 5 Early Childhood Education: Meeting the Challenge of Early Childhood Development in South Africa*. Pretoria: Department of Basic Education.

Department of Education (2001b). *Education White Paper 6 Special Needs Education: Building an Inclusive Education and Training System*. Pretoria: Department of Basic Education.

Dockett, S. & Perry, B. (2009). Readiness for school: A relational construct. *Australasian Journal of Early Childhood, 34(1)*, 20–26.

Engel, P. (1991). Tracking progress towards the school readiness goal. *Education Leadership, 48(5)*, 39–42.

Foxcroft, C., Paterson, H., Le Roux, N. & Herbst, D. (2004). *Psychological Assessment in South Africa: A Needs Analysis. The Test Use Patterns and Needs of Psychological Assessment Practitioners*. Pretoria: Human Sciences Research Council.

Foxcroft, C. & Roodt, G. (2008). *An Introduction to Psychological Assessment in the South African Context* (3rd edition). Cape Town: Oxford University Press.

Freeman, N. & Brown, M. (2008). An authentic approach to pre-kindergarten programs: Redefining readiness. *Childhood Education, 84(5)*, 267–274.

Goldblatt, A. (2004). A cross-cultural study of parent and teacher perceptions of school readiness. Unpublished Master's research report. University of the Witwatersrand, Johannesburg.

Graue, M. E. (2006). The answer is readiness – now what was the question? *Early Education and Development, 17(1)*, 43–54.

Guhn, M., Janus, M. & Hertzman, C. (2007). The Early Development Instrument: Translating school readiness assessment into community actions and policy planning. *Early Education and Development, 18(3)*, 369–374.

Kagan, S. L. (2003). Children's readiness for school: Issues in assessment. *International Journal of Early Childhood, 35(1/2)*, 114–117.

Kriegler, S. M. & Skuy, M. (1996). Perspectives on psychological assessment in South African schools. In P. Engelbrecht, S. M. Kriegler & M. I. Booysen (Eds), *Perspectives on Learning Difficulties: International Concerns and South African Realities* (pp. 109–122). Pretoria: Van Schaik.

La Paro, K. & Pianta, R. C. (2000). Predicting children's competence in the early school years: A meta-analytic review. *Review of Educational Research, 70(4)*, 443–484.

Maxwell, K. L. & Clifford, R. M. (2004). School readiness assessment. *Young Children, 59(1)*, 42–47.

Meisels, S. J. (1998). Assessing readiness. *Center for the Improvement of Early Reading Achievement*. Ciera Report No. 3-002.

Nell, V. (2000). *Cross-cultural Neuropsychological Assessment: Theory and Practice*. London: Lawrence Erlbaum Associates.

Ramey, C. T. & Ramey, S. L. (2004). Early learning and school readiness: Can early intervention make a difference? *Merill-Palmer Quarterly, 50(4)*, 471–491.

Rimm-Kaufman, S. (2004). School transition and school readiness: An outcome of early childhood development. In R. E. Tremblay, R. G. Barr & R. de V. Peters (Eds), *Encyclopedia on Early Childhood Development* (pp. 1–7). Montreal: Centre of Excellence for Early Childhood Development. Retrieved June 5, 2010, from http:/www.child-encyclopedia.com/documents/Rimm-KaufmanANGxp.pdf.

Scott-Little, C., Kagan, S. L. & Frelow, V. S. (2006). Conceptualisation of readiness and the content of early learning standards: The intersection of policy and research? *Early Childhood Research Quarterly, 21*, 153–173.

Sundelowitz, E. (2001). 'Coming ready or not': The hide and seek of school readiness in a historically 'Model C' school. Unpublished Master's research dissertation. University of the Witwatersrand, Johannesburg.

The Presidency, Republic of South Africa (2009). *Situational Analysis of Children in South Africa (2007–2008)*. Pretoria: The Presidency.

Van Zyl, E. (2004). The relation between perceptual development (as part of school readiness) and school success of Grade 1 learners. *Africa Educational Research, 70(4)*, 147–159.

Venter, A. (2000). Cross-cultural issues in child development and assessment within the South African context. *South African Journal of Child and Adolescent Mental Health, 12*, 162–177.

Vygotsky, L. S. (1978). *Mind in Society: The Development of Higher Psychological Processes*. Cambridge, MA: Harvard University Press.

Winter, S. M. (2009/2010). Interdisciplinary approaches to school readiness. *Childhood Education, 86(2)*, 96C.

Winter, S. M. & Kelley, M. F. (2008). Forty years of school readiness research: What have we learned? *Childhood Education, 84(5)*, 260–267.

Winter, S. M., Zurcher, R., Hernandez, A. & Zenong, Y. (2007). The Early ON school readiness project: A preliminary report. *Journal of Research in Childhood Education, 22(1)*, 55–69.

7 The Kaufman Assessment Battery in South Africa

K. Greenop, J. Rice and D. de Sousa

During the 1970s and 1980s, the dominance of intelligence quotient (IQ) tests, and users' dissatisfaction with their validity, led to the development of the Kaufman Assessment Battery for Children (K-ABC) in the USA to address cultural biases in assessments (Kaufman & Kaufman, 1983a; 1983b; Kaufman, Lichtenberger, Fletcher-Janzen & Kaufman, 2005; Miller & Reynolds, 1984). According to Clauss-Ehlers (2009, p.557), 'The K-ABC's theoretical underpinnings and its fairness in assessing children from diverse minority groups sets it apart from traditional IQ tests, notably those developed from the Binet and Wechsler traditions.' The test was designed to be used in psychological, psycho-educational and neuropsychological assessments (Kaufman & Kaufman, 2004). It is based on Sperry's cerebral lateralisation theory, as well as Luria's cognitive processing theory (Kaufman et al., 2005). The K-ABC was published in 1983 and the KABC-II in 2004. This second edition was developed in response to criticisms of a theoretical and conceptual nature (Kamphaus & Reynolds, 1987; Kaufman & Kaufman, 2004).

Kamphaus (1993) cites research (Bracken, 1989; Obringer, 1988) that demonstrates that the K-ABC has been a widely used instrument, second only to the Wechsler scales. This may be ascribed to various features of the battery: specifically, the inclusion of 'teaching items' in the subtests to ensure that the task is understood; a variety of developmental levels and novel test items; ease of administration; a strong theoretical basis; and the use of photographs in some items. Negative features of the K-ABC include floor and ceiling effects, and the debate surrounding whether the Mental Processing Composite (MPC) measures its intended processes (Kamphaus, 1993). These criticisms were addressed in the revised edition, the KABC-II (Kaufman & Kaufman, 2004).

Extensive research literature exists for the K-ABC, and focuses on both the psychometric properties of the measure as well as its use in an applied setting. In South Africa, from a psychological assessment perspective, the K-ABC is not a restricted test (HPCSA, no date) and it appears in a survey of instruments utilised by South African psychologists (Foxcroft, Paterson, Le Roux & Herbst, 2004). No research into the extent of the use of the K-ABC amongst psychologists, educationists and allied health professionals exists in this country. There is also little published international literature on the KABC-II; and the authors are not aware of any publications from South Africa focusing on this edition of the battery at the time of writing. The research on the KABC-II that has been published internationally is predominantly focused on the application of the KABC-II to clinical settings.

Description of the K-ABC and KABC-II

The K-ABC was designed to measure how children receive and process information, and outlines their strengths and weaknesses. The cognitive processing scales in the instrument include the Sequential Processing scale, the Simultaneous Processing scale, an MPC, a Nonverbal Composite and the Achievement scale (replaced by the Knowledge/Crystallised Ability scale in the KABC-II). The Achievement scale uses culturally specific images and items, and is only appropriate for US norm groups (Jansen & Greenop, 2008). The K-ABC was designed to assess a range of age groups (children aged 1:6–12:5 years for the K-ABC, and children aged 3:0–18:11 years for the KABC-II), minority groups and children with learning disabilities. It was designed for English-speaking and bilingual children, as well as children who are not verbal for a variety of reasons. Kaufman and Kaufman's (1983a) intention was to create a linguistically minimised and relatively culture-fair assessment, with norms available for different cultural groups and socio-economic levels. The degree to which this has succeeded is debatable, but the K-ABC remains one of the less culturally loaded tests available to professionals today. This is an essential point for South African professionals who work within linguistically and socio-economically diverse population groups.

Both Sperry's (1968) cerebral specialisation approach and Luria's (1973) clinical neuropsychological theory of the brain as three functional units, rather than mapping of areas and functions in a one-to-one manner, form the basis of the K-ABC. Both are dual processing approaches and form an important underpinning in both the K-ABC and the KABC-II. Luria's three functional units are:

- unit 1: responsible for cortical tone, arousal and attention, corresponding to the reticular activating system;
- unit 2: responsible for obtaining, analysing, coding and storing information from the outside world, corresponding to the anterior cortex and the temporal, parietal and occipital lobes;
- unit 3: responsible for executive planning, regulating and verifying conscious behaviour, and found anterior to the precentral gyrus.

Cognitive processing in unit 2 includes both sequential processing and simultaneous processing. However, it is essential that all three units work together during mental activity. As Kaufman and Kaufman (2004) point out for the KABC-II, all three units are measured by the subtests, and the expansion of the subtests to include learning and planning, and the increase in the age range, better reflect Luria's theory.

The KABC-II is a substantial revision of the original K-ABC, and an extension of the theoretical foundation to include both the Cattell-Horn-Carroll (CHC) theory of fluid-crystallised intelligence (Flanagan & Harrison, 2008) and Luria's neuropsychological theory (Kaufman & Kaufman, 2004). This allows interpretations to be made from either perspective. The CHC is a psychometric theory that merges Carroll's psychometric research and Raymond Cattell's *Gf-Gc* theory. The latter theory was later refined by Horn 'to include an array of abilities beyond *Gf* and *Gc*' (Kaufman & Kaufman, 2004, p.13). Cattell's theory is based on Spearman's *g*-factor theory, which outlines a general factor of intelligence, as well as smaller, specific factors. Cattell theorised that there two types of *g*:

- *Gf* – fluid intelligence. This requires reasoning to solve novel problems and is largely biologically determined.
- *Gc* – crystallised intelligence. This type of intelligence is knowledge-based and is determined by environment and education.

Horn then extended these two types of *g* to include the following, which are included in the KABC-II:

- *Gsm* – short-term acquisition and retrieval;
- *Gv* – visual processing;
- *Glr* – long-term storage and retrieval (Kaufman & Kaufman, 2004).

The CHC theory allows for the categorisation of cognitive abilities, including verbal ability, and produces a measure of cognitive intelligence. The Luria model excludes verbal ability from the score to generate the Mental Processing Index (MPI), and results in a neuropsychological measure. The Nonverbal Composite has the fewest verbal ability measures. The Nonverbal scale can be acted out and responded to with actions, enabling assessment of children with hearing impairments, and those with limited English proficiency (Flanagan, 1995; Flanagan & Harrison, 2008).

Table 7.1 Choice of model (CHC or Luria) based on the contexts of administration

CHC Model (FCI)	Luria Model (MPC)
Default cases – the first choice for interpretation unless other features in column 2 are present	Bilingual and multilingual background
Suspected reading, written expression or mathematical disability	If non-mainstream cultural background may have affected his or her knowledge acquisition and verbal development
Mental retardation	Language disorders (expressive, receptive or mixed)
Attention-Deficit/Hyperactivity Disorder	Suspected autism
Emotional or behavioural disturbance	Deaf or hard of hearing
Giftedness	Examiner firmly aligned with Luria processing model, and believes acquired knowledge should be excluded from any cognitive score

Source: Adapted from Kaufman et al. (2005).

Note: FCI = Fluid Crystallised Index; MPC = Mental Processing Composite.

Either the CHC theory or the Luria model can be used to interpret the battery, and the assessor makes this decision based on the particular child being assessed (see Table 7.1). The CHC model is recommended as the first choice, unless circumstances dictate that the knowledge levels or crystallised intelligence levels of the child would affect the validity of the measure. In those cases the Luria model should be used (Kaufman & Kaufman, 2004). The CHC theory has a global scale, the Fluid-Crystallised Index (FCI), which specifically examines crystallised intelligence levels.

The entire K-ABC battery is individually administered and takes 35–80 minutes to complete (the KABC-II takes 25–70 minutes), depending on which scales or theoretical model are used. The subtests that are included in both the K-ABC and the KABC-II can be found in the appendix to this chapter, in Table 7.A1. The KABC- II has eight of the original subtests, and ten new subtests have been added. The remaining subtests were revised because of the change in the age range, and to improve measurement (Kaufman & Kaufman, 2004). Revisions addressed the main criticisms of floor and ceiling effects, as well as theoretical and conceptual problems (Kamphaus, 1993). The MPI and FCI scales are both standard scores with a mean of 100 and a standard deviation of 15. The subtests of each of the standard scales have a mean of 10 and a standard deviation of 3. Table 7.2 outlines the correspondence between the Lurian and CHC scales and their descriptions.

Table 7.2 The KABC-II scales for each theoretical orientation

KABC-II scale name	Lurian model	CHC model
Memory/*Gsm*	Sequential Processing Coding that requires sequencing of information to solve a problem	Short-term Memory (*Gsm*) Taking in information, holding it, then using it within a few seconds
Simultaneous/*Gv*	Simultaneous Processing Coding that requires information to be integrated and synthesised holistically to solve a problem	Visual Processing (*Gv*) Perceiving, storing, manipulating and thinking with visual patterns
Planning/*Gf*	Planning Ability High-level decision-making, executive processes	Fluid Reasoning (*Gf*) Reasoning, such as deductive and inductive reasoning, used to solve novel problems
Learning/*Glr*	Learning Ability Integration of the three units, especially attention and concentration, coding and strategy generation in order to learn	Long-term Storage/Retrieval (*Glr*) Storage and retrieval of information newly learnt or previously learnt
Knowledge/*Gc*	–	Knowledge/Crystallised Ability (*Gc*) Knowledge acquired from culture
	Global Scores/Composites	
–	Mental Processing Index (MPI)	Fluid-Crystallised Index (FCI)
–	Nonverbal Composite	Nonverbal Composite

Source: Adapted from Kaufman et al. (2005).

Reliability of the K-ABC and KABC-II

Reliability of the K-ABC

The K-ABC, as reported in the manual, has a split-half reliability of .89–.97 (Kaufman & Kaufman, 1983a). Table 7.3 lists the average reliability scores for each subtest for school-age children, as well as the loading on the Sequential factor, and the loading on the Simultaneous factor for the K-ABC (Kamphaus, 1993).

Table 7.3 Reliability and factor analytic results in the standardisation sample for the Sequential and Simultaneous subtests of the K-ABC

Sequential subtests			
Subtest	**Average reliability**	**Loading on Sequential factor**	**Loading on Simultaneous factor**
Hand Movements	.76	.46	.31
Number Recall	.81	.66	.16
Word Order	.82	.68	.22
Simultaneous subtests			
Subtest	**Average reliability**	**Loading on Sequential factor**	**Loading on Simultaneous factor**
Gestalt Closure	.71	.10	.49
Triangles	.84	.21	.63
Matrix Analogies	.85	.30	.50
Spatial Memory	.80	.26	.58
Photo Series	.82	.25	.64

Source: Kamphaus (1993).

Studies of black and white US children aged from 2:6 years to 12:5 years have not shown significantly different internal consistency reliability estimates, and the MPC has been found to have reliability coefficients ranging from .89 to .96 for both groups (Matazow, Kamphaus, Stanton & Reynolds, 1991). The reliability coefficients ranged from .84 to .95 on each of the individual scales. The authors concluded that 'the K-ABC is not suspect in respect to systematic bias in reliability for black and white children' (Matazow et al., 1991, p.40).

Reliability of the KABC-II

The KABC-II MPI and FCI (Global scales) reliability scores are reportedly high, with split-half reliability scores over .90 for all age groups. Scores over time have demonstrated a range of between .86 and .94 for the MPI and FCI (Flanagan & Harrison, 2008). Kaufman et al. (2005) note that the average internal consistency coefficient for all age groups is .95 for the MPI and .96 and .97 for the FCI for age groups 3–6 and 7–18 years respectively. Table 7.4 outlines the reliability scores for the KABC-II.

Table 7.4 Reliability of the KABC-II

	Internal reliability		Test-retest reliability	
Scale/subtest	Ages 3–6	Ages 7–18	Ages 3–6	Ages 7–18
Sequential/*Gsm*	.91	.89	.79	.80
Number Recall	.85	.79	.69	.82
Word Order	.87	.87	.72	.72
Hand Movements	.69	.78	.50	.60
Simultaneous/*Gv*	.92	.88	.74	.77
Block Counting	.90	.87		.63
Conceptual Thinking	.80		.55	
Face Recognition	.75		.56	
Rover	.83	.80		.64
Triangles	.86	.87	.79	.83
Gestalt Closure	.74	.74	.70	.81
Learning/*Glr*	.91	.93	.79	.79
Atlantis	.83	.86	.73	.70
Rebus	.92	.93	.70	.79
Delayed Recall	.82	.90		.80
Planning/*Gf*		.88		.81
Pattern Reasoning	.89	.90		.74
Story Completion	.82	.77		.72
Knowledge/*Gc*	.91	.92	.93	.92
Expressive Vocabulary	.84	.86	.86	.89
Riddles	.85	.86	.80	.89
Verbal Knowledge	.85	.89	.81	.83
MPI	.95	.95	.86	.90
FCI	.96	.97	.90	.93
NVI	.90	.92	.72	.87

Source: Kaufman et al. (2005, p.23).

Note: NVI = Nonverbal Index.

Reliability of the K-ABC and KABC-II in South Africa

At the time of writing this chapter, the authors were unaware of any research into internal consistency or test-retest reliability for either the K-ABC or the KABC-II in South Africa. However, a study on K-ABC performance by monolingual English-speaking and bilingual English-Afrikaans-speaking 9-year-old children found reliability scores of between .77 and .84 (see Table 7.5; De Sousa, 2006).

Table 7.5 Reliability results for monolingual and bilingual 9-year-old children on the K-ABC

Scale/subtest	Internal reliability in monolingual children	Internal reliability in bilingual children
Sequential scale	.80	.81
Hand Movements	.79	.81
Number Recall	.80	.81
Word Order	.81	.80
Simultaneous scale	.81	.80
Gestalt Closure	.77	.77
Triangles	.83	.80
Matrix Analogies	.84	.80
Spatial Memory	.81	.80
Photo Series	.80	.83

Source: Adapted from De Sousa (2006).

Validity of the K-ABC and KABC-II

Validity of the K-ABC

The K-ABC manual (Kaufman & Kaufman, 1983a) lists 43 validity studies, including predictive, construct and concurrent validity studies. Developmentally, Kamphaus (2005) concludes that ceiling and floor effects limit the test's validity (a significant change for the KABC-II), but it still differentiates ages well. In terms of correlations with other tests, the K-ABC MPC correlates with the Wechsler Intelligence Scale for Children – Revised (WISC-R) at .70 for children from regular classrooms, which demonstrates 49 per cent shared variance (Kaufman & Kaufman, 1983a; Kamphaus, 2005). Finally, the K-ABC shows predictive validity at a similar level to the WISC-III.

Naglieri (1986) compared a matched sample of black and white US children on their performance on the WISC-R and the K-ABC. On the WISC-R, the white children scored nine points higher than the black children, while on the K-ABC the score difference on the MPC was six. This was due to a significant difference on the Triangles subtest, as none of the other subtests showed a significant difference in scores.

In terms of ecological validity, a variety of studies have been undertaken with different cultural groups (for example, in Uganda, by Baganda et al., 2006; in Central Africa, by Boivin et al., 1996; in Egypt, by Elwan, 1996; and in Korea, by Moon, 1998) as the rationale of the K-ABC was that it could be used as a measure of reduced cultural bias (Kaufman et al., 2005). Overall, the K-ABC has reduced the 15–16 point difference between white and African-American children on the Wechsler scales to half of this. Kaufman et al. (2005) also cite research by numerous authors (Campbell, Bell & Keith, 2001; Davidson, 1992; Fourquean, 1987; Valencia, Rankin & Livingston, 1995; Vincent, 1991; Whitworth & Chrisman, 1987) to demonstrate that the K-ABC produces smaller differences in scores between white and Latino children than conventional measures.

An investigation into the performance of 130 Zairean children aged 7.7 to 9.2 years found that the distinction between the Simultaneous and Sequential scales was upheld. However, the Simultaneous scale demonstrated two clusters. Gestalt Closure, Matrix Analogies and Spatial Memory clustered together, as did Triangles, Matrix Analogies and Photo Series. The authors argued that this was due to task difficulty and lack of cultural familiarity. Overall, the Simultaneous scores (63.53; SD = 9.91) were significantly lower than the Sequential scores (80.56; SD = 13.84). In comparison, the US norms were not significantly different at 97.0 (SD = 14.9) for the Sequential scale and 92.8 (SD = 14.5) for the Simultaneous scale. The Global scores were also vastly different at 67.59 for the Zairean children and 93.7 for the African-American children. This discrepancy was due to the low Simultaneous subtest scores (Giordani, Boivin, Opel, Nseyila & Lauer, 1996).

Keith and Dunbar (1984), in an exploratory factor analysis on a sample of 585 referred children, found three factors and argued that the K-ABC may not be measuring the mental processes that it purports to measure. Simultaneous and sequential processing may actually be measuring semantic memory and nonverbal reasoning. The KABC-II developers took this consideration into account in the revision of the K-ABC.

Validity of the KABC-II

Little research exists at present on the validity of the KABC-II. The manual (Kaufman & Kaufman, 2004) outlines a confirmatory factor analysis which supports the construct validity of the KABC-II. Confirmatory factor analyses were conducted across age levels and the findings of these analyses supported the use of different batteries at different age levels. At age 3, a single-factor model is the basis for the KABC-II. However, confirmatory factor analyses yielded a distinction between the Sequential subtests and the rest of the battery for this age group. The Concept Formation subtest loaded substantially on both Knowledge and Simultaneous factors at age 4. This dual loading led to a non-significant distinction between Knowledge and Simultaneous factors. The final KABC-II battery separates Knowledge and Simultaneous factors into distinct scales on the basis of the distinct content in each of the scales. Both the Sequential and Learning factors were well supported and distinct at age 4 (Kaufman & Kaufman, 2004).

Separate analyses at ages 5, 6, 7 and 8 revealed that Simultaneous and Planning factors were not distinguishable at age 5 or 6; but they were at ages 7 and 8. As a result, the decision was taken to introduce the Planning scale at age 7 and to treat Story Completion as a supplementary Simultaneous subtest at age 6 (Kaufman & Kaufman, 2004).

Analyses of age ranges from 7 through 18 were conducted. Triangles and Rover differentiated Simultaneous and Planning factors in younger portions of this age range. From around age 13, Block Counting and Rover improved this differentiation (Kaufman & Kaufman, 2004).

Research into the validity of the K-ABC in the USA (Flanagan & Harrison, 2008) with a standardisation sample of 3 025 children includes a confirmatory factor analysis which found very good fit, with 'four factors for ages 4 and 5–6, and five factors for ages 7–12 and 13–18, with the factor structure supporting the scale structure for these broad age groups' (p.351). In addition, there was a correlation between the FCI and WISC-IV Full Scale IQ at .89, WISC-III at .77, and Woodcock-Johnson Third Edition (WJ-III) General Intelligence Ability. The MPI correlated with the WJ-III at .72 for preschool children and at .84 for school-age children.

Cross-culturally, Fletcher-Janzen (2003) investigated the performance on the KABC-II in Taos Pueblo Indian children in New Mexico and found a correlation between the WISC-IV and the FCI and MPC at .85 and above for Taos. In a separate study, Malda, Van de Vijver, Srinivasan, Transler, Sukumar and Rao (2008) adapted the KABC-II for 6–10-year-old Kannada-speaking children of low socio-economic status from Bangalore, South India. The authors found that the adapted version of KABC-II subtests showed high reliabilities and the CHC model was largely replicated. The findings of this study lend support to the use and validity of this KABC-II adaption.

In a separate validity study, Bangirana et al. (2009) investigated the KABC-II construct validity in 65 Ugandan children (7–16 years old) with a history of cerebral malaria. They were assessed 44 months after the malaria episode. A principal component analysis found five factors after administering the KABC-II: specifically, the Sequential scale, Simultaneous scale, Planning and Learning; the fifth factor was ascribed to immediate and delayed recall.

Validity of the K-ABC and KABC-II in South Africa

Jansen (1998) conducted a principal component factor analysis of the performance of 5-year-old black children's performance (N = 335) on the K-ABC's processing scales and found the two scales of Simultaneous and Sequential Processing were generally upheld. Jansen and Greenop (2008) followed a group of 199 children from the age of 5 to 10 years. At these two points, the children were assessed on the K-ABC. A principal component analysis supported a two-factor loading.

Developmentally, Krohn and Lamp (1999) found, in a longitudinal investigation of children at 3:6 and 9 years old, that the processing abilities assessed by the K-ABC may change over time. The sample included 65 African-American and white children from the Midwest of the USA from families of low socio-economic status. This is consistent with Kaufman and Kaufman's (1983a) assertion that before school entry, children are more simultaneous processing-dominant, but as they enter formal schooling this shifts as they become more sequential processing-dominant. Jansen and Greenop (2008) investigated this assertion in a group of 10-year-old, multilingual children of low socio-economic status and found both age and gender differences over time. These differences always supported the two-factor model of simultaneous and sequential processing, but the dominance of processing style changed with age as is shown in Table 7.6. These changes were at times different for each gender, as detailed in Table 7.7.

Table 7.6 Simultaneous and Sequential group factor structure at 5 and 10 years (N = 199)

	5 years		10 years	
SEQ*	**SEQ**	**SIM**	**SEQ**	**SIM**
Hand Movements	.46	.41	.70	.04
Number Recall	.85	.05	.79	.04
Word Order	.76	.21	.59	.33
SIM				
Spatial Memory	.11	.78	.29	.61
Gestalt Closure	.04	.79	.12	.86
Triangles	.42	.62	.31	.60
Matrix Analogies	.28	.61	.38	.47
Photo Series**			.61	.40

Source: Adapted from Jansen and Greenop (2008).

Notes: * SEQ = Sequential processing; SIM = Simultaneous processing ** Only administered at 10 years.

At 5 years, the Hand Movements subtest loaded almost equally on both processing styles, but at 10 years this task was unequivocally loaded on a Sequential factor. Number Recall, which is a Sequential subtest, showed high loadings at both age groups on the sequential processing style. Word Order, which is also a Sequential subtest, revealed a slightly different result. Specifically, at 5 years the factor loading was high on the Sequential scale, but this was reduced for the 10-year-olds. Conant et al. (2003) have suggested that Word Order taps into cross-modal memory; and this is seen more clearly with increasing age and the corresponding increasing use of verbal mediation strategies. Jansen and Greenop's (2008) study supports that suggestion.

The Gestalt Closure loading, which is a Simultaneous subtest, was consistently high on the Simultaneous factor for both age groups. The loading for Spatial Memory, which is also a Simultaneous subtest, was high on the Simultaneous factor at 5 years, but less pronounced at 10 years. For the other Simultaneous subtests, Triangles loaded more clearly on the Simultaneous factor at 10 years, while Matrix Analogies was less strongly loaded by 10 years and instead loaded on the Sequential scale. One possibility for this finding given by Jansen and Greenop (2008) is that a similar process may also be operating in cross-modal processing with verbal mediation strategies.

Jansen and Greenop (2008) also examined gender differences in the factor structure for each developmental period (see Table 7.7).

Table 7.7 Simultaneous and Sequential gender factor structure at 5 and 10 years

	5 years – boys		5 years – girls		10 years – boys		10 years – girls	
SEQ*	**SEQ**	**SIM**	**SEQ**	**SIM**	**SEQ**	**SIM**	**SEQ**	**SIM**
Hand Movements	.26	.45	.68	.29	.81	.02	.65	.22
Number Recall	.84	.00	.83	.06	.78	.15	.84	.01
Word Order	.70	.22	.79	.18	.47	.52	.67	.27
SIM								
Spatial Memory	.05	.78	.31	.67	.27	.53	.39	.58
Gestalt Closure	.00	.79	.11	.82	.16	.84	.16	.84
Triangles	.41	.60	.50	.56	.25	.55	.26	.69
Matrix Analogies	.46	.54	.10	.76	.56	.26	.34	.52
Photo Series**					.58	.48	.45	.56

Source: Adapted from Jansen and Greenop (2008).

Notes: * SEQ = Sequential processing; SIM = Simultaneous processing ** Only administered at 10 years.

On the Sequential scale, two subtests, Word Order and Number Recall, had similar loadings for both boys and girls at the 5-year-old stage. However, the girls showed a higher loading for Hand Movements on the Sequential Processing scale. In contrast, the boys loaded more highly on the Simultaneous Processing scale for Hand Movements.

On the Simultaneous scale, all subtests loaded higher on the Simultaneous factor. Specific findings revealed that boys showed a higher loading for Spatial Memory. Both boys and girls loaded almost equally highly for Gestalt Closure. Matrix Analogies was clearly loaded for girls at 5 years of age on the Simultaneous factor.

Jansen and Greenop (2008) found that at 10 years, the boys' scores loaded clearly on a Sequential factor for Hand Movement and Number Recall, but almost equally on both factors for Word Order. In contrast, at 10 years, girls' scores were clearly loaded on the Sequential factor for Number Recall, Word Order and Hand Movements.

On the Simultaneous Processing factor, 10-year-old boys showed strong loadings for three of the subtests: Triangles, Gestalt Closure and Spatial Memory. Matrix Analogies loaded on a Sequential Processing factor and Photo Series (not administered at 5 years) loaded on both factors. Girls at 10 years old showed clear Simultaneous loadings on two subtests – namely, Gestalt Closure and Triangles.

In order to investigate whether there were any differences between 5- and 10-year-olds, paired sample t-tests were calculated (Jansen & Greenop, 2008) (see Table 7.8).

Table 7.8 Means, standard deviations (in brackets) and paired sample t-test scores at 5 and 10 years

	5 years	10 years	t
SEQ tests	**Mean (SD)**	**Mean (SD)**	
Hand Movements	8.8 (2.4)	10.4 (2.6)	6.9****
Number Recall	8.6 (3.0)	13.2 (3.0)	20.4****
Word Order	7.7 (1.8)	8.5 (2.7)	2.1***
SIM tests	**Mean (SD)**	**Mean (SD)**	
Spatial Memory	9.5 (2.8)	8.7 (2.3)	4.3***
Gestalt Closure	6.3 (2.9)	6.3 (2.9)	.1 (ns)*
Triangles	8.2 (1.9)	9.7 (2.8)	8.2****
Matrix Analogies	11.0 (1.9)	10.5 (1.9)	2.9**

Source: Adapted from Jansen and Greenop (2008).

Notes: * ns = not significant ** p < .01 *** p < .001 **** p < .0001.

The score pattern showed significant changes within the group of children. Specifically, the 5-year-olds and 10-year-olds differed on all the subtests except Gestalt Closure. Overall, significant differences were found between the composite Sequential Processing scores at 5 years and at 10 years ($t = 14.3$, $p = .0000$) and the composite Simultaneous Processing scores at 5 and at 10 years ($t = 11.0$, $df = 198$, $p < .0001$). When the group was divided by gender, more specific differences were found, as shown in Table 7.9 (Jansen & Greenop, 2008).

Table 7.9 Boys' (N = 97) and girls' (N = 102) means, standard deviations (in brackets) and paired sample t-test scores at 5 and 10 years

	HM	NR	WO	SM	GC	TRI	MA
Boys 5 years	8.9 (2)	8.4 (2.5)	7.6 (1.9)	9.4 (2.7)	6.5 (2.9)	8.1 (1.9)	10.8 (2.1)
Boys 10 years	10.3 (2.6)	13.3 (3.6)	8.4 (2.8)	9.2 (2.3)	6.7 (3)	9.9 (2.7)	10.6 (1.8)
t-scores	4.3***	16.0****	2.6*	0.5	0.8	7.1***	0.6
Girls 5 years	8.7 (2.6)	8.9 (2.5)	7.8 (1.9)	9.7 (2.9)	6.1 (3)	8.3 (2)	11.3 (1.7)
Girls 10 years	10.5 (2.4)	13.1 (3.1)	8.6 (2.6)	8.1 (2.3)	5.9 (2.7)	9.6 (2.9)	10.4 (2)
t-scores	5.4***	13.2****	3.3**	5.8***	0.9	4.7***	3.5**

Source: Adapted from Jansen and Greenop (2008).

Notes: * p < .05 ** p < .01 *** p < .001 **** p < .0001

HM = Hand Movements; NR = Number Recall; WO = Word Order; SM = Spatial Memory; GC = Gestalt Closure; TRI = Triangles; MA = Matrix Analogies.

It is evident from these results that, on the Sequential subtests, boys differed at 5 and 10 years on Hand Movements ($t = 4.3$, $df = 96$, $p < .001$), Number Recall ($t = 16.0$, $df = 95$, $p < .0001$) and Word Order ($t = 2.6$, $df = 96$, $p < .05$). The same pattern was observed for the 5- and 10-year-old girls in terms of Hand Movements ($t = 5.4$, $df = 101$, $p < .001$), Number Recall ($t = 13.2$, $df = 100$, $p < .0001$) and Word Order ($t = 3.3$, $df = 101$, $p < .01$) (Jansen & Greenop, 2008).

On the Simultaneous subtests, 5- and 10-year-old boys differed on the Triangle subtest (t = 7.1, df = 95, p < .001). Five- and 10-year-old girls differed on Spatial Memory (t = 5.8, df = 101, p < .001), Triangles (t = 4.7, df = 101, p < .001) and Matrix Analogies (t = 3.5, df = 101, p < .01). Neither 5- nor 10-year-old girls and boys differed on the Gestalt Closure task (Jansen & Greenop, 2008).

Skuy, Taylor, O'Carroll, Fridjhon and Rosenthal (2000) assessed black and white South African children from a school for children with learning disabilities on the K-ABC and the WISC-R. No significant difference was found between the groups on the K-ABC. However, significant differences were found between the black and white children on the WISC-R. The authors concluded that 'the results support other studies which have shown the K-ABC may provide a more equitable measure of intelligence [than the WISC] in culturally, linguistically disadvantaged communities' (Skuy et al., 2000, p.736).

De Sousa, Greenop and Fry (2010) compared 30 English and 30 Afrikaans Grade 3 children on the K-ABC (see Table 7.10). No significant differences were found on the MPC scale. However, the English children performed significantly better on the Matrix Analogies (Simultaneous scale) subtest (which was subsequently changed in the KABC-II), while the Afrikaans children scored significantly better on the Hand Movements subtest (a Sequential subtest, which remained unchanged in the KABC-II). This was attributed to the cognitive processing styles children used in learning how to read. Orthography affects cognitive processing. Children learning to read in Afrikaans are learning in a language that is relatively transparent, with clear letter-to-sound relationships. This may account for their higher performance on the Hand Movements subtest. Children learning to read in English rely to a greater degree on simultaneous processing as the letter-to-sound relationships are opaque. This may explain the higher performance on the Matrix Analogies subtest.

Table 7.10 Comparison of monolingual and bilingual 9-year-old children on the K-ABC

Scale	Monolingual English children, age mean = 9:8 years Mean (SD)	Bilingual Afrikaans-English children, age mean = 9:9 years Mean (SD)
MPC	105.13 (9.22)	100.66 (11.10)
Sequential scale	101.53 (9.34)	103.73 (9.67)
Simultaneous scale	104.13 (9.00)	102.00 (9.69)
Hand Movements	9.00 (2.12)	11.00 (1.91) **
Gestalt Closure	10.56 (2.82)	9.76 (2.15)
Number Recall	10.66 (2.40)	10.13 (2.27)
Triangles	10.80 (1.99)	10.30 (2.36)
Word Order	10.96 (1.63)	10.83 (1.87)
Matrix Analogies	11.56 (2.50)	10.33 (1.66) *
Spatial Memory	10.76 (1.63)	10.73 (2.36)
Photo Series	10.20 (2.01)	9.56 (1.94)

Source: Adapted from De Sousa, Greenop and Fry (2010).

Notes: * p < .05 ** = significantly different at p < .001

The scale scores of monolingual and bilingual children fell within the average range (mean = 100, SD = 15) compared to the US norms. The same was true of their subtest scores, which were within the average range of 10 (SD = 3), and all but two subscales were not significantly different across the two groups. The two groups were of similar middle-class socio-economic status (De Sousa, Greenop & Fry, 2010).

In a separate study that examined socio-economic effects on the K-ABC, Greenop (2004) assessed 10-year-old multilingual South African learners of low socio-economic circumstance. Learners were classified according to the language they were being taught to read and write in, as this was the one that they were most exposed to academically. The results are presented in Table 7.11.

Table 7.11 Simultaneous and Sequential subtest means and standard deviations (SD) for entire sample, English, isiZulu and Sesotho groups

	All (N =198)	English (n = 83)	isiZulu (n = 61)	Sesotho (n = 54)
	Mean (SD)			
Hand Movements	10.44 (2.49)	10.42 (2.33)	10.3 (2.38)	10.63 (2.87)
Gestalt Closure	6.19 (2.87)	6.76 (3.02)	5.44 (2.8)	6.15 (2.55)
Number Recall	13.12 (3.24)	12.91 (3.57)	13.51 (2.6)	13.02 (3.37)
Triangles	9.69 (2.85)	9.51 (2.81)	9.66 (3.01)	10.2 (2.74)
Word Order	8.59 (2.74)	9.21 (2.72)	7.84 (2.6)	8.46 (2.75)
Matrix Analogies	10.5 (1.91)	10.69 (2.13)	10.18 (1.7)	10.57 (1.74)
Spatial Memory	8.64 (2.33)	8.92 (2.34)	8.21 (2.29)	8.70 (2.32)
Photo Series	9.27 (2.26)	9.6 (2.42)	8.71 (1.9)	9.39 (2.30)
Sequential scaled	104.45 (14.04)	105.26 (14.4)	103.3 (11.73)	104.48 (15.91)
Simultaneous scaled	92.08 (11.06)	93.44 (12.02)	89.52 (9.68)	92.83 (10.68)
MPC scaled	96.25 (12)	97.8 (13.22)	93.72 (9.78)	96.69 (12)

Source: Adapted from Greenop (2004).

Results demonstrated that all groups fell within average limits on the full scales. However, not all groups were within the average range for the subscales, with Gestalt Closure being significantly below the mean and Number Recall being significantly above the mean. This may indicate that reduced socio-economic status impacts on these aspects of functioning, and because both these subtests have been retained in the KABC-II, cognisance should be taken of this finding when interpreting results (Greenop, 2004).

Interestingly, the only gender difference found was on the Spatial Memory subtest (which was discarded in the KABC-II), with boys scoring 9.17 (SD = 2.3) and females 8.15 (SD = 2.25). Both scores were within normal limits, but demonstrate a significant difference statistically ($t(198) = 36.98$, $p < .001$). This resulted in the Simultaneous scale showing a gender difference in favour of boys: 93.57 (10.44) versus 90.66 (11.5) for girls. Again, the scaled score is not significantly different to the norm, but within this normal range there was a gender difference. The discrepancy in gender performance on this subtest may be due to differences in social learning (Greenop, 2004).

Conclusion

Reynolds and Kamphaus (2003) argue that the K-ABC is psychometrically and conceptually strong. However, revision of the K-ABC was deemed necessary due to floor and ceiling effects on some subtests, as well as validity issues on certain subtests, such as the criticism that the Sequential and Simultaneous Processing measures may measure other constructs, including Semantic Memory and Nonverbal Reasoning (Kaufman et al., 2005). Flanagan and Harrison (2008) argue that one of the strengths of the KABC-II is the flexibility it allows in choosing a theoretical foundation to suit the child being assessed. In addition, Bangirana et al. (2009) argue that with some modifications, such as removing the culturally inappropriate items and translating the instructions, the KABC-II retains its construct validity. However, these authors used the raw scores in a factor analysis to test validity, which limits the generalisation of their results to clinical assessment situations.

Cahan and Noyman (2001) conclude that the strength of the K-ABC in being able to accommodate bilingual and culturally diverse children is also its main weakness, since verbal intelligence is not well represented in this battery. Another criticism of the K-ABC has been the use of the terms 'Achievement' and 'Intelligence', which have subsequently been modified in the KABC-II. These authors advise caution in using the measure for intelligence testing.

Despite the criticisms levelled against it, the K-ABC appears to be a good measure of academic success. The subtests are sensitive to the nature of literacy instruction of first- and second-language children despite their nonverbal presentation. The implication of this, however, is that caution needs to be exercised when using only the K-ABC (1983) to predict academic achievement of children from diverse linguistic backgrounds. Importantly, the use of a test that is considered to be relatively culture-fair, such as the K-ABC or the KABC-II, should not equate to unquestioning administration, but must be undertaken with the child's linguistic and educational context in mind.

References

Baganda, D., Nassali, A., Kalyesubula, I., Sherman, B., Drotar, D., Boivan, M. J. & Olness, K. (2006). Health, neurologic, and cogntive status of HIV-infected long-term surviving and antiretroviral-naïve Ugandan children. *Pediatrics, 117*, 729–740.

Bangirana, P., Seggane-Musisi, P., Allebeck, P., Giordani, B., John, C. C., Opoka, O. R. et al. (2009). A preliminary examination of the construct validity of the KABC-II in Ugandan children with a history of cerebral malaria. *African Health Sciences, 9(3)*, 186–192.

Boivin, M. J., Chounramany, C., Giordani, B., Xaisida, S., Choulamountry, L., Pholsena, P., Crist, C. L. & Olness, K. (1996). Validating a cognitive ability protocol with Lao children for community development applications. *Neuropsychology, 10*, 588–599.

Cahan, S. & Noyman, A. (2001). The Kaufman Ability Battery for Children mental processing scale: A valid measure of 'pure' intelligence? *Educational and Psychological Measurement, 61(5)*, 827–840.

Clauss-Ehlers, C. (2009). *Encyclopedia of Cross-cultural School Psychology*. New York, NY: Springer Verlag.

Conant, L. L., Fasteau, P. S., Giordani, B., Boivin, M. J., Chouramany, C., Xaisida, S., Choulamountry, L. & Pholsena, P. (2003). Environmental influences on primary memory development: A cross-cultural study of memory span in Lao and American children. *Journal of Clinical and Experimental Neuropsychology, 25*, 1102–1116.

De Sousa, D. S. (2006). The bilingual mind: Simultaneous and sequential processing and spelling ability in monolingual English and bilingual Afrikaans-English children. Master's dissertation. University of the Witwatersrand, Johannesburg.

De Sousa, D. S., Greenop, K. & Fry, J. (2010). Simultaneous and sequential cognitive processing in monolingual and bilingual children in South Africa. *South African Journal of Psychology, 40(2)*, 165–173.

Elwan, F. Z. (1996). The factor structure of the Kaufman Assessment Battery for Children with Egyptian school children. *Perceptual and Motor Skills, 80*, 99–110.

Flanagan, R. (1995). The utility of the Kaufman Assessment Battery for Children (K-ABC) and the Weschler Intelligence Scales for linguistically different children: Clinical considerations. *Psychology in Schools, 32*, 5–11.

Flanagan, D. P. & Harrison, P. L. (2008). *Contemporary Intellectual Assessment: Theories, Tests and Issues* (2nd edition). New York, NY: The Guilford Press.

Fletcher-Janzen, E. (2003). *A Validity Study of the KABC-II and the Taos Pueblo Indian Children of New Mexico*. Circle Pines, MN: American Guidance Service.

Foxcroft, C., Paterson, H., Le Roux, N. & Herbst, D. (2004). *Psychological Assessment in South Africa: A Needs Analysis*. Pretoria: Human Sciences Research Council.

Giordani, B., Boivin, M. J., Opel, B., Nseyila, D. D. & Lauer, R. E. (1996). Use of the K-ABC with children in Zaire, Africa: An evaluation of the sequential-simultaneous processing distinction within an intercultural context. *International Journal of Disability, Development and Education, 43(1)*, 5–24.

Greenop, K. T. (2004). The development of literacy skills in Zulu and Northern Sotho speaking children: A cognitive-neuropsychological investigation. PhD dissertation. University of the Witwatersrand, Johannesburg.

HPCSA (Health Professions Council of South Africa) (no date). *The Professional Board for Psychology Health Professions Council of South Africa List of Tests Classified as Being Psychological Tests*. Retrieved March 2, 2010, from http://www.hpcsa.co.za/downloads/psychology/form_207.pdf.

Jansen, P. (1998). Early lateral preferences and mental processing trends in black preschoolers. PhD dissertation. University of the Witwatersrand, Johannesburg.

Jansen, P. & Greenop, K. (2008). Factor analyses of the Kaufman Assessment Battery for Children assessed longitudinally at 5 and 10 years. *South African Journal of Psychology, 38(2)*, 355–365.

Kamphaus, R. W. (1993). *Clinical Assessment of Children's Intelligence: A Handbook for Professional Practice*. Boston, MA: Allyn & Bacon.

Kamphaus, R. W. (2005). *Clinical Assessment of Child and Adolescent Intelligence*. New York, NY: Springer Verlag.

Kamphaus, R. W. & Reynolds, C. R. (1987). *Clinical and Research Applications of the K-ABC.* Circle Pines, MN: American Guidance Service.

Kaufman, A. S. & Kaufman, N. L. (1983a). *Kaufman Assessment Battery for Children (K-ABC): Administration and Scoring Manual.* Circle Pines, MN: American Guidance Service.

Kaufman, A. S. & Kaufman, N. L. (1983b). *K-ABC Interpretive Manual.* Circle Pines, MN: American Guidance Service.

Kaufman, A. S. & Kaufman, N. L. (2004). *Kaufman Assessment Battery for Children, Second Edition Manual.* Circle Pines, MN: American Guidance Service.

Kaufman, A. S., Lichtenberger, E. O., Fletcher-Janzen, E. & Kaufman, N. L. (2005). *Essentials of KABC-II Assessment.* Hoboken, NJ: John Wiley & Sons.

Keith, T. Z. & Dunbar, S. B. (1984). Hierarchical factor analysis of the K-ABC: Testing alternate models. *Journal of Special Education, 18,* 367–647.

Krohn, E. J. & Lamp, R. E. (1999). Stability of the SB:FE and K-ABC for young children from low-income families: A 5-year longitudinal study. *Journal of School Psychology, 37(3),* 315–332.

Luria, A. R. (1973). *The Working Brain: An Introduction to Neuropsychology.* New York, NY: Basic Books.

Malda, M., Van de Vijver, F. J., Srinivasan, K., Transler, C., Sukumar, P. & Rao, K. (2008). Adapting a cognitive test for a different culture: An illustration of qualitative procedures. *Psychology Science Quarterly, 50(4),* 451–468.

Matazow, G. S., Kamphaus, R. W., Stanton, H. C. & Reynolds, C. R. (1991). Reliability of the Kaufman Assessment Battery for Children for black and white students. *Journal of School Psychology, 29(1),* 37–41.

Miller, T. L. & Reynolds, C. R. (1984). Special issue: The K-ABC. *Journal of Special Education,* whole issue.

Moon, S. B. (1988). A cross-cultural validity study of the Kaufman Assessment Battery for Children with Korean children. PhD dissertation. University of Alabama. *Dissertation Abstracts International, 49,* 2158.

Naglieri, J. A. (1986). WISC-R and K-ABC comparison for matched samples of black and white children. *Journal of School Psychology, 24(1),* 81–88.

Reynolds, C. R. & Kamphaus, R. W. (2003). *Handbook of Psychological and Educational Assessment of Children.* New York, NY: The Guilford Press.

Skuy, M., Taylor, M., O'Carroll, S., Fridjhon, P. & Rosenthal, L. (2000). Performance of black and white South African children on the Wechsler Intelligence Scale for Children – Revised and the Kaufman Assessment Battery. *Psychological Reports, 86,* 727–737.

Sperry, R. W. (1968). Hemisphere deconnection and unity in conscious awareness. *American Psychologist, 23,* 723–733.

Appendix A

Table 7.A1 Comparison of the K-ABC and KABC-II subtests

	K-ABC	KABC-II
Scale	**Subtests**	**Subtests**
Simultaneous	Triangles	Triangles
	Face Recognition	Face Recognition
	–	Pattern Reasoning (ages 5 and 6)
	–	Block Counting
	–	Story Completion (ages 5 and 6)
	–	Conceptual Thinking
	–	Rover
	Gestalt Closure	Gestalt Closure
	Magic Window	–
	Matrix Analogies	–
	Spatial Memory	–
	Photo Series	–
Sequential	Word Order	Word Order
	Number Recall	Number Recall
	Hand Movements	Hand Movements
Planning	–	Pattern Reasoning (ages 7–18)
	–	Story Completion (ages 7–18)
Learning	–	Atlantis
	–	Atlantis Delayed
	–	Rebus
	–	Rebus Delayed
Knowledge/Achievement	Riddles	Riddles
	Expressive Vocabulary	Expressive Vocabulary
		Verbal Knowledge
	Faces and Places	–
	Arithmetic*	–
	Reading/Decoding*	–
	Reading/Understanding*	–

Source: Adapted from Kaufman et al. (2005).

Note: *Reading, writing and arithmetic were excluded from the K-ABC as they were deemed more appropriate to achievement tests (Flanagan & Harrison, 2008).

8 The Das-Naglieri Cognitive Assessment System

Z. Amod

> Psychologists who missed the cognitive revolution entirely may not even suspect the great chasm between their testing methods and a theoretical framework needed to drive practice. (Das, Naglieri & Kirby, 1994, p.4)

The value of conventional intelligence quotient (IQ) testing, which is widely used on a global level, has been acknowledged and demonstrated over the years as it provides a structured method of evaluating achievement and an individual's acquisition of knowledge (Naglieri & Kaufman, 2001; Sattler, 2008). IQ testing has also shown its merit within education systems throughout the world (Kaufman, 1979). However, since what is described as the 'cognitive revolution' in the field of psychology in the 1960s (Miller, 2003; Naglieri, 1999a), there have been ongoing controversies about issues such as the definition and assessment of intelligence, as well as cultural and racial differences in IQ test results. Some have argued that IQ tests such as the Binet and Wechsler Scales, which were first developed in the early part of the last century, are based on a narrow and outmoded conceptualisation of intelligence as a general intellectual construct ('*g*') which is fixed and immutable (Das & Abbott, 1995; Naglieri, 1989). This argument can also be applied to the currently used standardised South African IQ tests, such as the Junior South African Individual Scales and the Senior South African Individual Scales which were first published in the 1980s.

A major criticism of traditional approaches to intelligence testing is that they place individuals with limited language or academic skills at an unfair disadvantage. Naglieri and Kaufman (2001) assert that the verbal subtests of conventional IQ measures could be conceived more as measures of achievement and acquired knowledge, rather than of underlying ability. The difficulty arises as acquired knowledge is influenced by the individual's formal learning experiences and cultural exposure. These issues are of vital importance within the multilingual South African context, where children have vastly different cultural experiences and a legacy of unequal early learning and schooling opportunities.

Over the years, major concerns have also been raised internationally and in South Africa about the validity of conventional IQ tests when used with cultural groups that differ from those for whom these tests were normed (Chan, Shum & Cheung, 2003; Fagan & Holland, 2007; Foxcroft & Roodt, 2005; Naglieri &

Rojahn, 2001; Skuy, Gewer, Osrin, Khunou, Fridjhon & Rushton, 2002; Tollman & Msengana, 1990). Researchers such as Naglieri and Rojahn (2001) have asserted that traditional IQ test measures tend to identify disproportionately more African-American children as having mental retardation, resulting in their over-representation within special education programmes. Similarly in South Africa, Skuy, Taylor, O'Carroll, Fridjhon and Rosenthal (2000) reported that the Wechsler Intelligence Scale for Children – Revised (WISC-R) scores of black South African children were considerably lower than those of their white counterparts. These researchers concluded that the difference in scores between the two groups was related to the cultural bias inherent in traditional IQ measures, rather than to actual differences in cognitive ability.

It has also been argued that IQ scores have a limited capacity to predict achievement differences (Das et al., 1994). As highlighted by Das (2000, p.29), 'a child with an IQ of 80 is as likely to show up in a reading disability class or clinic as a child whose IQ is 120'. A further argument is that general intelligence scores are not sensitive to the underlying cognitive processes that hamper the individual's functioning, which limits their value in providing guidelines for intervention (Das & Abbott, 1995; Kirby & Williams, 1991; Lidz, Jepsen & Miller, 1997).

In the last few decades, theorists, researchers and practitioners have proposed alternative conceptualisations of intelligence and its measurement which they assert are better aligned to developments in the fields of neuropsychology, cognitive psychology and information processing (Fagan & Holland, 2007; Feuerstein, Rand & Hoffman, 1979; Gardner, 1993; Kaufman & Kaufman, 1983; 2004; Naglieri & Das, 1990; Sternberg, 1985; Vygotsky, 1978). Information processing models of assessment embodied in the work of Luria (1966; 1973; 1980; 1982), Kaufman and Kaufman (1983; 2004) and Naglieri and Das (1997a), for instance, are in the forefront of some of the developments in cognitive psychology. These assessment approaches differ from traditional measures in that they are designed to evaluate the cognitive processes underlying general intellectual functioning. They are purportedly less influenced by verbal abilities and acquired knowledge (Das et al.,1994; Kaufman & Kaufman, 1983; 2004), are more intrinsically related to cognitive improvement (Das & Naglieri, 1992) and are more equitable in that they yield smaller differences between race groups (Fagan & Holland, 2007; Naglieri, Matto & Aqilino, 2005). In this chapter, the Das-Naglieri Cognitive Assessment System (CAS), which was developed by Naglieri and Das (1997a), is discussed in relation to its theoretical and research base, as well as its practical application within the South African context.

The underlying theoretical framework

The Planning, Attention, Simultaneous and Successive (PASS) cognitive processing model was proposed by Das et al. (1994) as an alternative view of intelligence. This model is rooted in the conceptual framework developed by the Soviet neuropsychologist Luria (1966; 1973; 1980; 1982) and the cognitive psychological work of others, such as Broadbent (1958) and Hunt (1980). Broadbent elucidated a theory of auditory attention, while Hunt argued for the location of intelligent behaviour within the context of information processing. Based on Luria's groundwork and the extensive research conducted by Das and his colleagues, each of Luria's proposed functional units has been operationalised (Das & Abbott, 1995) and these can be measured using the CAS assessment instrument. According to the PASS model, the focus of assessment is on *how* information is processed rather than on *how much* or *what* information an individual possesses (Das & Abbott, 1995).

Luria (1966; 1973), who conducted clinical work and research for about 40 years, viewed the brain as an autoplastic system which is able to change and adapt to the environment. He proposed (1973, p.43) that there are three functional units in the brain that 'work in concert' and are regarded as 'necessary for any type of mental activity'. These units are dynamic and interrelated, and they rely on and are influenced by the individual's knowledge base and experience. The first unit entails the regulation of cortical arousal and attention; the second unit codes information using simultaneous and successive processes; while the third unit provides planning, self-monitoring and structuring of cognitive ability (Das, Kar & Parilla, 1996).

The first functional unit, Arousal-Attention, is associated with the brainstem, diencephalon and medial regions of the brain and it is the foundation of mental activity. Maintaining an appropriate level of mental activity is necessary for information coding (simultaneous and successive processing) and planning. Arousal is a state of being active or alert, while attention regulates and maintains appropriate cortical tone/arousal so that other cortical activity can occur (Naglieri & Das, 1988).

The second functional unit, which includes Simultaneous-Successive coding, receives, analyses and stores information. This unit's functions are regulated by the occipital, parietal, and temporal lobes posterior to the central sulcus. Simultaneous processing involves the grouping of stimuli or recognition of a common characteristic or interrelationship amongst stimuli. The kinds of scholastic tasks that simultaneous processing is related to include sight word reading, reading comprehension, creative writing and solving geometry problems in mathematics.

Successive processing, on the other hand, involves the integration of stimuli into a specific sequential order where the elements form a chain-like progression (Das & Naglieri, 1992). While in simultaneous processing the elements are related in various ways, in successive processing only a linear relationship is found between the elements. Some of the school-related tasks associated with successive processing are spelling, writing, and the formation of syllable, letter and word recall. Naglieri (1989) highlights the point that the relationship between simultaneous and successive processing and school learning places the CAS at an advantage over a general intellectual ability measure, since it assists in the identification of underlying processes that may hamper learning and provides a guideline for intervention.

The functions of the third functional unit, Planning, are regulated by the frontal lobes, especially the prefrontal region of the brain. This unit allows the individual to formulate plans of action, implement them, evaluate the effectiveness of a solution and modify these plans if necessary (Luria, 1973). It is also responsible for the regulation of voluntary actions, impulse control and linguistic functions such as spontaneous speech (Luria, 1980). Das et al. (1994) also discuss the concept of meta-cognition and its role in planning. Meta-cognition involves 'the conscious awareness of ways of approaching tasks, of processing information and of monitoring success' (Kirby & Williams, 1991, p.70). The close relationship between planning and attention has been highlighted by Luria (1980).

According to the PASS model, the mode of input into the brain can be through the senses or it can be kinaesthetic (Das, 1992). This input is processed in the three functional units identified by Luria and the information is used in the performance or output phase. Particular tasks presented to an individual may be related to all of the cognitive processes in varying degrees, or may be more related to some cognitive processes and not to others. For example, when reading a new word a child may decode the word phonetically (using successive processing), look at the picture in the book and try to use the context of the story to make sense of the word (simultaneous processing and planning) or use all of these processes.

The theory-based PASS Remedial Programme (Das et al., 1994) has been developed to address deficient cognitive processing and to provide a link between assessment and intervention. In brief, this training programme attempts to address PASS processes, especially successive or simultaneous processing, that are related to the child's difficulty in acquiring reading skills.

The Cognitive Assessment System

Background and standardisation

Guided by the PASS theory, the CAS was developed as a norm-referenced, individually administered measure designed to evaluate the cognitive functioning of individuals between 5 and 17 years of age. The stipulated requirement for the use of this test is graduate training in the administration, scoring and interpretation of individual intelligence tests (Naglieri & Das, 1997c). While the CAS is not listed as a registered or classified test by the Health Professions Council of South Africa, it is used by psychological practitioners in this country to assess the cognitive processes underlying an individual's functioning (Foxcroft, Paterson, Le Roux & Herbst, 2004).

The CAS was standardised on 2 200 US children aged 5 to 17 years, using stratified random sampling (Naglieri & Das, 1997c). The sample was selected to represent several variables including age, gender, race, ethnicity, geographic location, classroom placement (special education or regular classroom), educational classification (for example, learning disabled, gifted, non-special education), parent education and community setting (urban/suburban, rural). An additional 872 children who participated in the reliability and validity studies were included in the CAS testing.

A description of the CAS instrument

The two versions of the CAS include a Standard Battery of twelve subtests and an eight-subtest Basic Battery. Each of the PASS scales in the Standard Battery consists of three subtests, while the Basic Battery consists of two subtests each. The CAS yields scaled scores for the PASS scales, as well as a composite Full Scale score which gives an indication of overall cognitive functioning. These scales provide standard scores with a normative mean of 100 and a standard deviation of 15 to identify specific strengths and weaknesses in cognitive processing. The subtests yield a scaled score with a mean of 10 and a standard deviation of 3.

The CAS structure is tabulated in Table 8.1, which is followed by a description of the CAS scales and subtests. These are fully detailed in Naglieri and Das's (1997b; 1997c) scoring manual and interpretive handbook.

Table 8.1 Structure of the CAS scales and subtests (Standard Battery)

Full Scale			
Subscales			
Planning	*Attention*	*Successive Processing*	*Simultaneous Processing*
*Matching Numbers	*Expressive Attention	*Word Series	*Nonverbal Matrices
*Planned Codes	*Number Detection	*Sentence Repetition	*Verbal-Spatial Relations
Planned Connections	Receptive Attention	Speech Rate (ages 5–7) or Sentence Questions (ages 8–17)	Figure Memory

Note: * These are the subtests included in the Basic Battery.

i) The Planning Scale

The purpose of the pencil-and-paper subtests on this scale is to find or develop an effective strategy to solve the timed tasks, which are of a novel nature. The Planning Scale score is based on performance on the subtests Matching Numbers, Planned Codes and Planned Connections, and the time that it takes the testee to complete each item. The cognitive skills that are needed to complete the tasks are the generation and use of efficient strategies, execution of plans, anticipation of consequences, impulse control, organisation of action, self-control, self-monitoring, strategy use and the use of feedback.

In the Matching Numbers subtest, the testee has to find and underline two numbers that are the same in each row. The Planned Codes subtest contains two items, each having its own set of codes. At the top of the page is a legend, which shows which letters correspond to which codes (for example, A with OX), and the testee has to write the corresponding codes in boxes, below each of the letters. On the Planned Connections subtest, testees are required to connect numbers in sequential order and then to connect both numbers and letters in sequential order, alternating between numbers and letters (for example, 1-A-2-B-3-C).

ii) The Attention Scale

The tasks on the Attention Scale require the testee to attend selectively to a particular stimulus and inhibit his or her attention to distracting stimuli. Both receptive and expressive aspects of selective attention are tested. The Attention score is based on measures of Expressive Attention, Number Detection and Receptive Attention, and the time it takes the subject to complete each item.

The Expressive Attention subtest consists of two different types of items. The first is administered only to children aged 5–7 years. The testee is asked to identify pictures of animals as either large or small based on their actual size, regardless of their relative size on the page. The second set of items is administered to children between 8 and 17 years. The testee is first asked to read words, such as 'blue' and 'yellow', then to identify colours, and finally is expected to focus on the colour and not to read the word. In the Number Detection subtest, the testee is presented with rows of numbers that contain both targets (numbers that match stimuli at the top of the page) and distracters (numbers that do not match the stimuli). The testee has to underline the numbers on the page that match the stimuli at the top of the page. In the Receptive Attention subtest, the testee has to find and underline pairs of pictures or letters that match on each page.

iii) The Successive Processing Scale

The tasks of the Successive Processing Scale require the testee to integrate stimuli in a specific linear/serial order, where each element or stimulus is related only to the one preceding it and there is little opportunity to integrate the parts. The stimuli range in difficulty from very easy (spans of two) to very difficult (spans of nine). Successive measures include Word Series, Sentence Repetition, Speech Rate (ages 5–7 only) and Sentence Questions (ages 8–17 only).

In the Word Series subtest, the task of the testee is to repeat a series of single-syllable, high-imagery words in order. Sentence Repetition requires the testee to repeat a series of sentences given by the examiner that have syntax, but reduced meaning. Each of the sentences contains colour names instead of content words. Speech Rate (for ages 5–7 years) requires the testee to repeat three-word series 10 times, and in Sentence Questions (for ages 8–17 years) the testee has to answer questions about sentences read aloud by the examiner. The questions in the latter subtest, like the Sentence Repetition subtest, contain colour names instead of content words.

iv) The Simultaneous Processing Scale

The subtests of this scale require the testee to integrate several pieces of information, and to comprehend them as a whole in order to arrive at the correct answer. Measures of simultaneous processing in the CAS are Nonverbal Matrices, Verbal-Spatial Relations and Figure Memory.

The Nonverbal Matrices task involves the selection of one of six options that best completes a matrix shape that is spatially or logically arranged. Verbal-Spatial Relations is a subtest in which the testee is required to comprehend logical and grammatical descriptions of spatial relations. In the Figure Memory subtest, the testee is presented with two- or three-dimensional figures that are shown for five seconds. The testee has to then find and trace these figures, which are embedded within a larger, more complex design.

v) The Full Scale

The CAS Full Scale score, which is based on an equally weighted aggregate of the PASS subtests, provides an estimate of overall cognitive functioning.

Administration, scoring and interpretation

The Standard Battery takes about an hour to administer, while the Basic Battery takes 45 minutes. The Planning and Attention subtests as well as the Speech Rate subtest are timed. While test instructions are given verbally, several of the CAS subtests require the assessor to show by gesture (for example, by the use of pointing) what is required of the testee. This test administration approach is very useful for children with hearing difficulties, and in the South African context where language issues are often a barrier in the assessment process.

An aspect that is unique to the CAS in comparison to most other tests is that guidelines are given to the assessor on a checklist, which is used to record the strategies that the testee is using to complete the tasks on the Planning subscale. For instance, on the Matching Numbers subtest of this scale, the checklist includes strategies such as a verbalisation of the numbers and looking at the last digit for a match. The testee's approach to the allotted tasks is observed, and he or she is also asked about the strategy used to complete the task. Gaining insight into the testee's underlying planning and problem-solving skills provides invaluable guidance for intervention. It also illustrates the value of a process- rather than product-based assessment procedure. Furthermore, it taps the testee's meta-cognitive and critical thinking skills.

As in intelligence testing by others such as Kaufman (1994), a dual set of criteria is used for the analysis of CAS results. The testee's cognitive strengths and weaknesses are identified by looking at intra-individual differences between each of the PASS scores, as well as by looking at the individual's performance in relation to the standardisation sample. Scaled PASS scores, rather than individual subtests, are focused upon in the interpretation of CAS results. Detailed guidelines for the scoring, analysis and interpretation of CAS results, as well as implications for intervention, are provided by Naglieri and Das (1997b; 1997c) and Naglieri (1999a).

While the CAS is relatively less linguistically loaded than some of the traditional intelligence tests, it does still require verbal reasoning and expression (for example, in the Sentence Questions subtest) and cultural and educational familiarity (such as using pencil and paper to complete the Planning subtests). Furthermore, research has shown that cultural differences can influence performance on nonverbal tasks and measures of fluid reasoning such as the completion of matrices (Fagan & Holland, 2007; Skuy et al., 2002).

Reliability

Internal consistency reliabilities and test reliability coefficients were computed for the CAS Full Scale, each PASS scale and the individual subtests (Naglieri & Das, 1997c). The Full Scale reliability coefficients ranged from .95 to .97 on the Standard Battery. Similarly, the average reliability coefficients for the other PASS scales were .88 (Planning), .88 (Attention), .93 (Simultaneous Scale) and .93 (Successive Scale). On the Basic Battery, Full Scale reliabilities ranged from .85 to .90.

Test-retest reliability and stability of the CAS standard scores were examined in a sample of 215 children from the standardisation sample. The CAS was administered to each child twice over in an interval ranging from 9 to 73 days. The stability coefficients were corrected for the variability of the standardisation sample using Guilford and Frucher's (1978, in Naglieri & Das, 1997c) formula for restriction in range. The median corrected stability coefficients across all ages was .73 for the CAS subtests and .82 for the PASS scales of the Standard and Basic batteries. On the basis of their findings, Naglieri and Das (1997c) concluded that the CAS demonstrates good stability across age groups over time. However, it can be argued that the period between the test administrations was very short, which may have affected the validity of these results.

Validity

There is a large body of international work and research that supports the PASS model of information processing (Das et al., 1994; Savage & Wolcott, 1994; Weyanat & Willis, 1994); the CAS as a measuring instrument of cognitive ability (Naglieri & Das 1997c; Naglieri et al., 2005; Van Luit, Kroesbergen & Naglieri, 2005); and the links between the CAS instrument and academic achievement (Naglieri, De Lauder, Goldstein & Schwebech, 2006; Powell, 2000). Naglieri and Das (1997c) and Naglieri (1999a) have reported extensive research that provides construct-, criterion- and content-related validity evidence for the CAS.

Criterion-related validity of the CAS has been supported by the strong relationships between PASS scale scores and educational achievement test scores; by correlations with academic achievement as related to special populations (such as mentally challenged children); and by studying the profiles of specialised groupings of children (for instance, children experiencing Attention Deficit/ Hyperactivity Disorder (ADHD) or reading disabilities, and gifted children). Naglieri and Das (1997c) conducted a study in which the CAS and the Woodcock Johnson Tests of Achievement – Revised (WJ-R) (Woodcock & Johnson, 1989) were administered to a representative sample consisting of 1 600 US children aged between 5 and 17 years. The WJ-R is a measure of academic achievement in reading, mathematics, written language and oral language. The correlation between the CAS Full Scale score and the WJ-R was reported to be high (.73 for the Standard Battery and .74 for the Basic Battery). Naglieri and Das concluded that the PASS theory could be considered a predictor of achievement and that it accounted for about 50 per cent of the variance in achievement, although the CAS does not have items that are directly reliant on achievement.

In a recent study related to the construct validity of the CAS, Naglieri et al. (2006) explored the relationship between the Wechsler Intelligence Scale for Children – Third Edition (WISC-III) and the CAS with the Woodcock Johnson Tests of Achievement – Third Edition (WJ-III) (Woodcock, McGrew & Mather, 2001) in a sample of 119 children referred to a clinic setting for assessment. The results of this study showed that the CAS Full Scale score had a significant correlation with achievement on the WJ-III and that this correlation was significantly higher (.80) than that between the WISC-III and WJ-III (.65). However, the researchers acknowledged that the small sample size used in a particular geographical location limits the generalisation of these findings. It would be informative to replicate this study using the revised Wechsler Intelligence Scale for Children – Fourth Edition (WISC-IV) (Wechsler, 2003), which aims to provide an improved measurement of working memory, fluid reasoning and processing speed.

The criterion-related validity of the CAS was supported by the findings of Van Luit et al. (2005). In this study the scores of 20 Dutch children with ADHD were compared to those of 51 children without ADHD (the control group). The children with ADHD reportedly achieved lowered scores on the Planning scale (mean = 81.8) and the Attention scale (mean = 87.3). The scores were average on the Simultaneous Processing (mean = 95.3) and Successive Processing (mean = 93.5) scales. The mean scores for the control group were within the average range of functioning (Planning – mean = 95.6; Attention – mean = 102.2; Simultaneous Processing – mean = 101.2; and Successive Processing – mean = 103). These findings were consistent with the results reported in earlier research by Naglieri and Das (1997c). It would be useful to conduct similar studies in South Africa, as there are limited psychoeducational assessment tools to evaluate individuals with ADHD in this country.

Issues relating to the factor structure of the PASS model

Two main criticisms of the PASS theory and the CAS were expressed by Carroll (1995). He suggested that the Planning scale is more an assessment of perceptual speed than of planning, and that there was insufficient factorial support for the PASS model. Subsequently, a group of researchers further challenged the construct validity of the CAS (Keith & Kranzler, 1999; Keith, Kranzler & Flanagan, 2001; Kranzler & Keith, 1999; Kranzler & Weng, 1995). Kranzler and Keith (1999) used confirmatory factor analysis to re-examine the original CAS standardisation data presented by Naglieri and Das (1997c). Keith et al. (2001) also conducted a joint confirmatory factor analysis of the CAS instrument and the WJ-III on a sample of 155 US children. These authors concluded that the constructs measured by the CAS overlap, and that the Planning and Attention scales measure processing speed and are part of the same construct. The average correlation between factors reflecting planning and attention exceeded .90 across all age groups (Kranzler & Keith, 1999).

Kranzler and Keith (1999) further suggested that the Successive Processing scale of the CAS measures short-term memory span rather than successive mental processing, and that the Simultaneous Processing scale may be viewed as a measure of fluid intelligence and broad visualisation rather than simultaneous mental processing. Their overall conclusion was that the Cattell-Horn-Carroll (CHC) theory of cognitive ability would provide a clearer framework for the interpretation of the CAS structure. They suggested that the CAS scales would be better understood as constituting one general factor (the psychometric '*g*'), processing speed (which combines planning and attention), short-term memory span and fluid intelligence/broad visualisation. The implication of the work conducted by Keith and his colleagues is that the CAS is not broader in scope than other intelligence tests, and that it is comparable to most other IQ tests (Keith et al., 2001).

In an invited commentary on the issues raised by Kranzler and Keith (1999), Naglieri (1999b) argued that Kranzler and Keith had over-relied on one aspect of factor analysis (a single statistical technique), which led to their rejection of the PASS model and of the CAS. He also pointed out (1999b, p.154) that Kranzler and Keith's claim that the CAS fit statistics were not strong in relation to other tests was based on 'trivial differences' in fit statistics, and that they had ignored the large amount of evidence on CAS content, predictive, construct and treatment validity presented by its developers, which extends beyond factor analysis.

Broad-scale, well-designed studies on the CAS could further address the debate regarding the structure of the CAS and its fit with the PASS model, as well as its use for the identification of learning strengths and weaknesses. Such research investigations could provide support for the wider use of the CAS within the South African context.

A sample of South African research on the CAS

There is a paucity of published research on measures of cognitive assessment in South Africa, especially in the past few decades. A few pilot studies conducted in recent years in this country suggest that the CAS is a relatively culture-fair instrument that can be used to assess cognitive functioning and educational needs (Churches, Skuy & Das, 2002; Fairon, 2007; Floquet, 2008; Reid, Kok & Van der Merwe, 2002; Von Ludwig, 2000).

Von Ludwig (2000) conducted a pilot study to investigate the usefulness of the CAS and WISC-R for assessing the scholastic difficulties of 48 Grade 6 learners who were placed in classes for children who were experiencing barriers to learning. The sample constituted both white and black children with a mean age of 12 years. The CAS and WISC-R were administered to each of these learners and the results were compared to their scholastic achievement. The findings of this study suggested that the WISC-R scores correlated with scholastic performance more strongly than the CAS scores did. Significant correlations were found between the WISC-R Full Scale scores and overall scholastic performance ($r = .36$, $p < .05$) and between the WISC-R Full Scale scores and scores on reading comprehension, grammar, mathematics as well as all scholastic language tests combined ($r = .41$, $p < .01$; $r = .53$, $p < .01$; $r = .34$, $p < .05$, $r = .33$, $p < .01$; respectively).

On the other hand, significant relationships were not found between the CAS Full Scale scores or the four PASS scales and overall scholastic performance, in the Von Ludwig (2000) study. Nevertheless, a significant relationship was found between the CAS Full Scale scores and scholastic performance in reading comprehension as well as creative writing ($r = .33$, $p < .05$ and $r = .43$, $p < .05$, respectively). Scores on the Successive Processing scale were significantly related to performance in reading comprehension ($r = .31$, $p < .05$), while the Simultaneous Processing scale was significantly related to scores in grammar

($r = .30$, $p < .05$) and the Planning scale was significantly correlated with scores in mathematics ($r = .30$, $p < .05$).

Von Ludwig (2000) concluded that, while the WISC-R was more predictive of scholastic performance than the CAS, the CAS based on PASS theory added an understanding of important dimensions of cognitive ability (such as planning) that influence academic performance. The results of this study suggest that a conventional cognitive assessment tool such as the Wechsler Scales, used in conjunction with the CAS, may provide an optimal understanding of a child's functioning. A limitation of this study is that the small sample size limits the generalisation of the findings. Furthermore, results of school performance were based on teacher-directed measures. Any further studies in this area of research need to use a standardised educational battery of tests to assess scholastic performance.

In a further South African study by Reid et al. (2002), Full Scale scores on the CAS, Woodcock Diagnostic Reading Battery (WDRB) (Woodcock, 1987) scores and school results were correlated. The study was conducted in an urban state school and the sample consisted of 32 randomly selected learners from the Grade 6 classes. The learners were all black, and English was their second language. In this study, a statistically significant relationship was found between the CAS and the WDRB ($r = .72$, $p < .01$) and between the CAS and the learners' year average marks ($r = .60$, $p < .01$). The researchers concluded that the CAS Full Scale score was related to achievement on the WDRB, implying that the PASS cognitive processes are linked to success or failure at reading. This finding is useful for the planning of intervention programmes. Unfortunately, the sample size in this study was small and the researchers did not elaborate on their reasons for selecting their sample. Further broad-scale studies need to be conducted that can make it possible to generalise findings regarding the use of the CAS in South Africa, and to establish its link with reading and scholastic achievement.

Moonsamy, Jordaan and Greenop (2009) investigated the relationship between cognitive processing as assessed on the CAS and narrative discourse production in children with ADHD. Their sample consisted of 30 English-speaking males between the ages of 9 and 11 years. A non-probability convenience sampling procedure was used in this study. According to the school records, the participants had all been diagnosed with ADHD by a medical practitioner, and they were of average intelligence. Children with co-morbid diagnoses other than ADHD, with or without related language difficulties, were not included in this study, to reduce the effect of extraneous variables. The researchers concluded that the subjects' lowered Planning scale scores (mean of 85.2) and Attention scale scores (mean of 80.7) as compared to their average Simultaneous and Successive scale scores (with means of 100.9 and 102.5, respectively), across all ages, supported the validity of the diagnostic value of the CAS for ADHD. Naglieri and Das (1997c) reported similar results when assessing children with ADHD. A significant relationship was not found in the Moonsamy et al. (2009) study between the CAS and the participants' oral narrative production. This study is limited by its failure to compare the functioning of the children with ADHD to a typically developing comparison group.

The CAS and dynamic assessment

Some international work has been conducted by Lidz et al. (1997) and Lidz and Greenberg (1997), combining the CAS with group dynamic assessment procedures. (See chapter 9 of this volume for a discussion of dynamic assessment.) The CAS was selected by Lidz and her colleagues for use as part of their group dynamic assessment screening approach because of its focus on cognitive processes, which have demonstrated a relationship to academic achievement, especially reading and mathematics, and its emphasis on intervention. They made minor adaptations to the CAS instrument to facilitate its administration within a group context. Using their CAS/Group Dynamic Modification (CAS/GDM) approach, they conducted pre- and post-testing on the CAS and used activities which tapped the same processes as the CAS (although they did not duplicate the CAS), to conduct the teaching and mediation process. The sample used in the study conducted by Lidz et al. constituted 66 adolescents from a special needs school. They reported significantly higher post-test scores, after mediation, in the CAS Attention ($t = 7.38$, $p < .001$), Successive Processing ($t = 3.43$, $p < .001$) and Planning ($t = 2.35$, $p < .05$) scales. Lidz et al. suggested that significant gains were not made in the tests of Simultaneous Processing, possibly as a result of insufficient mediated intervention in this area of functioning. The interpretation of these results is, however, limited by the absence of a control group to exclude practice effects.

In South Africa, pilot studies conducted by Fairon (2007) and Floquet (2008) have illustrated the potential usefulness of the CAS within a dynamic assessment approach. Fairon (2007) implemented a cognitive mediated intervention programme with first-year university students in an attempt to improve their academic performance. The CAS was selected for this study as it is an assessment tool which is based on the notion that cognitive processes can change, evolve and develop, and this conceptualisation of intelligence is consistent with the dynamic assessment view of the modifiability of cognitive structures. The results of this study showed that the mediation programme significantly improved the cognitive functioning of the 20 students, as measured by pre- and post-test scores of the CAS Planning and Simultaneous Processing scales ($t = 3.37$, $p < .05$ and $t = 2.04$, $p < .05$, respectively). The Attention and Successive Processing scales were not administered in the study. The 12-week mediated intervention programme was, however, not sufficient to significantly improve the students' academic performance, as assessed by their end-of-year examination results. Limitations of this study included the small sample size and the absence of a control group to rule out the effects of extraneous variables.

In a novel approach used by Floquet (2008), the dynamic assessment approach was combined with the PASS model of cognitive processing. The main aim of this study was to investigate the effectiveness of a mediated intervention programme in improving the planning abilities of learners. The sample consisted of 51 Grade 4 and Grade 5 learners who were attending a remedial school. A quasi-experimental pre-test post-test control group design was used in this study. A significant improvement was found in the experimental group's planning ability, following the intervention ($t = -8.09$, $p < .05$), suggesting that the CAS is useful for assessing planning and strategy use.

Concluding remarks

The CAS has been recognised for its clear theoretical base and empirical foundation, as well as for the adequacy of its psychometric properties (Sattler, 2008; Sparrow & Davis, 2000). Furthermore, as the tasks of the CAS are novel and nonverbal in nature, they are less reliant on expressive language and learned information, which are variables that can disadvantage certain groups of children. The CAS lends itself to use with language-impaired and bilingual children, where the examiner is able to give directions nonverbally or to augment the instructions through other means, such as translating the instructions or allowing children to read them. For example, the flexibility of the CAS instrument was demonstrated by its translation and successful adaptation in the Netherlands (Van Luit et al., 2005). It would be worthwhile to conduct similar studies in the multilingual and socio-culturally diverse South African context.

There is a dire need to explore context-appropriate assessment approaches in South Africa. The CAS is designed to be relatively fair cross-culturally, as it is purportedly less reliant on learned information than other tests, and incorporates more fluid reasoning skills in an attempt to understand cognitive processes. The potential value and application of this assessment tool, which can be used at least as an adjunct to conventional tests, needs to be further explored through empirical research. The innovation of combining information processing approaches to assessment with dynamic assessment methods needs to be further explored in the interest of using more equitable procedures in assessment and intervention.

References

Broadbent, D. M. (1958). *Perception and Communication*. London: Pergamon.

Carroll, J. B. (1995). Review of the book: *Assessment of Cognitive Processes: The PASS Theory of Intelligence. Journal of Psychoeducational Assessment, 13*, 397–409.

Chan, A. S., Shum, D. & Cheung, R. W. Y. (2003). Recent development of cognitive and neuropsychological assessment in Asian countries. *Psychological Assessment, 15(3)*, 257–267.

Churches, M., Skuy, M. & Das, J. P. (2002). Identification and remediation of reading difficulties based on successive processing deficits and delay in general reading. *Psychological Reports, 91*, 813–824.

Das, J. P. (1992). Beyond a unidimensional scale of merit. *Intelligence, 16*, 137–149.

Das, J. P. (2000). *Reading Difficulties and Dyslexia*. Oakhurst, NJ: Sarka Educational Resources.

Das, J. P. & Abbott, J. (1995). PASS: An alternative approach to intelligence. *Psychology and Developing Societies, 7(2)*, 155–184.

Das, J. P., Kar, B. C. & Parrila, R. K. (1996). *Cognitive Planning: The Psychological Basis for Intelligent Behaviour*. London: Sage.

Das, J. P. & Naglieri, J. A. (1992). Assessment of Attention, Simultaneous Successive Coding and Planning. In C. H. Haywood & D. Tzuriel (Eds), *Interactive Assessment* (pp. 207–299). New York, NY: Springer Verlag.

Das, J. P., Naglieri, J. A. & Kirby, J. R. (1994). *Assessment of Cognitive Processes: The PASS Theory of Intelligence*. Boston, MA: Allyn & Bacon.

Fagan, J. F. & Holland, C. R. (2007). Racial equality in intelligence: Predictions from a theory of intelligence as processing. *Intelligence, 35*, 319–334.

Fairon, K. T. (2007). Design and implementation of a cognitive mediated intervention programme with first-year metallurgy students. Unpublished Master's research report. University of the Witwatersrand, Johannesburg.

Feuerstein, R., Rand, Y. & Hoffman, M. B. (1979). *The Dynamic Assessment of Retarded Performers: The Learning Potential Assessment Device, Theory, Instruments and Techniques*. Baltimore, MD: University Park Press.

Floquet, D. (2008). Using the planning subtests of the CAS dynamically to assess the learning potential of children with barriers to learning. Unpublished Master's research report. University of the Witwatersrand, Johannesburg.

Foxcroft, C., Paterson, H., Le Roux, N. & Herbst, D. (2004). *Psychological Assessment in South Africa: A Needs Analysis. The Test Use Patterns and Needs of Psychological Assessment Practitioners*. Pretoria: Human Sciences Research Council.

Foxcroft, C. & Roodt, G. (2005). *An Introduction to Psychological Assessment in the South African Context* (2nd edition). Cape Town: Oxford University Press.

Gardner, H. (1993). *Multiple Intelligences: The Theory in Practice*. New York, NY: Basic Books.

Hunt, E. B. (1980). Intelligence as an information-processing concept. *British Journal of Psychology, 71*, 449–474.

Kaufman, A. S. (1979). *Intelligent Testing with the WISC-R*. New York, NY: John Wiley & Sons.

Kaufman, A. S. (1994). *Intelligence Testing with the WISC-III*. New York, NY: John Wiley & Sons.

Kaufman, A. S. & Kaufman, N. L. (1983). *Kaufman Assessment Battery for Children (K-ABC): Administration and Scoring Manual*. Circle Pines, MN: American Guidance Service.

Kaufman, A. S. & Kaufman, N. L. (2004). *Kaufman Assessment Battery for Children: Second Edition Manual*. Circle Pines, MN: American Guidance Service.

Keith, T. Z. & Kranzler, J. H. (1999). The absence of structural fidelity precludes construct validity: Rejoinder to Naglieri on what the Cognitive Assessment System does and does not measure. *School Psychology Review, 28(2)*, 303–321.

Keith, T. Z., Kranzler, J. H. & Flanagan, D. P. (2001). What does the Cognitive Assessment System (CAS) measure? Joint confirmatory factor analysis of the CAS and the Woodcock Johnson Tests of Cognitive Ability (3rd edition). *School Psychology Review, 30(1)*, 89–117.

Kirby, J. R. & Williams, N. H. (1991). *Learning Problems: A Cognitive Approach*. Toronto: Kagan & Woc.

Kranzler, J. H. & Keith, T. Z. (1999). Independent confirmatory factor analysis of the Cognitive Assessment System (CAS): What does the CAS measure? *School Psychology Review, 28(1)*, 117–144.

Kranzler, J. H. & Weng, L. (1995). The factor structure of the PASS cognitive tasks: A re-examination of Naglieri et al. *Journal of School Psychology, 33*, 143–157.

Lidz, C. S. & Greenberg, K. H. (1997). Criterion validity of a group dynamic assessment procedure with rural first grade regular education students. *Journal of Cognitive Education, 6(2)*, 89–99.

Lidz, C. S., Jepsen, R. H. & Miller, H. B. (1997). Relationships between cognitive processes and academic achievement: Application of a group dynamic assessment procedure with multiply handicapped adolescents. *Educational and Child Psychology, 14(4)*, 56–67.

Luria, A. R. (1966). *Human Brain and Psychological Processes*. New York, NY: Harper and Row.

Luria, A. R. (1973). *The Working Brain: An Introduction to Neuropsychology*. New York, NY: Basic Books.

Luria, A. R. (1980). *Higher Cortical Functions in Man* (2nd edition). New York, NY: Basic Books.

Luria, A. R. (1982). *Language and Cognition*. New York, NY: John Wiley.

Miller, G. A. (2003). The cognitive revolution: A historical perspective. *Trends in Cognitive Sciences, 7(3),* 141–144.

Moonsamy, S., Jordaan, H. & Greenop, K. (2009). Cognitive processing and narrative discourse in children with ADHD. *South African Journal of Psychology, 39(3),* 326–335.

Naglieri, J. A. (1989). A cognitive processing theory for the measurement of intelligence. *Educational Psychologist, 24,* 185–206.

Naglieri, J. A. (1999a). *Essentials of CAS Assessment.* New York, NY: John Wiley.

Naglieri, J. A. (1999b). How valid is the PASS theory and CAS? *School Psychology Review, 28(1),* 145–162.

Naglieri, J. A. & Das, J. P. (1988). Planning-Arousal Simultaneous-Successive (PASS): A model for assessment. *Journal of School Psychology, 26,* 35–48.

Naglieri, J. A. & Das, J. P. (1990). Planning, Attention, Simultaneous and Successive (PASS) cognitive processes as a model for intelligence. *Journal of Psychoeducational Assessment, 8,* 303–337.

Naglieri, J. A. & Das, J. P. (1997a). *Cognitive Assessment System.* Itasca, IL: Riverside Publishing.

Naglieri, J. A. & Das, J. P. (1997b). *Cognitive Assessment System Administration and Scoring Manual.* Itasca, IL: Riverside Publishing.

Naglieri, J. A. & Das, J. P. (1997c). *Cognitive Assessment System Interpretive Handbook.* Itasca, IL: Riverside Publishing.

Naglieri, J. A., De Lauder, B. Y., Goldstein, S. & Schwebech, A. (2006). WISC-III and CAS: Which correlates higher with achievement for a clinical sample? *School Psychology Quarterly, 21(1),* 62–77.

Naglieri, J. A. & Kaufman, J. C. (2001). Understanding intelligence, giftedness and creativity. *Roeper Review, 23(3),* 151–156.

Naglieri, J. A., Matto, H. C. & Aqilino, S. A. (2005). Black-white differences in cognitive processing: A study of planning, attention, simultaneous and successive theory of intelligence. *Journal of Psychoeducational Assessment, 23,* 146–160.

Naglieri, J. A. & Rojahn, J. (2001). Intellectual classification of black and white children in special education programs using the WISC-III and the Cognitive Assessment System. *American Journal of Mental Retardation, 106(4),* 359–367.

Powell, S. D. (2000). Assessing learning disabilities in reading: A validity study of the Cognitive Assessment System. Unpublished PhD dissertation. University of Colorado, Boulder.

Reid, K. D., Kok, J. C. & Van der Merwe, M. D. (2002). The PASS model for the assessment of cognitive functioning in South African schools: A first probe. *South African Journal of Education, 22(3),* 246–252.

Sattler, J. M. (2008). *Assessment of Children: Cognitive Foundations* (5th edition). San Diego, CA: Jerome M. Sattler.

Savage, R. C. & Wolcott, G. F. (1994). Overview of acquired brain injury. In R. C. Savage & G. F. Wolcott (Eds), *Educational Dimensions of Acquired Brain Injury* (pp. 3–12). Austin, TX: Pro-Ed.

Skuy, M., Gewer, A., Osrin, Y., Khunou, D., Fridjhon, P. & Rushton, J. P. (2002). Effects of mediated learning experiences on Raven's Matrices scores of African and non-African university students in South Africa. *Intelligence, 30,* 221–232.

Skuy, M., Taylor, M., O'Carroll, S., Fridjhon, P. & Rosenthal, L. (2000). Performance of black and white South African children on the Wechsler Intelligence Scale for Children – Revised and the Kaufman Assessment Battery. *Psychological Reports, 86,* 727–737.

Sparrow, S. S. & Davis, S. M. (2000). Recent advances in the assessment of intelligence and cognition. *Journal of Child Psychology and Psychiatry, 41(10),* 117–131.

Sternberg, R. J. (1985). *Beyond IQ: A Triarchic Theory of Human Intelligence.* New York, NY: Cambridge University Press.

Tollman, S. G. & Msengana, N. B. (1990). Neuropsychological assessment problems in evaluating the higher mental functioning of Zulu-speaking people using traditional Western techniques. *South African Journal of Psychology, 20(1),* 20–24.

Van Luit, J. E. H., Kroesbergen, E. H. & Naglieri, J. A. (2005). Utility of the PASS theory and Cognitive Assessment System for Dutch children with and without ADHD. *Journal of Learning Disabilities, 38(5),* 434–440.

Von Ludwig, H. A. I. (2000). A comparison of the WISC-R and the DN: CAS instruments for the assessment of academic performance of South African children. Unpublished Master's research report. University of the Witwatersrand, Johannesburg.

Vygotsky, L. S. (1978). *Mind in Society: The Development of Higher Psychological Processes.* Cambridge, MA: Harvard University Press.

Wechsler, D. (2003). *Wechsler Intelligence Scale for Children – Fourth Edition Technical and Interpretive Manual.* San Antonio, TX: Psychological Corporation.

Weyanat, L. L. & Willis, W. G. (1994). Executive functions in school-aged children: Potential efficacy of tasks in discriminating clinical groups. *Developmental Neuropsychology, 10,* 27–38.

Woodcock, R. W. (1987). *Woodcock Reading Mastery Tests – Revised.* Circle Pines, MN: American Guidance Service.

Woodcock, R. W. & Johnson, M. B. (1989). *Woodcock-Johnson Psychoeducational Battery Revised: Tests of Cognitive Ability.* Itasca, IL: Riverside.

Woodcock, R. W., McGrew, K. S. & Mather, N. (2001*). Woodcock-Johnson III Tests of Cognitive Abilities*. Itasca, IL: Riverside.

9 Dynamic assessment in South Africa

Z. Amod and J. Seabi

This chapter outlines current developments in relation to dynamic assessment (DA), an interactive assessment procedure that uses deliberate and planned mediational teaching and assesses the impact of that teaching on subsequent performance. The objective of the chapter is to critically review the major criticisms of the traditional 'static' testing approach, discuss the theoretical basis of the DA approach and its relevance within the South African context, and present an overview of current empirical research on DA.

There has been an increased demand worldwide for nondiscriminatory assessment procedures (Haywood & Tzuriel, 1992; Hessels & Hessels-Schlatter, 2002; Nell, 2000; Seabi & Amod, 2009; Skuy, Gewer, Osrin, Khunou, Fridjhon & Rushton, 2002; Tzuriel & Kaufman, 1999). The major criticism regarding the use of standardised intelligence tests is that they primarily reflect Eurocentric, middle-class values and attitudes (Nell, 2000). It is argued that they do not accommodate diversity in relation to culture, language, values, experiential background and cognitive styles. Given the political, socio-economic and educational conditions that have prevailed in South Africa under the apartheid regime and as an effect of its legacy, the application of traditional assessment procedures may be unfair to certain groups of people. Alternative, more equitable forms of assessment such as the DA approach have been proposed by several theorists and researchers for use within the multilingual and multicultural South African context (Amod, 2003; De Beer, 2005; Fairon, 2007; Floquet, 2008; Gewer, 1998; Lipson, 1992; Murphy & Maree, 2006; Seabi & Amod, 2009; Skuy et al., 2002).

A further criticism directed at the use of traditional intelligence tests/psychometric evaluations is that the scores are derived from a 'static' testing situation which provides minimal information regarding the individual's learning potential or potential to respond to intervention. 'Static' testing refers to the administration of tests in a standardised manner as stipulated in test manuals. Intervention which could include feedback, training and teaching is refrained from in the traditional static testing approach (Hessels-Schlatter & Hessels, 2009). The limitation of this approach is that the knowledge and skills needed to fulfil the requirements of tests have not necessarily been taught to the child, and this will undoubtedly limit his or her ability to perform well on these tests. In essence, the emphasis in DA is on intra-individual change rather than inter-individual difference. A number of theorists also argue that traditional/static testing provides a limited link between assessment and educational instruction, thus limiting the guidance given to teachers on the extent and type of intervention needed to promote learning (Ashman & Conway, 1993; Campione, 1989; Elliot, 2000; Haywood & Lidz, 2007).

In response to the disenchantment with traditional approaches, alternative forms of assessment have been proposed, such as the DA approach espoused by Feuerstein and his colleagues (Feuerstein, Feuerstein, Falik & Rand, 2002). This approach, which regards cognition as a modifiable construct, offers a fair way of assessing children within the South African context. It also offers the potential to integrate assessment findings with classroom intervention. This is related to current education policy, with its emphasis on the role of the teacher in the assessment process and on bridging assessment and instruction.

Interactive/dynamic assessment

Interactive assessment is a term used to encompass the variety of approaches to assessment that have in common a more active relationship between assessor and testee than is found in normative, standardised assessment (Haywood & Tzuriel, 1992). The assessor engages in 'deliberate and planned mediational teaching' and assesses 'the effects of that teaching on subsequent performance' (Haywood & Tzuriel, 2002, p.40). Campione (1989) has distinguished dynamic assessment from traditional assessment according to the following dimensions: focus – the way in which potential for change can be assessed; interaction – the nature of the interaction between assessor and testee; and target – the nature of the assessed task.

In relation to focus, Sternberg and Grigorenko (2001) describe two methods for assessing potential for change – namely, the 'sandwich' and 'cake' formats. The 'sandwich' format comprises an initial pre-test, a teaching phase and a post-test phase to assess the improvement achieved. On the other hand, the 'cake' format presents prompts and assistance during an initial assessment phase, gauging 'online' the individual's need for assistance. Although the 'sandwich' format may make use of standardised tests during the pre- and post-tests, the 'cake' format may use a non-standardised procedure. Lidz (1991, p.4) emphasises that DA must be viewed as an approach that is distinct from traditional static assessment, as it focuses on 'learning processes' in contrast to 'already learned products'. This goal of assessment is relevant to the South African situation, where diversity exists in individuals' educational backgrounds, and is a moderating factor in relation to test performance. In DA, the interaction between the assessor and the testee is altered so that the assessor can act as a mediator to facilitate learning, rather than assessing objectively without influencing the procedure. The collaborative interaction between assessor and testee has as its goal the assessment of potential, rather than current performance.

Numerous models of DA which differ in format and content are described in the literature. Most DA procedures have been developed for use on an in-depth, one-to-one basis with individual testees. However, attempts have been made to use them as a screening approach within group contexts (Floquet, 2008; Lidz, 2002; Lidz & Greenberg, 1997; Lidz, Jepsen & Miller, 1997; Seabi & Amod, 2009; Tzuriel & Feuerstein, 1992). The two subdivisions within the DA paradigm include global and domain-specific approaches. As an example of the former approach, the Learning Potential Assessment Device (LPAD) (Feuerstein et al., 2002) concentrates on general cognitive skills and processes, providing a qualitative and holistic picture of the child's ability to learn through a variety of tasks. On the other hand, Campione and Brown (1987), for example, use DA within the context of domain-specific skills. Their assessments relate to particular academic content areas such as reading. A further example of a domain-specific approach is that of Lidz's (1991) curriculum-based approach. Her approach uses actual curriculum content as the assessment task. An instrument designed by Lidz and Jepsen (1999) is the Application of the Cognitive Functions Scale, which is appropriate for preschool children. The content of this scale is strongly related to typical preschool curriculum demands.

The theoretical background of the dynamic assessment approach

DA is rooted in a socio-cultural and bio-ecocultural model of a socially constructed reality which emphasises environmental change, although the role of heredity is recognised (Murphy & Maree, 2009). Intelligence is defined within the DA approach as being a modifiable construct. This assumption is based on the belief that human beings have the potential for meaningful, permanent and pervasive change (Feuerstein, Rand & Rynders, 1988). The historical and theoretical foundation of the DA movement rests largely on the work of Lev Vygotsky (1978) and his concept of the 'zone of proximal development' (ZPD), and of Reuven Feuerstein (Feuerstein, Rand, Hoffman & Miller, 1980) and his theories of structural cognitive modifiability and mediated learning experience (MLE).

Vygotsky and the zone of proximal development

Vygotsky was one of the earliest critics of psychometric approaches to assessment. He suggested that learning and interaction were more valid bases for determining a child's cognitive functioning (Guthke & Wingenfeld, 1992). He emphasised the importance of cultural factors and, more specifically, the role of adult–child interactions in the development of the child's values, information and understanding. One of the most profound contributions by Vygotsky is his concept of the ZPD. This refers to the 'distance between a child's actual developmental level as determined by independent problem solving and the higher level of potential development as determined through problem solving under adult guidance or in collaboration with more capable peers' (Vygotsky, 1978, p.86). Vygotsky viewed the ZPD as a tool that psychologists and educators could use to understand children's mental and educational functioning. His writings have had a substantial impact on the theory and practice of cognitive psychology and its application to education (Ashman & Conway, 1997).

Feuerstein's model of dynamic assessment

Structural cognitive modifiability

Feuerstein's dynamic approach to assessment is based on his theory of structural cognitive modifiability (Feuerstein et al., 2002) and is the most influential of the DA models (Lidz, 2002). This theory is based on the assumption that human beings are dynamic and changing, and that they have the unique capacity to modify their cognitive functions and adapt to changing demands in life situations (Haywood & Tzuriel, 1992). While Feuerstein's theory of structural cognitive modifiability evolved out of his studies of children, it is understood to be applicable to individuals of different ages and cultural groups.

The theoretical roots of Feuerstein's approach to assessment, as well as his Instrumental Enrichment (IE) programme (Feuerstein et al., 1980), are in Piagetian structuralism. IE is the thinking skills programme derived from the theory of structural cognitive modifiability. While Piaget focused on the process of acquiring knowledge through stages of cognitive development, Feuerstein extended this view of the learning process. For Feuerstein, it is the MLE between a 'primary caregiver' and the child which accounts for the outcomes of the learning process (Feuerstein et al., 2002). Kozulin (1994) notes that, while Vygotsky proposed that adults and more competent peers introduce symbolic tools to the child in the course of learning, he did not fully elaborate on the role of the human mediator in his theoretical framework. This theoretical goal is addressed by Feuerstein's construct of MLE (Kozulin, 1994).

One of the most controversial issues in the field of psychology has been how intelligence is defined and what factors affect it. A fundamental question that remains at the centre of the debate is whether intelligence is static or modifiable. Feuerstein conceives of intelligence not as a fixed and unitary characteristic, but in terms of cognitive structures and processes that can be developed through learning. Feuerstein's concept of modifiability suggests that assessment should investigate and address a child's potential to change and to develop his or her cognitive skills. Several researchers support Feuerstein's assertion that there are many obstacles that can mask an individual's ability, and that when these obstacles are removed greater ability than was suspected may be revealed (Haywood & Lidz, 2007; Skuy et al., 2002; Tzuriel & Kaufman, 1999).

Mediated learning experience

A central concept related to Feuerstein's notion of structural cognitive modifiability is that the development of cognitive structures and processes is dependent upon the individual's opportunity to benefit from MLE. Feuerstein, Rand and Hoffman (1979, p.71) define MLE as 'the interactional processes between the developing human organism and an experienced, intentional adult who, by interposing himself between the child and external sources of stimulation, "mediates" the world to the child'. This process of MLE is distinct from direct learning, in the sense that the environmental stimuli are mediated taking into consideration the child's capacities and needs. Feuerstein's concept of MLE explains how culture is transmitted and how autonomous functioning is promoted. Intergenerational transmission of culture provides the individual with the tools for further development, while the MLE received and the degree of modifiability that the individual becomes capable of ensure the optimal use of these tools (Skuy, 1996).

According to Feuerstein (1980), lack of adequate MLE (proximal condition) is considered to be the causal factor for inadequate cognitive development, while conditions such as poverty, neurological impairment and emotional disturbance in the child or parents, as well as low education of parents, are viewed as distal aetiological conditions. This implies that, although these conditions are commonly found in people with inadequate cognitive development, they are not necessarily the direct cause of cognitive deficiency but are, rather, the correlates of cognitive deficiencies (Feuerstein, 1980).

In part, these distal conditions reflect the reality of South Africa, especially before 1994, because parents from poor socio-economic backgrounds, who were mainly from black communities, often had to work far away from home. The absence of parents, as well as extremely limited physical and social environments, made it difficult, if not impossible, for the optimal transmission of culture or development of learning. Mentis (1997) argues that apartheid created an environment hostile to the transmission of MLE, and this absence deprived the individual of the prerequisites for higher mental processes, despite a potentially normal inherent capacity.

Feuerstein (1980) makes a distinction between cultural deprivation and cultural difference. He considers the way culture and learning are mediated to an individual to be a proximal condition. When the transmission of culture from one generation to the next is lacking – for instance, in situations of war or famine – cognitive performance tends to be hindered and Feuerstein refers to this as cultural deprivation. On the other hand, cultural difference is viewed as a lack of familiarity with another culture. Although the child may come from a different culture, he or she may adapt easily and cope well in an unfamiliar environment, provided that the essential elements of the child's own culture have been sufficiently mediated.

In order for effective mediation to take place, certain parameters of interaction have to be present. These parameters, which guide the mediator, are presented in Table 9.1. Research demonstrates that not all teaching and parenting interactions constitute mediation, although these interactions can be considered as being mediational if they encompass certain of the MLE parameters (Falik, 1999). All of the parameters presented in Table 9.1 are applicable to a variety of behavioural interactions, and are important for the successful creation of conditions of learning and the development of skills. (See Skuy (1996) for a detailed discussion on cross-cultural implications of Feuerstein's construct of MLE.)

In sum, according to Feuerstein, MLE plays a vital role in moderating aetiological factors such as socio-economic status. Individuals with similar difficulties show markedly different learning and performance abilities, depending on the type and amount of MLE they receive. Founded on this premise, MLE-based intervention has been used in assessment as well as in learning support programmes.

Table 9.1 Feuerstein's criteria for mediated learning experience

Parameters of interaction	Definition
Intentionality and reciprocity	Refers to the conscious and consistent attempts of the mediator to influence behaviour and maintain his/her involvement (Lidz, 1991).
Meaning	The relevance and importance of an activity are conveyed.
Transcendence	This entails going beyond the immediate interaction, and connecting to and widening the transfer of goals to future areas and expectations (Seokhoon, 2001).
Regulation and control of behaviour	Refers to self-monitoring, where the behaviour is related to what was planned or intended.
Feelings of competence	Instilling in the mediatee a positive sense of ability to succeed.
Sharing behaviour	Emphasises the value of the mediator and mediatee cooperating and interacting supportively and empathically with each other.
Individuation and psychological difference	The mediatee is accepted and made aware of his/her uniqueness.
Goal planning	Explicit involvement of the mediatee, and the structuring of processes related to goal-setting and planning to achieve these goals (Skuy, 1996).
Challenge	Instilling optimistic belief in the mediatee to approach an unknown situation with curiosity, enthusiasm and determination.
Human being as a changing entity	Instilling a belief in the mediatee of the possibility for self-change with expectations for potential growth (Falik, 1999).
Search for optimistic alternatives	Facilitation of an awareness of potential for change and of available opportunities to do so.
Feeling of belonging	Although people are unique and independent, they are also interdependent on each other.

The principles and procedure of dynamic assessment

The conceptualisation of intelligence in terms of cognitive structures and processes, which can be changed through MLE, led to the development of the dynamic approach to assessment. In this approach, the cognitive processes engaged in by testees during problem-solving and their use of particular thinking strategies in relation to particular cognitive tasks is assessed.

The basic principle of DA is that the performance level of the testee in the assessment situation can be modified by introducing materials and instructions into the assessment procedure which can aid performance. The nature and extent of the mediation will provide an indication of the learning potential of the testee, and also provide guidance for further educational intervention.

As the goal of the assessment process is to analyse cognitive modifiability rather than to identify the testee's stable characteristics, the test situation is reshaped from a rigidly standardised procedure to a flexible interaction between the tester, the testee and the task (Lidz, 1991). Using the learning potential paradigm, a test-teach-retest technique is applied. After obtaining some information on initial baseline functioning, the testee is provided with training experiences relevant to the problem-solving task, and the resulting performance on similar tasks is assessed on the basis of the learner's ability to profit from the strategies offered. Teaching and learning are thus incorporated into the assessment process. During the DA process, the tester as mediator not only makes the stimuli meaningful but also attempts to instil in the testee the importance of being able to apply and transfer the learning to other areas of life. As the DA approach rejects the notion of ability as a fixed entity, it attempts to identify the learner's best performance, recognising that with further intervention this performance could be further modified, despite certain intervening cognitive, motivational, situational or cultural factors.

Feuerstein et al. (2002) have devised a cognitive functions list which provides a basis for identifying the testee's strengths and weaknesses in the DA process, and for appropriately addressing the latter through the provision of MLE. They conceptualise these cognitive functions as falling into three phases of cognitive processing: the input (data gathering), elaboration (data processing) and output (data expression) phases. The area of deficiency may be in one or more of these three mental phases.

In addition to criteria for MLE, Feuerstein (1980) provides techniques for mediation, which are briefly defined. Process questioning involves questions that focus on the process of learning or performing the skill, but not on the final product. During process questioning, the mediator asks 'how' questions. Bridging involves the creation of opportunities to link new learning to previous knowledge and to similar situations. Modelling involves step-by-step demonstration of learning and problem-solving. During modelling, the mediator first demonstrates to the testee and afterwards the testee imitates him or her. By using the technique of challenging or justification, the testee learns to evaluate his or her outcome. During this process, the mediator challenges both correct and incorrect responses, thus building upon and extending the testee's existing knowledge. Teaching about rules involves the making of rules for particular situations. Having made a rule for solving a problem, the goal is to assist the testee to apply this knowledge to similar problems that he or she may encounter in the future.

The Learning Potential Assessment Device

The LPAD developed by Feuerstein and his colleagues (Feuerstein, Haywood, Rand, Hoffman & Jensen, 1986) is based on their theory of structural cognitive modifiability and its construct of MLE. The LPAD consists of assessment tasks which are administered dynamically, and the assessment process itself provides specific direction for intervention. Accredited training is necessary to use the LPAD instrument.

The LPAD comprises a battery of verbal and nonverbal tasks which seek to tap a variety of operations including categorisation, numerical reasoning, memory and analogical reasoning. Each test comprises an original task and a variation of the task for purposes of mediation. The tasks are novel in nature, so that the child has not had previous experience of them (Lidz, 1991). The assessment tasks nevertheless reflect similar cognitive demands to school tasks (Feuerstein et al., 2002).

The Instrumental Enrichment programme

The IE programme was developed by Feuerstein (1980) to provide a vehicle for the transmission of optimal MLE. This thinking skills programme consists of a series of paper-and-pencil exercises that are presented to the individual. The primary goal of IE is to facilitate meaningful structural change in an individual's cognitive functioning, through the process of MLE, as well as to develop his or her ability to think both autonomously and creatively (Feuerstein & Jensen, 1980). Feuerstein and Jensen describe a number of subgoals of IE, such as the increase in intrinsic motivation, the development of insight and awareness, changing self-perception and the acceptance of greater control over the learning situation.

Dynamic testing versus dynamic assessment

Sternberg and Grigorenko (2001) argue that all testing is dynamic testing because there is a learning component to most tests. Tzuriel (2001) refutes this argument by pointing out the major differences between standardised testing and DA in terms of goals, orientation, the context of testing, the interpretation of results and the nature of tasks. He points out that static tests do not contain implicit learning components, and he presents empirical evidence to support this view.

Haywood (2001) also refutes Sternberg and Grigorenko's claim that all testing is dynamic testing. He points out their misconception of the nature of the intervention in DA, and argues that whereas Sternberg and Grigorenko define dynamic testing in narrow psychometric terms, testing is not synonymous with assessment, which draws upon data from a broad range of sources (including tests). While it is probable that some learning will take place during most testing procedures, the salient difference between static and dynamic approaches is not the learning, but the teaching that is done according to a mediational style (Haywood, 2001). According to Haywood, through the DA process the examiner explores:

- the obstacles that impact on the examinee's performance;
- the kind and amount of teaching and mediation needed to address these obstacles; and
- the expected extent of generalisation of learned cognitive and meta-cognitive concepts and strategies.

Application of dynamic assessment and the MLE construct

Considerable international research supports the effectiveness of DA in improving the cognitive functioning of students (Feuerstein et al., 2002; Haywood, 1995; Lidz, 2002; Tzuriel & Kaufman, 1999). In South Africa, there has been an increase in research in this area since the 1980s. A few empirical studies conducted in South Africa are reviewed here.

Several studies have documented the effectiveness of MLE in improving cognitive functioning and academic performance of students in the South African context (Mehl, 1991; Russell, Amod & Rosenthal, 2008; Schur, Skuy, Zietsman & Fridjhon, 2002; Seabi, 2012; Seabi & Amod, 2009; Seabi & Cockcroft, 2006; Skuy et al., 2002; Skuy & Schmukler, 1987). These have been conducted on samples ranging from preschool children and remedial school learners through to university students.

Russell et al. (2008) investigated the effects of parent–child MLE interaction on the cognitive development of 14 preschool children who engaged with their caregivers (11 mothers, 2 fathers, 1 grandmother) in free-play (a form of play similar to play at home) and structured tasks (which included 15-piece puzzles and wooden apparatus with 5 sticks of different lengths). The purpose was to explore and to compare the impact of parents' MLE during structured tasks and informal play interactions. Three sessions for each parent–child dyad took place, comprising a parent interview, playtime and two sessions of individual assessment. The MLE Scale (Lidz, 1991) was used to measure parents' MLE interactions, while cognitive functioning was measured by the Kaufman Assessment Battery for Children (K-ABC). Significant correlations were found between mediation of Transcendence, Joint Regard, Praise and Encouragement, Competence, and mediation of Meaning with cognitive modifiability. The parents' MLE during play interactions yielded greater significant impact than their MLE interactions during structured tasks. These findings suggest that playful parent–child interactions may create a powerful medium for cognitive development. Specifically, the results suggest that sharing experiences, information, affect, attention and relating a feeling of competence are necessary in interactions with young children in order to effect cognitive development.

Recently, Seabi and Amod (2009) compared the effects of one-to-one mediation with group mediation on a sample of Grade 5 learners in a remedial school. It was proposed that participants within the Individual Mediation group (N = 10), who were given individualised intervention, would perform significantly better than those within the Group Mediation group (N = 10). Mediation instruments (namely, Set Variations B-8 to B-12 from Feuerstein's LPAD) served as a vehicle for mediating cognitive deficiencies. The intervention was geared towards correcting thinking patterns that impair learning, and developing accurate perception, insight and understanding of the participant's thought processes. Specifically, participants were encouraged to develop effective thinking strategies, refrain from impulsivity, be precise and systematic in data gathering, clearly identify and define problems, devise a plan of action, avoid trial-and-error responses, look for logical evidence and reflect before responding. Results revealed a significant improvement from pre-test scores only within the Individual Mediation group. Despite this, no statistically significant difference was found between the performance of the Individual Mediation and the Group Mediation samples. It was therefore concluded that provision of MLE enhances cognitive functions irrespective of the type of mediation, whether individual or group.

In a follow-up study with a different sample of remedial learners, Seabi (2012) argued that the Seabi and Amod (2009) study may have underestimated the effects of mediation, since the two groups that were exposed to MLE were compared to one another in the absence of a control group. Therefore, Seabi (2012) investigated the effects of MLE intervention (that is, one-to-one mediation similar to the type provided in Seabi and Amod's study) by comparing the performance of a control group and an experimental group on the Raven's Coloured Progressive Matrices (RCPM), a nonverbal measure of intelligence. The sample comprised 67 participants (males = 35; females = 32; mean age = 11.8) from Grades 4 to 7. Participants were given the RCPM on two occasions, and inbetween, a non-randomly constituted experimental group was exposed to MLE intervention. The experimental group comprised Grade 4 and 5 learners, whilst the control group consisted of Grade 6 and 7 learners. The control group demonstrated superior performance over the experimental group in the pre-test RCPM scores, as an effect of grade level. However, the experimental group improved their performance significantly from pre- to post-test, presumably as an effect of the mediation, and the discrepancy in RCPM scores between the groups was narrowed at post-test. Analysis of between-group post-test differences revealed non-significant results. This suggests that provision of MLE is valuable for learners with special educational needs, and that these learners may have greater potential ability than is estimated by traditional intelligence tests.

At high school level, Schur et al. (2002) investigated the effectiveness of teaching an experimental astronomy curriculum (EAC) to a group of low-functioning learners based on a combination of MLE and a constructivist approach. This study included an experimental and a control group, each of which comprised 16 Grade 9 learners. Although learners within these groups received lessons focused on the concept of the earth for three hours per week, the experimental group did so within the framework of the EAC, while the control group was exposed to the conventional approach within the earth studies curriculum. The results revealed that the experimental group (receiving the curriculum through a combination of MLE and constructivism) improved their cognitive functions (as measured by Test of Understanding Science) and learnt astronomy (Nussbaum's test) to a significantly greater degree than a comparable control group. This suggests that the combination of MLE and constructivism can be used to produce domain-specific curricula, and that it is possible to use science teaching as a means of enhancing students' cognitive skills.

Several other studies (Mehl, 1991; Seabi & Cockcroft, 2006; Skuy et al., 2002; Skuy & Shmukler, 1987) were carried out at a university level. Mehl conducted a study with physics students to determine whether they displayed any cognitive deficiencies such as blurred and sweeping perception and impulsive exploration of a learning situation, documented by Feuerstein (1980). MLE was used as a vehicle for mediating the cognitive deficiencies identified. The sample comprised an experimental group that received a programme of MLE applied to the teaching of different aspects of physics, and a control group that received regular instruction. No statistically significant differences were found in the performance of the experimental and control groups in the two sections of the course – namely, optics and thermodynamics. However, a significant difference was found in the mechanics section of the course, in favour of the MLE group.

Skuy and Shmukler (1987) investigated the effectiveness of DA approaches among groups of socio-politically and educationally disadvantaged South African adolescents. The sample, comprising 60 Indian and 60 coloured adolescents from the top and bottom of their respective academic spectra, were assigned to experimental and control groups. Two sets of instruments were used – namely, several tasks (including Set Variations I and II, Complex Figure Drawing and Comparisons) from the LPAD and a set of independent measures of cognitive functioning (including the Raven's Standard Progressive Matrices (RSPM), Equivalent Complex Figure and the Similarities subset of the Wechsler Intelligence Scale for Children – Revised). Although pre-test–post-test measurements were conducted for the control and experimental groups, only the latter group was exposed to MLE intervention. The LPAD involved approximately six hours of interaction between the mediator and mediatee. The Set Variations I and II were presented in a group setting, since group interaction in these tasks is regarded as facilitative of mediation (Tzuriel, 2001). Following the intervention, improvements were found on the LPAD tasks. Although mediation was not generally effective in yielding change on the conventional measures of cognitive functioning, there was a mediation effect in interaction with academic performance and race. These results suggest the potential value of mediation with socio-politically disadvantaged groups in South Africa.

In another study, Skuy et al. (2002) investigated the effects of MLE on improving the cognitive functioning of psychology students. A sample of 98 students (70 black and 28 white) volunteered to participate in this study, and 55 were randomly assigned to the experimental group, while 43 were allocated to the control group. RSPM served as a pre- and post-test measurement of intellectual ability. Mediation was only provided to the experimental group, which was divided into two subgroups for purposes of the intervention. A two-way Analysis of Covariance (ANCOVA) was conducted with the two groups (black experimental, black control, white experimental, white control) as variables. Although analysis of the pre-test scores yielded significant differences due to the effect of race, the post-test results yielded significant difference as an effect of the mediation and non-significant results as an effect of race. The results of this study support the importance of mediation in improving the cognitive functioning of students.

A similar study was conducted with 111 first-year engineering students (Seabi & Cockcroft, 2006). The purpose was to compare the effectiveness of MLE, tutor support and peer collaborative learning on academic courses and intellectual tests. Of the 111 students, 45 constituted the experimental MLE group, which was compared to two groups of 36 and 30 students each, and which constituted the tutor and peer groups respectively. The participants were exposed to pre- and post-test measurements of intellectual ability – namely, the Raven's Advanced Progressive Matrices (RAPM) and the LPAD Organiser subtest, and academic courses (which included chemistry, mathematics, physics, an introductory course in engineering, mechanics, core courses and the overall course). While the mediator for the MLE group was guided by the MLE parameters of intentionally, consciously and actively eliciting cognitive functions, by initiating discussions and responding to the participants within the mediation group, the tutor served as a bystander to assist those students who experienced difficulties in solving engineering problems within the tutor group. In contrast, participants within the peer group were only able to consult one another for assistance. The intervention was conducted for 90 minutes over a five-week period.

Although significant improvements were found at post-test on the RAPM in all three groups, only the mediation group demonstrated significant improvement on the Organiser subtest of the LPAD. Of the seven academic variables assessed, six yielded significant post-test improvement within the mediation group, while two of these variables demonstrated significant improvement within the tutor group. No significant improvement was shown on any academic variables within the peer group. Consequently, it was concluded that exposure to adequate and appropriate MLE is effective in improving the academic achievement of students, thus supporting the existing research in this domain.

The reviewed studies suggest that students could benefit from interacting with a mediator, thereby enabling them to reach a level of cognitive functioning that they could not access without assistance from a knowledgeable adult. Given the years of educational and socio-political deprivation that black students have been exposed to, considerable mediation may be needed to overcome the cognitive deficits that they may display. The LPAD and the construct of MLE appear to provide valuable tools which can be applied in relation to psycho-educational assessment, intervention and research.

Criticisms of the dynamic assessment approach

DA, with its particular emphasis on learning potential, is a groundbreaking approach to assessment. Given its mediation of cognitive operations, this approach avoids the trap of taking acquired knowledge as the primary indicator of ability to accomplish future learning. However, DA is not widely applied, for several reasons. It is not yet taught in most of the institutions of higher learning; it is not cost-effective, given that it takes more time to administer than static tests; it requires more skill and experience than other forms of assessment, as well as suitable training; and the recipients of psychologists' reports typically do not expect a DA report and do not yet know how to interpret the data or the recommendations (Elliot, 2003; Karpov & Tzuriel, 2009; Tzuriel, 2001). While the theory and principles of DA have the potential to be widely applied to assessment practice in South Africa, use of the LPAD is very limited as the accredited training that is needed to implement this procedure is not easily accessible.

Some researchers (Grigorenko & Sternberg, 1998; Haywood & Tzuriel, 2002) criticise DA procedures as being highly clinical in nature and lacking in validity and reliability. For instance, Boeyens (1989a, cited in Du Plessis, 2008, p.35) maintains that the 'measurement of gain of post-mediation scores over pre-test scores is confounded by the fact that the reliability of a gain score is reduced by the error of measurement in the pre-test and post-test scores. The reliability of the difference score will thus always exhibit a lower reliability than that demonstrated by the pre-test and post-test scores.' Therefore, even when able to attest to acceptable levels of reliability for pre-test and post-test scores, it is not necessarily possible to attest to the reliability of the difference score (Murphy, 2002).

The issue of transfer of learning beyond the assessment situation (for example, to school subjects such as mathematics or reading) has also been cited as a concern (Karpov & Tzuriel, 2009). Furthermore, an evaluation of DA has been difficult, as various models have been postulated with each stipulating their own definitions, theoretical frameworks and requirements (Jitendra & Kameenui, 1993; Murphy & Maree, 2009).

Given both measurement and practical concerns relating to DA, computerised adaptive testing has been suggested as a possible solution. In South Africa, De Beer (2005) has conducted empirical studies on the Learning Potential Computerised Adaptive Test, a dynamic computer-based test, and a detailed review of this assessment procedure is provided in chapter 10 of this volume.

Conclusion

The current educational curriculum in South Africa, which was further revised for implementation starting in 2011, reflects the influence of concepts such as cognitive modifiability, the ZPD, process- rather than product-based education and assessment, and the enhancement of problem-solving and thinking skills. These are the principles and goals that need to be mirrored in psychological assessments conducted in South Africa, in response to the search for culturally fair tools. Local research suggests that DA, with its goal of enhancing learning potential, can make a notable contribution as an addition to the repertory of tests that are currently in use. Intensive and ongoing research needs to be conducted to develop viable ways of applying DA on a wider scale, and to ensure that the procedures used within this approach are valid and reliable, and adapted to meet local needs.

References

Amod, Z. O. (2003). A problem-solving psychoeducational assessment model for implementation by educators in South African schools. Unpublished PhD dissertation. University of the Witwatersrand, Johannesburg.

Ashman, A. F. & Conway, R. N. F. (1993). Examining the links between psychoeducational assessment instruction and remediation. *International Journal of Disability, Development and Education, 40*, 23–44.

Ashman, A. F. & Conway, R. N. F. (1997). *An Introduction to Cognitive Education*. London: Routledge.

Campione, J. C. (1989). Assisted assessment: A taxonomy of approaches and an outline of strengths and weaknesses. *Journal of Learning Disabilities, 22*, 151–165.

Campione, J. C. & Brown, A. L. (1987). Linking dynamic assessment with school achievement. In C. S. Lidz (Ed.), *Dynamic Assessment: An Interactional Approach to Evaluating Learning Potential* (pp. 85–115). New York, NY: The Guilford Press.

De Beer, M. (2005). Development of the Learning Potential Computerised Adaptive Test (LPCAT). *South African Journal of Psychology, 35(4)*, 717–747.

Du Plessis, G. A. (2008). Dynamic cognitive assessment: Investigating learning potential within the context of an academic institution. Unpublished Master's dissertation. University of Johannesburg, Johannesburg.

Elliot, J. G. (2000). The psychological assessment of children with learning difficulties. *British Journal of Special Education, 27(2)*, 59–65.

Elliott, J. G. (2003). Dynamic assessment in educational settings: Realizing potential. *Educational Review, 55(1)*, 15–32.

Fairon, K. T. (2007). Design and implementation of a cognitive mediated intervention programme with first-year metallurgy students. Unpublished Master's research report. University of the Witwatersrand, Johannesburg.

Falik, L. (1999). *Using Mediated Learning Experience Parameters to Change Children's Behavior: Techniques for Parents and Childcare Providers*. Retrieved May 7, 2004, from http://www.icelp.org/asp/Aspects_of_Mediated_Learning_Experience.shtm.

Feuerstein, R. (1980). *Instrumental Enrichment: An Intervention Programme for Cognitive Development*. Baltimore, MD: University Park Press.

Feuerstein, R., Feuerstein, R. S., Falik, L. H. & Rand, Y. (2002). *The Dynamic Assessment of Cognitive Modifiability: The Learning Propensity Assessment Device, Theory, Instruments and Techniques*. Jerusalem: ICELP Press.

Feuerstein, R., Haywood, H. C., Rand, Y., Hoffman, M. B. & Jensen, M. R. (1986). *Learning Potential Assessment Device Manual*. Jerusalem: Hadassah – WIZO – Canada Research Institute.

Feuerstein, R. & Jensen, M. R. (1980). Instrumental Enrichment: Theoretical basis, goals and instruments. *The Education Forum, 44*, 401–423.

Feuerstein, R., Rand, Y. & Hoffman, M. B. (1979). *The Dynamic Assessment of Retarded Performers: The Learning Potential Assessment Device, Theory, Instruments and Techniques*. Baltimore, MD: University Park Press.

Feuerstein, R., Rand, Y., Hoffman, M. B. & Miller, R. (1980). *Instrumental Enrichment: An Intervention Programme for Cognitive Modifiability*. Baltimore, MD: University Park Press.

Feuerstein, R., Rand, Y. & Rynders, J. E. (1988). *Don't Accept Me As I Am*. New York, NY: Plenum Press.

Floquet, D. (2008). Using the planning subtests of the CAS dynamically to assess the learning potential of children with barriers to learning. Unpublished Master's research report. University of the Witwatersrand, Johannesburg.

Gewer, A. (1998). Uncovering potential: Dynamic assessment of non-verbal reasoning ability in educationally disadvantaged children. Unpublished Master's research report. University of the Witwatersrand, Johannesburg.

Grigorenko, E. L. & Sternberg, R. J. (1998). Dynamic testing. *Psychological Bulletin, 124(1),* 75–111.

Guthke, J. & Wingenfeld, S. (1992). The learning test concept: Origins, state of the art and trends. In H. C. Haywood & D. Tzuriel (Eds), *Interactive Assessment* (pp. 64–93). New York, NY: Springer Verlag.

Haywood, H. C. (1995). Mediated learning: A unique way to level the playing field. *The Thinking Teacher, 10(1),* 2–9.

Haywood, H. C. (2001). What is dynamic 'testing'? A response to Sternberg and Grigorenko. *Issues in Education, 7(2),* 201–210.

Haywood, H. C. & Lidz, C. S. (2007). *Dynamic Assessment in Practice: Clinical and Educational Applications.* New York, NY: Cambridge University Press.

Haywood, H. C. & Tzuriel, D. (1992). Policy implications of psychological assessment of minority children. In H. C. Haywood & D. Tzuriel (Eds), *Interactive Assessment* (pp. 445–469). New York, NY: Springer Verlag.

Haywood, H. C. & Tzuriel, D. (2002). Application and challenges in dynamic assessment. *Peabody Journal of Education, 77(2),* 40–63.

Hessels, M. G. P. & Hessels-Schlatter, C. (2002). Learning potential in immigrant children in two countries: The Dutch and the Swiss-French version of the Learning Potential Test for ethnic minorities. In D. G. M. van der Aalsvoort, W. C. M. Resing & A. J. J. M. Ruijssenaars (Eds), *Learning Potential Assessment and Cognitive Training* Volume 7 (pp. 227–245). New York, NY: Elsevier.

Hessels-Schlatter, C. & Hessels, M. G. P. (2009). Clarifying some issues in dynamic assessment: Comments on Karpov and Tzuriel. *Journal of Cognitive Education and Psychology, 8(3),* 246–251.

Jitendra, A. K. & Kameenui, E. J. (1993). Dynamic assessment as a compensatory assessment approach: A description and analysis. *Remedial and Special Education, 33(2),* 93–102.

Karpov, Y. V. & Tzuriel, D. (2009). Dynamic assessment: Progress, problems and prospects. *Journal of Cognitive Education and Psychology, 8(3),* 228–237.

Kozulin, A. (1994). The cognitive revolution in learning: Piaget and Vygotsky. In J. N. Mangieri & C. Collins Block (Eds), *Creating Powerful Thinking in Teachers and Students* (pp. 269–286). London: Harcourt Brace College.

Lidz, C. S. (1991). *Practitioner's Guide to Dynamic Assessment.* New York, NY: The Guilford Press.

Lidz, C. S. (2002). Mediated Learning Experience (MLE) as a basis for an alternative approach to assessment. *School Psychology International, 23(1),* 68–84.

Lidz, C. S. & Greenberg, K. H. (1997). Criterion validity of a group dynamic assessment procedure with rural first-grade regular education students. *Journal of Cognitive Education, 6(2),* 89–99.

Lidz, C. S. & Jepsen, R. H. (1999). *Application of Cognitive Functions Scale (ACFS).* New York, NY: Touro College.

Lidz, C. S., Jepsen, R. H. & Miller, H. B. (1997). Relationships between cognitive processes and academic achievement: Application of a group dynamic assessment procedure with multiply handicapped adolescents. *Educational and Child Psychology, 14(4),* 56–67.

Lipson, L. E. (1992). Relationship of static and dynamic measures to scholastic achievement of black pupils. Unpublished Master's research report. University of the Witwatersrand, Johannesburg.

Mehl, M. C. (1991). Mediated learning experience at university level – a case study. In R. Feuerstein, P. Klein & A. Tannebaum (Eds), *Mediated Learning Experience: Theoretical, Psychological Learning Implications* (pp. 157–178). London: Freund.

Mentis, M. (1997). An integrated perspective on applications of Feuerstein's theories to a curriculum. Unpublished Master's research report. University of the Witwatersrand, Johannesburg.

Murphy, R. (2002). A review of South African research in the field of dynamic assessment. Unpublished Master's dissertation. University of Pretoria, Pretoria.

Murphy, R. & Maree, D. J. F. (2006). A review of South African research in the field of dynamic assessment. *South African Journal of Psychology, 36(1)*, 168–191.

Murphy, R. & Maree, D. J. F. (2009). Revisiting core issues in dynamic assessment. *South African Journal of Psychology, 39(4)*, 420–431.

Nell, V. (2000). *Cross-cultural Neuropsychological Assessment: Theory and Practice*. London: Lawrence Erlbaum Associates.

Russell, C., Amod, Z. & Rosenthal, L. (2008). The effects of parent–child mediated learning experience (MLE) interaction on young children's cognitive development. *Perspectives in Education, 26(4)*, 1–14.

Schur, Y., Skuy, M., Zietsman, A. & Fridjhon, P. (2002). A thinking journey based on constructivism and mediated learning experience as a vehicle for teaching science to low-functioning students and enhancing their cognitive skills. *School Psychology International, 23(1)*, 36–67.

Seabi, J. (2012). Feuerstein's mediated learning experience as a vehicle for enhancing cognitive functioning of remedial school learners in South Africa. *Australian Journal of Educational and Developmental Psychology, 12*, 35-45.

Seabi, J. & Amod, Z. (2009). Effects of mediated intervention on cognitive functions: A pilot study with Grade 5 learners at a remedial school. *Australian Journal of Learning Difficulties, 14(2)*, 185–198.

Seabi, J. & Cockcroft, K. (2006). The implementation and evaluation of a cognitive programme for first-year engineering students. Paper presented at the 7th National Conference of the International Association for Cognitive Education in Southern Africa (IACESA). North-West University Conference Centre, Vanderbijlpark, April 3–5.

Seokhoon, A. S. (2001). Parental involvement in child assessment: A dynamic approach. Paper presented at the Australian Association for Research in Education International Conference, Freemantle, Western Australia, December 2–6.

Skuy, M. (1996). Cross-cultural and inter-dimensional implications of Feuerstein's construct of mediated learning experience. In P. Engelbrecht, S. M. Kriegler & M. I. Booysen (Eds), *Perspectives on Learning Difficulties: International Concerns and South African Realities* (pp. 185–198). Pretoria: Kagiso Publishers.

Skuy, M., Gewer, A., Osrin, Y., Khunou, D., Fridjhon, P. & Rushton, J. P. (2002). Effects of mediated learning experience on Raven's matrices scores of African and non-African university students in South Africa. *Intelligence, 30*, 221–232.

Skuy, M. & Schmukler, D. (1987). Effectiveness of the Learning Potential Assessment Device with Indian and coloured adolescents in South Africa. *International Journal of Special Education, 2,* 131–149.

Sternberg, R. J. & Grigorenko, E. L. (2001). All testing is dynamic testing. *Issues in Education, 7(2),* 137–170.

Tzuriel, D. (2001). Dynamic assessment is not dynamic testing. *Issues in Education, 7(2),* 237–249.

Tzuriel, D. & Feuerstein, R. (1992). Dynamic group assessment for prescriptive teaching: Differential effects of treatments. In H. C. Haywood & D. Tzuriel (Eds), *Interactive Assessment* (pp. 187– 206). New York, NY: Springer Verlag.

Tzuriel, D. & Kaufman, R. (1999). Mediated learning and cognitive modifiability: Dynamic assessment of young Ethiopian immigrant children to Israel. *Journal of Cross-Cultural Psychology, 30,* 359–380.

Vygotsky, L. S. (1978). *Mind in Society: The Development of Higher Psychological Processes.* Cambridge, MA: Harvard University Press.

10 The Learning Potential Computerised Adaptive Test in South Africa

M. de Beer

In the multicultural and multilingual South African context, differences in socio-economic and educational background and development opportunities complicate psychological assessment (Claassen, 1997; Foxcroft, 1997; 2004). In this complex context, the measurement of learning potential provides additional information in the cognitive domain and has shown positive results in terms of psychometric properties and practical utility (De Beer, 2006; 2010b; Lidz, 1987; Murphy & Maree, 2006). Measurement of learning potential implies that assessment includes a learning experience or assistance, and typically adopts a test-train-retest approach. Measurement is therefore expanded to include two sets of measures, as well as a learning opportunity relating to the test task. Such assessments are also referred to as dynamic assessment (DA). DA allows for learning experiences to take place during assessment with a view to measuring learning potential, thus measuring not only the present level of performance of individuals but also the projected or potential future levels of performance these individuals may be able to attain if relevant learning opportunities can be provided.

This approach to assessment is generally associated with Vygotsky's (1978) theory of the 'zone of proximal development' (ZPD). This theory distinguishes between current performance (without help) – also referred to as the 'zone of actual development' (ZAD) – and performance that can be attained when relevant learning opportunities are provided, the ZPD. In DA, this same distinction is made in terms of a focus on measures obtained in a pre-test (unassisted performance) and a post-test (performance after learning or with assistance). Of importance is the fact that in interpreting the results of learning potential assessment of persons with varying educational qualifications, and across a wide range of ability/performance levels, learning potential is defined as the *combination* of current and projected future (potential) performance, and not only in terms of the improvement score (De Beer, 2000a; 2010a). The focus is not only on whether the individual will generally be able to profit from learning, but more specifically on what level of learning/training he or she will be able to cope with – or alternatively, to what degree he or she seems able to cope with a *particular* level of training offered. At a practical level, current and projected future (potential) levels of performance can be compared to the opportunity to evaluate whether the individual is currently already at or close to the required level (that is, the target level of training), or shows the potential to perform at or close to the required level.

Traditionally, intelligence quotient (IQ) scores have been seen as immutable and static, a view which has contributed to the strong emotional reactions often associated with this domain. These scores are, however, subject to changes and improvement – generally referred to as the Flynn effect (Flynn, 1987) – where scores on tests have shown increases over time (Wicherts, Dolan, Carlson & Van der Maas, 2010). These changes – which occur without any purposeful intervention – are normally ascribed to various factors, such as increased test-wiseness (Rushton & Jensen, 2010) and other environmental factors (Flynn, 1987) – for example, improvement of educational opportunities and socio-economic standing. Furthermore, IQ gains over time have shown the largest gains to occur in culturally reduced tests and tests of fluid intelligence (Flynn, 1987).

At the heart of DA or the measurement of learning potential is the provision of a learning experience within the assessment. Dynamic testing or learning potential testing focuses on providing learning experiences that might improve performance, and scores have been reported to increase by 0.5 to 0.7 standard deviations (Te Nijenhuis, Van Vianen & Van der Flier, 2007). In DA, the aim of providing a learning experience to allow for improvement in the level of performance by focusing on measurement of fluid ability could therefore allow for optimal improvement in an environment where further hints, guidelines and strategies focused on improving performance are provided.

Although the concept of dynamic testing is generally well supported, its practical use has been hampered by problems concerning, *inter alia*, lengthy testing times, high costs, a lack of standardised procedures, problems with measurement accuracy, a limiting focus on underachieving populations and a sparseness of validity information available (Grigorenko & Sternberg, 1998; Sternberg & Grigorenko, 2002).

This chapter begins with a brief history of DA, and then provides specific information on the Learning Potential Computerised Adaptive Test (LPCAT), as an example of a South African learning potential test that uses modern psychometric and assessment techniques to overcome some of the limitations and problems generally associated with DA (Kim-Kang & Weiss, 2008). The development of the LPCAT is described, and typical strategies for use of the scores obtained from it are explained. Furthermore, empirical psychometric results for the LPCAT in the South African context are presented. Lastly, the features and challenges of the LPCAT are discussed.

A short history of DA and the development of the LPCAT

The history of learning potential (or dynamic) assessment goes back quite far (Wolf, 1973). The well-known Binet-Simon test developed around the turn of the 20th century can be regarded as the very first learning potential test

(Binet & Simon, 1915). Its aim was to identify individuals who could improve their performance when they were afforded a relevant learning opportunity. This kind of assessment again became prominent in the 1970s and 1980s. Since then, numerous researchers have been involved in DA and various approaches to DA have evolved. Lidz (1987), Murphy and Maree (2006) and Haywood (2008) provide more detail of the history of, and different approaches to, DA. Two broad approaches can be identified – on the one hand, the more clinically and diagnostically oriented approach, with remediation as the main aim, and on the other hand, the more measurement- or psychometrically oriented approach, with accurate assessment and obtaining good psychometric properties as the main aim (De Beer, 2010a). The LPCAT falls within the latter of these two broad categories.

Assessment research in the South African context has shown that individuals from disadvantaged educational and socio-economic backgrounds often under-perform on standard cognitive tests (Claassen, 1997; Owen, 1998). These standard cognitive tests often include a large proportion of language-based questions, as well as education-related content such as numerical reasoning. Research has furthermore shown that nonverbal figural item content is fairer to disadvantaged individuals (Hugo & Claassen, 1991). Learning potential assessment – using nonverbal figural content only – provides an alternative measurement approach that can provide additional information to that which can be obtained from standard static tests.

A focus on learning potential is important in the South African context, where the vast majority (72 per cent) of the population aged 20 years and older have completed less than secondary education (Statistics South Africa, 2008). This means that a large number of individuals who may need to be assessed are at some disadvantage when measures rely on language proficiency and educational material – as is often the case in standard cognitive assessments. Learning potential assessment is not intended to replace any other assessments, but can provide additional information not available in standard tests to improve decision-making relating to the training and development of individuals, screening for selection and vocational appointments or for training opportunities, and career-related assessment and guidance. For specific aptitudes or choices of particular fields of study, other measures can provide the relevant information (such as aptitude, intelligence, personality and interest-related assessments, amongst others). Learning potential assessment results indicate the level of reasoning (albeit nonverbal figural reasoning) that the individual is currently capable of, as well as the potential future levels of such reasoning that the individual is likely to attain if he or she is afforded relevant learning opportunities. Hence, if the focus is on the development of individuals and improvement of their educational levels, or identification of the appropriate levels of training to provide for future development, learning potential assessment results provide useful additional information.

The concept of learning potential is in line with legislation (the Employment Equity Act No. 55 of 1998) regarding psychological assessment in South Africa. It makes allowance for the fact that not everyone has had the same educational and socio-economic opportunities, and acknowledges the research that has shown that these factors are related to performance in standard cognitive tests.

In the case of the LPCAT, instructions to administer the test have been translated and are available in the *User's Manual* in all 11 official South African languages (De Beer, 2000a), which allows for administration to individuals who may have limited English proficiency, provided that test administrators are fluent in the particular language of the individual being tested.

An overview of the LPCAT

The LPCAT is a dynamic and adaptive learning potential test focused on the measurement of learning potential within the general fluid reasoning ability or 'g_f' domain. It is 'intended to serve as a screening instrument that can be used mainly to counter inadvertent discrimination against disadvantaged groups' (De Beer, 2000b, p.1). It uses nonverbal figural material (Figure Series, Figure Analogies and Pattern Completion) in the test items to exclude language and scholastic content, since these item types show less bias in multicultural assessment, whereas verbal scales in particular often underestimate the cognitive ability of African-language examinees (Claassen, De Beer, Hugo & Meyer, 1991; Hugo & Claassen, 1991; Owen, 1998). Responding to such nonverbal figural pattern items requires common reasoning skills such as identification, comparison and recognition of relations (see Figure 10.1 for an example item).

Figure 10.1 LPCAT example item

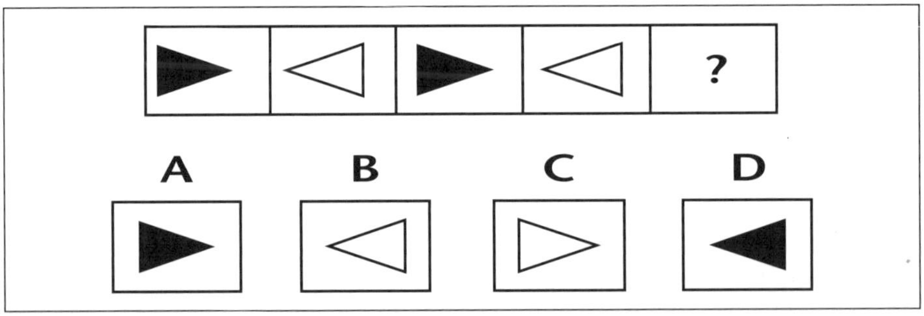

Because of the practical need in South Africa for instruments that can be group-administered, and used to identify (often disadvantaged) individuals over a broad spectrum of ability who show the potential to benefit from further training and development, a link was made between DA and Computerised Adaptive Testing (CAT) based on item response theory (IRT). These modern psychometric methods (IRT for item analysis and CAT in test administration) were employed in the development of the LPCAT (Embretson, 1996; 2004). At the core of IRT methods are three features: item difficulty and individual ability are measured on the same scale; item characteristics are sample-independent; and individual abilities are item-independent (Embretson, 1996; Weiss, 1983). This makes possible a form of CAT in which a unique set of items is selected for each individual during test administration, so that items presented to each individual are continually and interactively selected from the bank of available items to match the estimated ability of the individual at that point in time (Weiss, 1983). IRT furthermore allows for accurate measurement of difference scores, and CAT shortens the testing time (Kim-Kang & Weiss, 2008; Sijtsma, 1993a; 1993b; Van der Linden, 2008a; 2008b; Weiss, 1983).

IRT-based analysis was used to perform bias analysis of items (in terms of gender, culture, language and level of education) with a large (N = 2 450) representative sample (De Beer, 2000b). Classical test theory as well as IRT item analysis was performed, and items that did not meet the criteria in terms of measurement properties or differential item functioning (DIF) were discarded in the compilation of the final test (De Beer, 2000b; 2004). The item characteristic curves (ICCs) of different subgroups were compared to determine the extent of DIF (see Figure 10.2). The base scale in Figure 10.2 (indicated by theta (θ)) depicts both difficulty levels of items and ability levels of individuals, while on the Y-axis the probability of an individual at a specific level of ability answering this item correctly is shown as P(theta). The difficulty level of the item (indicated by the letter b) is determined by the theta-level (ability level) where the probability of a correct response is 0.5 (Weiss, 1983).

Figure 10.2 DIF analysis – culture group comparison

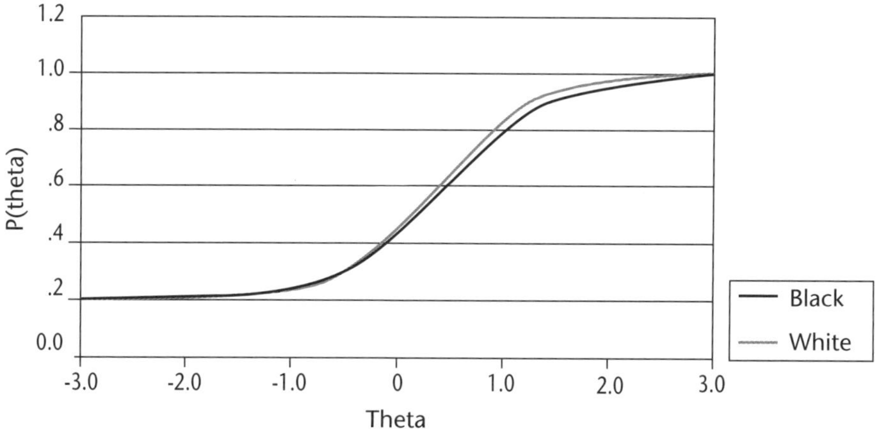

Two separate but linked adaptive tests were used for the pre-test and post-test respectively, and total testing time is approximately one hour (for details on the development of the LPCAT see De Beer, 2000b; 2005; 2010a). Advantages of using computerised adaptive methods are that testing time is shortened, and the results are available immediately after completion of the test. However, although the test is administered on a computer, candidates need to use only the space bar and enter key – hence computer literacy is not a requirement for its administration. The results are presented in graph form (see Figure 10.3) from which a report can be (manually) prepared. The levels of performance in both the pre-test and the post-test should be noted, as well as the pattern and gradients of the graphs. The training that is provided between the pre-test and the post-test is aimed at elucidating the applicable reasoning strategies, by providing more example questions in which the basic principles, building blocks and general strategies for answering the particular types of questions are provided. While practice with further questions might have some effect, use of IRT methods of measurement results in more accurate measurement of the latent trait concerned – in this case, level of fluid general reasoning ability. Furthermore, no questions are repeated in the pre-test and post-test, which precludes the undue effect of memory on performance in the post-test.

Figure 10.3 Example of LPCAT graphic output

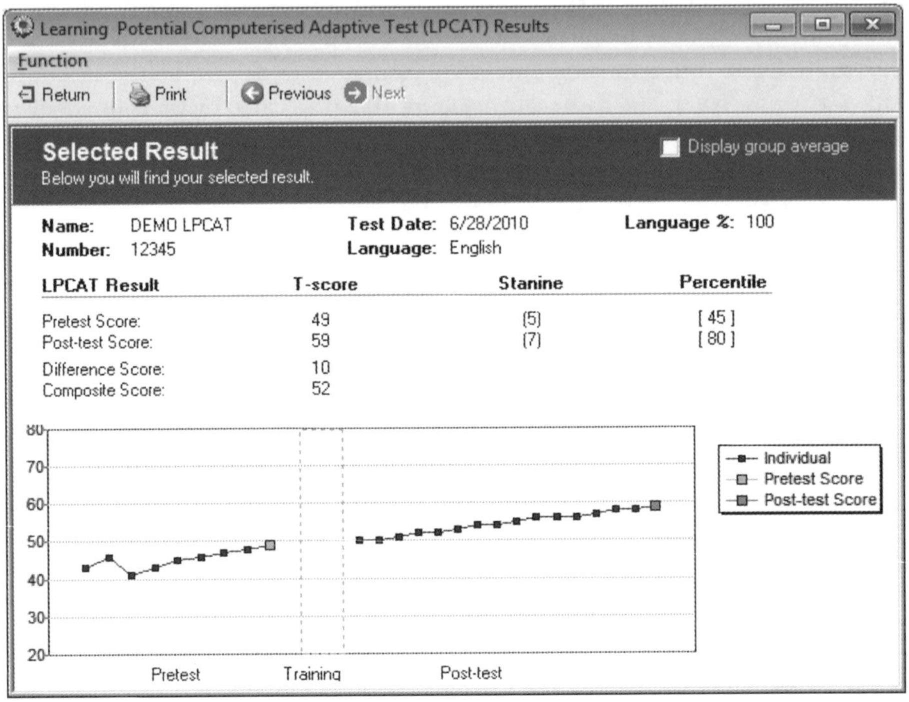

Administration of the LPCAT

As a dynamic CAT, the LPCAT has to be computer-administered to allow for the interactive selection of appropriate items for each individual, depending on the specific response pattern and the estimated performance level at the time. For ease of administration – in particular to persons with lower levels of formal qualification – only the space bar and the enter key are used to answer the multiple-choice questions. The use of the interactive CAT is possible, because in IRT the item difficulty levels and individual ability levels are measured on the same scale (Van der Linden, 2008a; 2008b; Weiss, 1983). In CAT, a bank of pre-calibrated items is available for presentation during the testing process. Unlike standard tests, in which all individuals who take the test complete exactly the same items in the same sequence, CAT presents a selection of items unique to each individual, continuously selecting items to be presented on the basis of their difficulty level, matching the individual's estimated ability level at that point in time. Not only can different items be presented to each individual, but candidates can also receive different numbers of items. A minimum and maximum number of items are pre-set to be used during test administration. No individual will receive fewer than the minimum number of items, and no individual will receive more than the maximum number of items. Test termination is only partially linked to the number of items; it is also linked to the accuracy of measurement, which in turn depends on the psychometric or measurement quality of items presented. Entry level to the pre-test is set, and thereafter the following steps are repeated until the testing is terminated:

- The first item presented is the item that measures best at the predetermined entry level (that is, the best psychometric quality item available in the bank that has a difficulty level closest to that particular level of ability).
- When the respondent answers the question, three things happen:
  - ~ If the item is answered correctly, the respondent's estimated ability level is readjusted upwards – assuming that since the question aimed at the entry level of ability was answered correctly, the respondent has a higher level of ability. If the item is answered incorrectly, the respondent's estimated ability level is adjusted downwards – assuming that since the question aimed at the entry level of ability was answered incorrectly, the respondent has a lower level of ability.
  - ~ The item characteristics of the item presented are also used to calculate an accuracy index, reflecting the accuracy of the ability estimation at that time. A check is done to determine whether the termination criteria are met – if they are, the test is terminated.
  - ~ If the test is not terminated, the next question selected will be the one in the bank that measures most accurately and provides the best information at the current newly estimated ability level.
- When the next item is presented, the process starts repeating – with a check for the number of items presented each time and a check for whether the required accuracy level has been achieved. All respondents will receive the minimum number of items. Thereafter, the test will terminate as soon as the required accuracy level (of the ability estimation) is attained, or as soon as the maximum number of items set have been administered – whichever comes first.

CAT has several positive features, including improving motivation by presenting items of appropriate difficulty level throughout testing, thereby not overwhelming or boring participants with items of an inappropriate difficulty level.

There is no fixed test administration time, due to the adaptive test process described above, but testing generally takes approximately one hour to complete. This includes the introduction, pre-test, training phase and post-test, and on completion the results are available immediately. When testing for various groups is arranged, it usually suffices if test sessions are arranged for one-and-a-half hours apart – since this should generally allow sufficient time for all examinees to complete the test.

Language versions of the LPCAT

There are two versions of the LPCAT – a version with either English or Afrikaans text on screen, and a version with no language on the screen – for which instructions to be read have been translated into all 11 official South African languages (De Beer, 2000a). In order to use the text-on-screen version, a reading proficiency level of at least Grade 6 or 7 in the language of administration is required. All software is installed during the installation process, and the selection of the language for testing is chosen per individual during the test administration process when entering the respondent's details (the options being 'English' or 'Afrikaans' or 'None'). When the 'None' (or 'no language') option is chosen, it implies that the instructions for administration have to be read from the *User's Manual* in the language chosen. For practical purposes in the case of the latter version, the group should be homogeneous in terms of the language to be used for test administration. In terms of age, it can be administered to respondents aged 11 years and older. In terms of educational level for adults, there is no minimum level required and it can be administered to illiterate adults too.

When the LPCAT is administered to groups, it is essential for all members of the group to complete the same version of the test – either all receiving full instructions and feedback on the example questions with text on the screen in the chosen language (English or Afrikaans) or, for the 'no language' or 'None' option, all seeing only the nonverbal figural patterns on their screens and having the instructions read aloud to them in the chosen appropriate language. Test administration sessions cannot allow for a mixture of the two versions, because those attempting to read instructions or feedback from the screen will be disturbed by the instructions being read aloud for the version in which no text appears on the screen.

The two versions of the LPCAT have different entry levels (in terms of the initial estimated ability level of the individual to start the adaptive testing process). For the version in which the instructions are provided on the screen, the entry level is at the mean level – that is, at a T-score of 50 – which is equivalent to a mid-secondary level (see Table 10.1). Once the first item has been answered, the adaptive process described earlier will commence. For the version of the LPCAT in which no instructions appear on the screen, and in which the instructions are read aloud to the respondents/candidates, the test commences at one standard deviation below the mean – that is, at a T-score level of 40 – which is equivalent to a senior primary level (see Table 10.1). It should be kept in mind that the entry level will not determine or influence the final levels attained in either the pre- or post-test, since the adaptive test administration will ensure that appropriately difficult (or easy) items are administered to match the individual's estimated ability level throughout the test session. Exactly the same introductory practice examples, and example items for the training between the pre- and the post-test, are used for the two versions. In the version in which the instructions and feedback are presented with the text appearing on the screen, the respondents can work independently through the introduction and initial practice examples, pre-test, training and post-test at their own pace. For the 'no language' version, instructions and feedback are read to the candidates, who should view the specific (and same) screens while the instructions for that screen are being read from the *User's Manual* (De Beer, 2000a).

Table 10.1 LPCAT score ranges in relation to NQF levels and educational levels

LPCAT T-score range	LPCAT Stanine score	ABET / NQF level	Educational level
20–32	1	ABET level 1	Grades 0–3 (Junior Primary)
33–37	2	ABET level 2	Grades 4–5 (Middle Primary)
38–42	3	ABET level 3	Grades 6–7 (Senior Primary)
43–47	4	ABET level 4/NQF 1	Grades 8–9 (Junior Secondary)
48–52	5	NQF levels 1–3	Grades 10–12 (Mid- to Senior Secondary)
53–54	6	NQF levels 4–5	Grade 12+ (Higher Certificate) (Junior Tertiary)
55–57	6	NQF level 6	Diploma/Advanced Certificate (Tertiary Diploma)
58–62	7	NQF level 7	3-year Degree/Adv. Diploma (First Degree)
63–68	8	NQF level 8	Honours/4-year Degree/Postgraduate Diploma
69–80 (65+)	9	NQF level 9	Advanced Degree (Master's Degree)
69–80 (65+)	9	NQF level 10	Advanced Degree (Doctoral Degree)

Results graph and scores of the LPCAT

The LPCAT pre- and post-test results are presented in graph form (see Figure 10.3). The estimated ability/performance levels after answering each question are plotted, and these levels, as well as the number of questions answered, can be seen in both the pre- and post-test plots. In the pre-test, between 8 and 12 questions are adaptively administered from an item bank of 63 questions, while in the post-test, between 10 and 18 questions are administered adaptively from a separate post-test item bank containing 125 questions. The performance level at the end of the pre-test is used as the entry level in the post-test, thereby further improving the accuracy of estimation in the post-test.

The following four scores are presented in the results graph in a T-test form:

- the pre-test score (performance level at the end of the pre-test);
- the post-test score (performance level at the end of the post-test);
- the difference score (numerical difference between pre- and post-tests);
- the composite score (a reasoned combination of the pre- and post-test scores).

Scores are also presented in stanine and percentile format, but these are less useful than the T-test scores. The latter are also used for the interpretation of the level of reasoning shown in the pre- and post-tests in relation to National Qualifications Framework (NQF) or academic levels (see Table 10.1).

Psychometric properties and fairness of the LPCAT

This section provides a summary of some empirical results on the psychometric properties of the LPCAT during its development and validation, as well as in the time since its release in 2000. Preference has been given to studies with larger sample sizes. Information on specific concerns referred to in the Employment Equity Act – that is, reliability, validity and fairness – is provided.

Reliability of the LPCAT

Reliability of CATs is not measured in the same way as that of standard static tests, since individuals completing the test can be given different items as well as different numbers of items to answer, although the scores obtained are on the same scale that measures the latent trait of the particular domain. McBride (1997) indicates that adaptive tests can achieve higher reliability compared with conventional tests in the upper and lower extremes of the ability scale, and at the same time reach a given level of precision, using substantially fewer items than standard tests. This is a result of the items being selected purposefully to match the estimated ability level of the respondent throughout the test. The IRT equivalent to test score reliability and standard error of measurement (SEM) of classical test theory is the test information function. This reflects the level of information available at a particular ability level, as a result of the number and quality of items available at that level in the item bank. The standard error is a function, which means that it is not a single measure over the entire ability range but is calculated at various ability levels, based on the amount of information at different ability levels (De Beer, 2000b).

LPCAT coefficient alpha reliability values range between 0.926 and 0.981 for subgroups based on gender, culture, language and level of education for the standardisation sample of 2 450 Grade 9 and Grade 11 learners, and are reported fully in the LPCAT *Technical Manual* (De Beer, 2000b). The detail of the test information function is also reported there.

Validity of the LPCAT

Determination of validity of a test generally entails ongoing gathering of information to evaluate the usefulness of test results for various groups in different contexts. It usually requires evidence of the relationships between performance on the test and other independently obtained scores which also reflect the behaviour of concern. Although DA was often criticised in the past for its lack of empirical psychometric evidence, this has changed in recent years (Caffrey, Fuchs & Fuchs, 2008).

The construct and predictive validity for the LPCAT are presented by reporting on results of samples at different educational levels, from low-literate adults to tertiary university levels. A short description of the sample groups is provided below.

i) Group 1: Low-literate adult group (Adult Basic Education and Training (ABET))
   A group of low-literate adults was assessed for the purpose of career guidance after their positions were made redundant. The sample (N = 194) was mostly

male and all black. Together with the LPCAT, the Paper-and-Pencil-Games (PPG) (Claassen, 1996) was also administered; this test provides a verbal, nonverbal and total score. For the criterion measure, ABET numeracy and literacy results (Level 1 and Level 3) were used (De Beer, 2000b).

ii) Group 2: Senior primary (Grade 6 and Grade 7 levels)
The longitudinal predictive validity results for two separate groups were investigated (De Beer, 2010b). The first sample group (N = 72) was all female (Grade 6) with a mean age of 11.18 years. The second sample (N = 79) was all male and in Grade 7, with a mean age of 12.44 years. An English proficiency test was also administered (Chamberlain & Reinecke, 1992) to the male sample, while two subtests of the Differential Aptitude Test (DAT) (Claassen, Van Heerden, Vosloo & Wheeler, 2000) were administered to the female sample. For both groups an aggregate score for school academic results was used as the criterion measure (De Beer, 2010b).

iii) Group 3: Junior secondary (Grade 8 level)
A sample group (N = 151) of junior secondary learners with a mean age of 13.2 years was assessed with the LPCAT as well as with the General Scholastic Aptitude Test (adaptive version) (GSAT-CAT) (Van Tonder & Claassen, 1992). An English proficiency measure (Chamberlain & Reinecke, 1992), as well as a test of basic numerical literacy (Venter, 1997), was also administered. School academic results were used as the criterion (De Beer, 2000b).

iv) Group 4: Junior secondary (Grade 9 level)
A group of 253 learners at Grade 9 level was assessed as part of a vocational guidance project. Of this sample group, 96 (37.9 per cent) were male and 157 (62.1 per cent) were female. Three subtests of the DAT Form R (Claassen et al., 2000) were also administered (Verbal Reasoning, Comparisons and 2-dimensional Spatial Reasoning). Academic results in English, Mathematics and Life Orientation were used as criterion measures.

v) Group 5: Senior secondary (Grade 11 level)
A group of 174 learners at a Grade 11 level was assessed as part of a vocational guidance project. For this sample, 63 were male (36.2 per cent) and 111 were female (63.8 per cent). Three subtests of the DAT Form K (Coetzee & Vosloo, 2000) were also administered (Verbal Reasoning, Comparisons and 3-dimensional Spatial Reasoning). Academic results in English, Mathematics and Life Orientation were used as criterion measures.

vi) Group 6: Junior tertiary (Further Education and Training (FET) college first-year level)
A sample group of 75 students was assessed for career guidance purposes. The DAT Form R (Claassen et al., 2000) was also administered. Academic results were used as criterion measures (De Beer, 2008).

vii) Group 7: Tertiary (first-year diploma level)
A first-year sample of engineering and technology students (N = 223) with a mean age of 19.9 years was tested with the LPCAT, as well as with the GSAT-CAT (Van Tonder & Claassen, 1992). Subtests of the Senior Aptitude Test (SAT) were also administered (Owen & Taljaard, 1989). Grade 12 academic results and first-year academic results were obtained, to be used for comparative predictive validity analyses respectively (De Beer, 2000b). (See also Van der Merwe and De Beer (2006) and Van Eeden, De Beer and Coetzee (2001), for other results at this level.)

viii) Group 8: Tertiary (first-year degree level)
A group of applicants for engineering studies at university (N = 382) was tested for screening and selection purposes. Their mean academic results were used as criterion data (De Beer & Mphokane, 2010).

ix) Group 9: Mixed (group from industry)
A sample group from industry (N = 150) was assessed with both the LPCAT and the Raven's Standard Progressive Matrices (Mann, 2007).

The mean LPCAT scores for the above groups are reported in Table 10.2.

Table 10.2 Mean LPCAT scores for groups at different educational levels

Group	Educational level	N	LPCAT pre-test	LPCAT post-test	LPCAT composite
Group 1	Adult low-literate	194	36.19	37.76	–
Group 2	Grade 6*	72	50.01	50.87	50.13
Group 2	Grade 7*	79	54.52	56.10	54.78
Group 3	Grade 8	128	45.67	47.83	–
Group 4	Grade 9	233	51.09	52.37	51.30
Group 5	Grade 11	119	52.50	53.34	52.60
Group 6	FET first year	74	48.82	49.43	49.00
Group 7	Diploma first year	159	55.21	56.47	–
Group 8	Degree first year	382	–	63.96	62.54
Group 9	Mixed (industry)	150	57.75	58.80	–

Note: * Private school. Sample sizes differ due to missing data.

Data obtained from the above sample groups are reported for construct and predictive validity in the next two subsections.

Construct validity of the LPCAT

To determine the construct validity of the LPCAT, its correlations with a variety of other cognitive measures for groups at various educational levels are summarised in Table 10.3.

Table 10.3 Construct validity of the LPCAT

Group	Educational level	Other measures	N	LPCAT post-test		LPCAT composite	
				r	p	r	p
Group 1	Adult	PPG Verbal	110	.408**	.000	.411**	.000
	low-literate	PPG NV	110	.543**	.000	.565**	.000
		PPG Total	110	.610**	.000	.552**	.000
Group 2	Grade 6	DAT English	72	.263*	.025	.213	.072
		DAT Calc	72	.278*	.018	.280*	.017
	Grade 7	English 1st prof.	79	.405*	.018	.328*	.003
Group 3	Grade 8	GSAT-CAT VB	120	.613**	.000	.574**	.000
		GSAT-CAT NV	120	.665**	.000	.653**	.000
		GSAT-CAT Total	120	.691**	.000	.664**	.000
Group 4	Grade 9	DAT Verbal	228	.544**	.000	.500**	.000
		DAT Comparisons	202	.335**	.000	.356**	.000
		DAT 2D	227	.500**	.000	.435**	.000
Group 5	Grade 11	DAT Verbal	114	.209*	.025	.114	.126
		DAT Comparisons	88	.111	.307	.051	.637
		DAT 3D	108	.524**	.000	.452	.000
Group 6	FET 1st year	DAT Language	74	.200	.088	.296**	.010
		DAT NV	74	.403**	.000	.363**	.001
		DAT Verbal	74	.389**	.001	.386**	.001
		DAT Calculations	74	.274*	.018	.298*	.010
		DAT Comparisons	74	.193	.100	.112	.334
Group 7	Diploma	GSAT-CAT VB	158	.571**	.000	.555**	.000
	1st year	GSAT-CAT NV	158	.645**	.000	.626**	.000
		GSAT-CAT Total	158	.668**	.000	.648**	.000
Group 8	Degree	ELSA Literacy	309	.481**	.000	–	–
	1st year	ELSA Numeracy	309	.418**	.000	–	–
		Maths test	309	.527**	.000	–	–
Group 9	Mixed	Raven's SPM (RS)	150	.585**	.000	–	–
	(industry)	Raven's SPM (TS)	150	.618**	.000	–	

Notes: * p < .05 ** p < .01. Sample sizes differ due to missing data.

The results indicate that the LPCAT, with its general measurement of 'g_f' fluid ability performance and potential, overlaps with abilities and domains measured by other (cognitive) tests.

Predictive validity of the LPCAT

The groups and different measures obtained are summarised in Table 10.4. Academic performance is generally used as it is easier to generalise from these measures.

Table 10.4 Predictive validity results for the LPCAT at different educational levels

Group	Educational level	Criterion measures	LPCAT score (highest corr.)	N	r	p
Group 1	Adult low-literate	ABET Literacy L1	Composite	110	.437**	.000
		ABET Literacy L3	Post-test	111	.461**	.000
		ABET Numeracy L1	Composite	182	.491**	.000
		ABET Numeracy L3	Post-test	26	.610**	.000
Group 2	Grade 6	Aggregate Academic	Post-test	72	.499**	.000
	Grade 7	Aggregate Academic	Composite	79	.482**	.000
Group 3	Grade 8	Academic (Sem. 2)	Post-test	118	.524**	.000
Group 4	Grade 9	English (Academic)	Post-test	233	.340**	.000
		Maths (Academic)	Post-test	233	.434**	.000
		Life Orient. (Academic)	Composite	233	.215**	.001
Group 5#	Grade 11	English (Academic)	Post-test	119	.025	.789#
		Maths (Academic)	Post-test	119	.005	.957#
		Life Orient. (Academic)	Post-test	119	–.063	.494#
Group 6	FET 1st year	Academic average	Composite	69	.350**	.004
Group 7	Diploma 1st year	Academic average	Composite	120	.218*	.017
Group 8	Degree 1st year	Academic average	Post-test	125	.333**	.000
Group 9	Mixed (industry)	None available			–	

Notes: For most of the above results, more detailed information and full results can be found in the sources referred to in the sample descriptions above.

* $p < .05$ ** $p < .01$. Sample sizes differ due to missing data.

Although the predictive validity results for the LPCAT have generally shown positive correlations of moderate to large practical effect sizes, the predictive validity correlation results for Group 5 show non-significant correlations. The Verbal Reasoning and Comparisons subtests of the DAT showed similar non-significant correlations with academic performance for this group, and only 3-dimensional Spatial Reasoning results showed statistically significant correlations with the academic results.

With the exception of one group (Group 5), the results show acceptable levels of predictive validity for academic results over a wide spectrum of academic levels.

Fairness of the LPCAT

The LPCAT is registered with the Health Professions Council of South Africa as a culture-fair test. The following features of the LPCAT can be deemed to contribute to its fairness in the multicultural and multilingual South African context:

- It focuses on the measurement of learning potential, addressing not only current level of performance but also the projected or potential future level that can be achieved if relevant learning opportunities are provided.

- The content of the test questions contains only nonverbal figural patterns, thereby not requiring language proficiency and not relying on mastery of scholastic content to measure reasoning ability.
- The test instructions have been translated into all official South African languages for the version in which no text appears on the screen and the instructions are read to the respondents, thereby not requiring them to read anything themselves (De Beer, 2000a; 2005). The text-on-screen version is available in English and Afrikaans.
- Computer literacy is not a requirement, since the easy use of only the space bar and the enter key to answer the multiple-choice questions presented simplifies the answering procedure. It allows for the measurement of learning potential of illiterate adults to ensure that appropriate learning and development opportunities are provided.
- During test development, a large and representative sample (N = 2 450) was used for the item analysis and standardisation. This sample was used to perform IRT-based DIF analysis on all new questions compiled with regard to subgroups based on level of education, language, culture and gender. Items not complying with the cut-off in terms of DIF for any one or more of the subgroups were discarded, and not used in the final test.
- CAT allows for items of suitable difficulty level in comparison with the performance (estimated ability) level of the respondent throughout the pre- and post-tests.
- The LPCAT is a power as opposed to a timed test, allowing sufficient time for each question that is presented to be answered, and with no overall set test time.

Practical use of the LPCAT

The LPCAT can be used in contexts in which decision-making involves obtaining information related to required future performance or development and training levels, in terms of the NQF level framework (see Table 10.1). It has shown statistically and practically significant predictive validity for academic results at different levels (basic education, primary, secondary and tertiary level academic results – see Table 10.4).

Practically, the process starts from the end, in the sense that the reason for assessment should be carefully considered first to determine what the required level of performance or the level of training to be completed is. Once this level has been identified (in terms of relevant NQF or educational levels), the LPCAT pre- and post-test results can be compared to this level to determine whether the individual currently (as reflected in the pre-test results) performs close to or at the required level or, if not, whether the individual shows that after a learning opportunity has been presented, he or she is able to function close to or at the required level (as reflected in the post-test results). Smaller improvement scores are an indication that the individual is, in future, likely to perform at similar levels to those currently shown. On the other hand, larger improvement scores indicate that the individual can be expected to perform at higher levels in the future than those currently shown, provided that relevant learning and development opportunities are provided. Table 10.1 indicates the interpretation of the LPCAT performance levels shown in terms of NQF and/or academic levels.

Other measures can be used to identify specific aptitudes, proficiencies or interests, but learning potential assessment can identify the appropriate level at which training and development should be currently targeted and aimed for over time. Due consideration should be given to actual academic attainment, to ensure that appropriate building blocks are put in place over time to assist with optimal development of the individual potential shown.

Measurement of learning potential on the LPCAT is not restricted to individuals of low formal education; it can also be administered to, and its results advantageously used for, individuals up to a postgraduate tertiary educational level. An important prerequisite is to ascertain whether the individual has obtained the specific formal level of academic qualification or training that is required to commence with the level of training offered. Once this has been verified, the difference between the LPCAT levels of performance and the level required for the training offered can be interpreted as the extent of effort that the individual will need to exert in order to achieve success at the required level. If the LPCAT level of performance is lower than the required level, it is interpreted as an indication that more effort will be needed from the individual to achieve success at the required level. The larger the difference, the greater the effort that will be required, or the longer the time it could take to achieve success. In such cases, it is recommended that a step-by-step approach be taken, with training broken down into smaller parts to allow for optimal levels of performance by not overloading the individual in terms of the magnitude (number of subjects) as well as the level of the challenge. If the individual's test performance is at a higher level than the required level, indications are that he or she should be able to achieve success with moderate effort and within the prescribed number of hours of study indicated.

Features and challenges of the LPCAT

Certain advantages and disadvantages are associated with psychological assessment in general. Some of the advantages include the information that it provides to promote better decision-making, the objective sample of behaviour it represents, and enhancement of a scientific approach to decision-making. The disadvantages include measurement error, the possible effect of poor testing conditions, and the fact that individuals may either try to manipulate results or not be appropriately motivated to ensure optimal results. When using any psychological assessment instrument, it is imperative to be aware of its particular features which may result in specific advantages and disadvantages being present.

Positive features of the LPCAT

As the preceding discussion of the LPCAT has indicated, it has a number of positive features:

- It is considered a culture-fair test. It was developed in South Africa, and has been used internationally, in Africa (South Africa, Mozambique, Namibia, Botswana, Zambia, Ethiopia, Uganda and Gambia), in a number of countries in the East (Sri-Lanka, Cambodia, Nepal and Vietnam) and in Europe (Finland and The Netherlands).
- It has shown satisfactory reliability, and its predictive validity results have compared favourably with those of standard tests.
- Standard training is provided to focus attention of the respondents on the relevant aspects of the task, so that intra- and inter-individual comparisons can be made.
- It allows for equal assessment opportunities, irrespective of the current level of formal qualification (from illiterate to postgraduate levels, with the test adapting to the performance level shown by the individual respondent).
- It can be administered individually or in groups. Instructions are available in all 11 official languages of South Africa (and in French).
- It is quick and easy to administer, and the results are immediately available on completion of the test. Results are presented graphically, which also allows for some qualitative analysis of performance during the pre- and post-tests (see Figure 10.4).
- It is in line with the Employment Equity Act, affording opportunities to those considered disadvantaged educationally and socio-economically and who may therefore not have had opportunities to reach their optimal level of development/qualification.

Figure 10.4 Example of LPCAT results

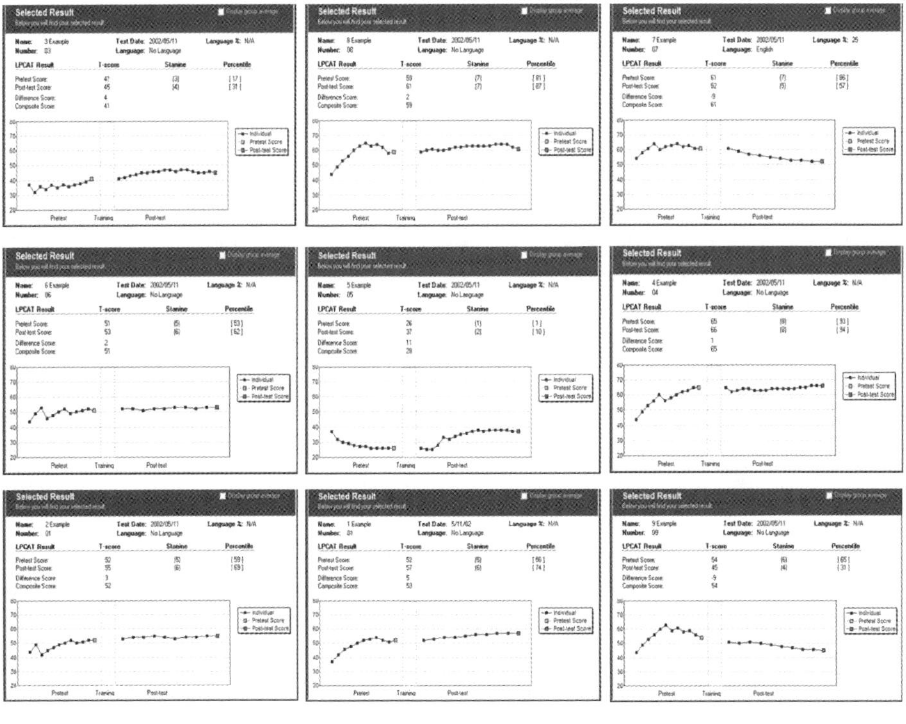

- It adds information that would not be available from static tests. It can therefore assist with the identification of individuals who may otherwise be overlooked (owing to current low levels of attained qualifications), but who have high potential for further development.

Challenges and problematic issues relating to the LPCAT

Notwithstanding all its positive features, this form of assessment does pose some challenges and raises problems that need to be addressed:

- The LPCAT could have limited face validity for individuals at higher educational levels, since its content is not related to job performance or training at higher levels. For such groups, it is therefore important to explain how the test works and to justify its inclusion in a particular assessment battery, to ensure that respondents remain motivated and perform to the best of their ability throughout.
- Reliance on computers, and thus on electricity, for administration and to ensure that results are saved could be a problem if power failures disrupt assessment.
- Information provided in the results is only linked to the current and projected levels of fluid reasoning ability shown, and does not provide a direct link to a particular career or job level. Other assessment information would be needed to provide information of the latter kind for career-related guidance and decisions.
- Newer test operating systems pose challenges for the current version of the test administration program. Ongoing updates of software required to maintain compatibility with new operating systems are required. This is discussed below.

Future developments

Demands for software programs (and computer-based tests and testing systems) to maintain compatibility with new technology and updated operating systems are ongoing. Interim challenges are addressed by means of bridging or patch programs, but major revisions and updates are also required from time to time. The current test administration program of the LPCAT will be updated in the near future to ensure improved compatibility with new operating systems.

An internet-based Results Analysis Program for processing LPCAT results has been developed. This allows different users from the same organisation to access the same database or specific subfolders of results remotely via the internet. The sharing of runs within a particular user group is also much easier with this program.

Internet-based adaptive test administration is the next development target; this will allow for the use of more automated processes. Other developments in the planning stages are the expansion of the item bank and recalculation of item parameters to ensure current relevance in terms of the interpretation of levels of performance.

Conclusion

As this chapter has shown, the LPCAT can provide a different kind of information than that obtained from standard cognitive tests. However, its results cannot answer all questions relating to the cognitive domain, as it only indicates current and potential levels of cognitive performance in the nonverbal figural domain. Nonetheless, it adds information that enriches the interpretation of individual results when used in an integrated manner with other tests and measures.

References

Binet, A. & Simon, T. (1915). *A Method of Measuring the Development of the Intelligence of Young Children*. Chicago, IL: Chicago Medical Book Co.

Caffrey, E., Fuchs, D. & Fuchs, L. S. (2008). The predictive validity of dynamic assessment. *Journal of Special Education, 41(4)*, 254–269.

Chamberlain, J. C. & Reinecke, S. (1992). *Manual: Proficiency Test English Second-Language Intermediate Level*. Pretoria: Human Sciences Research Council.

Claassen, N. C. W. (1996). *Paper-and-Pencil Games (PPG): Manual*. Pretoria: Human Sciences Research Council.

Claassen, N. C. W. (1997). Cultural differences, politics and test bias in South Africa. *European Review of Applied Psychology, 47(4)*, 297–307.

Claassen, N. C. W., De Beer, M., Hugo, H. L. E. & Meyer, H. M. (1991). *Manual for the General Scholastic Aptitude Test (GSAT) Senior Series*. Pretoria: Human Sciences Research Council.

Claassen, N. C. W, Van Heerden, J. S., Vosloo, H. N. & Wheeler, J. J. (2000). *Manual for the Differential Aptitude Test Form R (DAT-R)*. Pretoria: Human Sciences Research Council.

Coetzee, N. & Vosloo, H. N. (2000). *Manual for the Differential Aptitude Test (Form K)*. Pretoria: Human Sciences Research Council.

De Beer, M. (2000a). *Learning Potential Computerised Adaptive Test (LPCAT): User's Manual*. Pretoria: Unisa Press.

De Beer, M. (2000b). *Learning Potential Computerised Adaptive Test (LPCAT): Technical Manual*. Pretoria: Unisa Press.

De Beer, M. (2004). Use of differential item functioning (DIF) analysis for bias analysis in test construction. *South African Journal of Industrial Psychology, 30(4)*, 52–57.

De Beer, M. (2005). Development of the Learning Potential Computerised Adaptive Test (LPCAT). *South African Journal of Psychology, 35(4)*, 717–747.

De Beer, M. (2006). Dynamic testing: Practical solutions to some concerns. *South African Journal of Industrial Psychology, 32(4)*, 8–14.

De Beer, M. (2008). Predicting college academic results from aptitude and learning potential test scores. Poster presentation. British Psychological Society Annual Conference. Dublin, April 2–4.

De Beer, M. (2010a). A modern psychometric approach to dynamic assessment. *Journal of Psychology in Africa, 20(2)*, 225–231.

De Beer, M. (2010b). Longitudinal validity of a learning potential test. *Journal of Psychology in Africa, 20(2)*, 241–246.

De Beer, M. & Mphokane, A. (2010). Predictive validity of different measures for engineering student academic results. Poster presentation. Annual Conference of the Society for Industrial and Organisational Psychology. Pretoria, July 29–31.

Embretson, S. E. (1996). The new rules of measurement. *Psychological Assessment, 8(4)*, 341–349.

Embretson, S. E. (2004). The second century of ability testing: Some predictions and speculations. *Measurement and Interdisciplinary Research and Perspectives, 2(1)*, 1–32.

Flynn, J. R. (1987). Massive IQ gains in 14 nations: What IQ tests really measure. *Psychological Bulletin, 101(2)*, 171–191.

Foxcroft, C. D. (1997). Psychological testing in South Africa: Perspectives regarding ethical and fair practices. *European Journal of Psychological Assessment, 13(3)*, 229–235.

Foxcroft, C. D. (2004). Planning a psychological test in the multicultural South African context. *South African Journal of Industrial Psychology, 30(4)*, 8–15.

Grigorenko, E. L. & Sternberg, R. J. (1998). Dynamic testing. *Psychological Bulletin, 124(1)*, 75–111.

Haywood, H. C. (2008). Twenty years of IACEP, and a focus on dynamic assessment: Progress, problems, and prospects. *Journal of Cognitive Education and Psychology, 7(3)*, 419–442.

Hugo, H. L. E. & Claassen, N. C. W. (1991). *The Functioning of the GSAT Senior for Students of the Department of Education and Training*. Pretoria: Human Sciences Research Council.

Kim-Kang, G. & Weiss, D. J. (2008). Adaptive measurement of individual change. *Zeitschrift für Psychologie / Journal of Psychology, 216(1)*, 49–58.

Lidz, C. S. (1987). *Dynamic Assessment: An Interactional Approach to Evaluating Learning Potential*. New York, NY: The Guilford Press.

Mann, L. (2007). The relationship between learning potential and educative ability. Unpublished Master's dissertation. University of Pretoria, Pretoria.

McBride, J. R. (1997). Technical perspective. In W. A. Sands, B. K. Waters & J. R. McBride (Eds), *Computerized Adaptive Testing: From Inquiry to Operation* (pp. 29–44). Washington, DC: American Psychological Association.

Murphy, R. & Maree, D. J. F. (2006). A review of South African research in the field of dynamic assessment. *South African Journal of Psychology, 36(1)*, 168–191.

Owen, K. (1998). *The Role of Psychological Tests in Education in South Africa: Issues, Controversies and Benefits*. Pretoria: Human Sciences Research Council.

Owen, K. & Taljaard, J. J. (Eds) (1989). *Handbook for the Use of Psychological and Scholastic Tests of the IPER and the NIPR*. Pretoria: Human Sciences Research Council.

Rushton, J. P. & Jensen, A. R. (2010). Race and IQ: A theory-based review of the research in Richard Nisbett's *Intelligence and How to Get it. The Open Psychology Journal, 3*, 9–35.

Sijtsma, K. (1993a). Classical and modern test theory with an eye toward learning potential testing. In J. H. M. Hamers, K. Sijtsma & A. J. J. M. Ruijssenaars (Eds), *Learning Potential Assessment: Theoretical, Methodological and Practical Issues* (pp. 117–134). Amsterdam: Swets & Zeitlinger.

Sijtsma, K. (1993b). Psychometric issues in learning potential assessment. In J. H. M. Hamers, K. Sijtsma & A. J. J. M. Ruijssenaars (Eds), *Learning Potential Assessment: Theoretical, Methodological and Practical Issues* (pp. 175–194). Amsterdan: Swets & Zeitlinger.

Statistics South Africa (2008). *General Household Survey 2007*. Pretoria: Statistics South Africa.

Sternberg, R. J. & Grigorenko, E. L. (2002). *Dynamic Testing: The Nature and Measurement of Learning Potential*. Cambridge: Cambridge University Press.

Te Nijenhuis, J., Van Vianen, A. & Van der Flier, H. (2007). Score gains on *g*-loaded tests: No *g*. *Intelligence, 35*, 283–300.

Van der Linden, W. J. (2008a). Some new developments in adaptive testing technology. *Zeitschrift für Psychologie / Journal of Psychology, 216(1)*, 3–11.

Van der Linden, W. J. (2008b). Adaptive models of psychological testing. *Zeitschrift für Psychologie / Journal of Psychology, 216(1)*, 1–2.

Van der Merwe, D. & De Beer, M. (2006). Challenges of student selection: Predicting academic performance. *South African Journal of Higher Education, 20(4)*, 547–562.

Van Eeden, R., De Beer, M. & Coetzee, C. H. (2001). Cognitive ability, learning potential, and personality traits as predictors of academic achievement by engineering and other science and technology students. *South African Journal of Higher Education, 15(1)*, 171–179.

Van Tonder, M. & Claassen, N. C. W. (1992). *Manual for the General Scholastic Aptitude Test (Senior): Computerised Adaptive Test*. Pretoria: Human Sciences Research Council.

Venter, E. J. (1997). *Manual: Test of Basic Numerical Literacy*. Pretoria: Human Sciences Research Council.

Vygotsky, L. S. (1978). *Mind in Society: The Development of Higher Psychological Processes*. Cambridge, MA: Harvard University Press.

Weiss, D. J. (Ed.) (1983). *New Horizons in Testing: Latent Trait Test Theory and Computerised Adaptive Testing*. New York, NY: Academic Press.

Wicherts, J. M., Dolan, C. V., Carlson, J. S. & Van der Maas, H. L. J. (2010). Raven's test performance of sub-Saharan Africans: Average performance, psychometric properties and the Flynn effect. *Learning and Individual Differences, 20*, 135–151.

Wolf, T. (1973). *Alfred Binet*. Chicago, IL: University of Chicago Press.

11 APIL and TRAM learning potential assessment instruments

T. Taylor

APIL ((Conceptual) Ability, Processing of Information, and Learning), TRAM-2 and TRAM-1 (Transfer, Automatisation and Memory) are a suite of learning potential batteries designed for use over a wide educational spectrum, ranging from no education to tertiary level. All three produce multiple component scores as well as a global or overall learning potential score. All are based on a theoretical position broader than the one normally underpinning learning potential instruments.

This chapter presents an overview of these instruments. First, the theory on which they are based is presented. This is followed by a description of the structure of the batteries. Finally, information on the subscale intercorrelations, reliability, validity and bias of the three instruments is presented.

The theoretical basis of the instruments

The concept of learning potential originated with Vygotsky (1978; original Russian publication 1926). According to Vygotsky, intelligence has little or no genetic base and is, rather, a set of competencies passed on to others by parents, caregivers, educators and peers. Thus, it is primarily a social phenomenon and only secondarily a personal characteristic.

Vygotsky did, nevertheless, accept that there were differences in learning potential between individuals. This he operationalised in the concept 'zone of proximal development' (ZPD), which is the extent to which an individual can improve performance in an intellectual task given mediation by a skilled other. Learning potential is a difference between performance after mediation and performance before. Vygotsky does not explain how a person might ultimately excel beyond the level of his or her teachers and mentors (as did Mozart). In this regard, the difficulty of his conceptualisation of learning potential lies primarily in the almost exclusively social nature of his theory, which leaves little place for internal factors such as genetic endowment. Even individual differences in the magnitude of the ZPD seem difficult to explain in the absence of these factors.

The Israeli psychologist Feuerstein further developed Vygotsky's work, creating tools to assess and develop learning ability, the Learning Potential

Assessment Device for the former and the Instrumental Enrichment programme for the latter (Feuerstein, Rand & Hoffman, 1979; see also Grigorenko & Sternberg, 1998). Several other researchers have also developed learning potential assessment tools, but for the most part they remain close to the Vygotskyian idea of assessing learning potential through a difference score, assessed in a 'test-teach-test' procedure. The difference score, apart from its propensity for unreliability, is controversial, and it has been criticised by several researchers as psychometrically unsound (see Cronbach & Furby, 1970; Embretson, 1987; Glutting & McDermott, 1990; Sijtsma, 1996).

When considering the development of a learning potential assessment tool in the mid-1990s, it was the present author's contention that it was inappropriate to depend totally on the difference score as a measure of learning or developmental capacity. Thus it was argued that learning ability cannot be independent of certain fundamental constructs identified in cognitive psychology and information processing psychology. In Taylor (1994), the literature in three domains (learning theory, cognitive psychology and information processing psychology) was surveyed, and a broader model of developmental capacity was proposed, drawing on all three domains.

The work of Snow and colleagues (Snow, Kyllonen & Marshalek, 1984; Snow & Lohman, 1984; Snow, Marshalek & Lohman, 1976) and Ackerman (1988) was instrumental in the conceptualisation of the 1994 model (Taylor, 1994). Snow and his colleagues performed a radex analysis on subjects who had done a large variety of cognitive tests. They chose a two-dimensional representation of the data, which was effectively a disc. The disc could be split into three main sectors, verbal, numerical and spatial, with the more conceptual and abstract tests falling closer to the centre and the more specific and content-laden tasks more at the periphery.

The ability to solve novel conceptual problems has long been recognised as a fundamental aspect of intelligence. Spearman (1927) was the first to propose such a construct. Cattell (1971) named it 'fluid intelligence' and contrasted it with more specific and acquired skills and abilities, which he called 'crystallised intelligence'. Horn (1989) elaborated this theory. In Snow's research, the Raven's Progressive Matrices scores fell right at the centre of the radex. This test has long been recognised as a good measure of fluid intelligence or conceptual thinking, and has been widely used in cross-cultural contexts when researching this construct (Raven, Raven & Court, 1998). The centrality of fluid intelligence in Snow's radex and its prominence in other models such as Cattell's and Horn's led Taylor (1994) to conclude that it should be included in a battery measuring learning potential. It appeared to play a vital role in the acquisition of new competencies, as will be discussed in more detail shortly. Furthermore, it has the advantage of being measurable using stimulus material that is relatively free of cultural content.

Ackerman (1988), a learning theorist, pointed out that the Snow findings represented a 'static' situation: all tests were applied only once, so there was no information on how performance might have changed with repeated practice. In his own research with just a few tests, Ackerman (1988) found that as practice increased, correlations of the tests with fluid intelligence declined, whereas correlations with information processing variables increased. The results could be interpreted as indicating that there are two fundamental human capacities: power and processing efficiency. Both contribute to learning. If an individual understands the conceptual underpinnings of the material he or she is working with, and is also fast and accurate at carrying out steps required to perform a given task, learning proceeds swiftly. Apart from improving output, efficient information processing is beneficial in that essential information is not lost from working memory. Working memory has been shown to be significantly correlated with intelligence (Baddeley, 1986; Larson & Saccuzzo, 1989).

Ackerman's model is a three-dimensional extension of Snow's model. The circular radex acquires a vertical dimension, thus becoming a cylinder. The learning phenomena (at least with regard to the changes occurring as a result of repeated practice) are represented by the vertical dimension.

Taylor (1994) identified two basic forms of learning. The one that is represented by the vertical dimension of the Ackerman model has been called automatisation by Sternberg (1985; 1997). It is the process by which – with practice – performance becomes more proficient. In learning exercises of this type, the actual task that the person has to do remains the same and learning is revealed in the form of increased output and efficiency.

The other type of learning Taylor (1994) identified for inclusion in his assessment tools is typically called transfer. In this type of learning, the task changes and the individual is required to adapt knowledge and skill previously acquired in order to solve the new problems. Transfer may be simple, when the old and new problems are very similar, or challenging, when the new problems are very different or complex, needing to be broken down into subproblems that may be somewhat like problems previously encountered.

Transfer is the learning construct where fluid intelligence is most at play. Fluid intelligence powers the process whereby new competencies emerge out of established ones, and the radex becomes populated. For example, developing a competency in computer programming might involve adapting existing competencies in language, logic and mathematics. Conceptual thinking or fluid intelligence is required to effect these adaptations. In a way, transfer can be thought of as fluid intelligence applied in a learning context.

The model used by Taylor (1994) for the APIL and TRAM tests has four main components: fluid intelligence, information processing efficiency, transfer and automatisation. The first two are 'static' in that they can be measured in a non-learning way, whereas the last two are 'dynamic' – that is, direct measures of learning. Although the first two are static, they are not irrelevant to learning. Fluid intelligence underlies transfer, and information processing efficiency impacts on automatisation.

Although there are four components in the model, the APIL and TRAM learning potential instruments have more than four scores. This is because some of the components have been split into subcomponents.

The structure of the test batteries

The structure and contents of the three batteries will be dealt with in turn. A critical feature of all three is the sparing use of verbal material in the items, because verbal content has the propensity to introduce cultural bias. Where words are used, they are very high-frequency and emotionally neutral.

The APIL battery

The APIL, intended mainly for administration to individuals with tertiary education or aspirations towards tertiary education, is the longest of the batteries, producing eight scores. The full battery takes about 3 hours 45 minutes to administer; however, it is possible to administer only parts of the battery, the shortest recommended version consuming about 2 hours. A global score is available, irrespective of how many subtests have been administered.

If the full APIL is used, eight scores are produced – namely, fluid intelligence, speed of information processing, accuracy of information processing, flexibility of information processing, learning rate or automatisation, total amount of work done in the automatisation exercise, memory and understanding of the automatisation material, and transfer.

The fluid intelligence test, known as the Concept Formation Test (CFT), has an odd-man-out format and comprises six quasi-geometric drawings, one of which is conceptually anomalous.

Information processing efficiency is measured in a sub-battery of the APIL from which the second, third and fourth scores (as listed above) are derived. This sub-battery has three 'pure' subtests (called Series, Mirror and Transformations) and one mixed one (called Combined Problems). All problems consist of a row of symbols, one of which has been replaced with a question mark. The respondent has to say which symbol the question mark stands for, choosing his or her answer from a labelled set of symbols. Although the tasks are quite simple, very limited time is given, so that almost no one finishes. The speed score is the total output across the three pure tests. The accuracy score is a function of the error rates across all four subtests, and the cognitive flexibility score a function of performance in the Combined Problems test in comparison to performance on the pure subtests.

The three scores relevant to automatisation (learning rate, total amount of work done in the automatisation exercise, and memory and understanding of the automatisation material) are derived from another sub-battery of the APIL, called Curve of Learning (COL). It consists of four sessions in which the test-taker translates symbols into high-frequency words (such as 'cars', 'jackets', 'three' and 'red') using a 'Dictionary'. In fact, the task is a two-step one, requiring the translation of each symbol into another symbol, and then that symbol into a word. Interspersed between the working sessions are study periods. The individual's performance improves as he or she learns more of the Dictionary and does not have to look everything up. After the fourth work session, the Dictionary is removed and the subject is tested on his or her knowledge of the symbol-symbol and symbol-word equivalences.

The final dimension, transfer, is measured with a test that is named the Knowledge Transfer Test (KTT), and which requires the individual to associate shapes known as 'pieces' with symbols that represent them. Learning takes place through study and feedback. The universe of pieces and symbols grows as the test progresses, and so does the complexity of the relationships between them.

The TRAM-2 battery

The TRAM-2 battery is intended for administration to individuals with between 10 and 12 years of formal education. Unlike the APIL, this battery has to be administered in its entirety. Testing time is about 2 hours 45 minutes. The six scores it produces are fluid intelligence, learning rate or automatisation, transfer, memory and understanding, speed of information processing, and accuracy of information processing.

Fluid intelligence is measured with a test similar to the conceptual test in the APIL, but with easier items. Learning rate or automatisation is assessed by giving the individual a simplified version of the translation exercise of the APIL, where the symbols translate directly into words. There are only two sessions, separated by a lesson and study period. These two sessions with their learning intervention comprise what is called Phase A of the battery. The learning rate score is a function of performance in the second session relative to the first. Transfer is assessed by giving the person a second symbol translation exercise called Phase B, which has material related to but different from the Phase A material. The transfer score is a function of performance in Phase B relative to the first part of Phase A. The final test, Memory and Understanding, assesses knowledge of the Phase A and B Dictionaries. The speed and accuracy scores are based on the person's performance across both phases of the learning material.

The TRAM-1 battery

This battery is intended for individuals with zero to nine years of formal education. Whereas TRAM-2 requires a moderate level of literacy (the ability to follow written instructions in the test book as they are read out by the test administrator, and the ability to use a separate answer sheet), TRAM-1 requires no literacy, as the instructions are verbally given in one of six languages: English, isiZulu, isiXhosa, South Sotho (Sesotho), Setswana and Afrikaans. All material is pictorial and there is no separate answer sheet. To respond to an item, the subject places a cross over the picture or diagram of his or her choice in the test book.

TRAM-1 has a similar structure to TRAM-2, and produces the same scores, with the exception of the fluid intelligence score. The conceptual test has been omitted because of time considerations. At this low level of formal education, instructions have to be very explicit, and therefore very lengthy to ensure comprehension. Even with the conceptual test excluded, the battery typically takes almost three hours to administer.

Scale intercorrelations, reliability, validity and bias investigations

APIL

In the APIL manual (Taylor, 2007a), intercorrelations matrices are presented for six samples, although there are actually 13 norm groups for the battery. The intercorrelation matrix of the most general sample (537 working individuals with post-matric education, racially quite representative, average age 34) reveals that intercorrelations vary between 0.42 and 0.85, and there are only three correlations less than 0.5. Hence, it is defensible to combine the eight scores into a global score.

The reliabilities of the scores were calculated in various ways. The reader is referred to the APIL manual (Taylor, 2007a) for the actual techniques used. For the eight component scores, the mean reliabilities were 0.82 for the CFT, 0.88 for Speed, 0.79 for Accuracy, 0.79 for Flexibility, 0.95 for COLtot, 0.66 for COLdiff, 0.77 for Memory and 0.80 for the KTT.

A fairly large number of validity studies are reported in the APIL manual (Taylor, 2007a). Some of them are briefly reported on here. More detail can be found in the manual.

In a study at a beverage company using only the automatisation part of the APIL battery, COLtot, COLdiff and Memory correlated 0.32, 0.33, and 0.35 respectively with an overall performance rating. The sample size was 110.

The APIL was administered to over 2 400 first-year applicants at a South African university. Correlation with academic subjects varied between 0.14 and 0.69. A small subsample of 110 students also did the Human Sciences Research Council's General Scholastic Aptitude Test (Claassen, De Beer, Hugo & Meyer, 1991). The global score of the APIL correlated 0.70 with this test. Hence a test of learning potential seemed to share about 50 per cent of its variance with a test of more crystallised abilities.

The APIL was administered to 137 applicants for Bachelor of Commerce bursaries offered by a financial institution. Independent ratings of the applicants were done by a human resources manager on a four-point scale. The global score of the APIL correlated 0.53 with the rating.

In a study at another financial institution, the APIL was administered to 221 employees. The company had a three-point rating: above average, average and below average. The correlation between the APIL global score and the rating was 0.62.

Lopes, Roodt & Mauer (2001) did a predictive validity study in a financial institution involving 235 successful job applicants. Unfortunately, the criterion score, which was a five-point performance rating scale, was rather unsatisfactory, being highly peaked in the centre. Eventually the authors reduced it to a two-point scale, combining the bottom three and top two ratings. With this reduced rating scale, they were able to correctly classify over 72 per cent of the individuals using the APIL scores. The authors concluded (p.68): 'What has been shown is that despite concerns relating to the reliability of the criterion, the APIL-B is nevertheless able to predict the performance of employees in a financial institution at a level of accuracy that makes the test battery an important proposition in the field of human resources assessment.'

Three predictive bias studies have been performed using the APIL, two of which appear in Taylor (2007a). The psychology examination results, drawn from the large university study mentioned earlier, were used. The sample size was 466, of which 66 individuals were black and the remaining 400 white. In this group, the correlation of the examination results with the APIL global score was 0.48. Procedures outlined in Jensen (1980) were applied to investigate the similarity of the slopes and intercepts. No significant differences were found on either of these parameters. The other bias study reported on in Taylor (2007a) involved undergraduate commerce students (32 black and 72 white) who were bursars of a financial institution. The students were in various years of study and at four different universities. End-of-year marks were available for each student. The correlation between the APIL global score and university marks was 0.46. Again, no significant differences were found in the slope and intercept values obtained for the black and white students.

In an independent predictive bias and validity study undertaken by Makgoatha (2006), the sample consisted of 55 black, 10 coloured, 33 Indian and 155 white subjects, all employees of a financial institution (not the same one as in the study mentioned above). The criterion was performance ratings. No evidence of bias was found. The global score of the APIL correlated 0.53 with the performance ratings.

TRAM-2

The intercorrelations of the six TRAM-2 dimensions were examined based on a sample of 526 working individuals with between 10 and 12 years of formal education, tested across South Africa, drawn quite representatively from all race groups, and with an average age of 33. The reliabilities of the scales were calculated for all six samples. The samples varied in size from 282 to 5 225. The average reliabilities were 0.91, 0.93, 0.94, 0.79, 0.81 and 0.90 for, respectively, the CFT, Speed, Accuracy, Learning Rate, Transfer and Memory. Specifics of how these reliabilities were calculated may be found in the TRAM-2 manual (Taylor, 2007b).

Some of the validity studies done on TRAM-2 are now described. More details concerning these studies are to be found in Taylor (2007b).

TRAM-2 was administered to a sample of 151 municipal workers in Gauteng. These individuals were apprentice applicants. The municipality also had scores on these individuals from three other tests: the Mental Alertness Test (Roberts, 1968), the High Level Figure Classification Test (Taylor & Segal, 1978) and a test of technical knowledge developed by the municipality. A three-point rating was also devised which took the form of a recommendation ('Recommended', 'Marginal', 'Not Recommended') based on interview impressions and all tests excluding TRAM-2. The TRAM-2 component scores correlated between 0.14 and 0.66. The global TRAM-2 score correlated 0.66.

TRAM-2 was also administered to 112 young male military recruits from an intake in Bloemfontein. The average age was 20 and all were matriculated.

The instructors divided the trainees into two equal-sized groups based on their perception of their trainability, Group 1 being the superior group. The groups differed beyond the 0.001 level of significance on all TRAM-2 dimensions.

The trainees' scores were available on an examination of the theoretical aspects of their training. The intercorrelations between the TRAM-2 component scores, global score, group membership and the examination score were considered. The global TRAM-2 score correlated 0.61 with the exam result and 0.60 with group membership. Both of these correlations are highly significant.

TRAM-2 was administered to a sample of 378 clerical and administrative personnel who worked for an import-export company. Performance ratings of supervisors regarding the overall competence of these individuals were obtained, the ratings being on a five-point scale ranging from 'poor' to 'outstanding'. The correlation of the global score of TRAM-2 with the rating was 0.47.

Data on 292 (175 black and 117 white) clerks and administrative personnel were used for a predictive bias study on TRAM-2. These respondents constituted the black and white components of the sample mentioned immediately above. The correlation between TRAM-2 scores and the criterion was 0.52 for the black group and 0.43 for the white group. Jensen's (1980) procedures were used to examine the differences between the slopes and intercepts of the regression lines. No significant differences were found.

TRAM-1

TRAM-1 scale intercorrelations were calculated based on a sample of 902 working individuals with formal education ranging between zero and 9 years. Almost all respondents were black (98 per cent). The reliabilities of the component scales were calculated as Learning Rate: 0.87; Transfer: 0.91; Speed: 0.92; Accuracy: 0.68; Memory: 0.91. Details of how the reliabilities were obtained are given in the TRAM-1 manual (Taylor, 2006).

The validity of the instrument is now discussed. TRAM-1 was administered to 54 miners who were at the time attending an in-house Adult Basic Education (ABE) course. The test-takers had been highly pre-selected on other tests (especially the Raven's Progressive Matrices) as well as on other criteria such as work performance. These individuals did considerably better on TRAM-1 than unselected miners.

Four scores were available from the course for English and Mathematics, tested at the middle and end of the course. The following criteria were employed for the purposes of the concurrent validity study: English final, Maths final, English improvement from the middle to end of the course, Maths improvement from the middle to the end of the course, and the sum of the English and Maths final course. The TRAM-1 global score correlated well with the overall ABE score (0.59). The improvement scores had quite restricted ranges, but a very creditable correlation of 0.38 was obtained between Maths improvement and the TRAM-1 score. This finding offers some justification for characterising TRAM-1 as a genuine learning potential assessment instrument.

In a study done by Van Aswegen (1997), TRAM-1 was used to test semi-literate miners who had already been pre-selected using other techniques. These individuals (a different group from the one discussed above) were put through an ABE course and 101 were ultimately sponsored at a technical college. The TRAM-1 scores for this 'elite' group were very high. For example, the mean score on the Memory and Understanding Test was 42.75, with 10 per cent of the sample obtaining 53 or 54 out of 54. In a sample used for mine-worker norms, the mean for this dimension was found to be only 26.3.

As regards bias, no studies have been undertaken because almost all testees who do TRAM-1 are black.

Conclusion

With the advent of democracy in South Africa, there was some concern in the psychometric community that tests would be seen by the new government as a tool to maintain white dominance in the workplace and hence would be banned. The banning did not occur, although strict standards were put in place for tests, enshrined in law.

The Employment Equity Act No. 55 of 1998 states that a person be considered for a given position even if he or she lacks the requisite skills to do the job but has the potential to acquire those skills within a reasonable period of time. This clearly imposes a responsibility for training on an organisation, to a much greater extent than is the case in a first world country, where applicants are expected to arrive with the skills already in place. And of course, it places on the organisation the onus of identifying potential.

The assessment of learning potential seems to be the most defensible of the psychometric methods to use in South Africa, for this approach is in tune with the aspiration of uplifting people whose opportunities in the past have been limited – who have not had the opportunities of the more privileged to acquire valuable skills. And those inequalities persist in the new South Africa. Tests that measure specific skills or abilities are to a large extent an index of 'history', and history has not been fair in South Africa. But tests of learning potential can be used in a positive way, for they are a measure of 'the future'.

The damage of the past – such as poor schooling in the formative years – cannot be totally expunged by later developmental programmes, but these programmes can go a long way towards improving the situation. In the workplace, financial and other resources are limited, so not all employees will be given developmental opportunities – just those who are most likely to benefit from them, and thus become a greater asset for the organisation. Learning potential tests become a means of selecting people *for* development – a somewhat new application for tests, which have traditionally been used to disbar people at the gate who do not have the skills required for a given job.

The fluidity and dynamism of the modern workplace offers a further justification for the use of tests of learning potential. Jobs change rapidly, skills become outdated and organisations restructure themselves frequently. Hence, employees are on a constant learning curve. It is important to know whether a person is able to acquire new skills rapidly. Learning potential tests offer such information.

Given that learning potential assessment is a justifiable and appropriate psychometric approach, it is necessary to consider what sorts of activities a test of learning potential should incorporate. Since the work of Vygotsky, there has been a preference for assessing learning potential as an improvement score that reflects the degree to which a lesson or learning intervention has impacted positively on the person's performance in a given intellectual task. However, there are some psychometric objections to this approach, and there is also the issue of whether an improvement score is the only one that is relevant in the assessment of learning potential. As was discussed earlier in this chapter, a case can be made for a broader conception of learning potential. Transfer is a form of learning that is not explicitly assessed in the test-learn-test model. And there seems to be a place for certain constructs that are not actual learning phenomena, but are nevertheless fundamental to learning. The most important of these seem to be fluid intelligence and information processing efficiency.

The studies reported here are based on particular samples, and hence cannot be extrapolated to make extravagant claims regarding the appropriateness of the APIL and TRAM instruments for use in South Africa, but the results are encouraging. Strong predictive and concurrent validity correlations have been obtained, and there is evidence that the tests genuinely measure learning potential. The strength of the predictive power of APIL and TRAM tests might be partly due to the fact that they incorporate a motivational element. In both the automatisation and transfer elements of the test, the person has to learn new things – and this demands effort. Individuals who are willing to put in extra effort in the test situation are likely to do the same in real-life situations.

References

Ackerman, P. L. (1988). Determinants of individual differences during skill acquisition: Cognitive abilities and information processing. *Journal of Experimental Psychology: General, 117(3),* 288–318.

Baddeley, A. D. (1986). *Working Memory.* Oxford: Clarendon Press.

Cattell, R. B. (1971). *Abilities: Their Structure, Growth and Action.* Boston, MA: Houghton Mifflin.

Claassen, N. C. W., De Beer, M., Hugo, H. L. E. & Meyer, H. M. (1991). *Manual for the General Scholastic Aptitude Test (GSAT) Senior Series.* Pretoria: Human Sciences Research Council.

Cronbach, L. J. & Furby, L. (1970). How should we measure 'change' – or should we? *Psychological Bulletin, 74(1),* 68–80.

Embretson, S. E. (1987). Towards the development of a psychometric approach. In C. S. Lidz (Ed.), *Dynamic Assessment* (pp. 141–172). New York, NY: The Guilford Press.

Feuerstein, R., Rand, Y. & Hoffman, M. B. (1979). *The Dynamic Assessment of Retarded Performers: The Learning Potential Assessment Device, Theory, Instruments and Techniques.* Baltimore, MD: University Park Press.

Glutting, J. J. & McDermott, P. A. (1990). Principles and problems in learning potential. In C. R. Reynolds & R. W. Kamphaus (Eds), *Handbook of Psychological and Educational Assessment of Children* (pp. 277–295). New York, NY: The Guilford Press.

Grigorenko, E. L. & Sternberg, R. J. (1998). Dynamic testing. *Psychological Bulletin, 124(1),* 75–111.

Horn, J. L. (1989). Models of intelligence. In R. L. Linn (Ed.), *Intelligence* (pp. 29–73). Chicago, IL: University of Chicago Press.

Jensen, A. R. (1980). *Bias in Mental Testing*. London & New York, NY: Methuen & Free Press.

Larson, G. E. & Saccuzzo, G. E. (1989). Cognitive correlates of general intelligence: Towards a process theory of *g*. *Intelligence, 13(1)*, 5–31.

Lopes, A., Roodt, G. & Mauer, R. (2001). The predictive validity of the APIL-B in a financial institution. *South African Journal of Industrial Psychology, 27(1)*, 61–69.

Makgoatha, J. (2006). APIL-B: Cross-cultural predictive validity in a consulting environment. Unpublished Master's dissertation. University of Johannesburg, Johannesburg.

Raven, J., Raven, J. C. & Court, J. H. (1998). *Manual for Raven's Progressive Matrices and Vocabulary Scales. Section 1: General Overview*. San Antonio, TX: Harcourt Assessment.

Roberts, O. P. (1968). *User's Manual for the High Level Battery*. Johannesburg: National Institute for Personnel Research.

Sijtsma, K. (1996). Psychometric issues in learning potential assessment. In J. H. M. Hamers, K. Sijtsma & A. J. J M. Ruijssenaars (Eds), *Learning Potential Assessment: Theoretical, Methodological and Practical Issues* (pp. 175–194). Lisse: Swets & Zeitlinger.

Snow, R. E., Kyllonen, P. C. & Marshalek, B. (1984). The topography of ability and learning correlations. In R. J. Sternberg (Ed.), *Advances in the Psychology of Human Intelligence* Volume 2 (pp. 47–103). Hillsdale, NJ: Lawrence Erlbaum.

Snow, R. E. & Lohman, D. F. (1984). Towards a theory of cognitive aptitude for learning from instruction. *Journal of Educational Psychology, 76(3)*, 347–376.

Snow, R. E., Marshalek, B. & Lohman, D. F. (1976). Correlation of selected cognitive abilities and cognitive processing parameters: An exploratory study. Unpublished manuscript, School of Education, Stanford University, Palo Alto, CA.

Spearman, C. E. (1927). *The Abilities of Man: Their Nature and Measurement*. London: Macmillan.

Sternberg, R. J. (1985). *Beyond IQ: A Triarchic Theory of Human Intelligence*. New York, NY: Cambridge University Press.

Sternberg, R. J. (1997). The triarchic theory of intelligence. In D. P. Flanagan, J. L. Genshaft & P. L. Harrison (Eds), *Contemporary Intellectual Assessment: Theories, Tests and Issues* (pp. 92–104). New York: The Guilford Press.

Taylor, T. R. (1994). A review of three approaches to cognitive assessment and a proposed integrated approach based on a unifying theoretical framework. *South African Journal of Psychology, 24(4)*, 184–193.

Taylor, T. R. (2006). *Administrator's Manual for TRAM-1 Battery, Edition 3*. Johannesburg: Aprolab.

Taylor, T. R. (2007a). *Administrator's Manual for APIL Battery, Edition 3*. Johannesburg: Aprolab.

Taylor, T. R. (2007b). *Administrator's Manual for TRAM-2 Battery, Edition 3*. Johannesburg: Aprolab.

Taylor, T. R. & Segal, M. (1978). *Administrator's Manual for the High Level FCT*. Johannesburg: National Institute for Personnel Research.

Van Aswegen, M. (1997). The standardisation of a learning potential battery for the selection of poorly qualified employees. Unpublished Master's dissertation. University of Pretoria, Pretoria.

Vygotsky, L. S. (1978). *Mind in Society: The Development of Higher Psychological Processes*. Cambridge, MA: Harvard University Press.

12 The Griffiths Mental Developmental Scales: an overview and a consideration of their relevance for South Africa

L. Jacklin and K. Cockcroft

The Griffiths Mental Development Scales (GMDS) is one of a variety of tests available for assessing the development of young children. It consists of two separate developmental scales, one scale for infants and toddlers (aged 0–2 years) and the other for young children (aged 2–8 years), making it one of the few developmental tests that can be used to assess children from birth across all areas of their development.

The GMDS was developed in the UK in 1954 by Ruth Griffiths, who observed children in their natural environments while they were engaged in their everyday activities. Griffiths's purpose was to develop an instrument that contained a comparative profile of abilities across various domains of development, and which would facilitate early diagnosis of deficits in child development. Although standardised in the UK, the GMDS is widely used throughout the world and is especially popular in South Africa (Luiz, Oelofsen, Stewart & Michell, 1995).[1]

In South Africa, testing and assessment have been heavily criticised as possessing limited value for culturally diverse populations (Foxcroft, 1997; Nzimande, 1995; Sehlapelo & Terre Blanche, 1996). Despite these criticisms, it has also been pointed out that, regardless of its flaws, testing remains more reliable and valid than any of the limited number of alternatives. It is argued that since testing plays a crucial role within assessment internationally, the focus should be on valid and reliable tests for use within multicultural and multilingual societies (Plug in Foxcroft, 1997). Thus, one of the aims of this chapter is to determine the extent to which the GMDS is a valid and reliable measure for assessing the development of South African children.

The original GMDS has been extensively researched and compared to other commonly used developmental tests and shown to be valid (Luiz, Foxcroft & Stewart, 2001). Subsequent to the revision of the GMDS Infant Scales in 1996 and the Extended Scales for older children in 2004, research emerged that assessed the strengths and weaknesses of the revised scales, much of which has been done in South Africa (for example, Laughton et al., 2010b; Luiz, Foxcroft & Povey, 2006). What follows is an overview of this research, preceded by a brief description of the GMDS.

The development and structure of the GMDS

The GMDS was developed sequentially as two complementary tests – namely, 'The Abilities of Babies' (1954) for infants and toddlers (0–2 years) and 'The Abilities of Young Children' (1970) for older children (2–8 years – also referred to as the Extended Scales), a structure which is still in place. Subsequent to the development of the GMDS by Ruth Griffiths, substantial gains in the cognitive and developmental abilities of children have been noticed (Flynn & Weiss, 2007; Lynn, 2009). Referred to as the 'Flynn effect', these gains indicate that child development is dynamic and suggest that regular renorming of the GMDS is essential. The first revision of the GMDS commenced in 1996, when a comprehensive review of the infant and toddlers scales was undertaken (Huntley, 1996). In 2004, the GMDS Extended Scales were revised following extensive research, with key participation by South African researchers who led the process (Luiz, Barnard, Knoesen, Kotras, McAlinden & O'Connell, 2004). The descriptions of the scales below refer to these revised versions, unless otherwise indicated.

The GMDS Infant Scales

The Infant Scales consist of five scales (A–E), each evaluating an important dimension of early development. The Locomotor Scale (Scale A) measures developing gross motor skills important for an upright posture, walking, running and climbing. It allows for the observation of physical weakness or disability or defects of movement. The Personal-Social Scale (Scale B) requires more input from the primary caregiver than the other scales, as it measures early adaptive and self-help behaviour typically seen at home, as well as social behaviour that develops through early adult–child interactions. The Hearing and Speech Scale (Scale C) is considered to be the most intellectual scale and evaluates the development of language, by measuring responses to environmental sounds and speech as well as the production of sounds and words. The Eye and Hand Coordination Scale (Scale D) consists of items requiring fine motor handwork and visual ability. It assesses manipulative skills such as visual tracking, reaching and grasping, pen-and-paper skills and object manipulation. The Performance Scale (Scale E) evaluates manipulation skill, speed and precision of work. It assesses the application of developing skills in novel situations and examines simple object exploratory behaviour, object permanence and manipulation of form-board items (Huntley, 1996).

The GMDS is criterion-referenced in nature, and so the child is compared to an established criterion and not to another child. This is important for cross-cultural assessment, as it assesses the degree of mastery of the individual and serves to describe rather than to compare performance. The manual for the Infant Scales allows for raw scores to be converted into a subquotient for each of the five scales, an overall General Quotient (GQ), age in months or percentiles. Expressing the score as a percentile has a number of uses as it allows the professional to track a child's development over an extended time period using both versions of the GMDS.

Each scale is equally weighted, which allows for the generation of a developmental profile that can be used to produce a visual representation of the strengths and weaknesses of the child. This can be particularly useful when reporting the results to the layperson who may not otherwise understand them (Huntley, 1996). In resource-limited communities, the profile can also guide referral decisions, such as which of the allied medical disciplines will be of greatest assistance to the child. Profiles can also provide a description of a child with a particular disability or syndrome; for example, children with autism show characteristic weaknesses in the Personal-Social, Hearing and Practical Reasoning Scales, and relative strengths in the other scales (Gowar, 2003). A scale can be used in isolation by researchers wishing to investigate a particular developmental domain, as demonstrated by Giagazoglou, Kyparas, Fotiadou and Angelopoulou (2007), who studied the effect of maternal education on the motor development of a child.

In the selection of an assessment tool for research or for clinical practice, the validity and reliability of the tool are important, particularly with reference to the community of the child who is to be tested. The normative sample that was used for the Infant Scales was drawn from six regions in the UK, with the majority coming from an urban community (488:177; urban:rural) and an over-representation of boys (366:299; boys:girls). All the mothers of the sample spoke English to their children. Those children who were known to have a severe disability were excluded (Huntley, 1996). The socio-economic distribution was biased in favour of the higher classes when compared to the 1991 British national census. It must be borne in mind that the normative sample was therefore potentially biased in favour of a higher-functioning group of children (Reyes, Pacifico, Benitez, Villanueva-uy & Ostrea, 2010). The distribution curve of the normative scores for the Infant Scales showed a mean of 100.5 with a standard deviation of 11.8.

Statistical evaluation of the test found the reliability of the tool to be adequate. The internal consistency of the items was measured using a split-level method, and the resulting correlation coefficient, which was corrected using the Spearman-Brown formula, was 0.95. An average standard error of measurement (SEM) of 2.8 was obtained across all the ages and subscores of the Infant Scales, representing an acceptable level of accuracy (Huntley, 1996).

In children who are very young, the development of functional skills can vary widely from one construct to another; for example, one toddler may be more advanced in speaking but relatively slow to walk, whereas another may show the opposite development. It is therefore important to be able to ascertain when the variation in scores from one developmental skill or construct to another is significant, and equally important to ascertain whether the difference between the GQ and a subquotient is statistically significant. When the reliability was calculated for the Infant Scales, it was found that a difference as high as 22 points between subquotients is acceptable (1 per cent confidence) before further investigation or intervention is required (Huntley, 1996). For an illustration of this, see Table 12.1.

Table 12.1 GMDS Infant Scales minimum difference between subquotients, and between subquotient and GQ, required for statistical significance

Level of significance	Subquotient/GQ	Subquotients
5%	13	17
1%	18	22

Source: Adapted from Huntley (1996).

Confidence that the test can be trusted to accurately measure the same functional skills over a period of time in the same child is important. This test-retest stability is essential where any form of sequential evaluation is done, whether in research or in clinical practice. The test-retest reliability on the Infant Scales is low under one year of age (.28–.48), but highly reliable from the second year onwards (.82) (Huntley, 1996). This indicates some difficulties with the Infant Scales. In addition, for professionals working with significantly delayed children, the inability to convert raw scores into a meaningful score if the child's performance is more than two standard deviations below the norm limits the use of the scales in tracking the developmental progress of such children (personal experience and verbal communication with Laughton, 2010). The poor transition from the Infant Scales into the Extended Scales for older children is another weakness (Laughton et al., 2010b). This problem has been identified by the Association for Research in Infant and Child Development (ARICD), which is responsible for monitoring the quality of administration of the GMDS. The ARICD is undertaking a revision of the GMDS which will address the poor correlations between the Infant and the Extended Scales (personal communication with Elizabeth Julyan, 16 June 2010).

South African research on the GMDS Infant Scales

Most of the South African research on the GMDS has focused on the Extended Scales (for example, Allan, 1988; 1992; Bhamjee, 1991; Heimes, 1983; Luiz et al., 2006; Luiz et al., 2001; Mothule, 1990; Sweeney, 1994; Tukulu, 1996). To date, reliability and validity studies have not been conducted in South Africa on the 1996 revision of the Infant Scales, although preliminary studies of face and construct validity have been conducted on the Extended Scales (Barnard, 2003; Kotras, 2003; Luiz, 1994; Luiz et al., 2006; Luiz et al., 2001). Given the difficulty related to the use of appropriate assessment tools with South Africa's culturally diverse population, and since the British norms are currently used as an evaluation standard for the performance of South African infants, we report here on studies that attempted to determine the appropriateness of the Infant Scales for South African infants.

Amod, Cockcroft and Soellaart (2007) compared the performance of 40 black infants between 13 and 16 months, residing in Johannesburg, to the normative sample of the Infant Scales. Although the groups were not demographically identical, an attempt was made to control for extraneous variables which could influence the results – namely, age, developmental normality and urban or rural residence – by holding them constant in the analyses, while the variables gender and socio-economic status were controlled for by including them in the research design. The South African infants performed significantly better on the Eye-Hand Coordination and Performance Scales, but significantly poorer on the Personal-Social Scale relative to the normative sample, suggesting differences between the developmental rate of the British and South African infants, with each culture appearing to support a distinct aspect of development. A tentative explanation for the better performance of the local infants is the concept of African infant precocity, first advanced by Falade (1955), who found that Senegalese infants assessed on the Gesell Developmental Screening Inventory were significantly more advanced in areas of fine motor development, eye-hand coordination, problem-solving and object permanence than matched Caucasian American infants. Similar results were obtained with Ugandan infants (Gerber, 1958), Nigerian infants (Freedman, 1974) and African South African infants (Lynn, 2009; Richter-Strydom & Griesel, 1984).

The other main finding from the Amod et al. (2007) study was that the British sample performed significantly better than the local sample on the Personal-Social Scale. Since this scale may be influenced by socio-cultural and/or emotional differences (Griffiths, 1984), this difference could be related to varied child-rearing practices across the two cultural groups. Furthermore, the Personal-Social Scale is one of the least cognitive scales of the GMDS, and requires more input from primary caregivers than the other scales because it measures self-help behaviours typically seen at home, as well as social behaviour that develops through early adult–child interactions (McLean, McCormick & Baird, 1991). Aldridge Smith, Bidder, Gardner and Gray (1980) also found that the Personal-Social Scale of the 1970 version of the GMDS was more sensitive to use by different assessors when evaluating the development of infants from 6 months to 7.25 years, suggesting that results obtained from this scale should be interpreted with caution.

Some previously reported findings do not concur with those of Amod et al. (2007). For example, an investigation of the GMDS profiles of HIV-positive black South African infants found that their mean performance on the Personal-Social Scale was above average (Kotras, 2001). However, there was considerable variability among the infants' scores, with some infants performing extremely well and others performing well below the average range. Kotras suggested that infants raised in low socio-economic environments are sometimes left with little or no supervision, and hence become more independent at personal-social tasks such as dressing and undressing, holding a cup or using a spoon. The Personal-Social Scale from the Extended Scales shows the lowest correlation with the GQ, which may be indicative of that scale's cultural bias and of the possibility that it may be measuring attributes different from the other scales (Luiz et al., 2001). Whether this holds for infants as well needs to be determined, but this may be one of the reasons for the difference obtained on this scale by Amod et al. (2007).

In general, the results of Amod et al.'s (2007) study confirmed those of other local studies (Kotras, 2001; Luiz, 1988a; 1988b; 1988c; 1994; Luiz et al., 2001) that have shown the GMDS (for both infants and children) to be measuring a construct that is consistent across cultures. However, there were also some differences in performance between the South African sample and the norm group that could be attributed to cultural bias in the Infant Scales. Consequently, an examination of item bias or score comparability with a larger sample is necessary to determine whether members of different cultural groups demonstrate specific patterns of responses (Owen, 1991).

A major factor that has been found to affect test performance is level of education, both that of the testee and that of his or her parents (Kriegler & Skuy, 1996; Skuy, Schutte, Fridjhon & O'Carroll, 2001). This means that the use of available internationally relevant tests in South Africa would be a viable option, but only for educated and Westernised individuals, and that less literate, less Westernised and less educated groups may require the development of new and culturally appropriate measures (Nell, 1997). In this regard, Cockcroft, Amod and Soellaart (2008) compared the performance of infants with educated, professionally employed and less educated, nonprofessional mothers on the Infant Scales. The sample consisted of 40 black South African infants aged between 13 and 16 months (21 boys and 19 girls) residing in Johannesburg. The distinction between infants with highly educated, professional mothers and those with less educated, nonprofessional mothers was based on level of education and occupation of the infant's mother. Fifty per cent of the mothers had some tertiary education and were employed in professional occupations. Of the remainder, 27.5 per cent had received 12 years of formal education, while 20 per cent had completed 10 years of formal education and 2.5 per cent of the mothers had 7 years or less of formal education. None of the latter three groups of mothers were employed in professional occupations. The infants with highly educated, professional mothers performed significantly better than infants with less highly educated, nonprofessional mothers on the GQ and the Locomotor Scale. Allan (1988; 1992) found significant differences between high and low socio-economic English and Afrikaans groups on the GQ and the Hearing and Speech, Eye-Hand Coordination, Practical Reasoning and Performance Scales, although his sample consisted of 5-year-old children. The discrepancy in the ages of the samples in the Allan (1988; 1992) and Cockcroft et al. (2008) studies may partly account for the variation in scales of the GMDS in which differences were found. The effects of maternal level of education and, by association, socio-economic status may become more marked as the child develops, accounting for the more pervasive differences found by Allan.

While home environment plays an important role in the cognitive and academic outcome of high-risk infants, findings are inconsistent with regard to its influence on motor skills (Sommerfelt, Ellertsen & Markestad, 1995). The development of gross motor skills appears to be differentially influenced by the home environment, with infants from lower socio-economic groups performing significantly more poorly than their wealthier counterparts (Goyen & Lui, 2002). This may subsequently impact on their general intellectual functioning, as motor development during these formative years provides a foundation for subsequent development and optimises occupational performance in the areas of self-care, learning, recreation and play. Further evidence for the close connection between gross motor functioning and intellectual and social development is revealed by the findings of Luiz et al. (2006). Within their sample of 180 4–7-year-old South African children, the more discrete cognitive, motor and personal-social functions tapped by the GMDS were not clearly delineated when subjected to a factor analysis. With the exception of the Performance Scale, all of the scales seemed to tap complex skills or more than one construct, and aspects of the constructs tapped appeared to differ for the various age groups in the study. These findings would support the proposal that the differences found between the infants on the GMDS may become more pronounced and/or widespread with age, and/or that the Infant Scales may overestimate performance in the first year of life. The latter reflects the instability of development in the very young child, and is common to all developmental measures used on infants under one year old.

Further support for this proposal comes from Laughton et al.'s (2010a) longitudinal study of the developmental outcomes of Xhosa-speaking infants from low socio-economic backgrounds. The infants were assessed on the Infant Scales at 10–12 months and again at 20–22 months. Their performance was in the average range at the first assessment and decreased significantly to below age-appropriate levels by the second assessment. The decline in performance was unexpected, and is incongruous with the British norms which do not show such a decline. Possible reasons for this may include the instability of the GMDS in the first year of life, the use of a cohort from only low socio-economic circumstances, and cultural bias in the GMDS. The Hearing and Language Scale was the most affected, showing a decrease of more than one standard deviation. Since language development has been shown to be related to maternal education and socio-economic status (Magnuson, Sexton, Davis-Kean & Huston, 2009), the GMDS may be more discerning when testing language development as the child develops. For example, at 11 months a child is only expected to use 3 words meaningfully, identify 2 objects and try to sing, whereas at 21 months, the child is expected to use 20 words meaningfully, identify 7 objects and use word combinations. Decreases in performance were found on all of the other scales with the exception of the Locomotor Scale, suggesting that the Infant Scales may overestimate performance in the first year. This is due to the volatility in development in the first year of life, and indicates that it is critical to reassess the child after the first year in order to accurately predict functioning of children from disadvantaged circumstances.

The Infant Scales have also been used locally to assess the developmental ability of children with a range of neurodevelopmental disorders. Of these, HIV encephalopathy is currently the most common cause of developmental delay in South African children, with a prevalence of 2.5 per cent in children 12 years and younger. Laughton et al. (2009) compared the developmental outcome on the Infant Scales of four groups of children aged between 10 and 15 months. Group 1 comprised HIV-unexposed, uninfected children; Group 2 had HIV-exposed, uninfected children; Group 3 had HIV-infected children who were receiving antiretroviral treatment (ART) initiated before 12 weeks of age; and Group 4 consisted of HIV-infected children with ART deferred until immunological or clinical criteria could be determined. As shown in Figure 12.1, Group 4 showed a significant delay in development compared to the other groups, indicating the negative impact of delaying ART.

Figure 12.1 Developmental outcome in deferred treatment, early treatment, exposed and unexposed infants

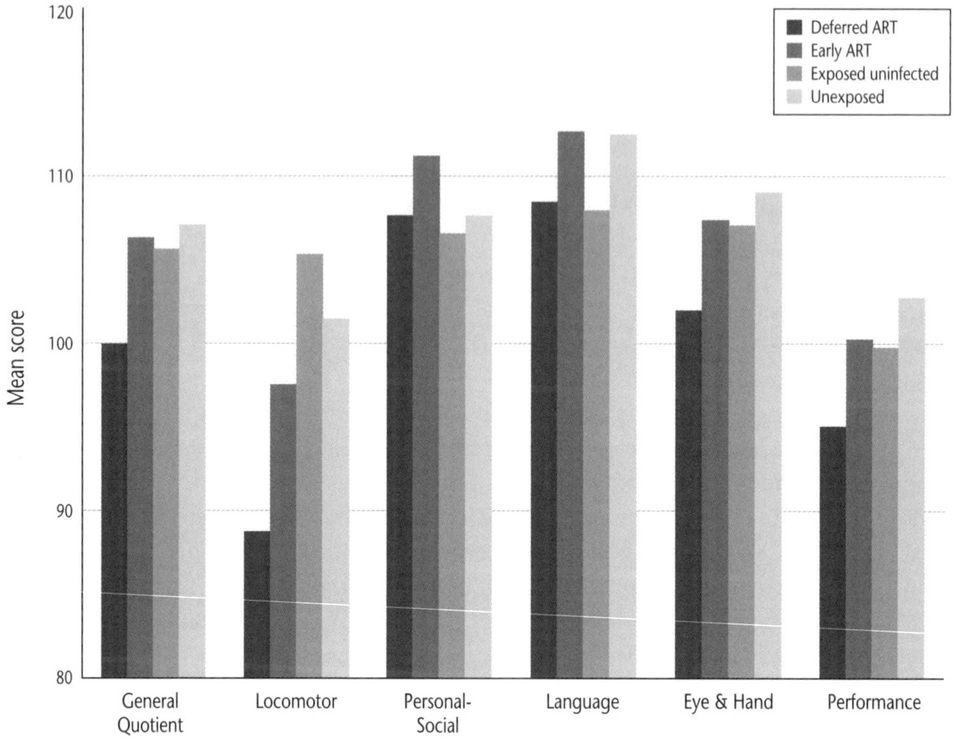

Source: Laughton et al. (2009), reproduced with permission.

Laughton et al. (2010a) also studied 37 HIV-affected children on ART treatment and 41 controls from the same community. The children were followed up over a period of 30 months and tested four times (at approximately 10-, 21-, 31- and 42-week intervals) using both the Infant and Extended Scales. It was found that the HIV-affected group's locomotor development was initially impaired, but improved to average levels at 42 months. In contrast, performance on the Personal-Social Scale deteriorated significantly in the HIV-affected children. Of significance is that there was a steady decline in the performance of both the HIV-affected children and the control group, again suggesting that the Infant Scales should be used with caution when predicting later developmental outcomes in local populations.

The Extended Scales

The Extended Scales for children aged 2–8 years differ in structure from the Infant Scales by the addition of the Practical Reasoning Scale, which appraises the child's arithmetical insight and problem-solving skills. The interpretation of the raw score in the 2006 revision of the Extended Scales is norm-based and is not represented as a coefficient, as it was in the first version of the test. The manual allows for scores to be presented as an age equivalent, z-score or percentile.

Prior to the revision of the Extended Scales, systematic research was conducted into the psychometric properties of the scales. It was found that they all tap the same underlying construct – namely, general intelligence, which appeared to be consistent across cultures (Luiz et al., 2001). The research was then extended to determine the construct validity of the items within each scale across three age groups – namely, 5, 6 and 7 years. The results showed that many of the scales tapped more than one construct, and some overlapped. Further, there was also evidence of a cultural bias in the Personal-Social Scale. Magongoa and Venter (2003) used the original version of the GMDS extended scales to examine potential developmental differences between rural black children with well-controlled clonic-tonic epilepsy and typically developing controls. Unsurprisingly, the children with epilepsy performed significantly lower than the controls. Interestingly, the controls obtained quotients between 113 and 120 on all but the Eye and Hand Coordination and Performance Scales. This better-than-average performance suggests that the developmental acceleration found by Flynn and Weiss (2007) and Lynn (2009) is also present in developing communities, and supported the need for restandardisation of the Extended Scales.

The research of Barnard (2003) was intrinsic to the restandardisation of the Extended Scales. It focused on the Practical Reasoning Scale and aimed to generate new items by means of a focus group, a facet analysis to investigate the comprehensiveness of the scale, and testing of the items. Three criteria were used for assessment of the items: negative responses to the items in a survey sent to GMDS users, an assessment of the items' reliability, and the difficulty of items. If there was a difference in passing the item by different cultural groups or genders, the item was rejected. Although the intention was to standardise the Extended Scales in Britain, the acceptability of the GMDS for use with white South African children was also emphasised because of previous research demonstrating their similarity to the British children (Barnard, 2003).

The normative sample for the Extended Scales consisted of 1 026 children from the UK. They ranged from 3 to 8 years and were evenly distributed across the ages and genders. Most (86 per cent) of the children were from an urban area and belonged to a middle or higher socio-economic group (upper, 32 per cent; middle, 44 per cent; lower, 24 per cent). The children were chosen on the basis of having English as a first language and generally normal development (Luiz, Barnard et al., 2004). Thus, as with the Infant Scales, there is possibly a bias towards a higher-functioning group of children.

The statistical basis for the restandardisation of the Extended Scales is described in the manual (Luiz, Faragher et al., 2006). The reliability of the scales was computed using the Cronbach alpha coefficient. The SEM was found to be very difficult to calculate and it was converted into a confidence range instead.

Once the Extended Scales had been restandardised, extensive research was undertaken to determine the validity of the constructs in each scale. In terms of local research, Kotras (2003) focused on the validation of the Language Scale. A construct analysis led to the identification of six constructs in this scale: receptive language, basic concepts/conceptualisation, knowledge, memory, reasoning and expressive language. The constructs were found to be equivalent across socio-economic groups and genders for English-speaking children. Knoesen (2005) demonstrated that the Locomotor Scale is made up of seven basic constructs – namely, balance, gross body coordination, visual motor coordination, rhythm, power and strength, agility and flexibility, and depth perception. She expressed concern about the under-representation of some other facets related to locomotor ability, such as speed of movement. Moosajee (2007) explored the construct validity of the Personal-Social Scale and also found that the tasks in the scale were multidimensional, comprising six main constructs (dressing, personal hygiene, feeding, cooperation, self-knowledge and sociability). These constructs were equivalent for all socio-economic groups and both genders. Although the facets in this scale covered an adequate range of items, certain important life skills were not addressed, such as personal safety and security. Povey (2008), on investigating the Eye-Hand Coordination Scale, found that each item in the scale had more than one underlying construct, but that there were underlying constructs that were common to all the items – namely, fine motor coordination, visual-motor integration and spatial orientation. Concern was expressed about the limited variety of skills tested in the Eye-Hand Coordination Scale for the older age group, and recommendations were made that more items be added to test a wider range of abilities. In order to assess the construct validity of the entire Extended Scales (first edition), Luiz et al. (Luiz, Foxcroft & Tukulu, 2004) investigated whether they correlated with performance on the Denver Developmental Screening Test II for 60 Xhosa-speaking children aged between 3 and 6 years. While there was a significant correlation between the measures, the Denver had more items which were culturally biased, and a much higher percentage of children were found to be developmentally delayed on the Denver than on the GMDS. (See Appendix 1 for further discussion of current research on South African use of the GMDS.)

In addition to construct validation studies, there has been interest in comparing the performance of South African children to that of the GMDS normative sample. Van Rooyen (2005) conducted the first such study on 129 children aged 4, 5, 6 and 7 years, across socio-economic and racial groups. He found that the South African children performed significantly better than the normative group on the Locomotor and Personal-Social Scales, while the British children performed significantly better on the more academic Language and Practical Reasoning Scales. The groups' performance was comparable on the Hand-Eye Coordination Scale, and too variable to be interpreted on the Performance Scale. Van Heerden (2007) conducted a similar study in which the performance of 31 black and white South African children, aged between 5 years and 6 years 11 months, was compared to the Extended Scale norms. The comparison groups were matched in terms of age, gender and socio-economic status. The local children performed significantly more poorly on the Language, Hand-Eye Coordination and Practical Reasoning Scales, while there were no significant differences between the groups on the Locomotor, Personal-Social and Performance Scales. Kheswa (2009) studied 20 Xhosa-speaking children aged between 3 and 8 years from a low socio-economic environment. The children were grouped according to age and whether they performed below, equivalent to, or above their chronological age on the Extended Scales. There was a trend towards strengths on the Locomotor and Personal-Social Scales, but underachievement on all the other scales. Kheswa (2009) also found that the South African children tended to underperform compared to the British norms on the more academic scales, suggesting a need for caution when using the scales with local populations. Further, there was a progressive deterioration in the scores as the children developed, which has also been observed in longitudinal studies using the Infant Scales and in other developing countries (Laughton et al., 2010b; Reyes et al., 2010). Unfortunately, Kheswa's (2009) sample was small, and repetition with a bigger sample is warranted to verify their findings. Although exploratory in nature, these differences suggest that the development of local children may be impeded by poor environmental circumstances, such as lack of stimulation and poor nutrition, and that there is a need for appropriate developmental interventions for South African children.

The predictive validity of the Extended Scales was explored by Knoesen (2003), who assessed 93 black, coloured, white and Indian South African preschool children and reviewed their school performance at the end of Grade 1. She found a significant relationship between the Language, Hand-Eye Coordination, Performance and Practical Reasoning Scales and the GQ and academic achievement in Literacy, Numeracy and Life Orientation. The Locomotor and Personal-Social Scales, which are the least intellectual of the six scales, were not significantly related to these academic areas. Limited support exists for idea that there is a relationship between motor skills and academic ability generally (Tramonta, Hooper & Selzer, 1988), while the Personal-Social Scale of the Extended Scales predominantly taps self-help behaviours which are different to the personal-social skills required in the early grades of schooling, the latter being related to the ability of the child to work cooperatively and sustain attention. In general, this study provided supportive evidence for the predictive value of the Extended Scales in identifying children at risk prior to entering formal education.

The possible influence of gender on the Extended Scales was explored by Jakins (2009), who compared the performance of preschool black, coloured and white girls (N = 32) and boys (N = 32) aged between five years and six years 11 months. The groups were matched for socio-economic status and ethnic group, and all had English as their home language. No significant differences were found between the genders, suggesting that the items in the Extended Scales have been appropriately selected to allow equal opportunities for girls and boys to perform.

Like the Infant Scales, the Extended Scales have also been used locally to assess the developmental ability of children with a range of neurodevelopmental disorders. Of these, Foetal Alcohol Spectrum Disorder is a major public health problem, with the highest prevalence rates reported in Wellington in the Western Cape (Viljoen et al., 2005). Adnams, Kodituwakku, Hay, Molteno, Viljoen and May (2001) compared the neurocognitive profiles on the Extended Scales of 34 Grade 1 children with Foetal Alcohol Syndrome (FAS) and 34 typically developing controls. The FAS children performed significantly more poorly than the controls on higher-order cognitive abilities, as assessed by the Speech and Hearing, Performance, Practical Reasoning and Eye-Hand Coordination Scales. There was a marginal effect on the Personal-Social Scale, which was relatively independent of the other cognitive competencies, suggesting that there is far less difference in adaptive functioning between the groups than on the other higher-order cognitive scales. This provides supportive evidence that FAS children experience difficulty with tasks involving sustained attention, fine motor coordination, problem-solving and verbal reasoning (Conry, 1990; Mattson & Riley, 1998), although studies of language function in such populations have produced inconsistent results. It also suggests that the GMDS – Extended Revised (GMDS-ER) is sensitive to discriminating these abilities in such a population, and may be useful in creating a developmental profile of functioning for children with FAS.

On the basis of the studies reported here, it has been recommended by many researchers that the GMDS be restandardised for South African children, which seems logical given the ever-increasing differences in standard of living between various sectors of South African society (Appel, 2011). However, this is a complicated issue as it raises questions regarding whether restandardising the GMDS implies that the mean should be dropped so that local children appear to be developing normally, when the South African norm may be far lower than the global norm, or whether a 'gold standard' should be maintained which clearly demonstrates the influence of poverty, malnutrition and a deteriorating level of education on local children. In addition, the need for developmental screening in South Africa has been widely debated, with substantial support from local researchers and practitioners (Povey, 2008; Van Heerden, 2007; Van Rooyen, 2005). The main arguments against screening are that there is a lack of resources to deal with the numbers of children with developmental delay, and that the identification of more children with difficulties, some of which are likely to be false positives, would further overload the system.

Conclusion

Of the 135 million infants born annually throughout the world, more than 90 per cent live in low-income or developing countries (Population Reference Bureau, 2010). Despite this, only a small percentage of published research addresses children who come from such backgrounds (Tomlinson, 2003). Tomlinson cautions that the typical infant lives in an environment that is very different from that inhabited by the typical child development researcher. It is important, therefore, that the different circumstances of infants be considered, particularly in the case of developmental assessment, since social factors such as parental education level and socio-economic status are among the strongest predictors of poor neurodevelopmental outcome in infants. However, the recommendation that the GMDS be restandardised in South Africa because of the poor performance of local children should be considered carefully, as there is a risk of producing a downgraded measure which will fail to identify the impact of poverty and poor socio-economic conditions on the development of our children.

Note

1 The use of the GMDS is controlled by ARICD, a registered charity administered by a group of paediatricians and child psychologists interested in increasing the understanding of early child development and thereby improving the welfare of children with disabilities. They are responsible for monitoring the quality of administration of the GMDS, by ensuring that users are suitably qualified and understand the psychological and developmental principles that underpin child development. In the past, the use of the GMDS was limited to psychologists with the minimum qualification of a Master's degree, or medical practitioners working in the field of child development. Recently this has been extended to allied medical practitioners such as occupational, speech and physiotherapists. All users are obliged to attend an intensive training course covering both the theoretical and practical aspects of administration of the GMDS.

References

Adnams, C., Kodituwakku, P. W., Hay, A., Molteno, C. D., Viljoen, D. & May, P. A. (2001). Patterns of cognitive-motor development in children with Foetal Alcohol Syndrome from a community in South Africa. *Alcoholism: Clinical and Experimental Research, 25(4),* 557–562.

Aldridge Smith, J., Bidder, R. T., Gardner, S. M. & Gray, O. P. (1980). Griffiths Scales of Mental Development and different users. *Child Care, Health and Development, 6,* 11–16.

Allan, M. M. (1988). A comparison of the performance of normal preschool South African and British children on the Griffiths Mental Development Scales. Unpublished Master's dissertation. University of Port Elizabeth, Port Elizabeth.

Allan, M. M. (1992). The performance of normal preschool South African children on the Griffith Scales of Mental Development: A comparative study. Unpublished PhD dissertation, University of Port Elizabeth, Port Elizabeth.

Amod, Z., Cockcroft, K. & Soellaart, B. (2007). Use of the 1996 Griffiths Mental Development Scales for infants: A pilot study with a black, South African sample. *Journal of Child and Adolescent Mental Health, 19(2),* 123–130.

Appel, M. (2011). *Social grants making an impact.* Retrieved March 30, 2011, from http://www.southafrica.info/about/social/ies-060308.htm.

Baradon, T. (2010). *The New Beginnings Programme Manual.* London: Anna Freud Centre.

Barnard, A. (2003). The Griffiths' Practical Reasoning Scale: A revision. Unpublished Master's dissertation. University of Port Elizabeth, Port Elizabeth.

Bhamjee, R. A. (1991). A comparison of the performance of normal British and South African children on the Griffiths Scales of Mental Development. Unpublished PhD dissertation. University of Port Elizabeth, Port Elizabeth.

Biringen, Z., Robinson, J. & Emde, R. (1998). *Emotional Availability (EA) Scales* (3rd edition). Retrieved June 30, 2010, from www.emotionalavailability.com.

Cockcroft, K., Amod, Z. & Soellaart, B. (2008). Maternal level of education and performance on the 1996 Griffiths Mental Development Scales. *African Journal of Psychiatry, 11,* 44–50.

Conry, J. (1990). Neuropsychological deficits in fetal alcohol syndrome and fetal alcohol effects. *Alcohol Clinical Experimental Research, 14,* 650–655.

Falade, S. (1955). *Contribution a une étude sur le développement de l'enfant d'Afrique noire.* Paris: Foulon.

Flynn, J. R. & Weiss, L. G. (2007). American IQ gains from 1932 to 2002: The WISC subtests and educational progress. *International Journal of Testing, 7(2),* 209–224.

Foxcroft, C. D. (1997). Psychological testing in South Africa: Perspectives regarding ethical and fair practices. *European Journal of Psychological Assessment, 13(3),* 229–235.

Freedman, D. G. (1974). *Human Infancy.* New York, NY: Halstead.

Gerber, M. (1958). The psychomotor development of African children in the first year, and the influence of maternal behaviour. *Journal of Social Psychology, 47,* 185–195.

Giagazoglou, P., Kyparas, A., Fotiadou, E. & Angelopoulou, N. (2007). The effect of residence area and mother's education on motor development of preschool-aged children in Greece. *Early Childhood Development and Care, 177(5),* 479–492.

Gowar, R. V. (2003). The performance of children with autism on the Revised Extended Griffiths Scales of Mental Development. Unpublished Master's dissertation. University of Port Elizabeth, Port Elizabeth.

Goyen, T. & Lui, K. (2002). Longitudinal motor development of 'apparently normal' high-risk infants at 18 months, 3 and 5 years. *Early Human Development, 70(1–2),* 103–115.

Griffiths, R. (1984). *The Abilities of Young Children.* Amersham: Association for Research in Infant and Child Development.

Heimes, L. (1983). The comparison of the JSAIS and the Griffiths Developmental Scale scores of 3–5-year-old boys and girls. Unpublished Master's dissertation. University of Port Elizabeth, Port Elizabeth.

Huntley, M. (1996). *The Griffiths Mental Developmental Scales: From Birth to 2 Years.* Amersham: Association for Research in Infant and Child Development.

Jakins, T. (2009). Comparing the development of a sample of South African pre-school boys and girls utilising the Griffiths Mental Development Scales – Extended Revised. Unpublished Master's dissertation. Nelson Mandela Metropolitan University, Port Elizabeth.

Kheswa, T. (2009). The Griffiths Mental Development Scales – Extended Revised: Profiles of children from a low socio-economic status. Unpublished Master's dissertation. Nelson Mandela Metropolitan University, Port Elizabeth.

Knoesen, N. (2003). An exploration of the relationship between the Revised Griffiths Scales and Grade One scholastic development. Unpublished Master's dissertation. University of Port Elizabeth, Port Elizabeth.

Knoesen, N. (2005). Exploring the reliability and construct-validity of the Locomotor Scale of the Griffiths Mental Development Scales – Extended Revised (GMDS-ER). Unpublished PhD dissertation. Nelson Mandela Metropolitan University, Port Elizabeth.

Kotras, H. (2001). Exploring a developmental profile of HIV-infected infants in the Eastern Province of South Africa, utilising the Revised Griffiths Scales of Mental Development. Unpublished Master's dissertation, University of Port Elizabeth, Port Elizabeth.

Kotras, N. (2003). Exploring the construct validity of the Revised Extended Griffiths Scales Language Scale in the British Isles. Unpublished PhD dissertation. University of Port Elizabeth, Port Elizabeth.

Kriegler, S. M. & Skuy, M. (1996). Perspectives on psychological assessment in South African schools. In P. Engelbrecht, S. Kriegler & M. I. Booysen (Eds), *Perspectives on Learning*

Difficulties: International Concerns and South African Realities (pp. 109–122). Pretoria: Van Schaik.

Laughton, B., Grove, D., Kidd, M., Springer, P. E., Dobbels, E., Janse van Rensburg, A., Violari, A., Babiker, A. G., Madhi, S. A., Jean-Philippe, P., Gibb, D. M. & Cotton, M. F. (2009). Early antiretroviral therapy is associated with improved neurodevelopmental outcome in HIV-infected infants: Evidence from the CHER (Children with HIV Early Antiretroviral Therapy). Poster presentation. Conference on HIV Pathogenesis, Treatment and Prevention. Cape Town, July 19–22.

Laughton, B., Kidd, M., Springer, P. E., Dobbels, E., Janse van Rensburg, A., Violari, A., Madhi, S. A., Jean-Philippe, P., Gibb, D. M. & Cotton, M. F. (2010a). The developmental outcome of HIV-infected infants on antiretroviral therapy. ARICD Scientific Conference. London, July 13.

Laughton, B., Springer, P. E., Grove, D., Seedat, S., Cornell, M., Kidd, M., Madhi, S. A. & Cotton, M. F. (2010b). Longitudinal developmental profile of children from low socio-economic circumstances in Cape Town, using the Griffiths Mental Development Scales. *South African Journal of Child Health, 4*, 106–111.

Luiz, D. M. (1988a). A child with a hearing loss: A longitudinal study. In D. M. Luiz (Ed.), *Griffiths Scales of Mental Development: South African Studies* (pp. 44–51). Research Papers No. C25. Port Elizabeth: University of Port Elizabeth.

Luiz, D. M. (1988b). A battered child: A follow up study. In D. M. Luiz (Ed.), *Griffiths Scales of Mental Development: South African Studies* (pp. 52–58). Research Papers No. C25. Port Elizabeth: University of Port Elizabeth.

Luiz, D. M. (1988c). A comparative study of two scales of language development: The Reynell and the Griffiths. In D. M. Luiz (Ed.), *Griffiths Scales of Mental Development: South African Studies* (pp. 16–20). Research Papers No. C25. Port Elizabeth: University of Port Elizabeth.

Luiz, D. M. (1994). Children of South Africa: In search of a developmental profile. Inaugural and Emeritus Address. University of Port Elizabeth, Port Elizabeth.

Luiz, D. M., Barnard, A., Knoesen, N., Kotras, H., McAlinden, P. & O'Connell, R. (2004). *Griffiths Mental Development Scales – Extended Revised. Administration Manual.* Oxford: Hogrefe, ARICD, The Test Agency.

Luiz, D. M., Faragher, B., Barnard, A., Knoesen, N., Kotras, N., Burns, L. E. & Challis, D. (2006). *Griffiths Mental Development Scales – Extended Revised. Analysis Manual.* Oxford: Hogrefe, ARICD, The Test Agency.

Luiz, D. M., Foxcroft, C. D. & Povey, J. (2006). The Griffiths Mental Development Scales: A factorial validity study. *South African Journal of Psychology, 36(1)*, 192–214.

Luiz, D. M., Foxcroft, C. D. & Stewart, R. (2001). The construct validity of the Griffiths Scales of Mental Development. *Child: Care, Health and Development, 27(1)*, 73–83.

Luiz, D. M., Foxcroft, C. D. & Tukulu, A. (2004). The Denver II Scales and the Griffiths Scales of Mental Development: A correlational study. *Journal of Child & Adolescent Mental Health, 16(2)*, 77–81.

Luiz, D. M., Oelofsen, N., Stewart, R. & Mitchell, S. (1995). An international survey of the Extended Griffiths Scales of Mental Development. Unpublished manuscript, University of Port Elizabeth, Port Elizabeth.

Lynn, R. (2009). What is the cause of the Flynn effect? Secular increases in the Developmental Quotient of infants. *Intelligence, 37*, 16–24.

Magnuson, K. A., Sexton, H. R., Davis-Kean, P. E. & Huston, A. C. (2009). Increases in maternal education and young children's language skills. *Merrill-Palmer Quarterly, 55(3)*, 319–350.

Magongoa, D. I. S. & Venter, A. (2003). The developmental profiles of children with idiopathic tonic-clonic epilepsy as measured on the Griffiths Mental Developmental Scales. *Journal of Child and Adolescent Mental Health, 15(2)*, 59–63.

Mattson, S. N. & Riley, E. P. (1998). A review of neurobehavioural deficits in children with fetal alcohol syndrome and prenatal exposure to alcohol. *Alcohol Clinical Experimental Research, 24*, 279–294.

McLean, M. E., McCormick, K. & Baird, S. M. (1991). Concurrent validity of the Griffiths' Mental Development Scales with a population of children under 24 months. *Journal of Early Intervention, 15(4)*, 338–344.

Moosajee, S. (2007). Exploring the construct-related validity of the Personal-Social Scale of the Griffiths Mental Developmental Scales – Extended Revised (GMDS-ER). Unpublished PhD dissertation. Nelson Mandela Metropolitan University, Port Elizabeth.

Mothule, V. B. (1990). The Aptitude Test for Beginners and the Griffiths Scales of Mental Development: An investigation into the assessment of the cognitive abilities of Grade 1 children. Unpublished Master's dissertation, Medical University of South Africa, Pretoria.

Nell, V. (1997). Science and politics meet at last: The insurance industry and neuropsychological norms. *South African Journal of Psychology, 27*, 43–49.

Nzimande, B. (1995). To test or not to test. Paper presented at the Congress on Psychometrics for Psychologists and Personnel Practitioners. Council for Scientific and Industrial Research, Pretoria, June 13–14.

Owen, K. (1991). Test bias: The validity of the Junior Aptitude Tests for various population groups in South Africa regarding constructs measured. *South African Journal of Psychology, 21(2)*, 113–118.

Population Reference Bureau (2010). *World Population Data Sheet*. Retrieved April 1, 2011, from http://www.prb.org/Publications/Datasheets/2010/2010wpds.aspx.

Povey, J.-L. (2008). Exploring the construct-related validity of the Eye and Hand Coordination Scale of the Griffiths Mental Development Scales – Extended Revised (GMDS-ER). Unpublished PhD dissertation. Nelson Mandela Metropolitan University, Port Elizabeth.

Reyes, A., Pacifico, R., Benitez, B., Villanueva-uy, E. & Ostrea, E. (2010). Use of the Griffiths Mental Developmental Scales in an agro-industrial province in the Philippines. *Child: Care, Health and Development, 36(3)*, 354–360.

Richter-Strydom, L. M. & Griesel, R. D. (1984). African infant precocity: A study of a group of South African infants from two to fifteen months of age. Internal report, Institute for Behavioural Sciences, University of South Africa, Pretoria.

Sehlapelo, M. & Terrre Blanche, M. (1996). Psychometric testing in South Africa: Views from above and below. *Psychology in Society, 21*, 49–59.

Skuy, M. S., Schutte, E., Fridjhon, P. & O'Carroll, S. (2001). Suitability of published neuropsychological test norms for urban, African secondary school students in South Africa. *Personality and Individual Differences, 30*, 1413–1425.

Sommerfelt, K., Ellertsen, B. & Markestad, T. (1995). Parental factors in cognitive outcome of non-handicapped low birthweight infants. *Archives of Disability in Children, 73*, 135–142.

Sweeney, K. (1994). Cluster analysis of the Griffiths profiles of a white South African clinical population. Unpublished Master's dissertation, University of Port Elizabeth, Port Elizabeth.

Tomlinson, M. (2003). Culture and infancy: A critical examination. *South African Journal of Child and Adolescent Mental Health, 15(1)*, 45–48.

Tramonta, M. G., Hooper, S. R. & Selzer, S. C. (1988). Research on the preschool prediction of later academic achievement: A review. *Developmental Review, 8*, 89–146.

Tukulu, A. N. (1996). The Denver II Scale and the Griffiths Scales of Mental Development: A correlational study. Unpublished Master's dissertation. University of Port Elizabeth, Port Elizabeth.

Van Heerden, R. (2007). Exploring normal South African and British children: A comparative study utilising the Griffiths Mental Development Scales – Extended Revised. Unpublished Master's dissertation. Nelson Mandela Metropolitan University, Port Elizabeth.

Van Rooyen, K. (2005). The performance of South African and British children on the Griffiths Mental Development Scales – Extended Revised: A comparative study. Unpublished Master's dissertation. Nelson Mandela Metropolitan University, Port Elizabeth.

Viljoen, D. L., Gossage, J. P., Brooke, L., Adnams, C. M., Jones, K. L., Robinson, L. K. et al. (2005). Foetal alcohol syndrome epidemiology in a South African community: A second study of a very high prevalence area. *Journal of Studies on Alcohol, 66*, 593–604.

Appendix 1

Current research: use of the GMDS with South African infants and young children

A study is in progress using the GMDS to test the efficacy of a UK-developed group psychotherapy programme for mother–baby dyads (Baradon, 2010). The programme aims to intervene in mother–baby dyads with disrupted attachment patterns and has been piloted by Dr Katherine Bain, a researcher from the University of the Witwatersrand, in collaboration with a Johannesburg non-governmental organisation, Ububele, and the Anna Freud Centre in London. In the pilot study, in which groups were run in Johannesburg shelters for mothers and their infants (personal communication, Bain, 2011), the GMDS was used to measure the overall development of the infants, who ranged in age from nine days to three years. The results revealed significant correlations between the GMDS Personal-Social Scale and measures of child responsiveness and how much the child involves the mother in their play (using the Emotional Availability Scales) (Biringen, Robinson & Emde, 1998). This provides further evidence for the cross-cultural applicability of the GMDS.

13 Neuropsychological assessment in South Africa

M. Lucas

> What neuropsychologists do best is describe behaviour – as it was in the past, as it is now, and as the individual is likely to behave in the future.
> (Nell, 2000, p.104)

This chapter is devoted to the current position of neuropsychological assessment in the South African context. With this in mind, a short overview defining the field and the profession is presented, followed by a review of neuropsychological assessment. A discussion follows of the major issues facing neuropsychological assessment in the South African context, including test adaptation. A brief discussion of the way forward concludes the chapter.

Defining neuropsychology

The term 'neuropsychology' may have its origins in the 16th century (Boeglin & Thomas, 1996), but general consensus is that the first modern use of the term can be attributed to William Osler in 1931 and later Donald Hebb in 1949 (Kolb & Whishaw, 1996). Neuropsychology is frequently defined as the relationship between brain functioning and behaviour, but with the collapse of Cartesian dualism, this focus has been expanded to include the study of the mind (Wilkinson, 2004). With the mind today seen as the output of the brain's neuronal connectivity (Le Doux, 2002), it is therefore available for objective consideration as well. Although open to debate, modern neuropsychology thus encompasses not only the understanding and interpretation of structural/functional brain systems, particularly in neuropathology, but includes broader understandings such as the effect of psychotherapy on brain functioning (Gabbard, 2000; 2006), the neurobiology of personality (Bergvall, Nilsson & Hansen, 2003; Blair, 2003), and the neurobiology of sense of self (Solms, 2006).

There have been two dominant traditions in neuropsychology: a syndrome-based clinical approach and a cognitive neuroscientific approach. Clinical neuropsychology as understood today was first practised in the late 19th century with the cortical localisation of function by Dax, Broca, Wernicke and Charcot (Solms, 2008; Zillmer, Spiers & Culbertson, 2008). It is dependent upon a clinicoanatomical analysis, using the medical model as its theoretical basis. Cognitive neuropsychology, first named in the late 1970s (Gazzaniga, Ivry & Mangun, 2009), grew out of cognitive psychology and neuroscience and assumes that mental activities operate in terms of specialised subsystems or modules that can be separated out (dissociated) from each other (Gazzaniga et al., 2009; Sternberg, 2009). It maintains close links to information processing and artificial intelligence (Reed, 2010).

Both approaches are complementary, using basic experimental methods and quantitative analysis, augmented by case studies when appropriate. Each adds valuable information to the study of the brain and mind, and despite their different starting positions, they appear to be currently moving towards a more unified model.

Neuropsychology in clinical practice

Clinical neuropsychologists are concerned with assessment, diagnosis, management and rehabilitation of not only cognitive impairment but the emotional and behavioural consequences of the causal illness and injury, which is optimally assessed within the framework of a person's social and cultural background (Nell, 2000; Zillmer et al., 2008). Such impairment may be temporary or permanent, but is always measurable by either subjective complaint (for example, 'I am forgetful') or objective measures (such as psychometric test results, neurological assessment, psychiatric diagnosis, neuro-imaging investigations, etc.). As with clinical psychology, the discipline sets out to understand, prevent and relieve psychologically based distress or dysfunction, but specifically within a population that has measurable central nervous system impairment.

In first world countries, neuropsychology became a clinical speciality within psychology from the 1970s onward, although training was not formally introduced until later (Lezak, Howieson & Loring, 2004; Milberg & Hebben, 2006). In South Africa, interest in neuropsychology was formalised in 1953 with the instigation of a Division of Neuropsychology at the National Institute for Personnel Research. Later, in 1985, the South African Clinical Neuropsychological Association (SACNA) was inaugurated at the Third National Neuropsychology Conference. In the same year negotiations were initiated with the Professional Board for Psychology for a clinical neuropsychology registration (Watts, 2008). Official recognition of neuropsychology as a speciality was only promulgated by parliamentary process in 2011, after a new professional registration category was proposed and adopted by the Health Professions Council of South Africa (HPCSA).

Neuropsychological assessment is a core component of the discipline (Darby & Walsh, 2005; Lezak et al., 2004; Strauss, Sherman & Spreen, 2006) and must take place through use of triangulation utilising, firstly, personal narratives, collateral information, medical records and investigations such as neuro-imaging; secondly, the extensive knowledge on the part of the psychologist of mind/brain issues, neuro-anatomy, pathology and physiology; and thirdly, psychometric assessment, which includes the careful administration, scoring and interpretation of appropriate measures of cognitive, emotional and behavioural functioning. Thus, assessment marries changes in structure and subsequent changes in function (although research suggests that the directional reverse is also possible) (Cappas, Andres-Hyman & Davidson, 2005).

Psychometric measurement provides a formidable basis for neuropsychology, adding to the information gained through interviews rather than the other way around (Nell, 2000). Two main approaches to the psychometric assessment are used internationally: the standard battery approach and the process, or flexible, approach driven by hypothesis testing. Both approaches have strengths and limitations and typically a combination is used, which arguably could be called a third approach, whereby standardised tests are selectively chosen to evaluate the hypothesised areas of impairment (Zillmer et al., 2008).

Design of neuropsychological tests was originally aimed at the assessment of focal neurological injuries, reflecting the origins of neuropsychological knowledge (Marshall & Gurd, 2003, p.4). Careful observations of patients with focal injuries were the mainstay of the 20th-century Russian psychologist, Alexander Luria, often referred to as the father of modern neuropsychology (Goldberg, 2009), and clinicians such as Edith Kaplan and Norman Geschwind in the West (Milberg & Hebben, 2006). Through such observations the 'equipotential' hypotheses of brain function gave way to a 'hierarchical' approach in which different levels of functioning were observed in and localisable to specific brain structures (Milberg & Hebben, 2006). In the latter half of the 20th century there was a shift in the presentation of neuropsychological problems from focal injuries to diffuse injuries, typically secondary to traumatic brain injury from motor vehicle accidents and similar high-velocity events (Loring, 2006), a change also seen in South Africa (Nell, 2000), so that increasingly neuropsychologists in private practice are required to assess the impact of diffuse injuries (Nell, 2000).

Many excellent books have been written about neuropsychological assessment. In South Africa, Muriel Lezak's *Neuropsychological Assessment* (1995; Lezak et al., 2004) has always been favoured, as has Strauss and Spreen's *A Compendium of Neuropsychological Tests: Administration, Norms and Commentary* (1998; Strauss et al., 2006), although many other useful books exist. Generally, these textbooks list tests by functional domain (that is, attention, memory, etc.) rather than structures of brain. An exception to this is the idea of 'frontal lobe tests', a precursor label to that of executive functioning which has been developed in recent years to capture the generalised higher cognitive dysfunction often sustained after acquired brain injury. Halstead's Category Test of 1943 (Choca, Laatsch, Wetzel & Agresti, 1997) and the Wisconsin Card Sorting Test (Berg, 1948) are examples of such tests. Detailing specific tests for specific disorders is rare, although domains of impairment in disorders can be found (see Lezak, 1995; Lezak et al., 2004; Ogden, 2005).

It is not the aim of this chapter to reiterate what has already been written, and the reader is urged to refer to these texts for further information about neuropsychological assessment. In particular, Victor Nell's (2000) *Cross-cultural Neuropsychological Assessment: Theory and Practice* made a long overdue contribution to assessment in South Africa (Verster, 2001), and Stuart Anderson's

(2001) paper entitled 'On the importance of collecting local neuropsychological normative data' gives a comprehensive overview of the approaches to neuropsychological assessment.

The current status of neuropsychological assessment in South Africa

South African neuropsychologists have tended to focus on the assessment process, with less attention being devoted to rehabilitation, for a number of practical reasons including limited funding by managed health care for such longer-term interventions, few trained neuropsychologists and difficulty in sustaining sufficient rehabilitative facilities (Watts, 2008). In private practice it would appear that some neuropsychologists devote much of their time to medico-legal assessment (Watts, 2008). Psychometric testing forms the basis of most neuropsychological evaluations, in the form of either pencil-and-paper tasks or computerised versions of these tasks. Frequently, internationally developed tests and the standardised norms supplied by test manufacturers are used in the assessments, though this practice has limitations that will be discussed later.

According to Foxcroft, Paterson, Le Roux and Herbst (2004), who reported on psychological assessment in South Africa, approximately 10 per cent of psychologists use tests frequently to conduct neuropsychological assessment, and another 24 per cent use them less frequently. These tests are currently used primarily by clinical psychologists, but psychologists from all registered categories may use them to identify neuropsychological markers. The Bender Visual Motor Gestalt Test is the only 'neuropsychological' test featured in the top 20 most commonly used psychometric tests in South Africa (Foxcroft et al., 2004).

Challenges of psychometric assessment in South Africa

The challenges facing the neuropsychologist working in South Africa, a developing nation, are demanding. He or she needs to objectively assess the day-to-day functioning or dysfunctioning of a heterogeneous society, a problem currently facing many nations (Pedraza & Mungas, 2008). In South Africa, however, the greatest challenge is the complexity and diversity of the country's population, with 11 official languages, varying degrees of quality in its education, wide discrepancies in socio-economic status, differing cultures and rapidly occurring acculturation (Foxcroft et al., 2004; Jansen & Greenop, 2008; Jinabhai et al., 2004; Thomas, 2010; Watts, 2008), all against a historical backdrop of previous political and socio-economic inequality (Claassen, 1997).

As might be expected, given the complexity of the issue, there is no universal test battery that can accommodate such differences (Jinabhai et al., 2004). A considerable body of research has accumulated which shows that virtually no test of cognitive ability is culture-fair, and that both between and within cultures there are wide differences in test ability (Jinabhai et al., 2004; Nell, 2000; Shuttleworth-Edwards, Kemp, Rust, Muirhead, Hartman & Radloff, 2004). Standardised norms for one community cannot automatically be applied to another, nor can norms for one language group be applied to another group even though both groups are ethnically similar (Jinabhai et al., 2004; Shuttleworth-Edwards, Kemp et al., 2004; Skuy, Schutte, Fridjhon & O'Carroll, 2001), a finding that extends to other African countries (see, for example, Amponsah, 2000).

With minor exceptions (Shuttleworth-Edwards, Donnelly, Reid & Radloff, 2004; Skuy, Taylor, O'Carroll, Fridjhon & Rosenthal, 2000), the dominant theme when comparing South African scores to imported normative data is that locally produced norms continue to reflect scores that are lower than the original standardised scores (Anderson, 2001; Bethlehem, De Picciotto & Watt, 2003; Jinabhai et al., 2004; Knoetze, Bass & Steele, 2005; Skuy et al., 2001). The measure of such differences extends predominantly within two South African cultures, with, as a general rule, lower scores for black South Africans, when compared with their white counterparts (Jinabhai et al., 2004; Skuy et al., 2001).

For example, Skuy and colleagues (2000) administered, *inter alia*, the Wechsler Intelligence Scale for Children – Revised (WISC-R) to black and white South African children with learning problems and found that the black children performed significantly worse than the white children on the WISC-R battery, but not on the Kaufman Assessment Battery for Children.[1] Similarly, Jinabhai and colleagues (2004) adapted four tests (Raven's Coloured Progressive Matrices, Auditory Verbal Learning Test, Symbol Digit Modalities Test and a Group Mathematics Test) and administered them to 806 isiZulu-speaking rural primary school children in order to produce norms for this group. The scores they obtained were lower than the norms presented in test manuals. The researchers offered several reasons for this difference, emphasising educational deprivation rather than ethnic differences, as well as socio-economic factors such as unemployment and migration. Skuy et al. (2001) further administered a battery of regularly used neuropsychological tests to South African urban high school children (from Soweto, Johannesburg) and found that the scores of the school children were consistently significantly lower than the North American norms. The researchers attributed this discrepancy to educational status and cultural and socio-economic differences.

This is the typical pattern seen not only in the test performance of children from historically disadvantaged schools but in students from similarly disadvantaged universities (Grieve & Viljoen, 2000). When comparing students from a previously 'black' university in South Africa on the Austin Maze Test to international norms to scores from non-historically disadvantaged students, the former group 'required a greater number of trials to criterion and made more errors than subjects in other studies' (Grieve & Viljoen, 2000, p.16). These students also made more errors on the Halstead-Reitan Category Test and obtained a lower mean score on the Raven's Standard Progressive Matrices than the non-disadvantaged students. Quality of education was considered a primary explanation for these differences, an issue that is repeatedly mentioned in recent research papers (for example, Jinahbai et al., 2004; Skuy et al., 2001).

Currently, comprehensive sets of local norms for a broad battery of neuropsychological tests do not exist (Thomas, 2010). However, there is ongoing work by academics with an interest in neuropsychology to bridge this gap, and momentum is gathering to adapt test materials for the South African populations. An overview of this research is presented in the next section.[2]

Approaches to test adaptation

In Annexure 12 of the ethical code of the HPCSA (2006), it is acknowledged that cultural diversity has a multifaceted impact upon assessment instruments. The test user is required to know the limitations of test outcomes used for diagnostic purposes in populations for which the test was not originally standardised. That it might be necessary to adapt the administration, scoring or interpretation of test results is also acknowledged. Unfortunately, few guidelines exist for such adjustments (Van Widenfelt, Treffers, De Beurs, Siebelink & Koudijs, 2005). Changing or administering any psychological test in a manner different from the developer's intentions alters the reliability and validity of the test (Dalen, Jellestad & Kamaloodien, 2007; Nell, 2000) and has ethical implications (see Dalen et al., 2007 for further comments on the ethical considerations of altering a standardised test).

The above notwithstanding, a variety of approaches have been used in South Africa in an attempt to overcome the issue of using Western-developed test materials in a multicultural, developing society, including developing norms for local populations without changing the test content (Shuttleworth-Edwards, Kemp et al., 2004; Skuy et al., 2001), adapting test content for local populations and then developing local norms (Ferrett, Dowling, Conradie, Carey & Thomas, 2010a; 2010b; Jinabhai et al., 2004), or developing new tests (Thomas, 2010). The first and second approaches are obviously less expensive than the third approach.

Development of local norms

The most prominent standardisation process undertaken in the last ten years was that of Claassen, Krynauw, Paterson and Mathe (2001), and involved standardisation of the Wechsler Adult Intelligence Scale – Third Edition (WAIS-III) for English-speaking South Africans. Measures of intelligence are often included under the umbrella of neuropsychological testing. However, the complexity and scope of defining intelligence is beyond the scope of this chapter, and Jinabhai et al. (2004) offer a more in-depth discussion concerning the measurement of the intelligence quotient (IQ) in South Africa.

As mentioned earlier, the study by Skuy (Skuy et al., 2001) conducted at urban secondary schools in Soweto, Johannesburg, produced norms for a battery of regularly used neuropsychological tests (Rey Auditory Verbal Learning Test, Stroop Test, Wisconsin Card Sorting Test, Bender Visual Motor Gestalt Test, Rey Complex Figure, Trail Making Test, Spatial Memory Test and Draw-A-Person Test). The researchers compared the learners' scores to published norms, and found that it was necessary to provide alternative scores to these norms for this group.

Shuttleworth-Edwards and her colleagues have made valuable contributions to the South African arena. As mentioned above, they published WAIS-III norms for Eastern Cape South Africans aged 19–30 years, with at least Grade 12 education (Shuttleworth-Edwards, Kemp et al., 2004). Furthermore, having originally produced local norms for the Digit Symbol Test from the South African WAIS, first published in 1995 (Shuttleworth-Jordan & Bode, 1995a; 1995b), she has subsequently expanded upon these (Shuttleworth-Edwards, 2002; Shuttleworth-Edwards, Donnelly et al., 2004) to produce updated local norms for the WAIS-III Digit Symbol Test. Of interest in this work is the suggestion that this test may be relatively culture-independent, in the South African context at least. Another study from the Eastern Cape has produced norms for the Raven's Coloured Progressive Matrices for isiXhosa-speaking primary school learners (Knoetze et al., 2005).

Most recently, symposiums were presented at the 2010 SACNA biennial conference in Johannesburg addressing the issues of test development in the South African cross-cultural arena, primarily by researchers from the Eastern and Western Cape provinces. Normative data for unskilled workers who are isiXhosa-speaking (the predominant indigenous language of both these provinces) were supplied for a selection of neuropsychological tests (Trail Making Test, Stroop Test, Tests of Malingering, and visual and verbal memory subtests of the Wechsler Memory Scale) (Andrews, Fike & Wong, 2010). Provisional normative data were provided for the Controlled Oral Word Association Test and the Boston Naming Test for Afrikaans, English and isiXhosa speakers, stratified by years of completed education (Ferrett et al., 2010a; 2010b). A summary of normative data for the WAIS-III and Wechsler Intelligence Scale for Children – Revised Fourth Edition (WISC-IV) was provided by Shuttleworth-Edwards and colleagues (Shuttleworth-Edwards, Van der Merwe & Radloff, 2010).[3]

The abovementioned work presented at the SACNA 12th biennial conference highlights some of the challenges faced when developing local norms. Unfortunately, the original version of the Wechsler Memory Scale was used in the standardising exercise; this scale is now outdated and not widely used, although its strength is the brevity of the scale compared with later versions. This indicates the difficulty in South Africa of keeping abreast with different test battery versions. The cost alone of buying new tests is often prohibitive, for institutions and private practitioners alike, and the investment of time and energy in standardisation of each version is not practical. Moreover, the language grouping selected by Shuttleworth-Edwards and colleagues is not comprehensive: isiXhosa speakers are one of 11 different language groups (although admittedly one of the larger language-differentiated population groups), and unskilled workers are only part of the labour profile of the population (although again, a large part of the population). At the very least, the use of simultaneous development of tests in different languages would seem the preferred approach, but time constraints, shortages of funding and lack of expertise to do this are major limitations in the South African context (Bethlehem et al., 2003; Foxcroft et al., 2004).

Adaptation of tests for local use (complementarity)

Adaptation of tests is probably the most frequently adopted approach among neuropsychologists, but is not without substantial statistical challenges if the subsequent results are to be valid and reliable (Ferrett et al., 2010a; 2010b). Various approaches to adaptation have been explored in research projects, such as modification of tests either through item changes, replacing items with more locally appropriate examples (Ferrett et al., 2010a; 2010b; Jinabhai et al., 2004); translation, of the test itself or of the instructions to complete the test (Jinabhai et al., 2004; Dalen et al., 2007; Knoetze et al., 2005; Shanahan, Anderson & Mkhize, 2001); or omission of certain items (Jansen & Greenop, 2008). Tests with a dominant verbal component usually need considerable adaptation (Ferrett et al., 2010a; 2010b; Jansen & Greenop, 2008), and it is erroneous to believe that tests considered measures of nonverbal function are not influenced by language (Rosselli & Ardila, 2003; Shuttleworth, Kemp et al., 2004; Skuy et al., 2001).

Producing local norms leads to the problem of producing innumerable sets of norms that take into account a long list of confounding variables (see the ethical guidelines of the HPCSA (2006)). The task of standardising every test for every individual group is unrealistic in terms of time, expense and effort – especially in the current context, where rapid acculturation and urbanisation are taking place, implying that constant updating of locally produced norms would be required. The validity of the results would also be short-lived (Shuttleworth-Jordan, 1996). It makes better sense to utilise research efforts to establish trends in differences, such as the research that has found differential patterns in test scores across groups (Anderson, 2001; Jinabhai et al., 2004; Skuy et al., 2001), which is frequently attributed to socio-cultural, socio-economic and quality-of-education differences.

Developing new tests

Minimal development of local neuropsychological tests has taken place, probably because of costs (although in the arena of organisational psychology more local tests prevail). Government organisations such as the Human Sciences Research Council (HSRC) have tackled test development on a commercial scale in the past, but the work of the HSRC appears to have been redirected from test development in recent years (Foxcroft & Davies, 2008; Foxcroft & Roodt, 2001), which has seriously compromised this approach to adaptation. Locally devised tests also lack international generalisability, and consequently very few local researchers have attempted the task (Shuttleworth-Jordan, 1996; Van Wijk, 2010). There is some suggestion that this is changing. Foxcroft and Davies (2008) mention that international companies with South African representation are taking up the challenge of validating tests for local use.

A variant on new test development is to assess cognitive functioning indirectly by using developmental tasks. Levert and Jansen (2001) did this when they applied Piagetian tasks of conservation and seriation instead of neuropsychological tests to differentiate between historically disadvantaged students with (and without) learning difficulties.

Current important issues in South African neuropsychological test development

It is evident that the most well-researched areas of impact upon test proficiency are education, socio-economic status, language and culture (Levert & Jansen, 2001; Nell, 2000; Shuttleworth-Jordan, 1996; Skuy et al., 2001). These variables are interrelated, and Shuttleworth-Jordan (1996) has used the term 'socio-culture' to encompass them. Other issues such as practice trials, computer skills, translators and test comprehension have also been mentioned (Nell, 2000). Some of these factors are explored below.

Quality of education

Level of education, an integral part of socio-economic status, has always been an important variable when interpreting neuropsychological test scores (Skuy et al., 2001). One major recent development in the testing arena in South Africa is cognisance of the differences in quality of education, as well as level of education (Nell, 2000; Shuttleworth-Edwards, Kemp et al., 2004). Education, as an indicator of test performance, is an integral part of neuropsychological assessment, but in South Africa at least, it is not only the number of years a person spends in the classroom, but the quality of the teaching received and the reason for leaving school (not necessarily because of intellectual constraints), which influence test performance. Many injustices in quality of education existed in South Africa during the apartheid years, and sadly, there has been insufficient capacity and capability to combat this since the democratic changes of 1994 (Jinabhai et al., 2004).

Explanatory models of difference

In South Africa it is clear that the explanatory reason for major differences in test performance is environmental rather than biological (Jinabhai et al., 2004; Kamin, 2006; Turnbull & Bagus, 1991). Current explanatory models used to justify differences in intellectual capability no longer rely on archaic ideas of determinism (for example, Herrnstein & Murray, 1994), but understand that an individual's intellectual potential is dependent upon the socio-cultural context in which that person is born and resides (Grieve & Viljoen, 2000; Kamin, 2006). In support of this, Shuttleworth-Edwards, Kemp et al. (2004) noted that students of good-quality education performed comparably on the WAIS-III, regardless of cultural or ethnic grouping. Furthermore, it would seem from the studies by Skuy and other colleagues (see Kamin, 2006) that the purported low IQ of black South Africans is increasing. Presumably even though the quality of education may not yet be equivalent to that of Western countries, improvement is still happening as South Africans have greater exposure to a Western way of life through media such as television and the internet.

Theories such as those of Sternberg (1988) and Vygotsky (1978) offer good explanatory models for the socio-cultural approach (cited in Grieve & Viljoen, 2000). Emerging research in cultural neuroscience is beginning to explore the impact of culture upon brain functioning (Ames & Fiske, 2010; Zhou & Cacioppo, 2010). As a result, the Western ideas of certain structure/function alignments as universals are being disputed. Notably, differences in localised cortical functioning between Western and other cultures have been identified for functions as diverse as perception and understanding of self (Ames & Fiske, 2010). Future neuropsychologists may be provided with more demonstrable ways of understanding the impact culture can make on brain functioning (Ames & Fiske, 2010).

Practice trials

The concept of practice trials was first introduced in South Africa in 1949 by Simon Biesheuvel of the National Institute for Personnel Research, to help illiterate groups with psychometric testing (Foxcroft & Davies, 2008). Nell (2000) strongly advocated practice trials for those who are not test-wise, even with 12 years of education. Some researchers have included practice trials when adapting tests (for example, Jinabhai et al., 2004) and many tests include practice items in their standardised application (for example, the Trail Making Test). Although this is a laudable attempt to level the playing fields for those at a disadvantage, the amount and type of practice that should be supplied is contentious (Nell, 2000).

Computerised testing

With the advent of widespread computerised technology, the idea of computerised psychometric testing has followed and several tests are now sold in a computer version (for example, the Wisconsin Card Sorting Test (Heaton & PAR staff, no date)). Whilst this is now a commonplace assessment method in Europe and North America, it presents some issues when employed in the developing world. The primary issue for neuropsychologists when using computerised tests is the level of familiarity with computer technology. The exposure of South Africans to computers is so variable that the efficiency of computer test use by psychologists in South Africa is mixed (Foxcroft et al., 2004). On the one hand, internet use in South Africa has passed the five million mark (World Wide Worx, 2010), but this constitutes less than 10 per cent of the population. Organisations such as Computer Aid (2010) circulate computers from first world to developing nations and this should assist in the acculturation process. Although experience with technology is associated with the developed world, this is rapidly changing (Bangirana, Giordani, John, Page, Opoka & Boivin, 2009), and there is a sense that computerised neuropsychological testing is becoming an acceptable approach in South Africa, at least for those with some prior exposure to such technology (Foxcroft, Watson & Seymour, 2004 cited in Foxcroft & Davies, 2008; Grieve & Viljoen, 2000).

Test understanding

Understanding of the testing experience by non-test-wise participants is largely uncharted territory (Nell, 2000), but it is important to realise that the 'investment' in testing is not necessarily interpreted in a similar manner by all South Africans (Foxcroft & Davies, 2008; Grieve & Viljoen, 2000), and some find the experience more stressful than their more test-wise counterparts (Shanahan et al., 2001). Nell's (2000) book offers an extensive overview of the testing experience in South Africa.

The way forward

The use of neuropsychological assessments in developing countries is an important but underestimated and underutilised practice (Jinabhai et al., 2004). It should be clear from the above overview that conducting valid and useful neuropsychological assessments in a developing country such as South Africa is fraught with difficulties. Nevertheless, many assessments are conducted here, with valuable and informative outcomes. It is clear that a standardised battery approach has severe limitations in any developing country, and a good case can be made for a hypothesis-driven, process approach (Levert & Jansen, 2001; Ogden, 2005; Solms, 2008). A combination of syndrome analysis and an individualised test battery, using appropriate norms when available, is most commonly utilised by practitioners in South Africa (Nell, 2000), and this approach has worked well. Test scores can be interpreted using a differential score or pattern analytical approach (Zillmer et al., 2008), which allows the testee to be his or her own control or norm reference and reduces dependence on standardised norms (Jinabhai et al., 2004). Such assessments require the careful evaluation of the patient in his or her social and economic context, and the practitioner must have a broad general knowledge not only of neuropsychological structural and functional relationships and clinical psychology, but also of the environmental and cultural consequential experiences of South Africans (Nell, 2000).

Of course, several challenges face practitioners who use this approach, including possible subjective bias, limitations in terms of test validity and reliability, and an expectation that the neuropsychologist has a thorough understanding that the lives of others may differ from his or her own life experiences. Also, this approach can be difficult to teach as it requires a combination of skills on the part of the practitioner, and takes the field of neuropsychology beyond science (Zillmer et al., 2008). One way to combat such limitations is to discuss the results of an assessment within a team framework. Practitioners often emphasise the utility of bringing a neuropsychological report to a group of colleagues (preferably including those from different disciplines and cultural backgrounds) for discussion, and more generally of seeking supervision when interpreting their psychometric test results.

In conclusion, neuropsychological assessment in the South African context is challenging and potentially difficult, but the challenges are not insuperable. It is necessary, when training future neuropsychologists, to ensure that the reliability and validity of assessment is preserved while socio-cultural empathy and sensitivity is consistently maintained.

Notes

1 The terms 'black' and 'white' are used here as the descriptors cited in the original paper by Skuy et al. (2000).

2 This chapter focuses on South African developments in assessment over the past ten years. A study exists of psychometric research in South Africa up to 1997, undertaken by Nell and Kirkby and cited in Nell (2000).

3 This recent symposium follows similar presentations at previous SACNA conferences (Watts, 2008), reflecting the ongoing concerns of the neuropsychological community with regard to usage of non-locally developed test norms.

References

Ames, D. L. & Fiske, S. T. (2010). Cultural neuroscience. *Asian Journal of Social Psychology, 13*, 72–82.

Amponsah, B. (2000). A comparison of sex differences in visual-spatial performance from preadolescence to adulthood in Ghana and Norway. *South African Journal of Psychology, 30*, 25–31.

Anderson, S. J. (2001). On the importance of collecting local neuropsychological normative data. *South African Journal of Psychology, 31*, 29–34.

Andrews, K., Fike, L. & Wong, A. (2010). Normative indicators and malingering cut-off points for an isiXhosa-speaking unskilled population on selected neuropsychological tests. Symposium handout. 12th Biennial SACNA Conference. Johannesburg, March 10–12.

Bangirana, P., Giordani, B., John, C. C., Page, C., Opoka, R. O. & Boivin, M. J. (2009). Immediate neuropsychological and behavioural benefits of computerized cognitive rehabilitation in Ugandan pediatric cerebral malaria survivors. *Journal of Developmental and Behavioral Pediatrics, 30*, 310–318.

Berg, E. A. (1948). A simple objective treatment for measuring flexibility in thinking. *Journal of General Psychology, 39*, 15–22.

Bergvall, A. H., Nilsson, T. & Hansen, S. (2003). Exploring the link between character, personality disorder, and neuropsychological function. *European Psychiatry, 18*, 334–344.

Bethlehem, D., De Picciotto, J. & Watt, N. (2003). Assessment of verbal fluency in bilingual Zulu-English speakers. *South African Journal of Psychology, 33*, 236–240.

Blair, R. J. R. (2003). Neurobiological basis of psychopathy. *British Journal of Psychiatry, 182*, 5–7.

Boeglin, J. A. & Thomas, R. K. (1996). *On the origin of the term 'Neuropsychology': Redux*. Retrieved April 9, 2010, from http://rkthomas.myweb.uga.edu/TermNeuropsychology.htm.

Cappas, N., Andres-Hyman, R. & Davidson, L. (2005). What psychotherapists can begin to learn from neuroscience: Seven principles of a brain-based psychotherapy. *Psychotherapy: Theory, Research, Practice, Training, 42*, 374–383.

Choca, J. P., Laatsch, L., Wetzel, L. & Agresti, A. (1997). The Halstead Category Test: A fifty-year perspective. *Neuropsychology Review, 7*, 61–75.

Claassen, N. C. W. (1997). Cultural differences, politics and test bias in South Africa. *European Review of Applied Psychology, 47(4)*, 297–307.

Claassen, N. C. W., Krynauw, A. H., Paterson, H. & Mathe, M. (2001). *A Standardisation of the WAIS-III for English-speaking South Africans*. Pretoria: Human Sciences Research Council.

Computer Aid (2010). Untitled document. Retrieved April 21, 2010, from http://www.computeraid.org.

Dalen, K., Jellestad, F. & Kamaloodien, K. (2007). The translation of the NEPSY-II to Afrikaans: Some ethical reflections. *Cognition, Brain, & Behavior, 11*, 609–620.

Darby, D. & Walsh, K. W. (2005). *Neuropsychology: A Clinical Approach* (5th edition). Edinburgh: Churchill Livingstone.

Ferrett, H., Dowling, T., Conradie, S., Carey, P. & Thomas, K. (2010a). Provisional normative data for the Boston Naming Test Short Form (South African version). Handout. 12th Biennial SACNA Conference, Johannesburg, March 10–12.

Ferrett, H., Dowling, T., Conradie, S., Carey, P. & Thomas, K. (2010b). Provisional normative data for the Controlled Oral Word Association Test (South African version). Handout. 12th Biennial SACNA Conference. Johannesburg, March 10–12.

Foxcroft, C. & Davies, C. (2008). Historical perspectives on psychometric testing in South Africa. In C. van Ommen & D. Painter (Eds), *Interiors: A History of Psychology in South Africa* (pp. 152–181). Pretoria: Unisa Press.

Foxcroft, C., Paterson, H., Le Roux, N. & Herbst, D. (2004). *Psychological Assessment in South Africa: A Needs Analysis. The Test Use Patterns and Needs of Psychological Assessment Practitioners*. Pretoria: Human Sciences Research Council.

Foxcroft, C. D. & Roodt, G. (Eds) (2001). *An Introduction to Psychological Assessment in the South African Context*. Cape Town: Oxford University Press.

Gabbard, G. O. (2000). A neurobiologically informed perspective on psychotherapy. *British Journal of Psychiatry, 177*, 117–122.

Gabbard, G. O. (2006). A neuroscience perspective on transference. *Psychiatric Annals, 36*, 282–289.

Gazzaniga, M. S., Ivry, R. B. & Mangun, G. R. (2009). *Cognitive Neuroscience* (3rd edition). New York, NY: Norton.

Goldberg, E. (2009). *The New Executive Brain*. Oxford: Oxford University Press.

Grieve, K. & Viljoen, S. (2000). An exploratory study of the use of the Austin maze in South Africa. *South African Journal of Psychology, 30*, 14–18.

Heaton, R. & PAR staff (no date). *WCST-64: Computer Version 2 Research Edition (WCST-64™:CV2)*. Retrieved April 21, 2010, from http://www4.parinc.com/Products/Product.aspx?ProductID=WCST64C2.

Herrnstein, R. J. & Murray, C. (1994). *The Bell Curve: Intelligence and Class Structure in American Life*. New York, NY: Free Press.

HPCSA (Health Professions Council of South Africa) (2006). *Ethical Rules of Conduct for Practitioners Registered under the Health Professions Act, 1974*. Retrieved April 19, 2010, from http://www.hpcsa.co.za/downloads/conduct_ethics/rules/ethical_rules_psychology.pdf.

Jansen, P. & Greenop, K. (2008). Factor analyses of the Kaufman Assessment Battery for Children assessed longitudinally at 5 and 10 years. *South African Journal of Psychology, 38*, 355–365.

Jinabhai, C. C., Taylor, M., Rangongo, M. F., Mkhize, N. J., Anderson, S., Pillay, B. J. et al. (2004). Investigating the mental abilities of rural Zulu primary school children in South Africa. *Ethnicity and Health, 9*, 17–36.

Kamin, L. J. (2006). African IQ and mental retardation. *South African Journal of Psychology, 36*, 1–9.

Knoetze, J., Bass, N. & Steele, G. (2005). The Raven's Coloured Progressive Matrices: Pilot norms for isiXhosa-speaking primary school learners in peri-urban Eastern Cape. *South African Journal of Psychology, 35*, 175–194.

Kolb, B. & Whishaw, I. Q. (1996). *Fundamentals of Human Neuropsychology* (4th edition). New York, NY: W. H. Freeman.

Le Doux, J. E. (2002). *The Synaptic Self: How Our Brains Become Who We Are*. Middlesex: Viking Penguin.

Levert, T. & Jansen, P. (2001). A Lurian-Piagetian approach to assessment of historically disadvantaged black scholars in English-medium schools. *South African Journal of Psychology, 31*, 21–31.

Lezak, M. D. (1995). *Neuropsychological Assessment* (3rd edition). New York, NY: Oxford University Press.

Lezak, M. D., Howieson, D. B. & Loring, D. W. (2004). *Neuropsychological Assessment* (4th edition.). New York, NY: Oxford University Press.

Loring, D. W. (2006). Preface. In A. M. Poreh (Ed.), *The Quantified Process Approach to Neuropsychological Assessment* (pp. xxi–xxiii). New York, NY: Taylor & Francis.

Marshall, J. C. & Gurd, J. M. (2003). Neuropsychology: Past, present and future. In P. W. Halligan, U. Kischka & J. C. Marshall (Eds), *Handbook of Clinical Neuropsychology*. Oxford: Oxford University Press.

Milberg, W. & Hebben, N. (2006). The historical antecedents of the Boston Process Approach. In A. M. Poreh (Ed.), *The Quantified Process Approach to Neuropsychological Assessment* (pp. 17–25). New York, NY: Taylor & Francis.

Nell, V. (2000). *Cross-cultural Neuropsychological Assessment: Theory and Practice*. London & Mahwah, NJ: Lawrence Erlbaum.

Ogden, J. A. (2005). *Fractured Minds. A Case-Study Approach to Clinical Neuropsychology* (2nd edition). New York, NY: Oxford University Press.

Pedraza, O. & Mungas, D. (2008). Measurement in cross-cultural neuropsychology. *Neuropsychology Review, 18*, 184–193.

Reed, S. K. (2010). *Cognition Theories and Applications* (8th edition). Belmont, CA: Wadsworth.

Rosselli, M. & Ardila, A. (2003). The impact of culture and education on non-verbal neuropsychological measurements: A critical review. *Brain and Cognition, 52*, 326–333.

Shanahan, S., Anderson, S. J. & Mkhize, N. J. (2001). Assessing psychological distress in Zulu-speakers: Preliminary findings from an adaptation of the SCL-90R. *Journal of the International Neuropsychological Society, 31*, 1–12.

Shuttleworth-Edwards, A. B. (2002). Fine tuning of the Digit Symbol Paired Associate Recall test for practitioner purposes in clinical and research settings. *The Clinical Neuropsychologist, 16*, 232–241.

Shuttleworth-Edwards, A. B., Donnelly, M. J. R., Reid, I. & Radloff, S. E. (2004). A cross-cultural study with culture-fair normative indications on WAIS-III Digit Symbol-Incidental Learning. *Journal of Clinical and Experimental Neuropsychology, 26*, 921–932.

Shuttleworth-Edwards, A. B., Kemp, R. D., Rust, A. L., Muirhead, J. G. L., Hartman, N. P. & Radloff, S. E. (2004). Cross-cultural effects on IQ test performance: A review and preliminary normative indications on WAIS-III test performance. *Journal of Clinical and Experimental Neuropsychology, 26(7)*, 903–920.

Shuttleworth-Edwards, A. B., Van der Merwe, A. & Radloff, S. E. (2010). South African cross-cultural normative data for the WAIS-III, WISC-IV including Digit Symbol Incidental Recall. Handout. 12th Biennial SACNA Conference. Johannesburg, March 10–12.

Shuttleworth-Jordan, A. B. (1996). On not reinventing the wheel: A clinical perspective on culturally relevant test usage in South Africa. *South African Journal of Psychology, 26(2)*, 96–102.

Shuttleworth-Jordan, A. B & Bode, S. G. (1995a). Taking account of the age effect on Digit Symbol and Incidental Recall for diagnostic purposes. *Journal of Clinical and Experimental Neuropsychology, 17*, 439–448.

Shuttleworth-Jordan, A. B. & Bode, S. G. (1995b). Use of the SAWAIS Digit Symbol test of Incidental Recall. *South African Journal of Psychology, 25*, 57–60.

Skuy, M., Schutte, E., Fridjhon, P. & O'Carroll, S. (2001). Suitability of published neuropsychological test norms for urban African secondary school students in South Africa. *Personality and Individual Differences, 30*, 1413–1425.

Skuy, M. S., Taylor, M., O'Carroll, S., Fridjhon, P. & Rosenthal, L. (2000). Performance of black and white South African children on the Wechsler Intelligence Scale for Children – Revised and the Kaufman Assessment Battery. *Psychological Reports, 86*, 727–737.

Solms, M. (2006). Putting the psyche into neuropsychology. *The Psychologist, 19*, 538–539.

Solms, M. (2008). Neuropsychology. In L. Swartz, C. de la Rey, N. Duncan & L. Townsend (Eds), *Psychology: An Introduction* (pp. 174–183). Cape Town: Oxford University Press.

Sternberg, R. J. (2009). *Cognitive Psychology* (5th edition). Belmont, CA: Wadsworth.

Strauss, E., Sherman, E. M. S. & Spreen, O. (2006). *A Compendium of Neuropsychological Tests: Administration, Norms and Commentary* (3rd edition). New York, NY: Oxford University Press.

Strauss, E. & Spreen, O. (1998). *A Compendium of Neuropsychological Tests: Administration, Norms and Commentary* (2nd edition). New York, NY: Oxford University Press.

Thomas, K. (2010). *Test Development in the South African Cross-cultural Arena.* Conference proceedings of the 12th Biennial SACNA Conference. Johannesburg, March 10–12.

Turnbull, O. H. & Bagus, R. (1991). The translation of the *Luria Neuropsychological Investigation* into Zulu: Its relationship to the work of A. R. Luria and L. S. Vygotsky. *South African Journal of Psychology, 21*, 61–63.

Van Widenfelt, B. M., Treffers, P. D. A., De Beurs, E., Siebelink, B. M. & Koudijs, E. (2005). Translation and cross-cultural adaptation of assessment instruments used in psychological research with children and families. *Clinical Child and Family Psychology Review, 8*, 135–147.

Van Wijk, C. (2010). Towards developing the Tupper Neuropsychological Task (TNT) (because dynamite comes in small packages). Poster presentation. 12th Biennial SACNA Conference. Johannesburg, March 10–12.

Verster, J. M. (2001). Review of the book *Cross-cultural Neuropsychological Assessment: Theory and Practice. South African Journal of Psychology, 31*, 55–56.

Watts, A. D. (2008). Neuropsychology in South Africa: Past, present and future. In C. van Ommen & D. Painter (Eds), *Interiors: A History of Psychology in South Africa* (pp. 358–384). Pretoria: Unisa Press.

Wilkinson, M. (2004). The mind-brain relationship: The emergent self. *Journal of Analytical Psychology, 49*, 83–101.

World Wide Worx (2010). *SA Internet Growth Accelerates.* Retrieved April 21, 2010, from http://www.worldwideworx.com/?p=234.

Zhou, H. & Cacioppo, J. (2010). Culture and the brain: Opportunities and obstacles. *Asian Journal of Social Psychology, 13*, 59–71.

Zillmer, E. A., Spiers, M. V. & Culbertson, W. C. (2008). *Principles of Neuropsychology* (2nd edition). Belmont, CA: Wadsworth.

Section Two

Personality and projective tests: conceptual and practical applications

14 The Sixteen Personality Factor Questionnaire in South Africa

R. van Eeden, N. Taylor and C. H. Prinsloo

Extensive literature exists in psychology on understanding and assessing personality. This chapter cannot even begin to do justice to such contributions. Suffice it to say that the Sixteen Personality Factor Questionnaire (16PF®) originated from the so-called trait or factor theories of personality.[1] Early proponents include USA and English pioneers such as Eysenck, Allport and Spearman. According to these theories, rational, objective and mostly quantitative evidence and explanations, and not therapeutic or clinical experience or animal studies, underpin and account for a broad and complex understanding of human behaviour. Instruments such as the 16PF questionnaire have endeavoured to measure and assess underlying personality structures and dimensions within a holistic notion of motivation, predictability and behaviour. Interested readers can consult 'classical' sources on the origins of the 16PF questionnaire and its theoretical and empirical underpinnings produced by people such as Hall and Lindzey (1957), Hjelle and Ziegler (1976), and the father of the 16PF himself, Raymond B. Cattell (Cattell, 1989; Cattell, Eber & Tatsuoka, 1970). Recent developments and literature relating to the same themes come from the rapidly expanding field of cross-cultural studies and assessment.

In this chapter the 16PF questionnaire is described and detail is given on the current version of the questionnaire, the 16PF Fifth Edition (16PF5). In considering the history and development of the 16PF in South Africa, earlier versions are mentioned to contextualise the development of the 16PF5 (the only version presently available). Psychometric properties of the latter are also presented. A detailed discussion follows on the cross-cultural research with the 16PF South African 1992 version (SA92) that formed the basis for continued work with the 16PF5. The chapter concludes with discussion of the 16PF in practice, and consideration of the future of the 16PF internationally and in South Africa.

A description of the 16PF

The 16PF is a trait-based measure of normal personality that provides a picture of personality through 16 primary factors and 5 higher-order factors. The rationale for using the 16PF is that a questionnaire developed and structured on the basis of personality traits that had been identified in a scientific manner from a large number of (everyday) personality descriptions should provide a reliable and valid measurement of an individual's true personality. Once obtained, such a picture would enable the trained, qualified and experienced psychologist to understand and predict an individual's behaviour in a consistent manner.

The current version of the 16PF – namely, the 16PF5 – can be used with respondents aged 16 and above. It consists of a total of 185 items with three response options ('a', 'b' and 'c'). Scores for the 16 primary factor scales, 5 global factors and 3 validity scales are provided. Respondents are required to indicate their 'interests and attitudes' in an intuitive and natural way without pondering too long about their responses, and by avoiding middle options as much as possible. Norms are provided in the form of sten scores for 16 first-order and 5 second-order factors. The test is available in hand-scoring and electronic versions, and also has an online option.

The names of the primary factors, as well as descriptors for high and low scores, are presented in Table 14.1. The second-order factors are referred to as global factors, and are made up of clusters of primary scales. The 16PF5 also contains three validity scales – namely, Infrequency, Acquiescence, and Impression Management which replaces the Motivational Distortion scale of previous versions. The second-order factors and the validity scales are also presented in Table 14.1.

Table 14.1 The primary factors, second-order factors and validity scales of the 16PF5

Primary factors		Low-score descriptors	High-score descriptors
A	Warmth	More emotionally distant from people	Attentive and warm to others
B	Reasoning	Fewer reasoning items correct	More reasoning items correct
C	Emotional Stability	Reactive, emotionally changeable	Emotionally stable, adaptive
E	Dominance	Deferential, cooperative, avoids conflict	Dominant, forceful
F	Liveliness	Serious, cautious, careful	Lively, animated, spontaneous
G	Rule-Consciousness	Expedient, nonconforming	Rule-conscious, dutiful
H	Social Boldness	Shy, threat-sensitive, timid	Socially bold, venturesome, thick-skinned
I	Sensitivity	Objective, unsentimental	Subjective, sentimental
L	Vigilance	Trusting, unsuspecting, accepting	Vigilant, suspicious, sceptical, wary
M	Abstractedness	Grounded, practical, solution-oriented	Abstracted, theoretical, idea-oriented
N	Privateness	Forthright, straightforward	Private, discreet, non-disclosing
O	Apprehension	Self-assured, unworried	Apprehensive, self-doubting, worried
Q1	Openness to Change	Traditional, values the familiar	Open to change, experimenting
Q2	Self-Reliance	Group-oriented, affiliative	Self-reliant, individualistic

Primary factors		Low-score descriptors	High-score descriptors
Q3	Perfectionism	Tolerates disorder, unexacting, flexible	Perfectionistic, organised, self-disciplined
Q4	Tension	Relaxed, placid, patient	Tense, high-energy, impatient, driven
Second-order factors		**Low-score descriptors**	**High-score descriptors**
Extraversion		Introverted, socially inhibited	Extraverted, socially participating
Anxiety		Low anxiety, unperturbable	High anxiety, perturbable
Tough-Mindedness		Receptive, open-minded, intuitive	Tough-minded, resolute, unempathic
Independence		Accommodating, agreeable, selfless	Independent, persuasive, wilful
Self-Control		Unrestrained, follows urges	Self-controlled, inhibits urges
Validity scales		**Description**	
Infrequency		Over-selection of the '?' option	
Acquiescence		The tendency to agree with items regardless of their content	
Impression Management		An indicator of inflated positive impression	

Source: Adapted from IPAT (2009). Copyright 2009 by IPAT. Adapted with permission.

The development of the 16PF5 was based on the selection and update of the 'best items' in the five earlier US forms (Forms A, B, C, D and the Clinical Analysis Questionnaire). The main changes involved rewriting many of the items to reduce their ambiguity and simplify the grammar, in order to improve their readability. All items were revised so that the middle response option was '?', except for the Reasoning (Factor B) items. This allowed respondents to choose the middle response when they thought that both 'a' and 'b' responses were equally applicable and when they thought that neither 'a' nor 'b' applied to them. All the Reasoning (B) items were placed together at the end of the questionnaire, with separate administration instructions. Most of the psychological terms were revised. The names of the scales in the 16PF5 were updated to make it easier to give feedback (Conn & Rieke, 1998).

History and development of the 16PF in South Africa

The first version of the 16PF was developed in the USA in 1949 by Raymond B. Cattell (Cattell, 1989; Cattell et al., 1970). The then Institute for Psychological and Edumetric Research adapted and calculated South African norms for the US edition of Form A in the late 1960s, and for the US edition of Form B in 1975. New and additional South African norms were released in 1989 (Afrikaans publication) and 1991 (English publication) by Prinsloo (1989; 1991) under the auspices of the Human Sciences Research Council (HSRC). The US editions of Form C and Form D were known in South Africa at the time, but were never adapted or provided with local norms or standardised on South African samples, although some research was conducted on them. Form E was also adapted for South African use; the adaptation involved limited language adjustments and the initial calculation and release of some local norms in 1990. In 1992, additional norms and a new experimental version of this form were released (Prinsloo, 1992b). Form F was never adjusted for or released in South Africa. The initial forms were followed by the SA92 and the 16PF5, adapted for local use.

Making 16PF instruments available in South Africa before 1992 mainly comprised minimal language adaptations and calculating local norms to ensure that respondents who were sufficiently proficient in the two test languages, Afrikaans and English, and similar enough to the norm groups, would complete equivalent and appropriately scored versions. National representative samples always proved too costly to achieve. Selected psychometric and normative information on the local versions of the 16PF is provided in Table 14.2 as an indication of the confidence with and boundaries within which each version could or can be used.

The target group for Forms A and B was adults (18 years and above) and norm tables were provided for various sample groups (see Table 14.2). The target group for Form E was adults with reading proficiency in the test languages of English or Afrikaans (Prinsloo, 1992b). This form required relatively low reading proficiency, by virtue of language and format simplifications. In the case of the 1992 edition, the participants came from all four population groups, with black and white respondents making up 47 per cent and 38 per cent of the norm sample respectively. Specific sample-based formulae were released for calculating second-order factor scores. The 16PF-SA92 comprised items selected from an original pool of items taken from earlier South African forms of the 16PF, as well as from the US versions of the various forms (Prinsloo, 1992a). This version was standardised for individuals who were at least 18 years old and who understood Afrikaans or English well. Although statistical analyses did not show substantial differences for subgroups based on biographical variables, Abrahams and Mauer (1999b) questioned the use of this version for different race groups, especially in the light of the under-representation of black South Africans in the norm sample. Reliability coefficients for the various forms are presented in Table 14.2. In terms of instrument validity, the strongest evidence throughout came from the fact that it was possible to replicate the Institute for Personality and Ability Testing (IPAT) factor structure to a large extent.

The 16PF5 is the only version presently available, as the previous forms have been discontinued. The development of the 16PF5 began in the US in 1988, as it had evolved into a number of different adult forms as well as other forms for children and adolescents. The six-year project involved an initial pool of over 750 items and 6 220 participants in four similar studies. The standardisation form, which included approximately 14 items per factor, was administered to a representative US sample. The final items were selected so that they had higher correlations with items from their own scale than with those from the other scales; the items maximised scale reliabilities; and the scales had similar correlations for men and women (Conn & Rieke, 1998).

In 1996, the HSRC conducted an investigation into the feasibility of using the US version of the 16PF5 that was realised in 1994 (Conn & Rieke, 1998), with

Table 14.2 Psychometric and normative information for the local versions of the 16PF

Form	Items	Education level	Internal consistency	Test-retest reliability	Norm groups	
A & B	187	Grade 12	0.35–0.74		1978	First-year male students (899)
						First-year female students (912)
						General population (1 342)
						Rural population (105)
					1982	Administrative staff (8 239)
						Graduated employees (111)
					1985	Branch managers at banks (111)
					1987/1988	Afr. & Eng. Speakers (1 233)
					1983	Zulu males (160)
						Other African-language males (160)
E	128	Grades 6–11	0.30–0.75	0.20–0.70	1989/1990	Black males (223)
						Nonblack males (252)
						Heavy vehicle drivers (139)
						Total group (475)
					1992	Male group (1 135)
						Female group (256)
						Heavy vehicle operators (217)
						Combined group (1 487)
SA92	160	Grade 12	0.51–0.82	0.52–0.74	1992	Male group (3 400)
						Female group (3 448)
						Combined group (6 922)
16PF5	185	Grade 10	0.55–0.85		2005	First-year university students (2 538)
					2009	Working adults (478)

the South African population (Van Eeden, Taylor & Du Toit, 1996). The sample consisted of job applicants for various organisations, split by language group: namely, English- and Afrikaans-speaking applicants (N = 104), African language speakers from the private sector (N = 111), and African language speakers from the public sector (N = 138). Van Eeden et al. (1996) found evidence for item bias in only 8 out of the 185 items, and mean differences on 5 of the factors, which could be explained within the occupational context of the various groups. They evaluated the factorial similarity between groups and found that even though the five expected global factors (see Table 14.1) could be identified, the loading patterns for the three subgroups differed. On the basis of these findings, Van Eeden et al. (1996) recommended some language adaptations and cultural considerations of the 16PF5 before standardisation in South Africa. Larger and more representative samples were also required.

The US version of the 16PF5 was also used in a follow-up study by the HSRC (Prinsloo, 1998). Only slight changes were made to ten items, often in the form of explanatory additions. The aim was to explore the influence of the level of understanding of English as the test language. The sample comprised first-year university students from different population groups (approximately 8 per cent black, 5 per cent coloured, 2 per cent Indian and 85 per cent white) and language groups (58 per cent Afrikaans, 35 per cent English and 7 per cent other). Reasonably favourable results were found in terms of differential item analysis and factor analysis when controlling for language proficiency. Recommendations were made in terms of a more representative sample and the potential role of language proficiency.

A first norm sample in South Africa consisted of 1 525 students, of whom 692 were men and 833 were women (Maree, 2002). This research was done using the original US version of the 16PF5. The majority of respondents were white, and around 60 per cent of the respondents were between 18 and 19 years old. In terms of gender, Maree (2002) found large mean score differences on most of the scales except for Liveliness (F), Social Boldness (H), Vigilance (L), Perfectionism (Q_3) and Tension (Q_4). With regard to race, the research design was very unbalanced, but just in an exploratory fashion it was found that Reasoning (B) and Privateness (N) presented the greatest disparities between the groups, although this was not necessarily evidence of bias. It was noted that there were possible cultural influences when answering the US version of the 16PF5. Language competency also appeared to play a role, which supported the argument for the development of the South African version of the 16PF5 questionnaire.

The adaptation of the 16PF5 questionnaire for the South African population began in 2002, with initially only changes to spelling and minor language usage changes to a 263-item research form. An attempt to translate the questionnaire into both Afrikaans and Zulu then guided the selection of items from the extended research form, as it was the intention to have the same items for all three translations of the South African adaptation of the 16PF5 instrument. Independent translators translated the items into Afrikaans and isiZulu. Certain linguistic dilemmas arose from the isiZulu translation (such as having different isiZulu dialects, and no equivalent isiZulu word for the English), and it was decided to halt the isiZulu translation while the English and Afrikaans adaptations progressed. The difficulties encountered with the isiZulu translation are also reflected in a subsequent attempt at a Tshivenda translation (Van Eeden & Mantsha, 2007). The items in the Afrikaans version are the same as those in the South African English version.

The items included in the South African version of the 16PF5 questionnaire are very similar to those in the US version. Minor grammatical and spelling changes were made to 37 of the final 185 items. The overlap of items with the US version is very high, except for Reasoning (B) and Vigilance (L). The trial versions were administered to a group of 3 189 first-year university students in 2003, of which 100 cases were removed due to missing data. With regard to gender, 41.5 per cent were men and 55.3 per cent were women. The population groups were distributed as follows: black (17.8 per cent), coloured (4.3 per cent), Indian (6.2 per cent) and white (68.5 per cent). Further changes were made to the items in both the English and Afrikaans versions after reviewing the initial results. The process evolved, and the psychometric properties of this trial version are described by Schepers and Hassett (2006). The changes were reviewed by experts, who made final suggestions and changes to the items at the end of 2004. These final versions of the English and Afrikaans adaptations were administered to a student norm group early in 2005 (see Table 14.2). A working adult norm group for the South African English version was created in 2009 (IPAT, 2009) (see Table 14.2). The working adult norm sample consists of incumbents in various sectors across South Africa, and the population groups were represented as follows: black (N = 152), white (N = 122), Indian (N = 124) and coloured (N = 72). The size of this sample was seen to be sufficient for an itinerant norm group, and given that additional data would continue to be collected in order to increase the size of this norm group.

Psychometric properties of the South African version of the 16PF5

The South African version of the 16PF5 was administered to a group of first-year university students, as part of their intake assessment battery. This group formed the first standardisation sample for the 16PF5 questionnaire, with 42 per cent of the sample being men and 58 per cent women. Each of the population groups was represented, with white students making up 42 per cent of the sample and black students making up 36 per cent. Most of the scales had reliability coefficients between 0.60 and 0.70, which was lower than that found for the US normative sample, but higher than previous South African versions (see Table 14.2). The standard errors of measurement for the sten scores ranged from 0.65 to 1.55, which were in line with those found for other international adaptations of the 16PF5 questionnaire (IPAT, 2009).

The results of a factor analysis, where items were grouped into parcels for each scale, indicated that most of the item-parcel loadings corresponded to Cattell's primary factors in the US 16PF questionnaire (IPAT, 2009). Apprehension (O) did not exist as a separate factor, but rather loaded clearly onto the Emotional

Stability (C) factor, so that high Apprehension correlated with low Emotional Stability. Despite this anomaly, the majority of the factors were clearly defined, providing evidence for construct validity.

With regard to gender differences, the results showed that female students tended to score significantly higher than male students on Warmth (A), Rule-Consciousness (G), Social Boldness (H), Sensitivity (I), Vigilance (L), Apprehension (O) and Tension (Q4). Male students tended to score higher than female students on Emotional Stability (C), Dominance (E), Abstractedness (M) and Privateness (N). With regard to the four South African population groups, significant differences were found on all the scales, except for Warmth (A), Social Boldness (H) and Apprehension (O). However, the effect sizes for all of these differences were small, except for Reasoning (B) and Liveliness (F), which demonstrated medium effect sizes. These results and the norms are available in the *16PF5 South African Version: User's Manual* (IPAT, 2009).

Research on the applicability and utility of the 16PF in South Africa

Research on the multicultural use of the 16PF-SA92 is discussed below (see Prinsloo and Ebersöhn (2002) for studies related to the validity but not specifically the cultural applicability of the instrument). This research provides a methodological basis for continued research in terms of multicultural personality assessment, specifically when this involves the 16PF5. The studies furthermore contextualise cultural and especially language problems related to the use of the 16PF questionnaire (regardless of the version of the questionnaire) in the local context. Research on the 16PF5 has focused on construct validity, but some work has also been done on issues related to language.

The 16PF-SA92

In a study by Van Eeden and Prinsloo (1997) with 637 applicants at a multicultural financial institution, internal consistency values for an African-language group were mostly above 0.50 but were generally lower than those found for the norm sample. Reliability was also a major concern for Abrahams and Mauer (1999a). Their sample consisted of 983 students of psychology or industrial psychology from four South African universities, with an equal distribution across different population groups. They found that the reliability coefficients for only three primary factors (H, Q2 and Q3) were larger than 0.50 in the black subgroup. The value for Factor M was exceptionally low. The values for the coloured, Indian and white population groups were also relatively low, with the latter being closest to those found for the norm sample.

Results of research on the 16PF-SA92 intensified the debate on the acceptability of differences in the profiles of mean scores (Retief, 1992; Taylor & Boeyens, 1991). The factor structure and the primary factor mean scores were compared for subgroups in the norm group (home language, population group, gender, etc.). Differences mostly occurred at the level of the mean factor scores, and only in the case of gender did the level of significance of these differences imply a need for separate norm tables (Prinsloo, 1992a). In the study by Van Eeden and Prinsloo (1997) significant differences in mean raw scores were found on only four primary factors for gender, whereas more than half of the factors differed for language. Only three of the latter differences were regarded as substantial, and it was concluded that the results did not warrant separate norms but that group-specific trends should be considered when interpreting the scores on the traits. Abrahams and Mauer (1999b), however, contended that the cross-cultural use of the 16PF-SA92 could not be justified given these differences in factor means. The differences in response rates found by them led to significant raw score mean differences for ten of the first-order and all of the second-order factors, when compared across the four population groups (Abrahams & Mauer, 1999a). Differences were found on only three primary and two second-order factors for gender. Retief (1992) argued that consistent differences in response to items in a personality questionnaire that can be explained in terms of cultural factors are acceptable. Abrahams (2002, p.59), however, regarded the description of the black subsample in terms of the characteristics associated with differences in the scores on the factors highlighted in the preceding research as 'highly questionable'. Prinsloo and Ebersöhn (2002) nevertheless cautioned that the mean profile of a sample of respondents was hypothetical and evaluation of scores on the personality traits was application-specific, the latter impacting on the interpretation of a score as positive or negative.

Abrahams and Mauer (1999b) further explored the differences in response pattern using qualitative analyses (including a request for synonyms for a list of nouns and adjectives used in the 16PF-SA92). Based on this analysis, problematic items (in terms of response pattern) were categorised in terms of a cultural factors category and a syntactical and word connotation problem category (about half of the items). However, according to Prinsloo and Ebersöhn (2002), understanding isolated word lists is not a good predictor of understanding the whole item where the word is used in context. It implies producing meaning rather than recognising meaning.

Wallis and Birt (2003), replicating the study by Abrahams and Mauer (1999b), also concluded that methodological issues rather than language proficiency resulted in problems in understanding. Their sample comprised 131 students, 96 being native English speakers and 35 non-native English speakers. Neither group was able to provide acceptable synonyms most of the time when relying on dictionary descriptions, but with less rigid marking both groups understood the list of words.

The factor structures for subgroups of the norm sample were basically the same, but with slight trends observed for specific groups, especially in the case of the fifth factor – namely, Tough Poise. In the study by Van Eeden and Prinsloo (1997), the factor structure for the total sample and the norm group was found to be essentially the same when considering the coefficients of congruence. Emotional Sensitivity could, however, not be identified for the African language group or for the gender groups separately. There was also overlap between this factor and Anxiety for the Afrikaans/English group, and Compulsivity could not be extracted for this group. The possibility of culture as a moderator of the constructs measured was mentioned. However, Abrahams (2002) did not regard this explanation as sufficient (especially given the possible negative reflection on a specific group), and proposed that more attention be given to language proficiency as a potential source of bias. The impact of language was highlighted in other local studies with the 16PF (for example, Meiring, 2000).

The 16PF5

To demonstrate the 16PF5's construct validity internationally, the 16PF5 scales were compared to four measures of normal personality. They were the Personality Research Form (Jackson, 1984), the California Psychological Inventory (Gough, 1987), the NEO Personality Inventory – Revised (Costa & McCrae, 1992) and the Myers-Briggs Type Indicator (Myers & McCaulley, 1985). These personality inventories all had different scale construction strategies, so the correlations would not be contaminated by similar scale construction. The results clearly showed that the constructs of most of the scales of the 16PF5 were quite similar to those of the Fourth Edition (Conn & Rieke, 1998).

For the primary factors of the South African version of the 16PF5, construct validity was established using the Locus of Control Inventory (LCI). Schepers and Hassett (2006) investigated the relationship between the fourth edition LCI and the trial version of the South African English 16PF5. The LCI was administered jointly with the 16PF5 to a sample of 2 798 first-year university students. The 16PF5 yielded six global factors with reliability coefficients that ranged from 0.721 to 0.861. These factors were named Liveliness, Perfectionism, Dominance, Tension, Abstractedness and Warmth. These link conceptually to the 16PF5 Global Factors of Extraversion (Dominance and Liveliness), Self-Control (Perfectionism), Anxiety (Tension), Tough-Mindedness (Abstractedness) and Independence (Warmth).

Three significant canonical correlations of 0.659, 0.455 and 0.322 were obtained between the three scales of the LCI and the primary factors of the 16PF5. Schepers and Hassett (2006) interpreted the first factor as Ascendancy with Social Boldness and Autonomy. High scorers on this factor were described as well balanced, forceful, socially bold, open to change and confident that they can overcome problems on their own. The second factor was interpreted as Emotional Stability. High scorers on this factor were described as emotionally stable, self-assured, trusting and relaxed. They would normally have low scores on External Control. The third factor was interpreted as Rule-Consciousness. High scorers on this factor were described as rule-conscious, dutiful, perfectionistic, well organised and practical. They would normally have quite high scores on Internal Control. These findings show that the relationship between locus of control and personality as measured by these two instruments is in line with the theoretical underpinnings of locus of control.

De Bruin, Schepers and Taylor (2005) conducted a study which examined the relationship between the Basic Traits Inventory (BTI), a South African-developed measure of the Big Five factors of personality, and the South African English 16PF5. These two questionnaires were administered to 2 009 first-year university students.

A joint common factor analysis of the 24 BTI facets and 15 16PF5 personality scales produced a psychologically meaningful six-factor solution, which was determined based on inspection of the scree plot and parallel analysis. Five of the six factors corresponded closely with the Big Five factors, and the resulting six factors were labelled Extraversion, Conscientiousness, Neuroticism/Anxiety, Openness, Agreeableness and Tough-Mindedness. The Tough-Mindedness factor was made up of Excitement-Seeking on the BTI and lower scores on Warmth and Sensitivity from the 16PF5, indicating a lack of emotional sensitivity. These factors also manifested equivalently for black and white students.

Using a research form of the 16PF5, Van Eeden and Mantsha (2007) attempted to develop a Tshivenda translation of the questionnaire. The translated version was administered to a sample of 85 Tshivenda-speaking students, and items were scrutinised in terms of their contribution to the reliability of the 16 primary factors. The results indicated that even if items that lowered reliability were excluded, the reliability coefficients would remain low. Further investigation revealed that some of the items were ineffective due to the fact that translation changed the meaning of the items. This could have been a result of the absence of an equivalent concept in the Tshivenda language, difficulty in translating colloquial expressions, potential confusion due to the use of the negative form, and translation errors. These difficulties were similar to those found in translation of the 16PF5 into isiZulu (IPAT, 2009). Van Eeden and Mantsha (2007) also identified potential trends of cultural differences in the manifestation of constructs that were related to cultural norms and experiential factors. The results indicated that literal translation of the questionnaire is insufficient, and that a different approach would have to be taken for future translations of the 16PF5 and other personality questionnaires.

The appropriateness of the language used in the 16PF5 still remains the focus in South Africa. At the time of publication of this chapter, studies were being conducted on the South African version of the 16PF5 that replicated Abrahams and Mauer's (1999b) previous research on the use of language. The fact remains that, as with any other psychological questionnaire used in South Africa, language proficiency is vital for the respondent to be able to understand the content of any item. It is up to the practitioner to ensure that the respondent is able to understand the language of assessment; otherwise any assessment will be futile and perhaps even detrimental to the well-being of the respondent.

The 16PF in practice

Given that the 16PF questionnaire was developed as a measure of normal personality traits, it can be used in any context where an evaluation of personality is indicated. Some of the contexts discussed in this section have to do with areas where the 16PF is most often used, but this does not necessarily exclude the use of the 16PF questionnaire in other contexts.

An assessment is either initiated by the individual or from within an institutional setting. The first aim is assumed always to be for the benefit of the individual, although institutional and societal purposes become important as well. Evaluation of a respondent's personality profile guides feedback and decisions pertaining to behavioural outcomes in relevant practical domains of concern. These may include vocational guidance, occupational choices, admission into and readiness for study and training opportunities, selection for and placement in positions in the workplace, leadership and promotion, and the diagnosis of minor to more severe (or clinical) personal problems. Such problems may interfere with job performance, personal relationships or individual well-being, and assessment will centre on developing remedies or treatment – for instance, for depression or anxiety. Personality measurement also plays an important role in academic research and theory development.

The use of the 16PF questionnaire in clinical settings is well known. Although it was not developed for diagnosing pathology, research exists that shows the utility of using surveys of normal personality in the clinical context (for example, Quirk, Christiansen, Wagner & McNulty, 2003). Tests of normal personality can help to provide a picture of the individual's total personality functioning, and highlight strengths and development areas to help the clinician or counsellor to develop effective treatment and therapeutic interventions. The 16PF questionnaire should obviously never be used in isolation, and should only be used as a tool to help improve the client's self-awareness, facilitate dialogue, and aid clinicians in determining their approach to therapy.

A survey by Van der Merwe (2002) of the assessment practices in a number of organisations showed that the 16PF was the most widely used personality test. The organisations indicated that they used testing not only as part of the selection and placement process but also for career development, the identification of training needs, counselling and many other applications. It is, however, its use for selection and placement in industry that has been most controversial, given the public debate around culture-fairness sparked by Abrahams and Mauer (1999a; 1999b). However, the practitioner faces the same legal risk using any personality assessment in the workplace. It remains the responsibility of the practitioner to ensure that he or she has selected the correct test for the evaluation process, has done a thorough job analysis and follows best-practice procedures throughout the process. The research review published in this chapter is intended to provide practitioners with enough information to facilitate the responsible use of the 16PF questionnaire within their contexts. The research should not only be seen in the light of the usual professional best practice, but also contributes deliberately to enhanced test fairness as demanded by recent legislative amendments.

Outside of selection and placement practices in the workplace, the 16PF can prove exceptionally useful for individual and group development purposes. For leadership and management development, it identifies strengths and development areas to enhance the coaching process and add to self-awareness. The 16PF is also used in team development processes to address personality-style conflicts, and to help teams identify and address personality-related process issues.

The future of the 16PF

With the development of technology, social networking and interconnectivity, the face of personality assessment has changed from what we have known it to be over the years, and is also likely to change how we do things in future. For a start, the evaluation of the statistical properties of assessments is more accurate, more flexible and more easily accessible to psychologists than before, which increases the critical evaluation of assessments and demands higher standards. The use of methods based on item response theory to determine the suitability of tests also provides psychologists with better standards for judging bias and the actual construction of assessments.

Since its humble beginnings in the 1940s, the 16PF questionnaire has remained an important assessment of personality. Constant adaptation and research have maintained the quality and relevance of the 16PF in different contexts and countries, and this tradition is likely to continue into the foreseeable future. The 16PF5 is now available in a number of administration formats, including paper-and-pen, computer-based and online administration. Practitioners can opt to score the questionnaires themselves, or have electronic narrative reports generated for a number of different contexts. There is an option to have the 16 personality factors linked to an organisation's competency matrix for customised competency reports. Future editions of the 16PF are also likely to incorporate technological advances in the presentation of the questionnaire and the delivery of results.

Research on the 16PF in South Africa has had a largely narrow and superficial focus on matters such as the understanding of vocabulary taken from test items and studied devoid of context, or an over-emphasis on mean score differences pertaining to test scales for subgroups. Although this research has highlighted psychometric difficulties and language issues related to the local use of the questionnaire, the issue of providing for different cultures at a conceptual level still needs to be addressed (see, for example, Meiring, Van de Vijver, De Bruin & Rothmann, 2008). The focus should shift towards more substantive studies on the integrity of factor structures across groups, predictive validity and other criterion-related validity studies. This is the only way to ensure the continued relevance of the 16PF in a multicultural South African context, and to maintain the variety of personality assessment tools available to psychologists in this country.

Note

1 16PF® is a registered trademark of IPAT in the USA, the European Community and other countries. IPAT is a wholly owned subsidiary of OPP® Ltd. OPP® is a registered trademark of OPP Ltd in the European Community. OPP Ltd, Elsfield Hall, 15–17 Elsfield Way, Oxford OX2 8EP, United Kingdom (www.opp.eu.com).

References

Abrahams, F. (2002). The (un)fair usage of the 16PF (SA92) in South Africa: A response to C. H. Prinsloo and I. Ebersöhn. *South African Journal of Psychology, 32(3)*, 58–61.

Abrahams, F. & Mauer, K. F. (1999a). The comparability of the constructs of the 16PF in the South African context. *Journal of Industrial Psychology, 25(1)*, 53–59.

Abrahams, F. & Mauer, K. F. (1999b). Qualitative and statistical impacts of home language on responses to the items of the Sixteen Personality Factor Questionnaire (16PF) in South Africa. *South African Journal of Psychology, 29(2)*, 76–86.

Cattell, R. B. (1989). *The 16PF: Personality in Depth*. Champaign, IL: Institute for Personality and Ability Testing.

Cattell, R. B., Eber, H. W. & Tatsuoka, M. M. (1970). *Handbook for the Sixteen Personality Factor Questionnaire (16PF)*. Champaign, IL: Institute for Personality and Ability Testing.

Conn, S. R. & Rieke, M. L. (1998). *The 16PF Fifth Edition Technical Manual* (2nd edition). Champaign, IL: Institute for Personality and Ability Testing.

Costa, P. T., Jr & McCrae, R. R. (1992). *Revised NEO Personality Inventory (NEO-PI-R) and NEO Five-Factor Inventory (NEO-FFI): Professional Manual*. Odessa, FL: Psychological Assessment Resources.

De Bruin, G. P., Schepers, J. M. & Taylor, N. (2005). Construct validity of the 16PF 5th Edition and the Basic Traits Inventory. Paper presented at the 8th Annual Industrial Psychology Conference. Pretoria, June 8–10.

Gough, H. G. (1987). *California Personality Inventory Administrator's Guide*. Palo Alto, CA: Consulting Psychologists Press.

Hall, C. S. & Lindzey, G. (1957). *Theories of Personality*. New York, NY: John Wiley & Sons.

Hjelle, L. A. & Ziegler, D. J. (1976). *Personality Theories: Basic Assumptions, Research, and Applications*. Tokyo: McGraw-Hill Kogakusha.

IPAT (Institute for Personality and Ability Testing) (2009). *16PF5 South African Version: User's Manual* (2nd edition). Champaign, IL: Institute for Personality and Ability Testing.

Jackson, D. N. (1984). *Personality Research Form Manual*. Port Huron, MI: Research Psychologists Press.

Maree, D. J. F. (2002). *Properties of and South African Norms for the 16PF Fifth Edition: Technical Report*. Johannesburg: Jopie van Rooyen & Partners.

Meiring, D. (2000). Revisiting the cross-cultural comparability of the 16PF in the South African context. Paper presented at the Industrial Psychology Conference (incorporating the Psychometrics Conference). Pretoria, June 8–9.

Meiring, D., Van De Vijver, F. J. R., De Bruin, G. P. & Rothmann, S. (2008). Personality structure in South Africa: Commonalities of three comprehensive measures. Draft article.

Myers, I. B. & McCaulley, M. H. (1985). *Manual: A Guide to the Development and Use of the Myers-Briggs Type Indicator*. Palo Alto, CA: Consulting Psychologists Press.

Prinsloo, C. H. (1989). *Norms, Gemiddeldes, Standaardafwykings en Betroubaarheidskoëffisiënte vir die Sestien-Persoonlikheidsfaktorvraelys (Vorm A)*. Pretoria: Human Sciences Research Council.

Prinsloo, C. H. (1991). *Norms, Means, Standard Deviations and Reliability Coefficients for the Sixteen Personality Factor Questionnaire (Form A)*. Pretoria: Human Sciences Research Council.

Prinsloo, C. H. (1992a). *Manual for the Use of the Sixteen Personality Factor Questionnaire, South African 1992 Version (16PF, SA92)* (2nd edition). Pretoria: Human Sciences Research Council.

Prinsloo, C. H. (1992b). *Manual for the Use of the Sixteen Personality Factor Questionnaire, Form E (16PF, Form E)*. Pretoria: Human Sciences Research Council.

Prinsloo, C. H. (1998). *The Factor Structure and Readability of the South African English Version of the Fifth Edition of the American 16PF*. Report to the External Advisory Committee. Pretoria: Human Sciences Research Council.

Prinsloo, C. H. & Ebersöhn, I. (2002). Fair usage of the 16PF in personality assessment in South Africa: A response to Abrahams and Mauer with special reference to issues of research methodology. *South African Journal of Psychology, 32(3)*, 48–57.

Quirk, S. W., Christiansen, N. D., Wagner, S. H. & McNulty, J. (2003). On the usefulness of measures of normal personality for clinical assessment: Evidence of the incremental validity of the Revised NEO Personality Inventory. *Psychological Assessment, 15*, 311–325.

Retief, A. (1992). The cross-cultural utility of the SAPQ – bias or fruitful differences? *South African Journal of Psychology, 22*, 202–207.

Schepers, J. M. & Hassett, C. F. (2006). The relationship between the fourth edition (2003) of the Locus of Control Inventory and the Sixteen Personality Factor Questionnaire (Version 5). *South African Journal of Industrial Psychology, 32(2)*, 9–18.

Taylor, T. R. & Boeyens, J. C. A. (1991). The comparability of the scores of blacks and whites on the South African Personality Questionnaire: An exploratory study. *South African Journal of Psychology, 21*, 1–11.

Van der Merwe, R. (2002). Psychometric testing and human resource management. *South African Journal of Industrial Psychology, 28(2)*, 77–86.

Van Eeden, R. & Mantsha, T. R. (2007). Theoretical and methodological considerations in the translation of the 16PF5 into an African language. *South African Journal of Psychology, 37(1)*, 62–81.

Van Eeden, R. & Prinsloo, C. H. (1997). Using the South African version of the 16PF in a multicultural context. *South African Journal of Psychology, 27*, 151–159.

Van Eeden, R., Taylor, T. R. & Du Toit, R. (1996). *Adaptation and Standardisation of the Sixteen Personality Factor Questionnaire Fifth Edition (16PF5) in South Africa: A Feasibility Study*. Pretoria: Human Sciences Research Council.

Wallis, T. & Birt, M. (2003). A comparison of native and non-native English-speaking groups' understanding of the vocabulary contained in the 16PF (SA92). *South African Journal of Psychology, 33(3)*, 182–190.

15 Using the Fifteen Factor Questionnaire Plus in South Africa

N. Tredoux

When the Fifteen Factor Questionnaire Plus (15FQ+) was launched in South Africa in 2000, personality measurement was at a critical point in this country. Abrahams and Mauer (1999a; 1999b) had raised questions about the culture-fairness of the 16PF form SA92, which was the most widely used measure of Cattell's model at the time in South Africa. The original Fifteen Factor Questionnaire (15FQ), which the 15FQ+ was intended to replace, was not yet well known in South Africa. Results based on the standardisation sample indicated that the 15FQ+ was more reliable than other questionnaires measuring Cattell's factors, including the original 15FQ (Paltiel, 2000). Many psychologists had already been trained in the interpretation of Cattell's model, and this facilitated the adoption of the 15FQ+. The new questionnaire was implemented by several South African organisations and consulting psychologists, who collaborated on the collection of local standardisation data (Tredoux, 2002–2011). Whereas initially there was a tendency to use the questionnaire on groups for which it was not suitable, there is now enough information to support responsible decision-making regarding the use of the 15FQ+ in South Africa.

Development of the 15FQ+

The original 15FQ questionnaire, which preceded the 15FQ+, was developed for industrial and organisational use (Budd, 1992). It included all Cattell's scales except for Factor B (Intelligence). The scales were constructed using a rigorous item analysis methodology (Barrett & Paltiel, 1993; 1996), designed to yield a short and reliable questionnaire with items correlating substantially higher with the scale for which they are coded, rather than with any other scale in the questionnaire. This approach helped to ensure that the scales were unidimensional. The 15FQ was offered as an alternative to the 16PF, which some authors considered too unreliable for occupational use at the time (Barrett & Kline, 1982; Saville & Blinkhorn, 1981). The 15FQ was developed for use in the UK, but soon gained acceptance in Australia and New Zealand. Pilot studies conducted in South Africa indicated that the 15FQ was less reliable in this country than the Occupational Personality Profile (OPPro); hence the use of the OPPro, rather than the 15FQ, was encouraged here. A notable feature of the

15FQ was the capability of generating sophisticated narrative reports using the GeneSys software (Bonderowicz, 1992).

Eight years after the release of the 15FQ it was replaced by the 15FQ+, which was designed to be more robust than the original version, using simpler language and carefully avoiding items that might have been culture- or gender-biased (Budd, 2010). The questionnaire was also revised to make it more suitable for international use. Like its predecessor, the 15FQ+ is intended specifically for occupational use. The new questionnaire was developed in the UK, but the items were sent for review to psychologists in other countries, including South Africa, before the finalisation of the item set (Paltiel, 2000).

Although Cattell's model of personality was derived through factor-analytical research (Cattell, Eber & Tatsuoka, 1970), the 15FQ and the 15FQ+ were developed using a similar classical psychometric approach (Kline, 1986), employing Barrett's item analysis methodology (Barrett, 1996). Item-level factor analysis did not form part of the development process for the 15FQ+ (Budd, 2010), although a factor analysis on the scale scores yielded the same five second-order factors produced by the 16PF. Thus, instead of attempting to rediscover the factor structure of personality, the developers of the 15FQ+ accepted Cattell's scales and developed item sets to measure those scales, with the emphasis on reliability and unidimensionality of the scales.

Administration and scoring

The 15FQ+ can be administered using pencil and paper or using a computer. If computer-based administration is used, the questionnaire can be completed in one of three ways: directly on the GeneSys computer system, using the GeneSys Remote Questionnaire Administrator, or using the GeneSys Online system (supervised administration). The GeneSys computer system and Remote Administrator require the Windows operating system to run, while the GeneSys Online system can also run on other operating systems – for example, the different variants of Linux or the Macintosh operating system. In South Africa paper-based scoring is not recommended, because the self-scoring answer sheet developed for overseas use is based on UK norms. Scoring masks are not supplied, for copyright reasons. If pencil-and-paper test administration is used, the questionnaire can be scored on the GeneSys software or online. Users can do the scoring themselves by entering the responses into the software. Users specify the norm group to be used and the type of report they want, and the report is automatically produced as a word-processor document.

Scales measured by the 15FQ+

Validity scales

The15FQ+ includes five scales designed to indicate possible motivational distortion or other factors that could interfere with the honest and consistent answering of the questionnaire. These scales and their interpretation are described in Figure 15.1.

Figure 15.1 15FQ+ response style indicators

Impression management scale	Explanation	Interpretation
Social Desirability	The desire to present an unrealistically positive image of oneself. Denying minor failings and idiosyncrasies that are typical of most people. An eight-item scale specifically designed for the purpose.	Stens of 8–10 may reflect either a deliberate attempt at distortion or a highly over-idealised, possibly unrealistic self-image. Consider the respondent's motivation for responding in a socially desirable manner. Integrate information from the candidate's background and the verification interview.
Faking Good	Presenting oneself in a favourable light by denying a variety of problem behaviours and difficulties that apply to many people. Consists of items keyed to score other scales as well.	Only interpret extremely high scores. Interpret with caution if different from the Social Desirability score. Take the rest of the personality profile into account, as well as information from the verification interview.
Infrequency	The extent to which a respondent has failed to attend diligently to the questionnaire with due thought and consideration. Incidence of infrequency endorsed or responses are random.	Raw scores of 10 or more are significant. Consider whether the respondent understood the items and instructions or not. Random responding can sometimes indicate a non-cooperative or disinterested attitude when completing the questionnaire. High anxiety levels during testing can also interfere with the respondent's ability to attend to the questionnaire properly. (Verify during interview and check against scale scores.)
Central Tendency	The extent to which the respondent chose non-committal, middle responses and did not give decisive answers to the items.	Extremely high scores (sten score of 10) may invalidate the profile. Use the validation interview to consider the reasons why the respondent did not reveal much about himself or herself. Consider the context in which the assessment was done.
Faking Bad	The extent to which the respondent presented himself or herself in an unfavourable light, admitting to a variety of problem behaviours and difficulties that do not normally apply to himself or herself.	Consider whether the respondent had very high anxiety levels when the questionnaire was administered. This could contaminate and inflate the Faking Bad score. Interpret in the context of the overall personality profile and take interview information into account.

In considering the validity of a particular 15FQ+ profile, it is important to note how the validity scales or response style indicators are interpreted in the context of the setting in which the assessment is done (Budd, 2010). These scales should not be interpreted in isolation, but in relationship to the rest of the personality profile, and in the light of information obtained from an interview or from other appropriate sources. In the end, the decision as to whether or not to accept that a person answered the questionnaire honestly should be based on a holistic psychological judgement by a professional person, and not simply by applying cut-off scores.

It is important to note that motivational distortion of the 15FQ+ profile can be avoided by proper, professional administration procedure. It is important to establish rapport with the respondents and to ensure that they cooperate with the assessment process. This is in line with the requirement of the ethical code for psychologists that assessment should take place within the context of a defined professional relationship (Department of Health, 1974). After completion of the questionnaire, it is important to have an interview with the respondent during which the veracity of the profile can be compared to the assessor's observations, and where apparent contradictions or vagueness in the profile can be clarified. Basic feedback can also be given during this interview.

Primary scales

The 15FQ+ was designed to measure 15 of the 16 original scales contained in Cattell's (1957) model of personality. The exception is Cattell's Factor B (Intelligence), which was omitted for theoretical and practical reasons. In place of Factor B, the 15FQ+ introduced a new scale. The Intellectance scale, labelled ß, measures a person's confidence in his or her own intellectual ability, rather than attempting to measure the ability directly. Criterion-keyed scales for Work Attitude and Emotional Intelligence were also included, over and above the original scales (Budd, 2010). The 16 primary scales, and the meaning of their high and low scores, are set out in Figure 15.2.

Figure 15.2 15FQ+ primary scale definitions

15FQ+ Scale	Low score description	High score description
*f*A	**Distant-aloof** Lacking empathy, distant, detached, impersonal	**Empathic** Friendly, personable, participating, warm-hearted, caring
β	**Low intellectance** Lacking confidence in one's own intellectual abilities	**High intellectance** Confident of one's own intellectual abilities
*f*C	**Affected by feelings** Emotionally intense, changeable, labile, moody	**Emotionally stable** Mature, resilient, calm, phlegmatic, unemotional
*f*E	**Accommodating** Passive, mild, humble, deferential	**Dominant** Assertive, competitive, aggressive, forceful

continued

15FQ+ Scale	Low score description	High score description
*f*F	**Sober-serious** Restrained, taciturn, cautious	**Enthusiastic** Lively, cheerful, happy-go-lucky, carefree
*f*G	**Expedient** Spontaneous, disregarding of rules and obligations	**Conscientious** Persevering, dutiful, detail-conscious
*f*H	**Retiring** Timid, socially anxious, hesitant in social settings, shy	**Socially bold** Venturesome, talkative, socially confident
*f*I	**Hard-headed** Utilitarian, unsentimental, lacks aesthetic sensitivity, tough-minded	**Tender-minded** Sensitive, aesthetically aware, cultured, sentimental
*f*L	**Trusting** Accepting, unsuspecting, credulous	**Suspicious** Sceptical, cynical, doubting, critical
*f*M	**Concrete** Solution-focused, realistic, practical, down-to-earth	**Abstract** Imaginative, absent-minded, impractical, absorbed in thought
*f*N	**Direct** Genuine, artless, open, straightforward, forthright	**Restrained** Diplomatic, socially astute, shrewd, socially aware, restrained
*f*O	**Confident** Secure, self-assured, unworried, guilt-free	**Self-doubting** Worrying, insecure, apprehensive, guilt-prone
*f*Q1	**Conventional** Traditional, conservative, conforming, resistant to change	**Radical** Experimenting, progressive, open to change, unconventional
*f*Q2	**Group-orientated** Sociable, group dependent, consultative, a 'joiner'	**Self-sufficient** Solitary, self-reliant, individualistic, autonomous
*f*Q3	**Informal** Uncontrolled, lax, follows own urges, nonconforming, expedient	**Self-disciplined** Compulsive, meticulous, exacting willpower, socially conforming
*f*Q4	**Composed** Relaxed, placid, patient, steady, even-tempered	**Tense-driven** Impatient, low frustration tolerance, restless, irritable

Second-order factors

Once the primary scales have been scored and sten scores obtained using the selected norm group, the reporting software calculates estimates of the second-order factor scores (Figure 15.3).

Figure 15.3 15FQ+ global factors

Definitions of 15FQ+ global factors, with contributing primary scales

Introversion Orientated towards their own inner world of thoughts, perceptions and experiences. Not requiring much social contact and external stimulation *f*A– (Distant-aloof), fF– (Sober-serious), *f*H– (Retiring), fQ2+ (Self-sufficient)	**E**	**Extraversion** Orientated to the outer world of people, events and external activities. Needing social contact and external stimulation *f*A+ (Empathic), *f*F+ (Enthusiastic), *f*H+ (Socially bold), *f*Q2– (Group-orientated)
Low aNxiety Well adjusted, calm, resilient and able to cope with emotionally demanding situations *f*C+ (Emotionally stable), *f*L– (Trusting), *f*O– (Self-assured), *f*Q4– (Composed)	**N**	**High aNxiety** Vulnerably, touchy, sensitive, prone to mood swings, challenged by emotionally gruelling situations *f*C– (Affected by feelings), *f*L+ (Suspicious), *f*O+ (Apprehensive), *f*Q4+ (Tense-driven)
Pragmatism Influenced more by hard facts and tangible evidence than subjective experiences. May not be open to new ideas, and may be insensitive to subtleties and possibilities *f*A– (Distant-aloof), *f*I– (Hard-headed), *f*M– (Concrete), *f*Q1– (Conventional)	**O**	**Openness** Influenced more by ideas, feelings and sensations than tangible evidence and hard facts. Open to possibilities and subjective experiences *f*A+ (Empathic), *f*I+ (Tender-minded), *f*M+ (Abstract), *f*Q1+ (Radical)
Independence Self-determined with regard to own thoughts and actions. Independent-minded. May be intractable, strong-willed and confrontational β+ (High intellectance), *f*E+ (Dominant), *f*L+ (Suspicious), *f*Q1+ (Radical)	**A**	**Agreeableness** Agreeable, tolerant and obliging. Neither stubbom, disagreeable nor opinionated. Is likely to be happy to compromise β– (Low Intellectance), *f*E– (Accommodating), *f*L– (Trusting), *f*Q1– (Conventional)
Low self-Control Exhibiting low levels of self-control and restraint. Not influenced by social norms and internalised parental expectations *f*G– (Expedient), *f*N– (Direct), *f*Q3– (Informal)	**C**	**High self-Control** Exhibiting high levels of self-control. Influenced by social norms and internalised parental expectations *f*G+ (Conscientious), *f*N+ (Restrained), *f*Q3+ (Self-disciplined)

Adapted from the 15FQ+ Technical Manual with permission.

The technical manual for the 15FQ+ (Budd, 2010) contains a detailed discussion of every scale and second-order factor, with descriptions of the typical behaviour of people who obtain high and low scores on each scale. The technical manual can be downloaded at no cost from the test publisher's website (Psytech International Limited, no date).[1] This chapter is not intended to be a substitute for the technical manual, and responsible users of the 15FQ+ should always ensure that they have the manual available when interpreting the test.

Derived scores

Besides the scales and second-order factors directly measured by the 15FQ+, the reporting software can also calculate estimates of a number of derived scores that are particularly useful in occupational settings. These include team types based on the work of Belbin (2003), leadership styles, subordinate styles and selling and influencing styles based on the work of Bass (1985), and career themes based on the work of Holland (1985). This information is found in the extended computer-generated report of the 15FQ+ (this is the most popular report and usually the first report requested by users). It is important for users to realise that these derived scores are only estimates, calculated using logically constructed formulas based on an overview of the research literature (Budd, 2010). They should not be regarded as actual measures, and users should not set cut-off scores on derived scores for selection purposes. Derived scores can, however, be very helpful in integrating test result information, giving feedback or writing reports for relevant contexts.

Computer-generated reports for the 15FQ+

A large selection of computer-generated reports is available. The most popular is the extended report, which is lengthy, aimed at a trained interpreter of the questionnaire, and covers the core scales as well as several derived measures. It is now possible for users to acquire customised reports for specific needs, such as a particular selection or development project. Specialised reports are available to deal with emotional intelligence, counterproductive behaviour and managerial competencies. The ease of use and convenience of the computer-generated reports make the 15FQ+ very attractive to the busy professional. While these reports can save a lot of time and help an inexperienced user to get to grips with the questionnaire, they should never be treated as a substitute for professional judgement, and the user should always take personal responsibility for any report which is the output of a professional service. Where necessary, computer-generated reports should be edited, amended, expanded and put into the proper context of the purpose for which the assessment is being done.

Psychometric properties of the 15FQ+

Available documentation for users

The technical manual for the 15FQ+ reports the reliabilities of the primary scales, and their correlations with other scales in the 15FQ+ as well as with related scales in other questionnaires. It also reports on validity studies done internationally. Local research is summarised in the *South African User Guide and Research Reference*, which is updated periodically (Tredoux, 2002–2011).

Norms

A large number of different norm groups are available for South African users, covering South African language groups and race groups. Some occupation-specific norm groups are also available. Users of the 15FQ+ also have the facility of creating and updating their own norms using the software that administers and scores the 15FQ+. When reporting on the 15FQ+ and giving feedback, users should be aware of the nature of the norm group: is it a general population group, or is the respondent being compared to a more selected group that may have a typical personality profile? When in doubt, it is safest to choose a recent, large, population norm group unless there is a compelling reason not to do so.

Reliability

Between 2000 and 2004, the 15FQ+ was used in a selection battery for candidate police officers. Large numbers of candidates were tested, under less than ideal conditions. Testing groups were large, and to expedite scoring, a non-standard answer sheet was used that could be scanned by an optical mark reader. Many respondents could not fill in their biographical particulars on the answer sheet, and it can be assumed that they had even more difficulty answering the questionnaire items. Large numbers of answer sheets had to be discarded as unreadable. Language was clearly an obstacle to the completion of the questionnaire. The reliability coefficients were unsatisfactory, particularly for persons who had an African language as their home language. In an attempt to address this problem, the items were progressively simplified. Since changing the questionnaire items did not bring about the desired changes in reliability (Meiring, Van de Vijver & Rothmann, 2003), the South African distributor of the 15FQ+ decided not to distribute the changed version, but to remain true to the international version of the 15FQ+. However, important lessons were learnt as a result of the police recruitment project. The 15FQ+ was clearly unsuitable for mass screening of entry-level workers in South Africa. Users are now advised to be selective about the use of the 15FQ+, and particularly to pay attention to the English proficiency of the intended respondents, even going so far as to use a structured test of English proficiency prior to using a personality questionnaire.

Earlier reliability studies, including the ones based on which the 15FQ+ was classified, were done on samples comprising mixed race and language groups. However, the majority of these respondents were white (Tredoux, 2002–2011). Larger groups were available when reliabilities were calculated in 2008, and more people from formerly disadvantaged groups were included in the sample. These studies yielded reliability coefficients that were by and large around .7, indicating that the questionnaire could be used with caution. It appeared that scale M (Concrete vs Abstract) was probably difficult to understand for some groups of South Africans. This scale includes some items with difficult English words (for example, 'profound', 'philosophical', 'the nature of free will', etc.). Another scale where possible problems with reliability existed was scale E (Accommodating vs Dominant).

By 2010, a very large number of respondents had completed the 15FQ+. A comparison between the reliability coefficients for different race groups indicated that for whites, coloureds and Asians, the reliabilities were consistently higher than for the black group. Particular care needs to be exercised when interpreting the results of black respondents on scales A (Empathic), E (Dominance), M (Abstract) and Q3 (Self-disciplined). When comparing reliabilities across language groups, the same scales emerged with lower reliabilities for the indigenous language group, compared to the Afrikaans and English language groups. When comparing the reliabilities between groups who are formerly disadvantaged as opposed to not formerly disadvantaged, the differences are still there, although not as marked, and the scale most clearly requiring caution is scale M (Abstract). Proficiency in English is clearly a factor in determining whether a scale will be reliable or not. It is, however, worth noting that Afrikaans speakers generally answer the questionnaire most consistently, with even higher reliability coefficients than those found for English speakers.

To investigate the contribution that language proficiency made to this problem, respondents who had completed both the 15FQ+ and the General Verbal Reasoning Test were extracted from the database. Reliability coefficients were calculated separately for each race, and for five levels of verbal reasoning test score: stanines 1 and 2, stanines 3 and 4, stanine 5, stanines 6 and 7, and stanines 8 and 9. This was done wherever there were enough data to compute the reliabilities – it was not possible in all cases, and in some cases, particularly at the extremes of the ability spectrum, the sample sizes were quite small. From this analysis it was possible to discern what the reliability coefficients for the 15FQ+ scales are if verbal reasoning, or English verbal comprehension, is held constant. For most scales, it became apparent that when verbal reasoning scores were high, the reliability coefficients for the different race groups tended to converge. When verbal reasoning scores were low, reliability coefficients were low.

South Africa is still struggling to overcome the disparities in the socio-economic status of the different race groups. The formerly disadvantaged groups still labour under educational disadvantage that is a result of relative poverty. Additionally, people who are so affected also often do not speak English as a first or even second language. The responsible test user must realise that this has an influence on the respondents' ability to answer a personality questionnaire such as the 15FQ+ consistently. For instance, screening job applicants solely on the basis of personality scores is discouraged. The questionnaire should be followed up by a verification interview to confirm and further explore the questionnaire findings. This interview should be conducted by a trained 15FQ+ user and should focus on scales where reliabilities are known to be lower for the particular group to which the respondent belongs. In this regard the person-job match report produced by the Profiler module in the GeneSys system can help the user who is relatively inexperienced with the questionnaire with suggested supplementary interview questions that are related to the personality scales that need to be probed.

Validity

The correlation patterns between the 15FQ+ scales and the Occupational Personality Questionnaire, the OPPro and the Minnesota Multiphasic Personality Inventory (Tredoux, 2002–2011) provide supporting evidence for the construct validity of the 15FQ+.

The 15FQ+ scales correlate as expected with the other questionnaire scales, and hence one can conclude that the construct validity of the 15FQ+ scales has been established, even in South Africa. There is no doubt a need for further research, especially independent research and research involving tests from other publishers, on the construct validity of the 15FQ+.

The 15FQ+ has been included in a number of criterion-related validity studies. Success in insurance sales could be predicted using the 15FQ+ and the Critical Reasoning Test Battery (Tredoux, 2000). Managerial competencies in the insurance industry could be predicted using the 15FQ+ and the Values and Motives Inventory the Cognitive Process Profile and assessment centre exercises (Marais, Tredoux & Prinsloo, 2003; Tredoux, 2002–2011). Higher scores on *f*L (Suspicious) were associated with higher performance ratings. This could be explained because the managers were working in the financial industry and had to accomplish their performance through others. To be rated as having high potential, higher levels of intellectance and enthusiasm, as well as being direct rather than restrained, were important. Although the intricate and highly customised competency model used in this validation study limits generalisation of the results to other organisations, it was clear from the study that personality variables as measured by the 15FQ+ could make a meaningful contribution to the prediction of managerial competency ratings.

Validation studies that use performance appraisals or competency ratings as criterion variables can be difficult to generalise, because the competency definitions can be tied to the company culture and the nature of the business. In another study involving managers and supervisors in the manufacturing industry (Tredoux, 2002–2011), being pragmatic rather than abstract was overall the most important personality characteristic associated with higher performance appraisals. For the supervisor subgroup the important characteristics were enthusiastic, relaxed, affected by feelings, accommodating and retiring. For the formerly disadvantaged subgroup in this study, the important characteristics were informal, relaxed, self-assured, empathic, retiring, accommodating and trusting. Seen as a whole, one wonders if it is not possible that 'nice people' get higher performance ratings. When studying managerial performance via ratings it is almost impossible to distinguish between a likeable personality and real high performance. Performance ratings are also often skewed towards the high end of the scale and restricted in range, because managers do not like to give subordinates a low rating. Ratings tend to vary between 'Average' and 'High'. This limits the correlations that can be found. One should also consider the possibility that there might be more than one 'ideal' personality for a role. People may, knowingly or unknowingly, compensate for deficiencies in one area by developing their strengths in another. Using classification tree analysis, it is possible to identify groups of people who share common personality profile characteristics, who fall into either the low- or high-performance group (see Figure 15.4).

Figure 15.4 Classification tree showing personality profiles of groups of persons with either high or low performance as managers or supervisors

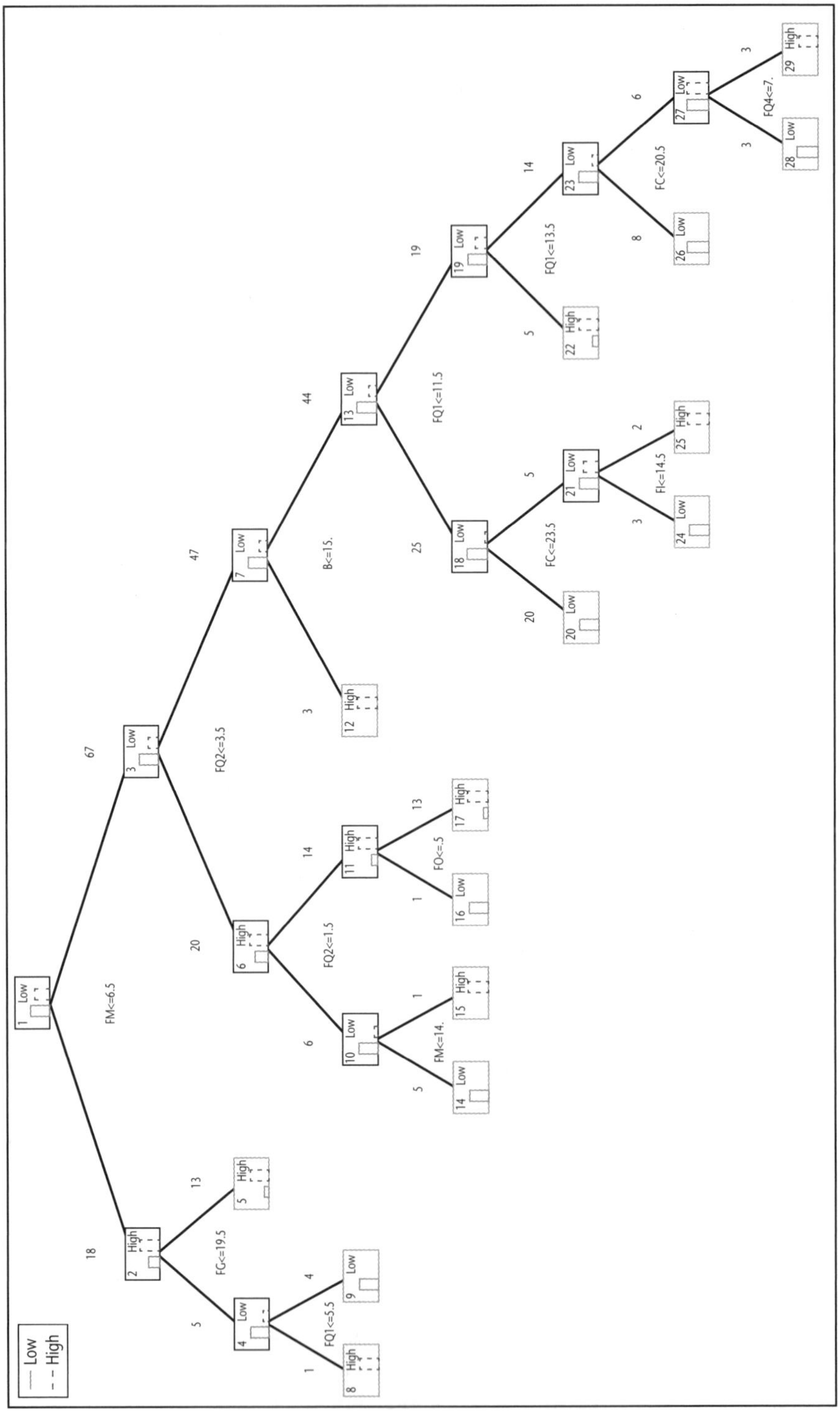

The diagram in Figure 15.4 shows the division of the abovementioned sample into groups based on cut-off scores (raw scores were used for this example but standardised scores can also be used). The cut-off condition for each branching is shown. Cells to the left meet the cut-off condition, whereas cells to the right do not. Using this strategy, one can choose the level of stringency to use when setting up desired profiles. This allows one to use a broad-banding approach and allow for possible alternative personality profile configurations that could be successful, as well as situations where the relationship between a personality characteristic and performance might not be linear. In another study (Tredoux, 2002–2011), where the 15FQ+ was used to predict work performance ratings in a chemical company, it was found that employees who were dominant, trusting, sober-serious, tense-driven and emotionally stable were more likely to obtain high performance ratings. When these data were analysed using classification trees, it was possible to identify different profiles that were associated with either high or low merit ratings.

In summary, there is considerable support for the construct validity of the 15FQ+. With regard to predicting performance at work, it appears that combinations of personality scales are more effective at predicting performance than single scales considered in isolation, and that the relationships between personality variables and success are dynamic and not always linear.

Bias and fairness

Although analysis of variance and t-tests demonstrated statistically significant effects for race, language and gender for almost all the scales (Tredoux, 2002–2011), it should be considered that because the samples are large, even a score difference that has no practical impact can reach statistical significance. When standardised effect sizes are calculated, it becomes clear that the differences in raw scores between groups on the 15FQ+ scales are small enough not to affect any particular group adversely (see Table 15.1).

Table 15.1 Standardised effect sizes for the differences in means on 15FQ+ scales between different South African groupings

Scale	Effect size for race	Effect size for gender	Effect size for language group
15FQ+_fA	0.12	–0.49	0.12
15FQ+_B	0.16	0.06	0.14
15FQ+_fC	0.07	0.13	0.08
15FQ+_fE	0.02	0.11	0.03
15FQ+_fF	0.13	–0.14	0.17
15FQ+_fG	0.14	–0.18	0.13
15FQ+_fH	0.15	–0.04	0.20
15FQ+_fI	0.07	–0.79	0.09
15FQ+_fL	0.20	–0.04	0.24
15FQ+_fM	0.02	0.07	0.04
15FQ+_fN	0.22	–0.05	0.25
15FQ+_fO	0.12	–0.04	0.12

continued →

Scale	Effect size for race	Effect size for gender	Effect size for language group
15FQ+_fQ1	0.04	–0.05	0.05
15FQ+_fQ2	0.15	0.03	0.18
15FQ+_fQ3	0.08	0.07	0.09
15FQ+_fQ4	0.28	–0.03	0.29
15FQ+_SD	0.26	–0.09	0.25
15FQ+_CT	0.04	0.04	0.04
15FQ+_INF	0.09	0.18	0.11
15FQ+_EIQ	0.21	–0.10	0.17
15FQ+_WA	0.10	0.03	0.00
15FQ+_fGOOD	0.22	–0.02	0.26
15FQ+_fBAD	0.13	–0.04	0.09

Notes: For differences between males and females, standardised effect sizes were calculated. For differences between race groups and language groups, the root mean square standardised errors were calculated.

It should, moreover, be borne in mind that the desired personality profile varies between job roles, depending on the nature of the work. Therefore, although groups may differ significantly, it is not possible to know whether these differences will be to the disadvantage of members of any particular group in a given situation. Thus the differences in mean scores between groups is not as big a concern as the differences between reliability coefficients.

Structural equivalence and differential item functioning of the 15FQ+ have also been examined. An investigation into the factor structure of the 15FQ+ for a sample of black South African managers concluded that low reliabilities were hampering structural equivalence (Moyo, 2009). Studies on larger samples found structural equivalence between groups with a point estimate of the root mean square error of approximation of 0.016 on a targeted varimax rotation (Tredoux, 2009).

It cannot be denied that language and culture probably affect the way respondents react to the items of the 15FQ+. Hence it is recommended that for all personality tests, not just the 15FQ+, questionnaire results not be interpreted in isolation. All test results should be placed in context using information obtained from interview observations, appropriate background information and other assessment measures.

Note

1 www.psytech.com.

References

Abrahams, F. & Mauer, K. F. (1999a). Qualitative and statistical impact of home language on responses to the items of the Sixteen Personality Factor Questionnaire (16PF) in South Africa. *South African Journal of Psychology, 29(2)*, 76–86.

Abrahams, F. & Mauer, K. F. (1999b). The comparability of the constructs of the 16PF in the South African context. *Journal of Industrial Psychology, 25(1)*, 53–59.

Barrett, P. T. (1996). PSWin psychometric software documentation. Unpublished document.

Barrett, P. T. & Kline, P. (1982). An item and radial parcel analysis of the 16PF questionnaire. *Personality and Individual Differences, 3(3)*, 259–270.

Barrett, P. T. & Paltiel, L. (1993). The concurrent and structural validity of the 15 Factor Personality Questionnaire. *International Journal of Recruitment Selection and Retention, 2(3)*, 30–36.

Barrett, P. T. & Paltiel, L. (1996). An evaluation of the psychometric properties of the Concept 5.2 OPQ Questionnaire. *Journal of Occupational and Organisational Psychology, 69(1)*, 1–19.

Bass, B. M. (1985). *Leadership and Performance Beyond Expectation*. New York, NY: Free Press.

Belbin, R. M. (2003). *Management Teams: Why They Succeed or Fail*. Oxford: Butterworth Heinemann.

Bonderowicz, S. (1992). *GeneSys Assessment and Profiling System Manual*. Letchworth: Psytech International Ltd.

Budd, R. (1992). *Fifteen Factor Questionnaire: The Technical Manual*. Letchworth: Psytech International Ltd.

Budd, R. (2010). *The 15FQ+ Technical Manual (Revised)*. Pulloxhill: Psytech International Ltd.

Cattell, R. B. (1957). *Personality and Motivation: Structure and Measurement*. Yonkers-on-Hudson, NY: World Book Co.

Cattell, R. B., Eber, H. W. & Tatsuoka, M. M. (1970). *Handbook for the Sixteen Personality Factor Questionnaire (16PF)*. Champaign, IL: Institute for Personality and Ability Testing.

Department of Health (1974). Genreg 197(c): Rules of conduct pertaining specifically to the profession of psychology. *Health Professions Act No. 56*. Pretoria: Government of the Republic of South Africa.

Holland, J. L. (1985). *Making Vocational Choices: A Theory of Vocational Personalities and Work Environments*. Odessa, FL: Psychological Assessment Resources.

Kline, P. (1986). *Handbook of Test Construction*. London: Routledge & Kegan Paul.

Marais, W., Tredoux, N. & Prinsloo, M. (2003). Assessment of leadership competencies. Paper presented at the Conference of the Society for Industrial and Organisational Psychology of South Africa. Johannesburg, June 25–27.

Meiring, D., Van de Vijver, F. & Rothmann, S. (2003). *Personality Tests: No More Controversial in South Africa: Weeding Out Bias*. Johannesburg: Society for Industrial and Organisational Psychology of South Africa.

Moyo, S. (2009). *A Preliminary Factor Analytic Investigation into the First-Order Factor Structure of the Fifteen Factor Questionnaire Plus on a Sample of Black South African Managers*. Department of Industrial Psychology, University of Stellenbosch, Stellenbosch.

Paltiel, L. (2000). 16PF – Industrial Seminar. Seminar presentation. Sunnyside Hotel, Johannesburg, March 21.

Psytech International Limited (no date). *The Fifteen Factor Questionnaire* +. Retrieved May 31, 2010, from http://www.psytech.com.

Saville, P. & Blinkhorn, S. (1981). Reliability, homogeneity and the construct validity of Cattell's 16PF. *Personality and Individual Differences, 2(4)*, 325–333.

Tredoux, N. (2000). Predicting insurance sales success. Paper presented at the Industrial Psychology Conference of the Society for Industrial and Organisational Psychology of South Africa. Pretoria, June 21.

Tredoux, N. (2002–2011). *The 15FQ+ South African User Guide and Research Reference*. Johannesburg: Psytech South Africa.

Tredoux, N. (2009). 15FQ+ best-use update. Presentation. Bryanston Country Club, Sandton, Gauteng, May 14.

16 The Basic Traits Inventory

N. Taylor and G. P. de Bruin

The emergence of the Five-Factor Model (FFM) of personality sparked an extensive amount of research in the area of personality theory and assessment. The FFM presents a structure for personality that is best described by five global domains or factors that characterise individual differences. These five domains are generally called Extraversion, Neuroticism, Openness to Experience, Agreeableness and Conscientiousness (Church, 2000; Costa & McCrae, 2008). This model is not based on any single theory of personality, and numerous factor analyses of existing personality instruments have returned very similar structures to that of the five factors (Allik & McCrae, 2004; McCrae, Terracciano & 79 Members of the Personality Profiles of Cultures Project, 2005).

The FFM of personality has its roots in the research that was done using the lexical approach to personality description. The lexical hypothesis assumes that most notable individual differences that are also socially relevant will become encoded as single words in natural language (Goldberg, 1990). In other words, the terms that are used in describing personality in this model are also the terms that people would use in everyday language in order to describe themselves and others. This research was followed by the development of the questionnaire tradition, which was led primarily by work on the NEO personality inventories as well as the work of Costa and McCrae (McCrae & Allik, 2002; Rolland, 2002).

The development of the Basic Traits Inventory (BTI) started in 2002, at which time no South African trait-based personality inventories were available. Taylor and De Bruin (2006) decided to create a new personality instrument for South Africa, using the FFM that has been shown to have cross-cultural applicability throughout the world (see McCrae et al., 2005). Some of the advantages of using this model as a framework are that it integrates a wide array of personality constructs, making it possible for researchers across different fields of study to communicate easily; it is comprehensive, providing a means to study relations between personality and other phenomena; and it is efficient, as it offers at least a global description of personality (McCrae & Costa, 2008). There is also a large body of evidence suggesting that the model can be applied successfully in different cultures (see Laher, 2008; 2011; McCrae et al., 2004; McCrae et al., 2005).

A description of the BTI

The intention to ensure construct validity of the BTI from the outset demanded the specification of precise definitions of the five factors. After an extensive literature review, Taylor (2004) provided definitions for the factors and the facets that would help define each factor. The five domains in the BTI each consist of five facets, apart from Neuroticism, which has four. The definitions used are provided in Table 16.1.

Table 16.1 Definitions of the factors and facets of the BTI

Factor	Descriptions of people with high scores
Extraversion (E)	Enjoys being around other people, likes excitement and is cheerful in disposition.
Gregariousness	Enjoys frequent social interaction.
Positive Affectivity	Frequently experiences positive emotions.
Ascendance	Enjoys entertaining and leading large groups of people.
Excitement-Seeking	Seeks out adrenaline-pumping experiences and intense stimulation.
Liveliness	Is bubbly, lively and energetic.
Neuroticism (N)	Experiences negative affects in response to his or her environment.
Anxiety	Is nervous, apprehensive and tense.
Depression	Frequently experiences guilt, sadness and hopelessness.
Self-consciousness	Is sensitive to criticism, and feels shame and embarrassment.
Affective instability	Is easily upset, emotionally volatile and feels anger or bitterness.
Conscientiousness (C)	Is effective and efficient in planning, organising and executing tasks.
Order	Is neat, tidy and methodical.
Self-discipline	Is able to start tasks and carry them through to completion.
Dutifulness	Sticks to principles, fulfils moral obligations and is reliable and dependable.
Effort	Sets ambitious goals and works hard to meet them.
Prudence	Thinks things through carefully, checks the facts and has good sense.
Openness to Experience (O)	Is willing to experience new or different things and is curious.
Aesthetics	Appreciates art, music, poetry and beauty.
Actions	Tries new and different activities.
Values	Is willing to re-examine social, political and religious values.
Ideas	Enjoys considering new or unconventional ideas.
Imagination	Has a vivid imagination and thinks creatively.
Agreeableness (A)	Is able to get along with other people and has compassion for others.
Straightforwardness	Is frank and sincere.
Compliance	Defers to others, inhibits aggression and forgives easily.
Modesty	Is humble and self-effacing.
Tender-mindedness	Has sympathy and concern for others.
Prosocial tendencies	Is kind, generous, helpful and considerate.

The BTI consists of 193 items written in the form of statements, where the respondent needs to indicate the degree to which he or she agrees with a statement on a five-point Likert-type scale, ranging from 'strongly agree' to 'strongly disagree'. It also includes a 13-item social desirability scale. The items were kept as short as possible, and the authors tried to follow closely the guidelines set out for writing items that would be used in translation (Van de Vijver & Leung, 1997).

Contrary to convention, the items are all keyed in the direction of their dimension. In addition, negative terms such as 'not', 'never' and 'no' are excluded from the inventory. The purpose of this is to allow for easy translatability, avoid confusion in deciding on a response, and keep items to the point. An item-sort revealed that conceptual confusion arose when negatively worded and negatively keyed items were included in the scale (Taylor & De Bruin, 2006).

The items of the BTI are grouped according to their respective facets, and these are presented together for each factor, instead of in random order. This is done in order to contextualise the items for the test-taker, and therefore attempt to remove any vagaries that might arise from a single item in a non-specific context. No formal demarcations are made between factors or their facets. The BTI is therefore presented as a single list of items. The social desirability items are placed between facets throughout the test. Research into whether the item order affected the psychometric properties of the test indicated that when the items were presented together there was more local dependence than when presented in random order, but this did not impact significantly on the reliability or structure of the BTI (De Bruin & Taylor, 2008).

The BTI is available as a pen-and-paper version or online. Electronic profile reports are generated for both versions. At present, norms are available for students, police applicants and working adults. The psychometric properties of the BTI in South Africa are discussed in the following section.

Psychometric properties of the BTI

There have been many studies investigating the reliability of the BTI across groups in South Africa. A summary table of the internal consistency reliability coefficients (Cronbach's alpha) across some of these studies is presented in Table 16.2.

Table 16.2 Summary of internal consistency reliability coefficients

Scale	Thomson (2007)	Govender (2008)	Taylor (2008)	Vogt & Laher (2009)	Desai (2010)
N	175	125	6112	176	130
Extraversion	0.89	0.89	0.90	0.89	0.86
Neuroticism	0.94	0.94	0.94	0.95	0.79
Conscientiousness	0.91	0.96	0.94	0.92	0.92
Openness to Experience	0.89	0.90	0.88	0.87	0.87
Agreeableness	0.90	0.93	0.88	0.90	0.92

Taylor (2008) investigated the psychometric properties of the BTI in a sample of 6 112 university students on which the student norms are based, using a combination of both classical test theory and item response theory methods. Comparisons across gender, population group and home language were done for all analyses. The comparison groups used were as follows: men and women; black and white respondents; and English, Afrikaans and indigenous African language speakers.

Internal consistency reliability was evaluated using both Cronbach's alpha reliability coefficient and the person separation index (PSI) from a Rasch analysis. Both methods revealed similar indices of internal consistency. For the five factors of the BTI, the reliability estimates were similar across methods, and deemed satisfactory for the Extraversion ($\alpha = 0.90$; PSI = 0.89), Neuroticism ($\alpha = 0.94$; PSI = 0.93), Conscientiousness ($\alpha = 0.94$; PSI = 0.92), Openness to Experience ($\alpha = 0.88$; PSI = 0.85), and Agreeableness ($\alpha = 0.88$; PSI = 0.86) scales. Three facet scales – namely, Openness to Values, Straightforwardness and Modesty – showed consistently lower than acceptable Cronbach alpha values across the comparison groups, indicating that scores on these facets should be interpreted with caution. From the Rasch analysis of each of the factors of the BTI, it emerged that 35 of the 180 items showed some evidence of misfit, and specifically underfit. Of the 35 misfitting items, only 10 items showed signs of extreme underfit (Taylor, 2008).

Taylor (2008) found very little evidence for item bias across all groups on each of the five factors of the BTI. In Rasch terminology, differential item functioning (DIF) is evident when there are differences in item location of greater than 0.5 logits. For the gender groups, there were three items with DIF contrast values larger than 0.5 logits across all five factors. For the population groups, eight of the items showed DIF contrast values larger than 0.5 logits. Only three items met the criteria for item bias in the language groups. Two of the Openness to Experience items were judged to show item bias in both the population groups and language groups, and Taylor (2008) recommended that they be removed from future versions of the BTI.

Taylor (2008) conducted a factor analysis and congruence analysis, and the results showed a regular pattern of factor loadings for all the comparison groups. Positive Affectivity consistently emerged with dual loadings on Extraversion and Agreeableness, an indication that the construct is not purely related to Extraversion. Openness to Actions also displayed a pattern of dual factor loadings on Openness to Experience and Extraversion, which showed that some element of Extraversion is captured in the Openness to Actions scale. However, this pattern seemed to be present in most of the comparison groups, and these two scales appear to have been interpreted similarly across the comparison groups. Openness to Values appeared to be a problematic facet, often failing to load meaningfully on its posited factor, and having slight discrepancies in meaning across comparison groups. On the whole, however, Taylor (2008) found good evidence for the structural equivalence of the scales of the BTI across the comparison groups.

With regard to mean score differences across groups, Taylor (2008) found that whilst consistent differences were reported, the effect sizes were negligible, or so small that they should not warrant serious concern. Whereas it would be irresponsible to ignore the differences found, it is unlikely that the mean differences found would impact on the interpretations of mean scores across groups. For the most part, the mean differences found in the comparison groups were consistent with those found in the literature.

As an additional test of construct validity, Taylor (2008) evaluated the test characteristic curves in each comparison group, and found no differences across gender in the functioning of the scales for the five factors of the BTI. However, some differences in functioning between the black student group and white student group emerged, consistent with the extreme response styles (consistently selecting the 'strongly disagree' and 'strongly agree' response options) that were identified in a subsequent analysis. The black student group was consistently more likely to use an extreme response style, and to avoid the 'disagree' option. Slight differences were also found across language groups, although these were less pronounced than for the population groups. The impact of non-uniform bias on the interpretation of mean scores across groups needs to be investigated to ensure that scores are not artefacts of responding to the instrument, but good indicators of an individual's true standing on the latent trait.

Research on the BTI

Using the BTI and a subtest of the 360-degree assessment called the Broad Band Competency Assessment Battery (BB-CAB) (Taylor, in press), Venter (2006) investigated the relationship between the Big Five and emotional intelligence (EI) competencies. Using a sample of 150 call centre employees, Venter (2006) found significant relationships between each of the Big Five factors and certain competencies of EI. Extraversion was positively related to the competencies Teamwork/Conflict Management and Influence/Leadership, and Conscientiousness was positively related to Self-confidence and Achievement Drive EI competencies. Venter (2006) also found positive correlations between Openness to Experience and Self-confidence, Initiative, Teamwork/Conflict Management and Influence/Leadership. Agreeableness was significantly positively correlated with Teamwork/Conflict Management.

Venter (2006) found that while Neuroticism was negatively correlated with Self-confidence, Persistence/Resilience, Teamwork/Conflict Management and Influence/Leadership, it was also positively correlated with Empathy and Conscientiousness. These findings are interesting, and could probably explain some of the underlying motivations behind EI competencies. Individuals who are more likely to experience a wider range of emotions may more easily recognise these in others, and a tendency towards worrying and self-consciousness may drive performance in trying to avoid trouble in a call centre environment (Venter, 2006).

De Bruin and Rudnick (2007) examined the relationship between Conscientiousness, Excitement-Seeking and academic cheating in a group of 683 second-year university students. The results showed that more Conscientious students were less likely to engage in cheating behaviour during examinations, and that students high on Excitement-Seeking were more likely to engage in cheating behaviour. De Bruin and Rudnick (2007) proposed a model to explain academic dishonesty based on these results. They suggested that students who are low on Conscientiousness are more likely to procrastinate on academic tasks and be less prepared for examinations. These students are also less likely to be mindful of rules and regulations, and this, combined with a tendency to rate the risks associated with cheating as low, would lead them to consider cheating as a potential solution to their problems. The application of these findings in the workplace would perhaps be useful in examining unethical behaviour in employees, although this is yet to be determined.

In order to determine whether Conscientiousness was related to job performance in a group of 101 information technology customer support service engineers in the banking sector, Sutherland, De Bruin and Crous (2007) used the Conscientiousness scale of the BTI, a measure of empowerment, and a performance evaluation questionnaire. There was no significant relationship found between supervisor ratings of job performance and Conscientiousness, although there was a weak curvilinear relationship between empowerment and performance. Conscientiousness and empowerment were also significantly correlated. The authors recommended further research with larger groups of individuals on more objective measures of job performance.

Thomson (2007) studied the relationship between personality traits and life balance in a sample of 175 corporate sector employees, using the BTI and a life-balance questionnaire. She found that Extraversion, Conscientiousness and Openness to Experience were positively related to life balance, while Neuroticism was negatively related to life balance. Thomson (2007) also found that personality accounted for approximately 15 per cent of the variance in life balance, with Conscientiousness and Openness to Experience being the most significant contributors.

The relationship between personality traits and coping in 125 police officers was investigated using a measure of coping styles, the Coping Orientations to Problems Experienced (COPE) scale (Carver, Scheier & Weintrab, 1989) and the BTI. Govender (2008) found statistically significant correlations between Conscientiousness, Agreeableness and Openness to Experience and Problem-focused Coping. This suggests that officers with these traits tend to actively address their problems by either talking to others, problem-solving or using physical exercise (Govender, 2008). Neuroticism was related to Dysfunctional Coping strategies, and Agreeableness and Openness to Experience were both related to Emotion-focused Coping strategies. Emotion-focused strategies tend to incorporate activities such as anger catharsis, sleeping, withdrawal and substance usage. Govender's (2008) results showed that police officers tended to use Problem-focused and Emotion-focused Coping strategies rather than Dysfunctional Coping strategies. These results have important implications for the process of selecting police officers so that those candidates with the best capacity to cope with the stark nature of police work are selected.

Ramsay, Taylor, De Bruin and Meiring (2008) conducted a test of measurement invariance of the BTI across three black language groups in 2 432 applicants for a clerical position. The language groups were made up respectively of Nguni (N = 496), Sesotho (N = 891), and Sepedi (N = 1 045) speakers. Ramsay et al. (2008) found that for practical purposes, the BTI was invariant across the three language groups. This suggests that combining black language groups would not introduce too much variance into cross-cultural comparisons.

Taylor (2008) conducted a study in order to evaluate the presence of differing response styles across groups, and used Rasch analysis as a way of investigating response style separately from the sample characteristics. A pattern of responding was identified that would not be picked up when investigating response styles using traditional methods. Taylor (2008) found that black students and indigenous African language-speaking groups appeared to endorse the 'disagree' category so infrequently or irregularly that it was hardly ever the most probable category across all five factors. In addition, a trend of extreme responding was found for women, black students and indigenous African language-speaking students on the scales of the BTI. Evidence for a midpoint response style was found for women, and only slight differences in response style were found for the English-speaking and Afrikaans-speaking students. For women, there is an indication of two response styles – namely, extreme and midpoint responding; this indicates an avoidance of the 'disagree' and 'agree' response options. Taylor (2008) recommended that the actual impact of these response styles on mean scores be investigated in order to determine whether steps should be taken towards controlling or removing the effects of response style in future.

Vogt and Laher (2009) investigated whether the five factors are related to individualism/collectivism in a sample of 176 students using the BTI and the Individualism/Collectivism scale. The results showed that there were no significant relationships between the five factors and individualism/collectivism. In addition, no significant difference was found between population groups and the five factors and individualism/collectivism. There were also no significant differences between home language and the five factors and individualism/collectivism. These results are important, as the construct of individualism/collectivism is often used to explain occasional group differences in personality assessment. This shows promise for the continued use of the BTI in cross-cultural settings.

Desai (2010) investigated the relationship between personality as measured by the BTI and team emotional and social intelligence in trainees in the South African Police Service. She found significant correlations between Agreeableness and team identity, motivation, emotional awareness, stress tolerance, conflict resolution and positive mood. Desai (2010) found the lack of a relationship between personality and team culture at the beginning of training and a slight relationship between the variables towards the end. She also commented that a significant increase in Neuroticism and decreases in Agreeableness and Openness to Experience were found over a six-month period. These results appear consistent with work done by Steyn (2006), which reported that successful socialisation of police trainees into the police force often required them to suppress certain personal characteristics in order to develop discipline and suspicion, as they would be consistently exposed to threats of imminent danger and uncertainty (Steyn, 2006).

The BTI-Short

The BTI-Short consists of 60 items and provides psychologists with a brief measure of the Big Five traits. Each trait is measured by 12 items, which were selected from the full-length BTI item pool. Six criteria were used in selecting the items for the short version: (a) each item should correlate strongly with the total scale; (b) each item should contribute towards the reliability of its respective scale (Cronbach alpha of at least 0.80 for each scale); (c) each item should saliently load on its intended factor but not on any other factors in a joint factor analysis of the items; (d) each item should be free of item bias across different language groups; (e) each of the original 24 facets must be represented by at least one item (but preferably three items); and (f) the total scores of the brief scales must correlate strongly with the total scores of the full-length scales. The item selection was performed using the responses to the full-length BTI of 1 000 persons representing four language groups (English, N = 250; Afrikaans, N = 250; Nguni, N = 250; and Sesotho, N = 250).

Reliability coefficients for the five scales were calculated for the calibration sample (N = 1 000) by means of Cronbach's alpha coefficient: Extraversion = 0.80, Neuroticism = 0.86, Conscientiousness = 0.85, Openness = 0.77 and Agreeableness = 0.75. Reliabilities were also calculated for a new data set containing the responses of 883 persons: Extraversion = 0.81, Neuroticism = 0.86, Conscientiousness = 0.87, Openness to Experience = 0.83 and Agreeableness = 0.81. Overall, the reliabilities were > 0.80 and indicate that the BTI-Short yields scores that might be profitably used for research and screening purposes. As expected, the reliability coefficients are lower than those of the full-length BTI. It is recommended that the full-length BTI be used when important decisions are to be made about individuals.

Factor analysis of the pooled data set yielded five well-defined factors that accord with the theoretical model underlying the BTI-Short. Each of the 60 items had a satisfactory loading on its expected factor. The factor analysis shows that the items measure the traits that they are intended to measure, and therefore provides support for the construct validity of the five BTI-Short scales.

Item analysis indicated that each of the 60 items correlated satisfactorily with the total score of the relevant scale. Rasch analysis showed that conditional on the latent traits measured by the BTI-Short, all the items elicited responses that accorded with theoretical expectation. These results show that the items appropriately discriminate between persons with different trait levels on each of the Big Five factors.

Overall, results suggest that the BTI-Short provides an alternative to the full-length BTI when time constraints prohibit the use of the latter. The BTI-Short contains the best items of the long version and may be expected to yield scores that adequately represent the Big Five personality traits.

Studies using the BTI-Short have looked at the relationship between the Big Five factors and other constructs such as career barriers, burnout and stress. Additional research is under way with regard to personality and self-directed learning, career decision-making and volunteering for HIV/AIDS testing. So far it has proved useful in research settings, although its usefulness in industry is yet to be demonstrated.

Critiques of the BTI

As with any measure of a psychological trait, there is always room for improvement, and certain criticisms can be levelled against the BTI. From a psychometric perspective, the fact that the questionnaire is a self-report measure could attract comments from critics who believe this to be an inferior form of assessment of psychological constructs. In addition, the BTI also shares the criticisms levelled against the FFM of personality as (amongst other criticisms) too simple a description of personality (see, for example, Block, 1995; 2001; Laher, 2011).

However, there have been few published criticisms levelled against the BTI itself. Ramsay et al. (2008) suggest that the straightforwardness and clustering of the items may create a more transparent questionnaire that could encourage faking. However, they allow that it is also possible that this format allows individuals with lesser English ability to understand the context and the item more easily, and therefore answer more consistently.

Research on the BTI has consistently found that some of the Openness to Experience facets (particularly Openness to Values and Openness to Actions) do not always perform as they should. While there is little empirical research as to why this happens, it is a pattern found by other research on the FFM in South Africa (see Heuchert, Parker, Stumpf & Myburgh, 2000; Laher, 2008; 2011; Laher & Quy, 2009; Taylor, 2000; Teferi, 2004). It is possible that this factor is affected by the type of language used, which is more abstract than some of the other scales, or is loaded with cultural content, such as acceptance of other people with different values. More research into the manifestation of this trait is needed in the South African context.

The future of the BTI

Much of the research to date has focused on the psychometric properties of the BTI, with a special focus on cross-cultural applications in the South African context. These results have been very satisfactory and hold promise for the continued use of the BTI. Some research has examined the construct validity of the BTI by focusing on its relations with relevant variables, such as burnout, self-directed learning, empowerment and health. These results have also been encouraging, and suggest that the BTI indeed measures the traits it purports to measure.

More work is needed on criterion-related validity in industrial and educational settings. In particular, future studies might focus more closely on the ability of the BTI to predict outcomes such as academic success, job performance and wellness in the workplace. The use of the BTI in counselling and clinical settings may also yield fruitful results.

In South Africa there is a dearth of suitable instruments for the measurement of personality in adolescence. This can hinder both research and practice in educational and learning environments. Against this background, a potentially fruitful area of research is the utility of the BTI with adolescents.

A final critique of the BTI stems from its use of the FFM as the benchmark against which to construct and measure personality in South Africa. The assumption inherent in this approach is that the FFM adequately maps personality in the South African context. This may be erroneous, in that both local and international research has shown the existence of factors additional to the FFM (see Cheung et al., 2001; Laher, 2008; Laher & Quy, 2009; MacDonald, 2000; Vogt & Laher, 2009). This is not to undermine the value of the BTI, since this instrument – by virtue of its local development – represents a significant step towards emic approaches in assessing and understanding personality in South Africa.

Conclusion

The BTI is a relatively new addition to the collection of personality instruments used in South Africa. It provides a measure of the five factors of personality – namely, Extraversion, Neuroticism, Conscientiousness, Openness to Experience, and Agreeableness. It is mostly used in research and organisational settings around the country, and it shows promise in counselling and wellness applications.

In summary, the BTI represents a successful attempt at developing a measure of the five-factor personality traits in South Africa. It has been shown to reliably and validly measure the five-factor personality traits across different cultural and language groups in this country. Because it was explicitly developed for the South African context, the BTI represents a viable alternative to imported measures of personality traits.

References

Allik, J. & McCrae, R. R. (2004). Toward a geography of personality traits: Patterns of profiles across 36 cultures. *Journal of Cross-Cultural Psychology, 35*, 13–28.

Block, J. (1995). A contrarian view of the five-factor approach to personality description. *Psychological Bulletin, 117*, 187–215.

Block, J. (2001). Millennial contrarianism: The five-factor approach to personality description five years later. *Journal of Research in Personality, 35*, 98–107.

Carver, C. S., Scheier, M. F. & Weintrab, J. K. (1989). Assessing coping strategies: A theoretically based approach. *Journal of Personality and Social Psychology, 56*, 267–283.

Cheung, F. M., Leung, K., Zhang, J. X., Sun, H. F., Gan, Y. Q., Song, W. Z. & Xie, D. (2001). Indigenous Chinese personality constructs: Is the Five-Factor Model complete? *Journal of Cross-Cultural Psychology, 32*, 407–433.

Church, A. T. (2000). Culture and personality: Toward an integrated cultural trait psychology. *Journal of Personality, 68*, 651–703.

Costa, P. T., Jr & McCrae, R. R. (2008). The Revised NEO Personality Inventory. In G. J. Boyle, G. Matthews & D. H. Saklofske (Eds), *The Sage Handbook of Personality Theory and Assessment* (pp. 179–198). London: Sage Publications.

De Bruin, G. P. & Rudnick, H. (2007). Examining the cheats: The role of conscientiousness and excitement seeking in academic dishonesty. *South African Journal of Psychology, 37(1)*, 153–164.

De Bruin, G. P. & Taylor, N. (2008). Block versus mixed-order item presentation in personality inventories: An IRT analysis. Paper presented at the 23rd International Congress of Psychology. Berlin, July 20–25.

Desai, F. (2010). The relationship between personality traits and team culture. Unpublished Master's dissertation. University of South Africa, Pretoria.

Goldberg, L. R. (1990). An alternative 'description of personality': The Big Five-factor structure. *Journal of Personality and Social Psychology, 59*, 1216–1229.

Govender, S. A. (2008). The relationship between personality and coping amongst members of the South African Police Service. Unpublished Master's dissertation. University of South Africa, Pretoria.

Heuchert, J. W. P., Parker, W. D., Stumpf, H. & Myburgh, C. P. H. (2000). The Five-Factor Model of personality in South African college students. *American Behavioral Scientist, 44(1)*, 112–125.

Laher, S. (2008). Structural equivalence and the NEO-PI-R: Implications for the applicability of the Five Factor Model of personality in an African context. *South African Journal of Industrial Psychology, 34(1)*, 76–80.

Laher, S. (2011). The applicability of the NEO-PI-R and the CPAI-2 in the South African context. Unpublished PhD dissertation. University of the Witwatersrand, Johannesburg.

Laher, S. & Quy, G. (2009). Exploring the role of spirituality in the context of the Five Factor Model of personality in a South African sample. *Journal of Psychology in Africa, 19(4)*, 513–521.

MacDonald, D. A. (2000). Spirituality: Description, measurement, and relation to the Five Factor Model of personality. *Journal of Personality, 68*, 153–197.

McCrae, R. R. & Allik, J. (2002). Introduction. In R. R. McCrae & J. Allik (Eds), *The Five-Factor Model of Personality across Cultures* (pp. 1–5). New York, NY: Kluwer Academic/Plenum.

McCrae, R. R. & Costa, P. T., Jr (2008). The Five Factor Theory of personality. In O. P. John, R. W. Robins & L. A. Pervin (Eds), *Handbook of Personality: Theory and Research* (3rd edition, pp. 157–180). New York, NY: The Guilford Press.

McCrae, R. R., Costa, P. T., Martin, T. A., Oryol, V. E., Rukavishnikov, A. A., Senin, I. G. et al. (2004). Consensual validation of personality traits across cultures. *Journal of Research in Personality, 38*, 179–201.

McCrae, R. R., Terracciano, A. & 79 members of the Personality Profiles of Cultures Project. (2005). Universal features of personality traits from the observer's perspective: Data from 50 cultures. *Journal of Personality and Social Psychology, 88*, 547–561.

Ramsay, L. J., Taylor, N., De Bruin, G. P. & Meiring, D. (2008). The Big Five personality factors at work: A South African validation study. In J. Deller (Ed.), *Research Contributions to Personality at Work* (pp. 99–114). Munich & Mering: Rainer Hampp Verlag.

Rolland, J. P. (2002). Cross-cultural generalizability of the Five-Factor Model of personality. In R. R. McCrae & J. Allik (Eds), *The Five-Factor Model of Personality across Cultures* (pp. 7–28). New York, NY: Kluwer Academic/Plenum.

Steyn, J. (2006). Venus versus Mars: An attitudinal comparison made at the start of South African police service basic training. *International Journal of Police Science and Management, 9(2)*, 145–163.

Sutherland, R., De Bruin, G. P. & Crous, F. (2007). The relation between conscientiousness, empowerment and performance. *South African Journal of Human Resource Management, 5(2)*, 60–67.

Taylor, I. A. (2000). The construct comparability of the NEO-PI-R questionnaire for black and white employees. Unpublished PhD dissertation. University of the Orange Free State, Bloemfontein.

Taylor, N. (2004). The construction of a South African five-factor personality questionnaire. Unpublished Master's dissertation. Rand Afrikaans University, Johannesburg.

Taylor, N. (2008). Construct, item, and response bias across cultures in personality measurement. Unpublished PhD dissertation. University of Johannesburg, Johannesburg.

Taylor, N. & De Bruin, G. P. (2006). *Basic Traits Inventory: Technical Manual.* Johannesburg: Jopie van Rooyen & Partners.

Taylor, T. (in press). *BB CAB Technical Manual.* Johannesburg: Aprolab.

Teferi, T. B. (2004). The application of the NEO-PI-R in the Eritrean context. Unpublished Master's dissertation. University of the Witwatersrand, Johannesburg.

Thomson, L.-A. (2007). The relationship between personality traits and life balance: A quantitative study in the South African corporate sector. Unpublished Master's dissertation. University of Johannesburg, Johannesburg.

Van de Vijver, F. J. R. & Leung, K. (1997). *Methods and Data-analysis for Cross-cultural Research.* Newbury Park, CA: Sage.

Venter, A. (2006). The relationship between the big five personality traits and emotional intelligence competencies among employees in a Durban-based medical aid administrator. Unpublished Master's dissertation. University of KwaZulu-Natal, Durban.

Vogt, L. & Laher, S. (2009). The relationship between individualism/collectivism and the Five Factor Model of personality: An exploratory study. *Psychology in Society, 37*, 39–54.

17 The Myers-Briggs Type Indicator® in South Africa

K. Knott, N. Taylor, Y. Oosthuizen and F. Bhabha

The story of the development of the Myers-Briggs Type Indicator® (MBTI®) instrument, as captured by Wright Saunders (1991), states that in 1929 Katharine Briggs read a review of Jung's *Psychological Types* (Jung, 1923/1971), which at that stage had just been translated into English.[1] She became a Jung enthusiast and spent the next 20 years studying his work and checking his theories against her own observations. She always had a strong and intuitive interest in children. It was this interest in the development and individuality of children, as well as in aspects of effective parenting, that led to her discovery and appreciation of Jung. She became convinced that what Jung had to say was of value to all people in understanding themselves and others.

Katharine shared her convictions with her daughter, Isabel Briggs Myers, and during World War II (1939–1945) the two women started developing an indicator that would enable people to gain access to their preferred Jungian type. They felt that if people could be placed in jobs which they would find satisfying, and in which they could rely on their gifts, it would not only give them greater work satisfaction but would also contribute to their increased productivity. Neither of these women were psychologists, nor had they even taken a course in psychology, but their own research had convinced them that Jung's theory was sound and practical (Wright Saunders, 1991).

Isabel formulated indicator items, and tried them out on friends and family. This was the beginning of a thorough and lengthy search for appropriate items that would more accurately enable the identification of a true type and the compilation of the Type Indicator (Wright Saunders, 1991). Over the years Isabel worked with large samples in order to validate the Indicator's use, including 15 000 nurses and 5 000 doctors. According to Van der Hoop (1970, cited in De Beer, 1997), a particular contribution that Briggs and Myers made to Jung's theory was the development of the Judging-Perceiving scale. Although Jung had mentioned that he observed differences between individuals relating to this preferred attitude to life, the Myers-Briggs team had to formulate and develop a scale to measure this attitude.

In the development of the Indicator, Myers and Briggs experienced a number of challenges. Primarily these were related to the attitudes among psychology professionals of their time, the constraints inherent in developing a self-report-format questionnaire, having to create an instrument that sorts rather than measures, keeping scales independent in order to create an instrument that would represent the dichotomous nature of Jung's theory, accepting that type variables do not reflect a normal curve distribution, having to attain precision at the midpoint of a dichotomous scale, and developing balanced and unbiased items (Lawrence, 1986). Further challenges were related to the need to use nonthreatening and nontheoretical language to make people feel comfortable in answering the questionnaire. Questions were to be written in such a manner that they could be used as 'observable "straws in the wind" to make inferences about the direction of the wind itself' (McCaulley & Myers, 1985, p.41). Thus they needed to take into account possible differences in the way each type might answer – dealing with, for instance, a difference in mindset influencing how extraverts and introverts might answer questions. Finally, the weighting of items, giving extra weight to items that discriminated well and ensuring that the Indicator also worked accurately for people who were less sophisticated or of lower general ability, was also debated (Lawrence, 1986).

Subsequent to the groundbreaking work done by Isabel and Katharine, and further development by CPP, Inc., the MBTI instrument has gone through many years of research and adaptations.[2] This is reflected in what is today known as Step I, Step II and Step III. Interestingly, these stages occurred concurrently. MBTI Step I involves knowing and understanding a person's type, and yields a four-letter code based on four dichotomous scales. MBTI Step II also gives the four-letter type, but in addition gives scores on 20 facets, which is particularly useful in coaching. MBTI Step III focuses on type development, an aspect of typology that Isabel began to study quite early in her development of the Indicator. Her overriding goal was not only to give people access to their Jungian type but also to help them make the most effective use of that type – to develop their type as fully as possible.

The development process therefore began in 1942 and culminated in the current publications of the MBTI Form M, the latest version of Step I (1998), the MBTI Form Q, the latest version of Step II (2001), and the MBTI Step III, the latest version of Step III (2009). For the purposes of this chapter we will be focusing on the MBTI Form M, or Step I, which is an international assessment used in most Fortune 100 companies, with more than two million people completing it worldwide each year. It has been translated into over 30 languages, and is used in over 70 different countries worldwide (Freeman, Kirby & Barger, 2009).

The MBTI model

The MBTI assessment provides a useful method for understanding people by looking at eight personality preferences that everyone uses at different times. These eight preferences are organised into four dichotomies, each made up of a pair of opposite preferences. When one completes the assessment, the four preferences an individual identifies as being most like him- or herself are combined into what is called a *type*. The four dichotomies are shown in Table 17.1.

Table 17.1 The four dichotomies of MBTI theory

Where you focus your attention	**E**	**Extraversion** Preference for drawing energy from the outside world of people, activities, and things.	**I**	**Introversion** Preference for drawing energy from one's inner world of ideas, emotions, and impressions.
The way you take in information	**S**	**Sensing** Preference for taking in information through the five senses and noticing what is actual.	**N**	**Intuition** Preference for taking in information through a 'sixth sense' and noticing what might be.
The way you make decisions	**T**	**Thinking** Preference for organising and structuring information to decide in a logical, objective way.	**F**	**Feeling** Preference for organising and structuring information to decide in a personal, values-based way.
How you deal with the outer world	**J**	**Judging** Preference for living a planned and organised life.	**P**	**Perceiving** Preference for living a spontaneous and flexible life.

Source: Myers and Myers (2005). Used with permission of CPP, Inc.

How an individual decides to answer each item on the MBTI assessment determines the reported MBTI type. Since each of the preferences can be represented by a letter, a four-letter code is used as shorthand for indicating type. For example, ISTJ represents an individual with a preference for Introversion, Sensing, Thinking and Judging, while ENFP represents an individual with a preference for Extraversion, Intuition, Feeling and Perceiving. When the four dichotomies are combined there are 16 possible permutations. These are often depicted in a type table, as in Table 17.2.

Table 17.2 The MBTI type table

ISTJ	ISFJ	INFJ	INTJ
ISTP	ISFP	INFP	INTP
ESTP	ESFP	ENFP	ENTP
ESTJ	ESFJ	ENFJ	ENTJ

Source: Myers and Myers (2005). Used with permission of CPP, Inc.

Type, as well as the insight that it provides, is used in numerous and diverse applications. Some examples include personal, team and leadership development, conflict resolution, team building, engagement, career choice and diversity work, to name but a few.

Criticisms of the MBTI

With the MBTI assessment being so widely used, it has been subject to criticisms which can be grouped into three areas of concern (Pittenger, 2005; Zemke, 1992):

- the purpose and benefits of the MBTI assessment;
- the validity and reliability of the MBTI assessment;
- the MBTI assessment's theoretical foundation.

Some critics comment that the MBTI assessment does not tell one anything that one does not already know (Pittenger, 2005). The full interpretation process, however, does provide numerous insights into the way individuals think and behave, shedding light on how they interact with others at work and in their personal life. Some critics are frustrated that the MBTI does not predict performance or measure pathology.

The MBTI instrument is also criticised for relying too heavily on the process of verification – the process whereby participants reflect on their placement into a type and identify whether it is the best fit (Pittenger, 2005). This is related to the Forer effect, in which individuals align or conform to a particular psychological description even when such a description is not theirs (Forer, 1949; Marks, 2000). In addition, one can 'fake' MBTI results if one really wants to. However, others will counter that the motivation to fake results is low when the instrument is used properly. When misapplied, such as when used for selection, people can feel that they have much at stake and may try to respond so as to achieve what they perceive to be the desired results.

Some feel that human personality, with all its complexities, cannot possibly fit into one of the 16 categories, and that it leads to stereotyping (Zemke, 1992). MBTI users will defend the instrument, saying that it does not purport to qualify every aspect of personality, nor does it claim that individuals of the same type are alike. However, the sorting of people into the 16 type categories allows for the identification of four dimensions of personality that are common among people of similar type, and provides useful and insightful information (CPP, 2010).

Psychometric properties of the MBTI

Internationally the *MBTI Manual* presents decades of evidence on the reliability of the MBTI instrument and the validity of the MBTI assessments when they are used for a broad range of purposes (Myers, McCaulley, Quenk & Hammer, 1998). For the purposes of this chapter, the focus will be on recent South African psychometric properties. The previous forms of the MBTI instrument (for example, Form G, which has been replaced by Form M) have been widely researched in South Africa, and their psychometric properties have been well established. The results of the research presented in this chapter are a summary of the *South African MBTI Form M Data Supplement* (Taylor & Yiannakis, 2007), which provides the latest psychometric information that is available on the MBTI Form M in South Africa at the time of writing.[3]

Taylor and Yiannakis (2007) carried out research in order to investigate the distribution of type in a South African context, with special focus on group differences. Their sample consisted of 1 538 South African respondents, of whom 661 were women and 850 were men, and who ranged in age from 14 to 68 years. In terms of ethnicity, 39.1 per cent indicated that they were Caucasian, 17.7 per cent indicated their ethnicity as African and 29.5 per cent did not specify their ethnicity.

Type tables are a useful way of presenting the proportion of each type within a particular group, as the percentage of each of the 16 type preferences can be indicated. For each of the 16 types in the South African sample, Taylor and Yiannakis (2007) found that the most common reported type preference was ESTJ (20.8 per cent), closely followed by ISTJ (19.8 per cent). The least common type preference for the South African sample was INFJ (1.7 per cent). The preference for Extraversion or for Introversion was fairly evenly distributed. However, it is clear that the South African group had a majority with preferences for Sensing, Thinking and Judging. Implications of this trend for South African culture can be seen in a focus on realistic, productive, established and profitable issues in a majority of situations, and conversely a frequent lack of focus on possibilities, people and flexibility that is sometimes required. While these results may not necessarily be generalisable to the entire South African population, due to the largely urbanised nature of the sample, they do provide some insights into the mindset of the South African workforce.

With reference to possible changes in type distribution over time, Taylor and Yiannakis (2007) compared their results with those that had been found ten years previously. The MBTI Form G type distribution (N = 6 452) was compiled by Jopie de Beer in 1997 as a doctoral study. De Beer (1997) found that the South African type distribution represented all 16 profiles, with ESTJ and ISTJ preferences being the most prevalent. The data from De Beer (1997) showed that the most common type preference for South Africans was ESTJ (23.22 per cent), followed by ISTJ (19.9 per cent), which was similar to that found by Taylor and Yiannakis (2007). De Beer (1997) reported that the least common type preference was ISFP (1.72 per cent), and in the new data the least common type preference was INFJ (1.70 per cent). When comparing the South African type distributions of the MBTI Form M to the research done by De Beer (1997), it is evident that South Africans continue to report preferences for Sensing, Thinking and Judging. Taylor and Yiannakis (2007) suggested that the type distribution for the South African population has remained fairly stable over time. There were, however, fewer INTJ, ENFP and ENTJ preferences, and more ESFP and ENFJ preferences, in the new South African sample compared to the previous type distribution.

Reliability and validity evidence

The internal consistency reliability coefficients for each of the MBTI dimensions were calculated using Cronbach's alpha coefficient (Cronbach, 1951). Table 17.3 shows the internal consistency reliability coefficients for the South African sample. Internal consistency reliability was considered to be excellent with Cronbach alpha coefficients of above .85 for each of the four dichotomies (Taylor & Yiannakis, 2007). In relation to international research done on the MBTI Form M, these reliabilities are comparable to those found in Africa in general and all other continents, where internal consistency reliabilities ranged from .81 to .91 (Schaubhut, Herk & Thompson, 2009).

Table 17.3 Internal consistency reliability

Dimension	Cronbach's alpha
Extraversion/Introversion	.91
Sensing/Intuition	.85
Thinking/Feeling	.88
Judging/Perceiving	.91

Source: Taylor and Yiannakis (2007). Used with permission of the publisher.

Validity evidence for the MBTI instrument is gathered through studies that compare an individual's type obtained on the instrument (reported type) to the type they feel best describes them ('best-fit' type). In addition, studies that look at the types of environments to which people with certain preferences are attracted, and studies that investigate correlations between the MBTI assessment and other tests of personality or interest, also add to the body of validity evidence. In terms of validity, the best-fit evidence is presented below, and the other kinds of studies are discussed later in the chapter.

The purpose of the MBTI instrument is to help individuals to identify their true or 'best-fit' type through a process called validation or verification of type. A good indication of the validity of the MBTI instrument is how well the results relate to an individual's best-fit type. Taylor and Yiannakis (2007) conducted a separate verification study with a sample of 89 South African individuals who completed the MBTI Form M self-scorable version before attending an MBTI accreditation course. The results need to be considered within the South African context, in that all these delegates were psychologists or psychometrists and it might be said that they are probably more self-aware than the general population, which could have an impact on the results obtained. The 89 training delegates' Form M reported type was matched to their verified best-fit type. The number of letters in their verified type that agreed with the Form M reported type was captured. Taylor and Yiannakis (2007) found that 74 per cent of respondents agreed with all four letters of their reported type, and that 96.6 per cent of respondents agreed with at least three letters. A very small percentage of the respondents only agreed with two letters (3.4 per cent), and there were none who agreed with only one or no letters of their reported type. These results are good evidence for the accuracy of the MBTI instrument in South Africa, and are comparable to those found internationally (Taylor & Yiannakis, 2007).

Group differences

Taylor and Yiannakis (2007) explored group differences according to age, gender and ethnic group in order to understand possible differences in type distribution across relevant groups. It is important to note that these differences are not necessarily indications of bias, and should not be interpreted as such. The MBTI Forms M and Q were developed using item response theory, which ensured that each item was selected on the basis that it could correctly sort a person into their preference category, and that the items functioned in the same way across gender, age and ethnic groups. Research into the presence of bias in the MBTI items in South Africa is under way, but it is expected that the results will reflect those found internationally.

Within the South African sample, Taylor and Yiannakis (2007) found statistically significant gender differences on the Thinking-Feeling scale for training delegates and individuals who completed the MBTI instrument for personal growth. The results showed that both men and women were more likely to prefer Thinking over Feeling. However, more men than women were likely to report a preference for Thinking. It is likely that one would find more women than men within groups of people with a preference for Feeling.

Statistically significant differences in the frequency of reported type were also found between black and white respondents in terms of the Sensing-Intuition and Judging-Perceiving type preferences (Taylor & Yiannakis, 2007). No differences were found between race groups for the Extraversion-Introversion and Thinking-Feeling dimensions. These results indicated that more black individuals reported Sensing and Judging preferences than white individuals, and that similar patterns are likely to be found in future studies. These findings are in line with those reported by De Beer (1997), although she also found differences in the Thinking-Feeling dimension with more black individuals reporting a preference for Thinking. It appears that the trend of group differences for Sensing and Judging preferences seems to be fairly stable. This combination often suggests that individuals are likely to have a strong sense of community, internalise their history and maintain traditions and customs (Myers et al., 1998), which is indicative of black South African culture. However, it is important to remember that both black and white individuals were more likely to report Sensing, Thinking and Judging preferences than Intuition, Feeling and Perceiving preferences, so these behaviours are also likely to be reflected in the wider community.

With regard to age, Taylor and Yiannakis (2007) found statistically significant differences in reported type for two of the preference categories. On the Thinking-Feeling dimension, the mean age was higher for individuals with a preference for Thinking. On the Judging-Perceiving dimension, the mean age was higher for individuals with a preference for Judging. In both cases the older sample had possibly been exposed to the ESTJ social forces for longer, thereby allowing the environment to affect their preferences more so than for the younger sample. This finding could also be explained by a change in society between different generations.

Very little research on the MBTI instrument was done in South Africa before 1990. Since then the use of and research on the MBTI instrument has become more prevalent. In those early years it was assumed that type distribution data in South Africa would be similar to results found in the US or the UK, based on the wide usage of English in South Africa. As part of Taylor and Yiannakis's (2007) study, a group of respondents from the USA (N = 1 502) similar in age and gender distribution was matched to the South African sample, in order to look at differences in type preferences across the two cultures.

In previous research done on the MBTI Form G in South Africa, De Beer (1997) found that when compared to the US normative sample, South Africans were found to be more Extraverted, and had a higher preference for Thinking and Judging. While Taylor and Yiannakis (2007) did not find differences in terms of Extraversion-Introversion, their results indicated that Sensing, Thinking and Judging preferences were over-represented in the South African sample when compared to the US sample. These differences in distribution could be linked to a number of factors, but one hypothesis could be that they are a reflection of the cultural values of high power-distance, individualism and masculinity as measured by Hofstede (2001). The Sensing, Thinking and Judging combination also links to a strong cultural identity, with emphasis on history, tradition and customs, which may resonate strongly with the majority of South Africans.

Research findings on the MBTI

There has been extensive research conducted with the MBTI instrument over the years. For example, the Center for the Application of Psychological Type's (CAPT®) bibliography for the MBTI instrument has been maintained since 1976. The growth in publications has been exponential, from the 1968 bibliography containing 81 references to the February 2011 bibliography containing approximately 12 006 references (CAPT, 2011). The MBTI instrument finds application in a variety of different contexts which provide individuals, families, teams and organisations with insight that can lead to personal and interpersonal growth and development. A search for published studies done using the MBTI instrument in Africa yields only 72 records, of which only 13 were published after 2000. In addition, most of the references to the MBTI instrument in Africa are presentations made at the fourth conference of the International Type Users' Organisation held in South Africa in 1996 (CAPT, 2011). There is a great need for additional peer-reviewed and published research on the MBTI assessment in South Africa. Some of the recent findings on the applicability and utility of the instrument, focusing specifically on the South African context, are summarised in the paragraphs below.

Employee wellness

A study by Du Toit, Coetzee and Visser (2005) focused on the relationship between an aspect of employee wellness – namely, sense of coherence as measured by the Orientation to Life Questionnaire, and personality type, as measured by the MBTI instrument. A convenience sample of 100 volunteer participants from the technical division of the Department of Defence was used. It was found that Sensing and Thinking types were predominant in the sample. Furthermore, individuals with the Sensing Judging and Extraverted Judging preference styles scored significantly higher on sense of coherence than individuals with the Sensing Perceiving or Introverted Perceiving preference styles. Multiple regression analysis revealed that the Extraversion–Introversion and Judging–Perceiving continuums were significant predictors of sense of coherence, where preferences for Extraversion and Judging scored significantly higher than those for Introversion and Perceiving. Despite the limitations in the nature and size of the sample, the study showed promise for investigations of the association between personality type, as conceptualised by the MBTI assessment, and ability to cope.

Leadership

Sieff and Carstens (2006) examined the relationship between personality type and leadership focus in a group of South African executives (N = 200). Personality type was assessed using the MBTI instrument, and leadership focus was explored through the development and application of a Leadership Focus Questionnaire. Results suggested that Extraverted personality types are more comfortable with the challenges of focus in the leadership role than are Introverted types, and Extraverted, Sensing, Thinking and Judging types experience a greater degree of fit with their organisations than do Introverted, Intuitive, Feeling and Perceiving types (Sieff & Carstens, 2006). These results should also be related to findings by Taylor and Yiannakis (2007) that more top executives tend to report a preference for Introversion than for Extraversion in South Africa. Sieff and Carstens (2006, p.61) have suggested that

> [t]he study findings present Human Resource (HR) professionals with important challenges in relation to those high-potential leaders with preferences for Introversion and Feeling. A strategic HR development role would be to assist such leaders to develop and balance their less preferred behaviours in order to find a more comfortable fit in dealing with the challenges of leadership focus, without letting go of the gift that their natural preference for Introversion and Feeling may bring to the leadership role. Equally, HR professionals need to encourage a more rounded set of behaviours that include more practice of Introversion (or introspection and reflection) and Feeling behaviours in those leaders who are comfortable with taking on the challenges of focus, who have a natural preference for Extraversion and Thinking.

Linde (2004) researched the relationship between transformational leadership and personality preferences. The transformational leaders' ratings, as identified by use of the Multifactor Leadership Questionnaire, were compared with personality preferences as indicated on the MBTI instrument. The research group was a convenience sample that consisted of 66 leaders chosen from two organisations in the financial and entertainment industries at the level of team leader or in a supervisory capacity. The findings suggested that personality preferences cannot be utilised to predict transformational leadership in, for instance, a selection process in a company. This is in line with the theory that while leaders may have certain personality type preferences, this does not prevent them from developing skills in the use of their opposite preference and using those to the benefit of the organisation, and is another reason why the MBTI should not be used in selection processes.

Emotional intelligence

Work by Roger Pearman explores parallels between type and emotional intelligence (EQ) and shows how MBTI results can be used to enhance emotional intelligence. Pearman (2002; 2007) highlight how developing EQ can enhance leadership ability, enrich relationships and extend influence. The *Bulletin for Psychological Type* (Association for Psychological Type International, 2006) lists a number of articles that investigate the link between EQ and MBTI preferences. South African studies that either support or challenge these findings have also been conducted. Differences found between the research studies could lie in the fact that different assessments of EQ were used in the various studies.

A study conducted by Du Toit et al. (2005) analysed the relationship between leaders' personality preferences, self-esteem and emotional competence in 107 South African leaders in the manufacturing industry. The MBTI instrument, the Culture-Free Self-Esteem Inventories for Adults (CFSEI-AD) and the 360° Emotional Competency Profiler (ECP) were administered. It appeared that others perceived Introverted types as more emotionally competent than Extraverted types, possibly due to their more introspective and quiet nature, which may lead to them being perceived as more in control of their emotions. Although positive relationships were found between the three constructs, the self-esteem construct appeared to be a more reliable predictor of emotional competence than the MBTI personality preferences. The correlations between the MBTI preferences and emotional competence scales show some relationships in accordance with the theory, although they are not large enough to imply that they measure the same thing. The findings of the study make an important contribution to the expanding body of knowledge concerned with the evaluation of personality variables that influence the effectiveness of leaders. The apparent lack of predictive ability could be due to the fact that the MBTI instrument is aimed not at predicting behaviour, but rather at explaining behaviour and being an aid towards personality development (Myers et al., 1998).

Another study by Rothmann, Scholtz, Sipsma and Sipsma (2002) focused on assessing the relationship between EQ and personality preferences in a group of management students at a business school (N = 71). The Emotional Quotient Inventory (EQ-i) and the MBTI instrument were used as measuring instruments. The results showed that there is a significant relationship between EQ and preferences for Extraversion, Intuition, Feeling and Perception. Rothmann et al.

(2002) suggest that lecturers should use the findings of this study in planning their educational strategies. Business students (who will be employees, managers and entrepreneurs in the future) need to adapt to changes, to tolerate stress and to be interpersonally effective.

Career choice

A study by Van Rensburg, Rothmann and Rothmann (2003) investigated the relationship between personality characteristics and career anchors in a sample of pharmacists (N = 56) in a corporate environment. The MBTI instrument, the Revised NEO Personality Inventory (NEO-PI-R) and the Career Anchor Inventory were used as measuring instruments. The results of the empirical study showed that personality characteristics of pharmacists were related to their career anchors. Extraversion and Emotional Stability were positively related to general management, service, pure challenge and entrepreneurial challenge. Introversion, Neuroticism and low Openness to Experience were related to technical/functional competence and security as career anchors.

The researchers made a few application-oriented suggestions, the main MBTI-related suggestion being that pharmacists should be trained in identifying their own and others' personality preferences, and described the development areas arising from these. Van Rensburg et al. (2003) felt that pharmacists should therefore learn not only to identify and accept their real personality preferences, but also to develop their skills in the opposite or shadow preference (Myers et al., 1998).

MBTI research and applications are diverse and ongoing, both internationally and in South Africa. The theory lends itself to many contexts, and the research boundaries are limited only by the curiosity and imagination of MBTI users.

Conclusion

The MBTI assessment is a well-researched and methodologically sound personality inventory. Professionals use it worldwide to assist people in gaining self-insight and awareness of how their preferred behaviour may complement or differ from the behaviour of others. Such insight can assist in personal development, and in dealing with and improving on interpersonal issues such as decision-making, conflict handling, communication and team functioning.

The MBTI assessment can also be of particular value in the southern African context when dealing with issues of diversity management, engagement, stress management and problem-solving. Its nonjudgemental approach to understanding personality adds to its unique applications, which set it apart from trait-based personality assessments. With an awareness of our adolescent democracy in South Africa, and our ongoing challenge of nation-building throughout Africa, Isabel Myers's words are particularly pertinent:

> When people differ, knowledge of type lessens friction and eases strain. In addition, it reveals the value of differences. No one has to be good at everything. By developing individual strengths, guarding against own

weaknesses, and appreciating the strengths of other types, life will be more amusing, more interesting, and more of a daily adventure than it could possibly be if everyone were alike. (Myers & Myers, 1980, p.201)

Notes

1 MBTI, Myers-Briggs, Myers-Briggs Type Indicator and the MBTI logo are trademarks or registered trademarks of the MBTI Trust, Inc., in the USA and other countries.

2 CPP, Inc., the company formerly known as Consulting Psychologists Press, became the exclusive publisher of the MBTI in 1975.

3 Full copies of the data supplement are available. Please send requests to research@ jvrafrica.co.za.

References

Association for Psychological Type International (2006). *Index to 2006 Bulletin of Psychological Type, (29)3*. Retrieved June 23, 2010, from http://www.aptinternational.org/Publications/Bulletin-of-Psychological-Type.aspx.

CAPT (Center for the Application of Psychological Type) (2011). *MBTI® Bibliography Search*. Retrieved February 11, 2011, from http://www.capt.org/research/MBTI-bibliography-search.htm.

CPP (2010). *Myers Briggs Type Indicator: Frequently Asked Questions*. Palo Alto, CA: CPP, Inc.

Cronbach, L. J. (1951). Coefficient alpha and the internal structure of tests. *Psychometrica, 16(3)*, 297–344.

De Beer, J. (1997). South African Myers-Briggs Type Indicator: A comparative study. Unpublished PhD dissertation. Rand Afrikaans University, Johannesburg.

Du Toit, F., Coetzee, S. & Visser, D. (2005). The relation between personality type and sense of coherence among technical workers. *Southern African Business Review, 9(1)*, 51–65.

Forer, B. R. (1949). The fallacy of personal validation: A classroom demonstration of gullibility. *Journal of Abnormal and Social Psychology, 44(1)*, 118–123.

Freeman, F., Kirby, L. & Barger, N. (2009). *Presenting Type in Organisations*. Palo Alto, CA: CPP, Inc.

Hofstede, G. (2001). *Culture's Consequences: Comparing Values, Behaviours, Institutions and Organisations across Nations* (2nd edition). Thousand Oaks, CA: Sage.

Jung, C. G. (1923/1971). *Psychological Types*. Princeton, NJ: Princeton University Press.

Lawrence, G. (1986). Issues in the development of the MBTI. *Journal of Psychological Type, 12*, 2–7.

Linde, T. (2004). Transformational leadership and its relationship with personality preferences in South African organisations. Unpublished Master's dissertation. University of Johannesburg, Johannesburg.

Marks, D. F. (2000). *The Psychology of the Psychic* (2nd edition). Amherst, NY: Prometheus Books.

McCaulley, M. H. & Myers, I. B. (1985). *A Guide to the Development and Use of the Myers-Briggs Type Indicator*. Palo Alto, CA: CPP, Inc.

Myers, I. B., McCaulley, M. H., Quenk, N. L. & Hammer, A. L. (1998). *MBTI Manual: A Guide to the Development and Use of the Myers-Briggs Type Indicator*. Palo Alto, CA: CPP, Inc.

Myers, I. B. & Myers, P. B. (1980). *Gifts Differing: Understanding Personality Type*. Palo Alto, CA: CPP, Inc.

Myers, P. B. & Myers, K. D. (2005). *Form M Interpretive Report for Organisations.* Palo Alto, CA: CPP, Inc.

Pearman, R. (2002). *Introduction to Type and Emotional Intelligence: Pathways to Performance.* Palo Alto, CA: CPP, Inc.

Pearman, R. (2007). *Using the MBTI Tool to Enrich Emotional Intelligence.* Palo Alto, CA: CPP, Inc.

Pittenger, D. J. (2005). Cautionary comments regarding the Myers-Briggs Type Indicator. *Consulting Psychology Journal: Practice and Research, 57(3),* 210–221.

Rothmann, S., Scholtz, P. E., Sipsma, J. F. & Sipsma, L. (2002). The relationship between personality preferences and the emotional intelligence of postgraduate management studies. *Business Dynamics, 11(1),* 2–12.

Schaubhut, N. A., Herk, N. & Thompson, R. C. (2009). *MBTI Form M Manual Supplement.* Palo Alto, CA: CPP, Inc.

Sieff, G. & Carstens, L. (2006). The relationship between personality type and leadership focus. *South African Journal of Human Resource Management, 4(1),* 52–62.

Taylor, N. & Yiannakis, C. (2007). *South African MBTI® Form M Data Supplement.* Johannesburg: Jopie van Rooyen & Partners.

Van Rensburg, S., Rothmann, J. C. & Rothmann, S. (2003). The relationship between personality characteristics and career anchors of pharmacists. *South African Journal of Human Resource Management, 12(3),* 24–33.

Wright Saunders, F. (1991). *Katharine and Isabel: The Story of the Making of the Myers-Briggs Type Indicator.* Palo Alto, CA: CPP, Inc.

Zemke, R. (1992). Second thoughts about MBTI training. *Training, 29(4),* 43–48.

18 The NEO-PI-R in South Africa

S. Laher

The first edition of the Neuroticism–Extraversion–Openness Inventory (NEO-I) was published in 1978. The NEO-I consisted of 3 domain scales (Neuroticism, Extraversion and Openness to Experience) and 18 facet scales. In 1983, 18 item domain scales measuring Agreeableness and Conscientiousness were added, and around 1985 a revised version was produced, the NEO Personality Inventory (NEO-PI).[1] The next revision occurred in the late 1980s and was published in 1990 as the Revised NEO Personality Inventory (NEO-PI-R). In 1990, the facet scales for Agreeableness and Conscientiousness were completed and 10 items in the original NEO were modified. The 30 facet scales of the NEO-PI-R were chosen to represent constructs frequently identified in the psychological literature that embody important distinctions in each of the 5 domains (Costa & McCrae, 1992). At this time another instrument was created, the NEO Five-Factor Inventory (NEO-FFI). Most recently the NEO-Personality Inventory-ÿ3 (NEO-PI-3) has been released.

The NEO-PI-R is based on the idea that personality traits are arranged in hierarchies from very broad to very narrow, and that both highly general (domain) and relatively specific (facet) traits should be assessed. The constructs measured by the NEO-PI-R are not original discoveries and were not intended as such. Rather, the developers searched the available psychological literature to identify traits and dispositions that were important to personality theorists, that were represented as trait terms in the natural English language and that appeared in personality research literature. Items were then developed to tap those constructs. Costa and McCrae (1992) employed a modified rational approach to scale construction. Although item analyses began with a pool of items constructed rationally, final item selection was based on extensive item analyses using factor analytic techniques.

The NEO-PI-R

The NEO-PI-R is a self-report instrument consisting of 240 items and requiring approximately 45 minutes to complete. It is available in two forms: Form S, which is an instrument for self-rating, and Form R, which is used for rating someone else. The items are the same except that the subject is changed from 'I' to 'he' or 'she'. The instrument measures each of the five factors postulated in the Five-Factor Model (FFM) – namely, Neuroticism, Extraversion, Openness to Experience, Agreeableness and Conscientiousness, but refers to these as domains. Each of the domains is measured by 48 items, which are subdivided into 6 sets of 8 items. These clusters of items are called facets, and were designed to provide more specific information about some important concepts within each of the domains. Table 18.1 summarises the domain and facet descriptions.

Table 18.1 NEO-PI-R domain and facet scale descriptions

NEO-PI-R scale	Scale description
Neuroticism	The tendency to experience negative affects such as fear, sadness, embarrassment, guilt and disgust.
Anxiety	Describes individuals who are apprehensive, fearful, prone to worry, nervous, tense and jittery.
Angry Hostility	The tendency to experience anger and related states such as frustration and bitterness.
Depression	Measures normal individual differences in the tendency to experience feelings of guilt, sadness, hopelessness and loneliness.
Self-Consciousness	The tendency to be uncomfortable around others, sensitive to ridicule, and prone to feelings of inferiority, usually characterised by the emotions of shame and embarrassment.
Impulsiveness	Refers to the ability to control cravings and urges and deals with levels of frustration tolerance.
Vulnerability	Measures ability to cope with stress, dependency issues and the tendency to feel hopeless or panicked when facing emergency situations.
Extraversion	A general tendency towards sociability, assertiveness, activeness and being talkative.
Warmth	Is associated with interpersonal intimacy in terms of general affectionate and friendly behaviour and capacity to form close attachments to others.
Gregariousness	Refers to the preference for other people's company.
Assertiveness	Measures the tendency to be dominant, forceful and socially ascendant.
Activity	Refers to general pace of life, with high scores suggesting a rapid tempo and vigorous movement and a need to keep busy.
Excitement-Seeking	Refers to the tendency to crave stimulation and excitement like bright colours and noisy environments.
Positive Emotions	Refers to the tendency to experience positive emotions such as joy, happiness, love and excitement.
Openness to Experience	Describes levels of willingness to entertain novel ideas and unconventional values, as well as the degree to which a person is imaginative and curious as opposed to concrete-minded and narrow-thinking.
Fantasy	Refers to having a vivid imagination and an active fantasy life.
Aesthetics	Deals with capacity for appreciation of art and beauty.

NEO-PI-R scale	Scale description
Feelings	Measures receptivity to one's own inner feelings and emotions.
Actions	Refers to willingness to try different activities, go to new places or try different foods.
Ideas	The tendency to be open-minded and to consider new and sometimes unconventional ways of thinking.
Values	Refers to the readiness to re-examine social, political and religious values.
Agreeableness	Encapsulates constructs of sympathy, cooperativeness and helpfulness towards others.
Trust	Measures the degree to which individuals believe that others are honest and well-intentioned.
Straightforwardness	Describes the level to which an individual is frank, sincere and ingenuous.
Altruism	Refers to an active concern for the welfare of others as demonstrated in generosity, consideration of others and a willingness to assist others in need of help.
Compliance	Measures the extent to which individuals defer to others, inhibit aggression and forgive and forget.
Modesty	Refers to the extent that an individual demonstrates humility.
Tender-Mindedness	Measures attitudes of sympathy and concern for others.
Conscientiousness	Refers to the degree to which a person is persevering, responsible and organised.
Competence	Refers to the sense that one is capable, sensible, prudent and effective.
Order	Measures the extent to which an individual is neat, tidy and well organised.
Dutifulness	Characterised by strict adherence to ethical principles and scrupulous fulfilment of moral obligations.
Achievement Striving	Refers to the tendency to be ambitious, driven to succeed, diligent and purposeful.
Self-Discipline	Measures the ability to begin tasks and carry them through to completion despite boredom and other distractions.
Deliberation	Refers to the tendency to be cautious and think carefully before acting, especially in decision-making.

NEO-PI-R items are answered on a 5-point scale ranging from strongly agree (4) to strongly disagree (0), and scales are balanced to control for the effects of acquiescence. No validity scales are included in the instrument, but three questions appear at the end of the questionnaire asking respondents whether they have answered all the questions, whether they have answered all the questions in the correctly numbered spaces and whether they have answered them honestly. The NEO-PI-R was standardised on over 1 000 individuals taken primarily from the Augmented Baltimore Longitudinal Study of Aging (ABLSA), the ABLSA Peer Sample, individuals in a large US national organisation and several clinical samples (Costa & McCrae, 1992).

Reliability of the NEO-PI-R

Internal consistency reliability coefficients range from .86 to .92 for the domain scales and from .56 to .81 for the facet scales. Test-retest reliability coefficients for the domain scales were between .79 and .91, while the facet scale reliabilities ranged between .66 and .92. These stability estimates remained virtually the same in various studies ranging from 1 month to 6 years. Stability estimates were better in adult samples than in adolescent or young adult (21 years or under) samples (Costa & McCrae, 1992).

More recently McCrae, Terracciano and 79 Members of the Personality Profiles Project (2005) conducted a study across 50 cultures representing 6 continents using translations into Indo-European, Hamito-Semitic, Sino-Tibetan, Daic, Uralic, Malayo-Polynesian, Dravidian and Altaic languages. Median internal consistency reliability coefficients of .90, .90, .88, .92 and .94 for Neuroticism, Extraversion, Openness to Experience, Agreeableness and Conscientiousness domains respectively were found in this study, suggesting that the NEO-PI-R has high reliability across cultures. However, closer examination of these coefficients indicates that the reliability for Asian and African cultures is slightly lower than the US standard. The USA had reliability coefficients of .91 for Neuroticism, .91 for Extraversion, .88 for Openness to Experience, .93 for Agreeableness and .94 for Conscientiousness (McCrae et al., 2005). Reliability coefficients of .87 for Neuroticism, .85 for Extraversion, .83 for Openness to Experience, .87 for Agreeableness and .90 for Conscientiousness were found in the Chinese group. While Japan, South Korea and Hong Kong exhibited internal consistency reliability coefficients that were similar to those of the US sample, or slightly below the US value but higher than the Chinese values. Other Asian countries such as Thailand, Indonesia, Malaysia and India exhibited reliability coefficients that were lower than the US values but more in line with the Chinese values. South American countries (for example, Peru) and Middle Eastern countries (for example, Kuwait) also have reliability coefficients that are more comparable with their Chinese rather than US counterparts (McCrae et al., 2005).

The lowest reliability coefficients were from the African countries. Burkina Faso and Botswana exhibited coefficients that closely resembled those found in Asian cultures, but Nigeria, Ethiopia, Uganda and Morocco were visibly lower (McCrae et al., 2005). Morocco had the lowest coefficients, with .54 for Neuroticism, .57 for Extraversion, .58 for Openness to Experience, .66 for Agreeableness and .82 for Conscientiousness. Conscientiousness appears to have the best internal consistency reliability across the 50 cultures. McCrae et al. (2005) attribute these results in part to poorer data quality from the Asian and African countries. Data quality was measured using six indicators: number of missing responses, number of acquiescent responses, number of substituted responses, language that the test was completed in, published or unpublished version of the test, and researchers' reports of problems experienced during administration. McCrae et al. (2005) also suggest that the results may indicate true differences in personality in these cultures as well as possible emic constructs that are untapped.

In an African context, Piedmont, Bain, McCrae and Costa (2002) reported alpha coefficients of .87 for Neuroticism, .92 for Extraversion, .77 for Openness to Experience, .80 for Agreeableness and .81 for Conscientiousness, using a Shona translation of the NEO-PI-R in a sample of 314 Zimbabweans. Only 14 of the 30 facet scales exhibited alpha coefficients between .50 and .65. The remainder of the facet scales exhibited coefficients below .50. Seven of the remaining 16 scales exhibited particularly low alpha coefficients. Values had the lowest alpha coefficient of .13, followed by Activity, .21; Ideas, .22; Feelings, .24; Self-Consciousness, .27; Modesty, .30; Excitement-Seeking, .36; and Tender-Mindedness, .38 (Piedmont et al., 2002).

Teferi (2004) reported alpha coefficients of .79 for Neuroticism, .50 for Extraversion, .45 for Openness to Experience, .73 for Agreeableness and .82 for Conscientiousness using a Tigrignan translation of the NEO-PI-R in a sample of 410 Eritrean individuals. Only 5 scales (Depression, Positive Emotions, Aesthetics, Dutifulness and Deliberation) exhibited alpha coefficients in the range of .51 to .61. All of the Neuroticism facets, with the exception of Depression, had alpha coefficients between .45 and .49. Extraversion facets, with the exception of Positive Emotions, ranged between .24 and .44. Excitement-Seeking had the worst coefficient of .24, followed by Activity with a coefficient of .29. Alpha coefficients on the Openness to Experience domain, with the exception of Aesthetics, were particularly poor. Actions had a coefficient of .02; Values, .10; Feelings, .22; Fantasy, .32; and Ideas, .45. Agreeableness facets were also poor, with Trust having an alpha coefficient of .30; Straightforwardness, .32; and Compliance, .37. The remaining facets (Altruism, Modesty, Tender-Mindedness) had coefficients in the range of .46 to .49. With the exception of Dutifulness and Deliberation, Conscientiousness facets (Competence, Order, Achievement Striving, Self-Discipline) had alpha coefficients ranging between .30 and .40 (Teferi, 2004).

Rossier, Dahourou and McCrae (2005) reported alpha coefficients for the 5 domains of between .71 and .85, with a median alpha coefficient of .79, in a sample of 470 French-speaking individuals in Burkina Faso. Facet scale coefficients ranged from .16 to .68, with a median alpha coefficient of .52. Impulsiveness (α = .33), Actions (α = .31) and Values (α = .16) exhibited the lowest internal consistency reliability coefficients (Rossier et al., 2005).

A final study conducted in an African context considered internal consistency reliability in a sample consisting of 50 Japanese students as well as 50 Egyptian students. However, Mohammed, Unher and Sugawara (2009) used the NEO-FFI, not the NEO-PI-R. Students completed the English version of the NEO-FFI. Cronbach alpha coefficients for the domains in the Japanese sample were .87 for Neuroticism, .89 for Extraversion, .86 for Openness to Experience, .81 for Agreeableness and .83 for Conscientiousness. In the Egyptian sample, on the other hand, Neuroticism had an alpha coefficient of .63; Extraversion had a coefficient of .76; Openness to Experience, .75; Agreeableness, .70; and Conscientiousness, .73 (Mohammed et al., 2009).

Reliability of the NEO-PI-R in South Africa

The most recent evidence for the reliability of the NEO-PI-R in a South African context comes from Laher (2010), who considered the applicability of the NEO-PI-R in a sample of 425 students at the University of the Witwatersrand. Reliability coefficients of .91, .89, .87, .87 and .92 were found for the NEO-PI-R domain scales of Neuroticism, Extraversion, Openness to Experience, Agreeableness and Conscientiousness respectively. Facet scale reliability coefficients ranged between .50 and .81, but with the exception of Tender-Mindedness (.50) and Actions (.55), all other facets had reliability coefficients at or exceeding .60. Contrary to the literature which suggested that alpha coefficients would be lower in African samples, Laher's (2010) study suggested that the internal consistency reliability of the NEO-PI-R is equivalent to that found in the USA and other Western and some Eastern countries (for example, Japan, South Korea, Hong Kong and Turkey) (see McCrae et al., 2005).

Also in the South African context, Laher and Quy (2009) reported reliability coefficients ranging from .89 to .92 on the domain scales and coefficients ranging from .52 to .82 for the facet scales, using a sample of 94 psychology undergraduate students at a university in Johannesburg. However, the facet scales of Activity (.45), Actions (.49), and Tender-Mindedness (.48) had alpha coefficients less than .5 (Laher & Quy, 2009).

Rothman and Coetzer (2003) reported Cronbach's alpha coefficients of .86 for Neuroticism, .83 for Extraversion, .77 for Openness to Experience, .76 for Agreeableness and .78 for Conscientiousness in a sample of 159 South African employees in a pharmaceutical organisation. Facet scales ranged between .55 and .83 for all facets, with the exception of Values (.48) and Tender-Mindedness (.34) (Rothman & Coetzer, 2003). Similarly, Storm and Rothman (2003), using a sample of 131 South African employees in a corporate pharmaceutical group, reported Cronbach's alpha coefficients of .86 for Neuroticism, .84 for Extraversion, .78 for Openness to Experience, .74 for Agreeableness and .76 for Conscientiousness, but no information was given on the facet scales in this study.

Zhang and Akande (2002) explored the reliability of the NEO-FFI in a sample of 368 students from 4 universities in South Africa. Coefficients below .5 were found for the Neuroticism and Openness to Experience domains. Seventeen items with poor item-total correlations were deleted as follows: four from Neuroticism, three from Extraversion, five from Openness to Experience, three from Agreeableness and two from Conscientiousness (see Zhang & Akande, 2002, p.74 for the items). Following item deletion, a .78 alpha coefficient was found for Neuroticism, .75 for Extraversion, .56 for Openness to Experience, .63 for Agreeableness and .79 for Conscientiousness (Zhang & Akande, 2002).

From the literature presented above, it is evident that internal consistency reliability is poorer in African countries. Reliability coefficients were particularly poor in African countries which used translated versions, adding weight to the argument about the poorer data quality of translated versions (see McCrae et al., 2005). Reliability coefficients were better with studies using the English version of the NEO-PI-R, particularly in the South African context, but with the exception of Laher's (2010) and Laher and Quy's (2009) study, they were still lower than the coefficients for other countries reported in McCrae et al. (2005).

Validity of the NEO-PI-R

Costa and McCrae (1992) provide a large body of evidence for construct and criterion validity. The NEO-PI-R factors loaded as expected, with the domain scales appearing clearly in all samples and the facet scales loading appropriately on the domains. Where cross-loading occurs on some facets, these, according to Costa and McCrae (1992), are due to the inherent relationships between the facets. For example, Altruism and Extraversion might load together since one would need to be sociable to be altruistic. Evidence is also provided that indicates that domain and facet scores from the NEO-PI-R have shown to relate in predictable ways to personality trait scores from a variety of personality measures, most notably the Personality Research Form, the Myers-Briggs Type Indicator, the California Personality Inventory, peer reports, adjective checklists, sentence-completion tests and the Thematic Apperception Test (Costa & McCrae, 1992).

Following these initial studies, research on the NEO-PI-R continued at a rapid rate across different contexts and in different cultures. A summary of these findings is beyond the scope of this study, but McCrae et al. (2005) undertook an examination of studies using the NEO-PI-R in 50 cultures, and found evidence for its reliability and validity across most of the studies examined. Also evident from McCrae et al. (2005) was the differential replicability of the Openness to Experience domain. This domain did not replicate well in Asian and African countries, with Thailand, Indonesia, India, Malaysia, Botswana, Nigeria, Ethiopia, Uganda and Morocco demonstrating congruence coefficients of .84 or less. The same was found in India and Malaysia.

McCrae et al. (2005) suggest that this may be due to poorer data quality from these countries, but they also allude to the possibility that Africans may have certain emic dimensions of personality that set them apart from non-Africans. McCrae et al. (2005) also argue that these results may be due to the fact that the NEO-PI-R was developed within a Western tradition, and completing it may be a more meaningful task for Westerners than for non-Westerners. The questionnaire format may also have been foreign to these cultures, resulting in artefactual results. In collectivistic cultures the possibility exists that this format of the questionnaire requires decontextualised trait assessments in a culture that is used to describing people within the context of an interpretive relationship. Furthermore, African cultures, according to McCrae et al. (2005), share certain features such as close bonds within the family and a traumatic history of European colonialism that may have led to similarities in personality structure. When the African cultures were combined (N = 940), better congruence coefficients were obtained. A congruence coefficient of .96 was found for Neuroticism, .91 for Extraversion, .88 for Openness to Experience, .95 for Agreeableness and .96 for Conscientiousness (McCrae et al., 2005).

Cheung et al. (2008) elaborate further on this by providing evidence of the low validity of the Actions, Values and, to a lesser extent, Feelings in Asian cultures. Cheung et al. (2008) also argue that Fantasy is an inappropriate facet in Chinese culture and could not be located in Chinese folk concepts. Cheung et al. (2001) also found Modesty and Straightforwardness in the Agreeableness domain to be problematic, whilst McCrae, Costa, Del Pilar, Rolland and Parker (1998) found Tender-Mindedness from the Agreeableness domain to be problematic.

In an African context, the construct validity of the NEO-PI-R has been variable. Piedmont et al. (2002), using a Shona translation of the NEO-PI-R in Zimbabwe, found that although the five-factor structure was obtained, Extraversion and Agreeableness did not replicate as well as Neuroticism and Conscientiousness, and Openness to Experience replicated poorly.

Teferi (2004), using a Tigrignan translation, found a five-factor solution, but it was only Conscientiousness that replicated as expected. Agreeableness replicated clearly on two factors, with one factor consisting of the Agreeableness facets of Modesty, Tender-Mindedness and Compliance, as well as negative loadings on the Extraversion facets of Assertiveness and Activity and a negative loading on the Openness to Experience facet of Values. The second Agreeableness factor consisted of positive loadings on Trust, Straightforwardness and Altruism, as well as the Extraversion facets of Positive Emotions and Warmth. Neuroticism replicated as expected, with the exception of the facets of Impulsiveness and Vulnerability, which loaded on the Conscientiousness factor. Openness to Experience replicated poorly, with only Aesthetics, Feelings and Ideas loading as expected. Extraversion did not replicate as a factor at all, with Extraversion facets loading across all five factors (Teferi, 2004).

Validity of the NEO-PI-R in South Africa

South African studies have found variable results in terms of construct validity. While the five factors are generally retrieved, differences in factor structure can be found across population and language groupings. Heaven and Pretorius (1998) found support for the five factors with an Afrikaans-speaking South African sample, but found that the five factors did not replicate well for a Sesotho-speaking South African sample. However, Heaven and Pretorius used adjective terms and principal components analysis with oblimin rotation.

A study by Heuchert, Parker and Stumpf (2000) indicated support for the Five-Factor Model on a sample of 408 South African university students. Heuchert et al. (2000) used exploratory factor analysis with varimax rotation. All 30 facet scores had a loading of at least .40 on the hypothesised domain. Only two facet scores showed secondary loadings at or above .40 on another domain in addition to the hypothesised domain. Angry Hostility loaded negatively and Warmth loaded positively on the Agreeableness domain. Congruence coefficients between the South African group and the US normative group (Costa & McCrae, 1992) were above .95 for all the domains except Openness to Experience, which had a congruence coefficient of .90. Heuchert et al. (2000) comment on the fact that methodological differences, particularly with regard to different factor rotation methods, may account for the differences in results found in South African research studies.

Zhang and Akande (2002) reported that a five-factor structure could be obtained in a South African sample using an exploratory principal component factor analysis with oblimin rotation, but this replicability was weak and differed as a function of gender, race, educational level and socio-economic status. In all the studies cited above, language proficiency in English is cited as playing a role in the observed differences. These studies do not, however, underestimate the role of true cultural differences. The possibility exists that there may be some underlying elemental differences based on cultural experience that have yet to be discovered and explored.

Piedmont et al. (2002) cite a number of reasons for the results obtained. The first of these has to do with the general quality of the translation, which may not have been adequate. (In their study, Piedmont et al. (2002) used a Shona translation of the NEO-PI-R.) Alternatively, Piedmont et al. (2002) suggest the possibility that the Shona language may lack equivalent terms for the English-language items. This concurs with findings by Teferi (2004) with the Tigrignan translation, as well as with those from an unpublished thesis which examined an isiXhosa translation of the NEO-PI-R (Horn, 1965). A common criticism levelled against the FFM is that it is an approach developed from the analysis of adjective terms in the English language.

Piedmont et al. (2002) also allude to the possibility that differences may occur in response styles and response biases in African samples. Allik and McCrae (2004) argue that acquiescent response biases, as well as a tendency to avoid extreme responses, are more prominent in collectivistic cultures, but this case of metric equivalence has yet to be fully explored in an African context. In a South African context, Laher (2010) found evidence for method bias across home language, which contradicts the findings of Allik and McCrae (2004) that English second-language speakers are more likely to endorse extreme responses.

Finally, Piedmont et al. (2002) posit the possibility that some of the constructs measured by the NEO-PI-R may have no counterpart in Shona culture, especially at the facet level. They cite the example of Excitement-Seeking (an essentially self-centred motivation), which is foreign in collectivistic cultures. Teferi (2004) also found Excitement-Seeking problematic in the Tigrignan translation, in terms of both translation and replication. However in Teferi's (2004) study, the five-factor solution yielded no consistent Extraversion factor. Extraversion facets loaded on all other factors. A similar result was obtained with Openness to Experience. Positive loadings above .40 on Feelings (O), Actions (O), Ideas (O), Gregariousness (E) and Excitement-Seeking (E), and a negative loading on Values (O, –.37), constituted the Openness factor in Teferi's (2004) study. The Openness facets of Fantasy, Aesthetics and Actions were highly problematic, while Values loaded negatively (–.37) on the Openness factor and the Agreeableness factor, with Modesty (A), Tender-Mindedness (A), Compliance (A), Positive Emotions (E) and Warmth (E). Thus Teferi (2004) concluded that Extraversion and Openness, as measured by the NEO-PI-R, were not adequate assessments of the manifestations of Extraversion and Openness to Experience in the Eritrean context.

Allik and McCrae (2004) suggest the possibility that traits such as Extraversion and Openness to Experience are more valued, and therefore more readily endorsed, in Western cultures, whereas cooperation and tradition are more valued in non-Western cultures. Piedmont et al. (2002) also discuss the weak replicability of Openness to Experience, suggesting that this is a heritable trait but that its development may be primarily in relation to urbanisation and industrialisation, and would therefore not feature in non-industrialised, agrarian cultures.

Whilst this may be a possibility for certain parts of Africa, it is certainly not the case for a large part of the continent, particularly South Africa, where the studies cited were conducted with relatively urbanised and industrialised individuals. In support of this, Okeke, Draguns, Sheku and Allen argued in 1999 (p.140) already that, despite the presentation of African cultures as 'slowly changing, rural, and small cultural groups untouched by the worldwide social, political, economic, and technological transformations of the 20th century ... the typical contemporary African is more likely to be resident of the urban conglomerates in and around Accra, Dakar, Johannesburg, Kinshasa, Lagos and Nairobi'.

This argument may assist in explaining Laher's (2010) results. According to Laher (2010), sufficient agreement with the normative sample was found to support evidence for the applicability of the NEO-PI-R, and by extension the FFM, in a sample of South African university students. Laher (2010) highlights some important issues in this regard. These are (a) the problematic nature of the Actions (Openness to Experience) facet, and (b) the order of the factor loadings. Openness to Actions is characterised by the willingness to try different activities, go to new places or try new foods (Costa & McCrae, 1992). According to Costa and MCrae (1992), high scorers on this scale prefer novelty and variety, while low scorers prefer familiarity and routine and find change difficult. It is evident from the reliability analysis that Actions had a moderate reliability coefficient in the normative sample (α = .58) as well as in this study (α = .55). Given this result, one has to question whether there are more implicit problems with the scale and its items. Certainly the definitions are clear enough, but perhaps the items do not come across clearly, or individuals cannot identify with the situations that the items depict.

Laher's (2010) second point refers to the order of factor loadings. Costa and MCrae (1992) suggest that the factors load with Neuroticism on Factor 1, Extraversion on Factor 2, Openness to Experience on Factor 3, Agreeableness on Factor 4 and Conscientiousness on Factor 5. In total the five-factor solution explained 56.73 per cent of the shared variance. In the five-factor solution for Laher's (2010) study, Factor 1 emerges as a Conscientiousness factor and explains 17.86 per cent of the variance. Factor 2 is defined by loadings on the Neuroticism factor and explains 12.78 per cent of the variance. The Agreeableness factor, Factor 3, explains 11.07 per cent of the variance. Factor 4 is the Extraversion factor and explains 9.19 per cent of the variance, while Factor 5 is the Openness factor and explains 5.83 per cent of the variance. Given the loadings and the percentage of variance explained by each of the domains, Laher (2010) concludes that it is possible that certain factors may contribute more towards personality, life and culture in the South African student sample explored in her research. She does caution that this claim requires more empirical research.

Bias and the NEO-PI-R in South Africa

Laher (2010) found that construct bias was operational for all three variables – gender, population group and home language – in the NEO-PI-R. These results were generally in line with other research found on systematic differences in personality across gender, population group and, to a lesser extent, home language (see Allik & McCrae, 2004; Costa, Terracciano & McCrae, 2001; Heuchert et al., 2000; McCrae et al., 2005; Zhang & Akande, 2002). Thus females were found to be higher in Neuroticism and Agreeableness than males, and non-white individuals were found to score lower on Extraversion and Openness to Experience than white individuals. With home language, it was possible to conclude that English second-language speakers were generally lower on Openness to Experience. However, effect sizes for these differences were small to moderate. Therefore this conclusion is drawn with caution, and future research is warranted. Evidence for item bias in the NEO-PI-R at both quantitative and qualitative levels corresponds to the construct bias findings, with items from the same problematic scales evidencing bias. A number of problematic items were identified, and these need to be explored further in the South African context to determine the nature and extent of the difficulties with the items. Linguistic difficulties, item construction difficulties, and the personal and cultural relevance of items were cited as possible reasons for this item bias.

Conclusion

In considering the utility of the NEO-PI-R in a South African sample of university students, it is possible to conclude that the NEO-PI-R is a reliable and valid instrument for use in the South African context, particularly with regard to university students. An interesting trend, observed in research conducted with South African student samples from 1994 to the present time, suggests that the FFM is becoming more replicable in a South African context. However, this may be because most of this research was conducted on university students, who represent a more acculturated sample.

Van Dyk and De Kock (2004) argued with regard to student samples in South Africa that student populations tend to be more individualist in nature, due in part to their shared exposure to similar education. In support of this view, Oyserman, Coon and Kemmelmeier (2002) have argued that the demands of an academic environment foster individualism, since the focus is on individual striving, competition and the realisation of one's potential. Eaton and Louw (2002) argue that acculturation, which can be occurring at both the individual and community level, could be influencing the extent to which cultural differences are expressed or even in fact exist. Mpofu (2001, p.342) has spoken of what is referred to as the 'African modernity trend', which represents a shift towards Western individualism. This ideological shift has been greatly influenced by Africa's participation in the global economy, where Western free-market economies emphasise individualist values. Studies of acculturation have shown that overt behaviours become oriented to those of the dominant culture, but that the 'invisible' elements of the individual's traditional culture remain intact (Mpofu, 2001). Whatever the case may be, it appears at present that the NEO-PI-R is not without flaws in terms of its applicability in the South African context, but evidence suggests that for educated samples that are conversant in English, the NEO-PI-R is a reliable and valid measure.

Note

1 At this time NEO was registered as the official name of the test.

References

Allik, J. & McCrae, R. R. (2004). Toward a geography of personality traits: Patterns of profiles across 36 cultures. *Journal of Cross-Cultural Psychology, 35*, 13–28.

Cheung, F. M., Cheung, S., Zhang, J., Leung, K., Leong, F. & Yeh, K. H. (2008). Relevance of Openness as a personality dimension in Chinese culture: Aspects of its cultural relevance. *Journal of Cross-Cultural Psychology, 39*, 81–108.

Cheung, F. M., Leung, K., Zhang, J. X., Sun, H., Gan, Y., Song, W. & Xie, D. (2001). Indigenous Chinese personality constructs: Is the Five-Factor Model complete? *Journal of Cross-Cultural Psychology, 32*, 407–433.

Costa, P. T. & McCrae, R. R. (1992). *Revised NEO Personality Inventory (NEO-PI-R) and NEO Five-Factor Inventory (NEO-FFI) Professional Manual*. Odessa, FL: Psychological Assessment Resources.

Costa, P. T., Jr, Terracciano, A. & McCrae, R. R. (2001). Gender differences in personality traits across cultures: Robust and surprising findings. *Journal of Personality and Social Psychology, 81*, 322–331.

Eaton, L. & Louw, J. (2002). Culture and self in SA: Individualism and collectivism predictions. *Journal of Social Psychology, 140*, 210–217.

Heaven, P. C. & Pretorius, A. (1998). Personality structure among black and white South Africans. *Journal of Social Psychology, 138*, 664–666.

Heuchert, J. W. P., Parker, W. D. & Stumpf, H. (2000). The Five-Factor Model of personality in South African college students. *American Behavioural Scientist, 44*, 112–125.

Horn, J. L. (1965). A rationale and test for the number of factors in factor analysis. *Psychometrika, 30*, 179–185.

Laher, S. (2010). Exploring the applicability of the NEO-PI-R and the CPAI-2 in the South African context. Unpublished PhD dissertation. University of the Witwatersrand, Johannesburg.

Laher, S. & Quy, G. (2009). Exploring the role of spirituality in the context of the Five-Factor Model of personality in a South African sample. *Journal of Psychology in Africa, 19*, 513–521.

McCrae, R. R., Costa, P. T., Del Pilar, G. H., Rolland, J. P. & Parker, W. D. (1998). Cross-cultural assessment of the Five-Factor Model. *Journal of Cross-Cultural Psychology, 29*, 171–188.

McCrae, R. R., Terracciano, A. & 79 Members of the Personality Profiles Project (2005). Universal features of personality traits from the observer's perspective: Data from 50 cultures. *Journal of Personality and Social Psychology, 88*, 547–561.

Mohammed, E. F., Unher, M. & Sugawara, M. (2009). Big Five personality factors: Cross-cultural comparison between Japanese and Egyptian students. *Acta Psychologica Sinica, 8*, 135–141.

Mpofu, E. (2001). Exploring the self-concept in African culture. *Journal of Genetic Psychology, 155*, 341–354.

Okeke, B. I., Draguns, J. G., Sheku, B. & Allen, W. (1999). Culture, self and personality in Africa. In Y. T. Lee, C. R. McCauley & J. G. Draguns (Eds), *Personality and Person Perception across Cultures* (pp. 139–162). Mahwah, NJ: Lawrence Erlbaum Associates.

Oyserman, D., Coon, H. M. & Kemmelmeier, M. (2002). Rethinking Individualism and Collectivism: Evaluation of theoretical assumptions and meta-analyses. *Psychological Bulletin, 128*, 3–72.

Piedmont, R. L., Bain, E., McCrae, R. R. & Costa, P. T., Jr (2002). The applicability of the Five-Factor Model in a sub-Saharan culture: The NEO-PI-R in Shona. In R. R. McCrae & J. Allik (Eds), *The Five-Factor Model of Personality across Cultures* (pp. 155–175). New York, NY: Kluwer Academic.

Rossier, J., Dahourou, D. & McCrae, R. R. (2005). Structural and mean level analyses of the Five-Factor Model and locus of control: Further evidence from Africa. *Journal of Cross-Cultural Psychology, 36*, 227–246.

Rothman, S. & Coetzer, E. P. (2003). The Big Five personality dimensions and job performance. *South African Journal of Industrial Psychology, 29*, 68–74.

Storm, K. & Rothman, S. (2003). The relationship between burnout, personality traits and coping strategies in a corporate pharmaceutical group. *South African Journal of Industrial Psychology, 29*, 35–42.

Teferi, T. B. (2004). The application of the NEO-PI-R in the Eritrean context. Unpublished Master's dissertation. University of the Witwatersrand, Johannesburg.

Van Dyk, G. A. J. & De Kock, F. S. (2004). The relevance of the Individualism-Collectivism (IC) factor for the management of diversity in the South African National Defence Force. *South African Journal of Industrial Psychology, 30*, 90–95.

Zhang, L.-F. & Akande, A. (2002). What relates to the Big Five among South African university students? *IFE PsychologIA: An International Journal, 10*, 49–74.

19 Using the Occupational Personality Profile in South Africa

N. Tredoux

The Occupational Personality Profile (OPPro) was developed by Paltiel and Budd in 1990 and was introduced to South Africa in 1994. Initially the questionnaire did not receive a great deal of attention because users of the Psytech range of tests preferred the Fifteen Factor Questionnaire (15FQ), since the 15FQ was based on a model with which most psychologists had become familiar in the course of their professional training. However, once comparative analyses had been done between the 15FQ and the OPPro, the South Africa distributor felt more comfortable recommending the OPPro for South African use since it was shorter and less expensive to use, and the initial reliability coefficients were better than those of the 15FQ. Users have tended to select the OPPro for large-scale projects, and for respondents who have lower levels of English proficiency or education than those who have completed the 15FQ+. The name of the questionnaire was originally abbreviated as OPP; this was subsequently changed to the abbreviation OPPro.

Rationale for the development of the OPPro

The OPPro was not developed according to a general theory of personality. This does not mean that there is no theoretical basis for the questionnaire, because every individual scale does have a theoretical rationale. The choice of constructs to be included in the OPPro was based on an overview of the research literature in the late 1980s. Dimensions were included if they could be shown to be associated with work performance (Budd, 2009). The goal was to develop a questionnaire that tapped into dimensions that predicted work performance according to the knowledge available at the time. The OPPro scales are summarised in Table 19.1.

Even though the scales were considered on individual merit rather than in relation to a general theory of personality, there is sufficient information in these nine scales to generate a comprehensive report on an individual. Derived estimates of the 'Big Five' personality factors are also calculated from the OPPro's scales. In practice the OPPro has proved extremely useful, yielding a remarkably comprehensive description of a person within a short administration time of usually less than half an hour.

Table 19.1 Summary of the scales measured by the OPPro

Accommodating Empathic, people-orientated, accepting, sensitive to people's feelings, avoiding confrontation.	**Assertive** Dominant, task-orientated, challenging, unconcerned about others' feelings, confrontative.
Important at work, influences leadership style.	
Detail-conscious Deliberating, controlled, rigid, enjoying attending to detail, conscientious.	**Flexible** Spontaneous, lacking self-discipline and self-control, flexible, dislikes attending to detail, disregards rules and obligations.
Relevant to the authoritarian personality style (Adorno, Frenkel-Brunswik, Levinson & Sanford, 1950).	
Cynical Suspicious, inclined to questions others' motives, cautious and guarded, may distrust other people.	**Trusting** Philanthropic, takes people at face value, has faith in others' honesty, sometimes a little credulous, naïve.
Based on the work of Christie and Geiss (1970) on the Machiavellian personality, this dimension is important because of its emphasis on political expediency, which is relevant to many work roles.	
Emotional Prone to worry, moody, inclined to be anxious in social settings, troubled by feelings of anxiety and self-doubt, easily takes offence.	**Phlegmatic** Self-assured, emotionally stable, socially confident, secure, resilient.
Eysenck and Eysenck (1969) argued that anxiety is an important personality factor, and that it may have a biological basis. Included because of its implications for emotional resilience and stress tolerance.	
Reserved Cool and introspective, prefers to work alone, enjoys own company, aloof and detached.	**Gregarious** Outgoing and sociable, lively and talkative, enjoys working with others, high need for affiliation, warm and participating.
The need for affiliation has been described as one of the most basic human motives (Maslow, 1970), and gregariousness as one of the most important and stable aspects of the human character (Eysenck & Eysenck, 1969). It is clearly relevant to many occupations.	
Genuine Bases behaviour on own feelings and attitudes, forthright, honest and open, sincere, lacking social awareness, may lack tact and diplomacy.	**Persuasive** Behaviour is determined by the demands of the situation, diplomatic, manipulating and expedient, shrewd and calculating, sensitive to 'political' issues.
According to Snyder (1974), people base their behaviour either on the demands of the situation or on their own attitudes and opinions. This dimension is relevant to roles that require tact and diplomacy.	
Composed Calm, able to delegate, keeps work separate from home life, able to unwind and relax, tolerant, able to distance himself/herself from work pressures.	**Contesting** Ambitious and competitive, may take on too much work, works long hours, has difficulty relaxing, impatient, may be prone to stress-related illnesses.
'Type A' behaviour (Contesting) has been related to coronary disease (Jenkins, 1971). This tense, competitive and hard-driving approach to work may have short-term benefits but could be self-defeating in the long term.	

continued →

Optimistic Achieving and striving, believes his/her own actions determine outcomes, positive approach to setbacks, believes he/she is in control of his/her own destiny.	**Pessimistic** Resigned, prone to feelings of helplessness, inclined to pessimism, fatalistic, has little faith in his/her ability to determine events, may give up easily.
This dimension is based on the concept of internal and external locus of control (Rotter, 1966). It has important implications for self-motivation and influences the way people react to setbacks.	
Abstract Imaginative, aesthetically sensitive, creative and artistic, intellectual, has a theoretical orientation.	**Pragmatic** Down to earth and concrete, not interested in artistic matters, practical and realistic, more concerned with 'how' than 'why'.
Originated in Jung's concept of thinking-extraversion vs thinking-introversion. This dimension will be important for selection decisions in roles that require either a practical, pragmatic or a theoretical, abstract approach.	
Low social conformity Low distortion due to social desirability responding.	**High social conformity** High distortion due to social desirability responding.
A typical social desirability scale based on the work of Crowne and Marlow (1964).	

Source: Adapted from Budd (2009), with permission.

Administration and reporting

The OPPro can be administered using pencil and paper, onscreen using the GeneSys system (Agnew, 2003) or via the internet. Test users can score the answer sheets themselves by entering the responses into the software or the online system, selecting the appropriate norm group, and producing one of several computer-generated reports. The extended report describes the respondent's interpersonal style and thinking and problem-solving style, and discusses how the individual is likely to cope with stressful situations. Descriptions of the individual's likely behaviour in a team, how he or she would function as a manager or a subordinate, and his or her style of influencing others follow. Finally, a summary of the respondent's strengths and development areas is given. A feedback report is also available, summarising the findings in non-technical terms for the respondent. An interview schedule customised for the particular respondent is also available. This highlights areas that need to be probed, and gives suggested lines of questioning. This is particularly useful for users who are new to the questionnaire, and helps the user develop a 'feel' for the interpretation of the OPPro.

It is possible to use the software to specify an 'ideal' profile for a role, or for a specific competency, and to compare respondents in terms of their degree of similarity to this profile. This can be a very useful way of making sense of large volumes of information, but users should never let a computer make selection decisions. They should moderate the findings suggested by the computer using their own personal judgement and information from other sources, such as interviews.

Documentation

The *Technical Manual* for the OPPro (Budd, 2009) explains the development of the questionnaire and the rationale for every scale, as well as some international research demonstrating reliability and validity of the questionnaire. The *South African User Guide and Research Reference* (Tredoux, 2002–2011) documents the South African research done on the questionnaire, including revisions made to some items, and makes recommendations regarding the use of the questionnaire in South Africa.

Psychometric properties of the OPPro

Reliability

The OPPro has lower reliabilities for people from disadvantaged groups than for white, educated persons with high English proficiency (see Figure 19.1).

Figure 19.1 Comparison of reliabilities of the OPPro for different South African language groups

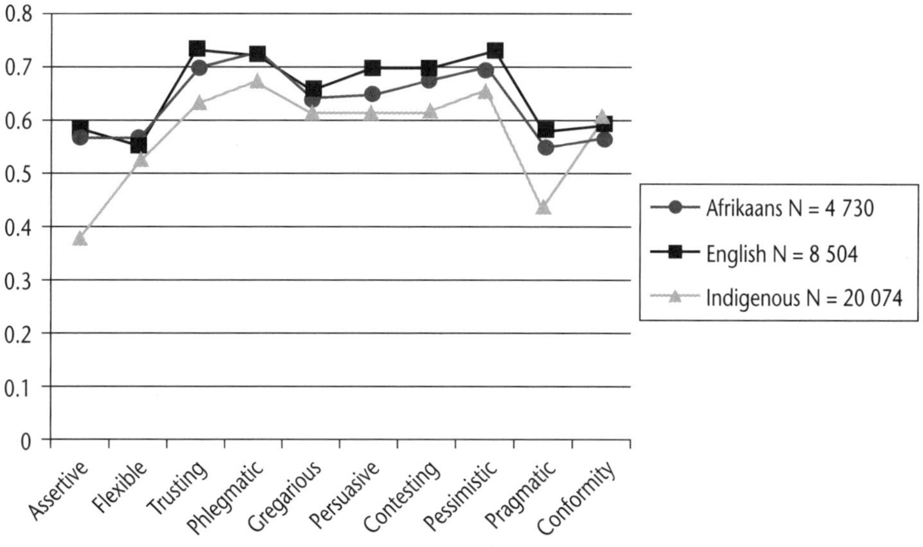

Note: Reliabilities are Cronbach's alpha coefficient (unstandardised).

With greater levels of education and English-language proficiency, the differences in reliabilities between the race groups become less apparent (Tredoux, 2002–2011). Users should exercise caution when considering the use of the OPPro on groups where the educational level and the proficiency in the language of the questionnaire are such that the respondents may have difficulty understanding the items. The verification and feedback interview then becomes very important, and this is where the interview questions that can be generated as a report from the personality profile become very useful.

Validity

The *Technical Manual* and *South African User Guide* (Budd, 2009; Tredoux, 2002–2011) summarise various international and local studies illustrating the correlations between the OPPro scales and various other instruments, for the purpose of determining construct validity. For this chapter, new correlations were calculated on larger samples, and these are presented in Table 19.2.

Table 19.2 Summary of correlations between the OPPro scales and various other tests, recalculated in 2010

Scale	Test	Correlating scales
Assertive	15FQ+	Dominant .46
	OPPro	Persuasive .37
	OIP	Need for control .45
Flexible	15FQ+	Conscientious –.34, Self-disciplined –.33, Work Attitude –.35
	OIP	Need for variety .45, Administrative interest –.33
Trusting	15FQ+	Suspicious –.49
	OPPro	Phlegmatic .43, Contesting –.37, Pessimistic –.47
Phlegmatic	15FQ+	Intellectance .3, Emotionally stable .46, Apprehensive –.43, Tense-driven –.32, Emotional Intelligence .34, Faking Good .41, Faking Bad –.37
	OPPro	Trusting .43, Gregarious .34, Contesting –.32, Pessimistic –.52
	OIP	Stability .53
Gregarious	15FQ+	Assertive .32, Enthusiastic .48, Socially Bold .42, Self-sufficient –.50
	JTI	Introverted –.54
	OIP	Need for people .55
	VMI	Affiliation .40, Affection .30
Persuasive	15FQ+	Dominant .47
	JTI	Introverted –.43
	OPPro	Pragmatic –.36
	OIP	Need for control .40, Persuasive interest .61
Contesting	OPPro	Trusting –.37, Phlegmatic –.32, Pessimistic .38
External	15FQ+	Suspicious .35
	OPPro	Trusting –.47, Phlegmatic –.52, Contesting .38
Pragmatic	15FQ+	Tender-Minded –.48, Abstract –.32
	JTI	Introverted .31, Intuitive –.57
	OPPro	Persuasive –.36
	OIP	Artistic –.60
	VMI	Aesthetic –.5
Conformity	15FQ+	Emotionally stable .3, Tense-driven –.35, Social desirability .44, Faking Good .37,
	VMI	Social desirability .54

Notes: 15FQ+ = Fifteen Factor Questionnaire Plus; JTI = Jung Type Indicator; OPPro = Occupational Personality Profile; OIP = Occupational Interest Profile; VMI = Values and Motives Inventory.

The accumulated evidence, and the pattern of the correlations, support the construct validity of the OPPro scales.

The OPPro was successfully used to predict competencies in the retail industry, and also to select candidates for postgraduate business school courses (Tredoux, 2002–2011). It was also used with success in a study predicting safety-related behaviour in the electricity supply industry.

Differences between groups

Table 19.3 summarises the standardised effect sizes for the differences in mean scale scores between males and females and between race groups on the OPPro scales. The differences between the groups are remarkably small even when statistically significant, suggesting that the main concern in using the OPPro should be whether the respondents understand the items, rather than expected differences between groups.

Table 19.3 Effect sizes for differences in mean OPPro scale scores for gender and race

	Gender	Race
Assertive	–0.24	0.17
Flexible	–0.22	0.26
Trusting	–0.02	0.13
Phlegmatic	–0.22	0.19
Gregarious	–0.04	0.24
Persuasive	–0.22	0.19
Contesting	0.21	0.19
Pessimistic	0.3	0.27
Pragmatic	–0.09	0.19
Conformity	0.06	0.19
	Males N = 25 064 Females N = 35 386	African N = 26 174 European N = 2 850 Coloured N = 8 097 Asian N = 3 553

Available norms

Substantial norm groups are available for all major groupings in South Africa. Users can also create their own norms using the GeneSys software. 'Custom norms' or 'in-house norms', as these are sometimes called, should be used with caution, because with repeated updating on such norm calculations the group can become progressively more restricted, especially if the questionnaire also forms part of the selection battery. All things considered, it is probably better to compare respondent scores with large population norm groups when using a personality questionnaire for selection purposes.

Recommendations

The OPPro is a classified psychological test and should be used only by psychologists and psychometrists. Users are strongly advised to undergo the appropriate training, and to seek mentorship from the test publisher and experienced OPPro users when they are still learning how to use the questionnaire. Users should also remember that although the questionnaire is supported by very useful computer-generated reports, they are still personally and professionally responsible for the reporting. The reports should be used judiciously, and integrated with biographical information, observed behaviour, other measures and interview data.

References

Adorno, T. W., Frenkel-Brunswik, E., Levinson, D. J. & Sanford, R. N. (1950). *The Authoritarian Personality*. New York, NY: Harper and Row.

Agnew, M. (2003). *Manual for the GeneSys Integrated Assessment System Version 3*. Pulloxhill: Psytech International.

Budd, R. (2009). *Occupational Personality Profile Technical Manual*. Pulloxhill: Psytech International.

Christie, R. & Geiss, F. L. (1970). *Studies in Machiavellianism*. New York, NY: Academic Press.

Crowne, D. P. & Marlow, D. (1964). *The Approval Motive*. New York, NY: Wiley.

Eysenck, H. J. & Eysenck, S. B. (1969). *Personality Structure and Measurement*. London: Routledge Kegan Paul.

Jenkins, C. D. (1971). Psychological and social precursors of coronary disease. *New England Journal of Medicine, 284*, 244–255.

Maslow, A. (1970). *Motivation and Personality*. New York, NY: Harper and Row.

Rotter, J. B. (1966). Generalised expectancies for internal versus external control of reinforcement. *Psychological Monographs, 80*.

Snyder, M. (1974). Self-monitoring of expressive behaviour. *Journal of Personality and Social Psychology, 30*, 526–537.

Tredoux, N. (2002–2011). *Occupational Personality Profile South African User Guide and Research Reference*. Johannesburg: Psytech South Africa.

20 The Occupational Personality Questionnaire

T. Joubert and N. Venter

The Occupational Personality Questionnaire (OPQ) is a family of personality questionnaires designed to give information on an individual's preferred behaviour on a number of work-related characteristics. The questionnaires were developed by SHL for use in the workplace, and only item content which is directly related to the world of work has been included. The OPQ questionnaires have been designed for a range of applications involving the individual, the team as well as the organisation (SHL, 1999a). The OPQ is particularly appropriate for use with graduate, professional and managerial groups, although the content is applicable to a variety of roles. A number of other OPQ versions have been developed over the years for particular occupational groups, such as the Customer Contact Styles Questionnaire (SHL, 1997) for those in customer service and sales roles and the Work Styles Questionnaire (SHL, 1999b) for use in production and manufacturing. Other, shorter versions of the OPQ were also developed to accommodate those who prefer less detail. These questionnaires provide a summary of an individual's personality based on factor principles, and include a Factor Model with 16 scales and a 6-scale model (Bartram, Brown, Fleck, Inceoglu & Ward, 2006).

The latest model of the OPQ, the OPQ32, has evolved into an international model of personality with 32 dimensions, reflecting the changing nature of work at the beginning of the 21st century. The OPQ32 model of personality breaks personality into three domains – namely, Relationships with People, Thinking Style, and Feelings and Emotions. According to SHL (1999a) the design of the OPQ32 was guided by five criteria: is designed specifically for the world of work; avoids clinical or obscure psychological constructs; is comprehensive in terms of personality scales measured; can be used by human resource professionals and psychologists; and is based on sound psychometric principles.

The OPQ32 consists of 32 scales or dimensions. These are illustrated in Table 20.1. The questionnaire was originally developed in two versions: a normative rating scale version (OPQ32n) and a forced-choice format ipsative scale (OPQ32i). The ipsative scale version (OPQ32i) has now been replaced by a forced-choice format version, using item response theory to generate normative scale scores (OPQ32r).

Table 20.1 OPQ32 scale descriptions

Relationships with people		
Persuasive	Enjoys selling, comfortable using negotiation, likes to change other people's views.	Influence
Controlling	Likes to be in charge, takes the lead, tells others what to do, takes control.	Influence
Outspoken	Freely expresses opinions, makes disagreement clear, prepared to criticise others.	Influence
Independent Minded	Prefers to follow own approach, prepared to disregard majority decisions.	Influence
Outgoing	Lively and animated in groups, talkative, enjoys attention.	Sociability
Affiliative	Enjoys others' company, likes to be around people, can miss the company of others.	Sociability
Socially Confident	Feels comfortable when first meeting people, at ease in formal situations.	Sociability
Modest	Dislikes discussing achievements, keeps quiet about personal success.	Empathy
Democratic	Consults widely, involves others in decision-making, less likely to make decisions alone.	Empathy
Caring	Sympathetic and considerate towards others, helpful and supportive, gets involved in others' problems.	Empathy
Thinking styles		
Data Rational	Likes working with numbers, enjoys analysing statistical information, bases decisions on facts and figures.	Analysis
Evaluative	Critically evaluates information, looks for potential limitations, focuses upon errors.	Analysis
Behavioural	Tries to understand motives and behaviour, enjoys analysing people.	Analysis
Conventional	Prefers well-established methods, favours a more conventional approach.	Creativity & Change
Conceptual	Interested in theories, enjoys discussing abstract concepts.	Creativity & Change
Innovative	Generates new ideas, enjoys being creative, thinks of original solutions.	Creativity & Change
Variety Seeking	Prefers variety, tries out new things, likes changes to regular routine, can become bored by repetitive work.	Creativity & Change
Adaptable	Changes behaviour to suit the situation, adapts approach to different people.	Creativity & Change
Forward Thinking	Takes a long-term view, sets goals for the future, more likely to take a strategic perspective.	Structure
Detail Conscious	Focuses on detail, likes to be methodical, organised and systematic, may become preoccupied with detail.	Structure
Conscientious	Focuses on getting things finished, persists until the job is done.	Structure
Rule Following	Follows rules and regulations, prefers clear guidelines, finds it difficult to break rules.	Structure
Feelings and emotions		
Relaxed	Finds it easy to relax, rarely feels tense, generally calm and untroubled.	Emotion
Worrying	Feels nervous before important occasions, worries about things going wrong.	Emotion

Feelings and emotions		
Tough Minded	Not easily offended, can ignore insults, may be insensitive to personal criticism.	Emotion
Optimistic	Expects things will turn out well, looks to the positive aspects of a situation, has an optimistic view of the future.	
Trusting	Trusts people, sees others as reliable and honest, believes what others say.	
Emotionally controlled	Can conceal feelings from others, rarely displays emotion.	
Vigorous	Thrives on activity, likes to be busy, enjoys having a lot to do.	Dynamism
Competitive	Has a need to win, enjoys competitive activities, dislikes losing.	
Achieving	Ambitious and career-centred, likes to work to demanding goals and targets.	
Decisive	Makes fast decisions, reaches conclusions quickly, less cautious.	

Source: Bartram et al. (2006, p.9). Reprinted with permission.

The normative version (OPQ32n)

This version of the OPQ32 requires that respondents rate each statement on a 1 to 5 Likert scale, ranging from Strongly Disagree (1), Disagree (2), Unsure (3), Agree (4) to Strongly Agree (5). Apart from 32 dimensions/scales, the OPQ32n questionnaire also includes a Social Desirability scale, which reflects the extent to which a respondent has given socially desirable answers. This scale can provide an indication that a respondent is 'faking' responses to the statements (Bartram et al., 2006).

The item response theory version (OPQ32r)

The OPQ32r takes on a forced-choice format, and asks respondents to consider three statements from which they have to choose the statement that they consider 'most' like them and the statement they consider 'least' like them. Apart from 32 dimensions/scales, the OPQ32r questionnaire also includes a Consistency scale. This Consistency scale has been designed to measure 'the probability that an individual's true scores are higher than the chance level' (Brown & Bartram, 2009a, p.25). The more the choices between statements diverge from what one would expect, given the person's estimated trait levels for the scales, the lower the Consistency score.

Both the OPQ32n and the OPQ32r are available in South Africa to be administered via an online system, the PC-based Expert system, and paper and pencil. A wide range of reports are available in a variety of languages. The reports include a sten score profile and/or detailed narrative reports. These narrative reports include, amongst others, concepts such as leadership, team impact, emotional and social competence, and stress. Integrated competency-based and other specialised reports can also be produced. There is also an OPQ32-based person-job match report designed for use by end users, using job analysis information together with assessment data to match the applicant to a specific job (Bartram et al., 2006).

Development of the OPQ

The development of the initial OPQ model of personality started in 1981, with a team of experts identifying Adjective Construct Checklists (ACLs) relevant to the world of work. These ACLs were identified by reviewing all existing questionnaires (for example, the California Psychology Inventory, Myers-Briggs Type Indicator, Gordon Personal Profile and Inventory, Kostic Personality and Preference Inventory) and models of personality, such as the work by Cattell and Eysenck, relevant to the field of work (SHL, 1993). Validation data on the relationship between personality and job performance were also reviewed, as well as documentation from client organisations to determine which aspects of personality were relevant to them. Approximately 100 Repertory Grids were completed to investigate the constructs used by managers for selection in the working environment. The ACLs were then trialled and the resulting data were analysed and refined, and the Amended Conceptual Model of personality was developed. Full items were then written to represent this model (SHL, 2009a). The data were again trialled and analysed, and the OPQ Concept Model of personality originated (SHL, 2009a).

Bartram et al. (2006, p.26) explain that '[i]n response to the changing nature of work and the accumulating amount of validation research combined with input from OPQ users around the world, SHL embarked on the OPQ32 Development Programme to update the OPQ Concept Model.' The impetus for this was primarily to develop a model that is applicable in a wide range of countries and cultures, improve the questionnaires' relevance and face validity, improve the reliabilities of some of the scales, reduce any overlap that might exist between scales, and keep the questionnaires' length to a minimum without losing reliability and variance (Bartram et al., 2006).

The two original versions of the OPQ32, normative and ipsative, were designed to cater for various stakeholders and to make the most of the advantages of both questionnaire formats. The OPQ32n has been favoured by traditional research practices and is used in South Africa mostly for development purposes. The normative questionnaire, however, is subject to various response biases such as acquiescence, leniency, halo effects and socially desirable responding. To counter these disadvantages, the ipsative version of the OPQ (OPQ32i) was developed to create a questionnaire that was free from response bias and more robust to impression management distortion (Brown & Bartram, 2009a). The OPQ32i contains forced-choice items, which reduces socially desirable responding, as respondents cannot endorse all items (Brown & Dowdeswell, 2008).

The disadvantage of using the OPQ32i, however, is that it does not have the same variability on the scale scores as the normative version. This limitation is not a result of the forced-choice format of the questionnaire, but rather a result of the classical test theory (CTT) scoring methodology that is used. According to Brown and Bartram (2009a, p.11), '[t]he CTT scoring methodology cannot adequately describe the decision-making process behind responding to multidimensional forced-choice items. Modelling this decision process correctly is the key to making the most of this response format.'

It was for this reason that the OPQ32r was developed and launched in 2009. This latest version of the OPQ32 combines the advantages of the forced-choice item format with multidimensional item response theory (IRT). The OPQ32r makes it possible to get 'normative' data from forced-choice questionnaires (Brown & Bartram, 2009b).

Standardisation and reliability of the OPQ32

Norms

The OPQ32 has various national and international norms that assign meaning to the raw scores obtained from the questionnaire. Each country where the OPQ32 is being used, including South Africa, has various OPQ32 norms applicable to its language and unique circumstances (Bartram et al., 2006). According to Bartram et al. (2006), the norms are also regularly updated by adopting SHL Test Development Guidelines to ensure that the samples used for the norms are representative of the population for which it is intended. The current OPQ32r norm update (SHL, 2011) includes 92 norms spanning 24 languages and 37 countries or regions. This includes a South African General Population norm (N = 4 880) and a Managerial and Professional norm (N = 1 267).

SHL has also developed OPQ32 international norms. As a result of globalisation and pan-geographical operations by many organisations, a need was identified to assess candidates across countries, while being able to compare these individuals against the same norm (Burke, Bartram & Philpott, 2009). An international norm was produced for OPQ32i in 2009. More recently, three OPQ32r international norms were created based on data collected from over 118 324 individuals across 43 countries (including South Africa) and 23 languages: a General Population norm, a Managerial & Professional norm and a Graduate norm (SHL, 2012).

Reliability

According to SHL (2004, p.7), '[i]nternal consistency coefficients pose interesting issues for developing personality questionnaires. If the coefficient is too low it suggests that the scale has very mixed or even ambiguous items, whereas too high a coefficient implies a very narrow factor with items that repeat essentially the same idea.' A case is therefore made for an optimum range of 0.70 to 0.80, neither too high nor too low.

Various South African and international reliability studies have been performed on OPQ32 data sets (Bartram et al., 2006). Eleven different South African reliability studies have been performed on the OPQ32 since its introduction in 1999.

In one of these studies the OPQ32n was used. This sample consists of a composite group of 1 181 employees and students from various industry sectors. There were 454 (38.44 per cent) females and 727 (61.56 per cent) males in this sample, with a mean age of 32.35 years (SD = 9.07). The sample included 232 (19.64 per cent) Africans, 32 (2.71 per cent) Indians, 27 (2.29 per cent) coloureds and 390 (33.02 per cent) whites. Five hundred (42.34 per cent) of the respondents did not indicate their ethnicity. The qualifications of the sample ranged from Grade 10 to a postgraduate degree (SHL, 2002a). In this study, the alpha coefficients ranged between 0.69 and 0.88, with 20 of the scales' alpha coefficients exceeding 0.80 (SHL, 2002a).

Reliabilities were also calculated on the OPQ32r. The reliabilities presented in Table 20.2 are based on the calibration sample used for developing the OPQ32r. The sample (N = 518) consists of mainly university students from the USA, the UK and the West Indies, and includes 68.9 per cent females and 30.3 per cent males (0.8 per cent did not indicate their gender). The ages ranged from 18 to 55. Ethnicity was indicated by 57 per cent of the participants, and of these, 36 per cent were white and 48 per cent were black (Brown & Bartram, 2009a).

OPQ32r reliabilities were also calculated for a South African sample. However, due to the size of the sample, the item parameters established with the calibration sample were used. The South African sample consisted of 87 males and 99 females, with ages ranging from 18 to 59. The ethnic composition of the sample was Africans (N = 59), coloureds (N = 36), Indians (N = 14) and whites (N = 71). The educational level of the sample ranged from Grade 10 (N = 2) to postgraduate degrees (N = 81) (SHL, 2009b). The results are also presented in Table 20.2.

Table 20.2 Internal consistency reliability estimates for the OPQ32r

OPQ32 scale	IRT composite reliability		Standard error (theta = 0 for all scales)
	Calibration sample (N = 518)	South African sample (N = 185)	
RP1 Persuasive	0.83	0.82	0.36
RP2 Controlling	0.91	0.93	0.22
RP3 Outspoken	0.86	0.87	0.31
RP4 Independent Minded	0.77	0.78	0.41
RP5 Outgoing	0.89	0.88	0.25
RP6 Affiliative	0.84	0.86	0.33
RP7 Socially Confident	0.87	0.89	0.29
RP8 Modest	0.81	0.83	0.34
RP9 Democratic	0.74	0.75	0.43
RP10 Caring	0.81	0.83	0.37
TS1 Data Rational	0.88	0.89	0.26
TS2 Evaluative	0.80	0.79	0.39
TS3 Behavioural	0.79	0.80	0.39
TS4 Conventional	0.68	0.69	0.49
TS5 Conceptual	0.78	0.77	0.40
TS6 Innovative	0.89	0.89	0.27
TS7 Variety Seeking	0.77	0.78	0.40
TS8 Adaptable	0.87	0.88	0.28
TS9 Forward Thinking	0.87	0.88	0.30

OPQ32 scale	IRT composite reliability		Standard error (theta = 0 for all scales)
	Calibration sample (N = 518)	South African sample (N = 185)	
TS10 Detail Conscious	0.89	0.89	0.24
TS11 Conscientious	0.84	0.82	0.35
TS12 Rule Following	0.89	0.89	0.26
FE1 Relaxed	0.87	0.89	0.28
FE2 Worrying	0.78	0.80	0.37
FE3 Tough Minded	0.80	0.80	0.39
FE4 Optimistic	0.81	0.81	0.37
FE5 Trusting	0.88	0.89	0.28
FE6 Emotionally Controlled	0.86	0.88	0.29
FE7 Vigorous	0.88	0.90	0.27
FE8 Competitive	0.87	0.86	0.30
FE9 Achieving	0.79	0.79	0.41
FE10 Decisive	0.83	0.85	0.35

Source: OPQ reliabilities adapted from Brown and Bartram (2009a, p.23) and SHL (2009b, p.4). Adapted with permission.

The IRT composite reliabilities for the OPQ32r range from 0.68 to 0.91 with a median of 0.84 on the calibration sample, and from 0.69 to 0.93 with a median reliability of 0.85 on the South African sample. However, the real strength of IRT modelling is that standard errors are obtained for individual theta scores on each scale. These standard errors can be used to provide good estimates of scale reliability. The IRT preference model on which the OPQ32r is based produces normative trait level scores from forced-choice responses, by finding 'the most probable combination of scale scores to explain the individual choices made in blocks of statements' (Brown & Bartram, 2009a, p.16). The raw scores resulting from this process are theta scores produced by a multidimensional IRT optimisation algorithm.

Validity of the OPQ32

A large body of evidence has been collected over the years to support the validity of the OPQ32, both internationally as well as in South Africa (Bartram et al., 2006). In South Africa various studies support the construct as well as criterion-related validity of the OPQ32 (Bartram et al., 2006).

Construct validity

Factor structure of the OPQ32

In terms of the assessment of personality, 'the Five Factor Model (FFM) is well established and it could be expected that scales which, in terms of content, relate to the same factor of the FFM would correlate more strongly than they correlate with scales which relate to other FFM factors' (Bartram et al., 2006, p.124). This means that when performing exploratory factor analysis, a factor model fairly similar to the FFM should be found. It should be noted that in developing the OPQ model of personality, a deductive approach was followed rather than a factor analytic approach. The OPQ model of personality is comprehensive in terms of the personality measured, even at the risk of slight redundancy of measurement. It was not developed specifically to fit the FFM. However, as the OPQ32 scales cover the full range of the personality domain, it is possible to create scale composites that measure the FFM. According to Bartram et al. (2006), there are no clear internationally accepted definitions of the five factors. For this reason the research reported on below uses the most widely used FFM, the NEO by Costa and McRae (1992), as an operational basis for defining the FFM constructs (Bartram et al., 2006).

A South African sample (N = 644) from the mining industry was used in an exploratory factor analysis study. Principal components extraction with orthogonal varimax rotation was performed. The number of factors to be extracted was set based on Cattell's scree test. The data yielded six factors with 51 per cent of the variance explained. The sixth factor related to adaptability. The factor analysis was rerun, constraining five factors to be extracted to enable comparisons with factor analyses from other countries (Bartram et al., 2006).

OPQ32 scales hypothesised to relate to the FFM are listed in Table 20.3. The factor loadings obtained in the abovementioned rotation are listed in brackets.

Table 20.3 Conceptual mappings between the FFM and the OPQ32

Level	Extraversion	Agreeableness	Conscientiousness	Emotional Stability	Openness
Strong	Outgoing (0.76) Affiliative (0.62) Socially Confident (0.50)	Caring (0.66) Trusting	Forward Thinking (0.58) Detail Conscious (0.72) Conscientious (0.69)	Relaxed (0.67) Worrying (–) (–0.60) Tough Minded (0.68)	Conventional (–) (–0.71) Conceptual (0.47) Innovative (0.58)
Moderate	Persuasive (0.49) Controlling (0.45) Emotionally Controlled (–) (–0.68)	Outspoken (–) Independent Minded (–) (–0.52) Democratic (0.73) Competitive (–)	Vigorous (0.47) Achieving (0.65)	Socially Confident (0.55) Optimistic (0.57)	Behavioural Variety Seeking (0.73)
Weak	Variety Seeking Optimistic Vigorous	Modest	Decisive (–)		

Source: Adapted from Bartram et al. (2006, p.120). Adapted with permission.

It can be seen from the table that the scales that clustered together to form the five factors are interpretable in terms of the FFM. However, there are OPQ32 scales that were hypothesised but do not relate empirically to any of the FFM factors. These include Modest (in Agreeableness), Vigorous, Variety Seeking and Optimistic (in Extraversion) and Decisive (in Conscientiousness). The results of the South African sample were also compared to British and US samples, and the majority of scales showed consistently strong loadings on the factors (Bartram et al., 2006). There were almost no scales which were specific to a particular data set. The South African sample obtained higher loadings than the other countries on Trusting (in Emotional Stability) and Independent Minded (in Openness). The OPQ32 measures a broader personality domain than the five factors (Bartram et al., 2006). This can be related back to the development of the OPQ model of personality, in that it was developed to provide a detailed description of personality based on a 'rational analysis of the important personality characteristics in the world of work' (SHL, 1999a, p.1). Optimal measurement of the Big Five personality scales is obtained when just 26 of the 32 scales are used (Bartram & Brown, 2005).

The OPQ32 in relation to other personality questionnaires

The construct validity of the OPQ32 was also investigated by examining the OPQ32 scores in relation to other inventories that assess personality. The OPQ32 was correlated with various questionnaires including the 16PF, Occupational Personality Profile, Hogan Personality Inventory, Minnesota Multiphasic Personality Inventory and Myers-Briggs Type Indicator. The relationship between the OPQ32 and other personality questionnaires supports the validity of the constructs in the OPQ32. For more detail on these international as well as South African studies, refer to the *OPQ32 Technical Manual* by Bartram et al. (2006).

Criterion-related validity

The relationship between the OPQ32 and job and training performance is well proven through international as well as South African research. Internationally, various meta-analytic studies (Bartram, 2005; Robertson & Kinder, 1993) have been reported indicating the linear relationship between OPQ-based predictions and measures of successful job performance. In South Africa, more than ten validation studies demonstrate the relationship between the OPQ32 and job and training performance. These include studies in various industry sectors as well as in tertiary institutions. One of these studies was done to identify valid predictors and measures of the academic performance of Master of Business Administration (MBA) students. The sample consisted of 135 MBA students from a South African school of management, of which 65 per cent were male and 35 per cent female. The average age of the students was 38.20 (SD = 7.26). Seventy per cent of the sample was black (as defined by the Employment Equity Act No. 55 of 1998), and 30 per cent white. Significant correlations of moderate effect size were found between academic performance and numerical ability and competencies derived from the OPQ32i. Regression analysis indicated that 25 per cent of academic success can be predicted by numerical ability and personality (Kotzé & Griessel, 2008).

Another study was done on broker consultants in the insurance industry. Production data (in rand value) was collected for 234 broker consultants for a two-year period. The sample included 166 (70.94 per cent) males and 68 (29.06 per cent) females, with a mean age of 32.59 years (SD = 6.57). The sample comprised 17 (7.33 per cent) Africans, 24 (10.34 per cent) Indians, 13 (5.60 per cent) coloureds and 177 (76.29 per cent) whites. Significant correlations with a medium effect size were found between certain OPQ32 scales (Persuasiveness, Controlling, Data Rational, Innovative, Decisive, Modest(–), Democratic(–), Caring(–), Variety Seeking(–), Worrying(–) and Tough Minded(–)) and the production data. Regression analysis indicated that a total of 40 per cent of the criterion variance could be explained by the OPQ32 scales (SHL, 2002b).

Equivalence across administration modes

Different versions of the OPQ32 can be administered through various modes of administration (paper and pencil, personal computer and online) with or without direct supervision. It is important to establish whether the same constructs are being measured regardless of the different modes.

Bartram and Brown (2004) investigated the measurement equivalence of the OPQ32i when administered supervised using paper and pencil, and unsupervised via the internet. Sample data were collected and matched in terms of industry sector, assessment purpose and candidate category. The effect of the different modes of administration was investigated by examining their influence on the pattern of scale intercorrelations and scale means. The analysis indicated that neither the relationships between scales nor the scale means were affected by mode of supervision or administration (Bartram & Brown, 2004).

Two South African studies were performed investigating the equivalence of online unsupervised and paper-and-pencil supervised administration of the OPQ32n and the OPQ32i (Holtzhausen, 2004; Joubert & Kriek, 2009). In the first study, a group of managers (N = 322) in a mining company that completed the OPQ32n online and unsupervised was compared with a mixed group (N = 322) that completed the OPQ32n supervised and with paper and pencil. In order to ensure that certain biographical variables (age, ethnicity, education and gender) did not act as moderators, the paper-and-pencil sample was randomly selected to reflect the biographical data of the online sample. The groups were compared by examining the mean differences and reliabilities of the two groups. The effect of mode of administration as well as of supervision was also investigated, by examining the pattern of scale intercorrelations using structural equation modelling (SEM). The model tested was that all the samples were drawn from the same population (Bartram et al., 2006).

The results indicated that the paper-and-pencil supervised administration had comparable psychometric properties to the online unsupervised administration. Only small differences in the sample means were found. The largest effect size was d = 0.35 for the scale Affiliative, where people from the online sample were less Affiliative than people from the paper-and-pencil sample. The average reliability coefficient of 0.80 was the same for both samples. The SEM analysis obtained a CFI = 0.976 with RMSEA = 0.021, indicating an exceptionally good fit (Holtzhausen, 2004).

The second study was performed using the OPQ32i, comparing supervised paper-and-pencil administration with online unsupervised administration. The methodology that was followed was similar to that of the OPQ32n study, where mean differences (based on Cohen's measure of effect size, d-statistic), reliabilities and patterns of scale intercorrelations were investigated using SEM. For this study two separate investigations were conducted. One investigation used a graduate sample that completed the OPQ32i online and unsupervised, in a high-stakes selection setting (N = 1 091), compared with a randomly selected sample that completed the OPQ32i supervised and with paper and pencil (N = 1 136), also in a high-stakes selection setting. The other investigation used a group of managers that completed the OPQ32i online and unsupervised, in a high-stakes selection setting (N = 1 159), comparing them with a randomly selected sample that completed the OPQ32i supervised and with paper and pencil (N = 950). For both these studies the supervised paper-and-pencil samples were randomly selected from a bigger database to reflect the biographical data of their respective online samples. This was once again done to ensure that age, gender, ethnicity and education had no moderator effect on the results (Joubert & Kriek, 2009).

For the graduate sample, the median internal consistency was 0.73 for the paper-and-pencil supervised sample and 0.74 for the online unsupervised sample. For the managerial sample, the median internal consistency was 0.75 for the paper-and-pencil supervised sample and 0.75 for the online unsupervised sample (Joubert & Kriek, 2009).

The effect sizes (d-statistic) for the first group (the graduates sample) range from a small 0.02 to a medium 0.57, and for the second group (the sample comprising managers) from a small 0.01 to a medium 0.41. The scales that obtained medium effect size differences in the first group (the graduates sample) included Conscientious, Worrying, Emotional Control and Consistency. Joubert and Kriek (2009, p.7) state that '[a]lthough great care was taken to equate the samples in terms of their biographical information, no previous work experience data were available. The internet-based sample consisted solely of young graduates with possibly no work experience applying for positions, whereas the paper-and-pencil sample more likely consisted of candidates with previous work experience.'

In order to compare the scale covariance of the samples, one scale was deleted from the correlation matrix to free variance, so that the number of scales became equal to the degrees of freedom. The models tested were that the covariance matrices were identical. The CFI obtained for Study 1 (graduates) was 0.985 and the RMSEA was equal to 0.015. The CFI obtained for Study 2 (managers) was equal to 0.993 and the RMSEA was 0.012. It can be seen that relationships between the OPQ32i scales were not affected by mode of administration or supervision (Joubert & Kriek, 2009).

Applicability and utility of the OPQ32 in the South African context

The development of the OPQ32 has been a project involving widespread international collaboration between multiple countries, including South Africa. South Africa provided input into the OPQ32 model of personality as well as into the writing of the items (SHL, 2004). South Africa had, for example, a direct impact on changing the name of the 'Traditional' scale to 'Conventional', due to the negative political connotations attached to the word 'traditional'. With its involvement, South Africa made sure that from the development phase the instrument was applicable to the local environment. Since the launch of the OPQ32 in South Africa, various research studies on the utility and applicability of the instrument, specifically on different ethnic groups, have been performed, supporting this notion.

Group comparisons

With the development of the OPQ32, special attention was paid to ensuring that the item content was appropriate for all the people who might respond to each item (Bartram et al., 2006). Group differences in the South African environment, with its diverse workforce, were also analysed.

In the first study, a sample of 13 523 applicants to and incumbents of various positions in various industry sectors that had completed the OPQ32i since 2006 was used to investigate the mean differences, by gender and ethnicity. The gender split for the sample included 7 432 (55.0 per cent) males and 6 091 (45.0 per cent) females, with an average age of 32.47 (SD = 8.773). The ethnic composition of the group included 52.4 per cent Africans, 9.6 per cent coloureds, 8.5 per cent Indians and 29.1 per cent whites. There were 53 candidates who indicated another ethnicity. In terms of level of education, the sample included Grade 10 (2.6 per cent), Grade 12 (28.5 per cent), postmatriculation certificate (15.4 per cent), degree (34.5 per cent) and postgraduate (18.7 per cent), with 0.30 per cent missing (SHL, 2008).

The effect sizes for significant differences between the male and female groups ranged from very small (0.02) for Adaptable to small (0.33) for Caring and (0.36) for Innovative (SHL, 2008). The moderate size of these differences makes adverse impact unlikely, but users should always monitor the results to ensure that neither gender group is unjustifiably excluded.

The same sample was used to investigate the mean differences in terms of ethnicity. Four ethnic groups were used: African, coloured, Indian and white. The biggest mean differences were found between the African and white groups (SHL, 2008). Although many of the differences reach statistical significance due to the large sample sizes, the magnitude of these differences is mostly small. There is only one scale that obtained a medium effect size, and that is 0.54 for Forward Thinking. The African group seems to take more of a long-term view, and is more likely to set goals for the future than the white group (SHL, 2008).

Equivalence across ethnicity

Visser and Viviers (2010) published a study in which the construct equivalence of the OPQ32n was investigated for black and white people in South Africa. The sample consisted of 248 blacks and 476 whites. SEM was used to compare the scale intercorrelations between the black and white groups. The comparison of correlation matrices yielded positive results, with a CFI = 0.961 and a RMSEA = 0.041. The comparison of covariance matrices yielded similar results, with the CFI = 0.942 and the RMSEA = 0.048. Visser and Viviers (2010, p.1) state that '[a] good fit regarding factor correlations and covariances on the 32 scales was obtained, partially supporting the structural equivalence of the questionnaire for the two groups.'

Utility of the OPQ32

It is fundamental for running a successful business that the investment in objective selection techniques can be justified in financial return on investment (ROI) terms. It is important to also look specifically at personality. Burke (2005, p.4) writes that

> in the 'knowledge economy' of today, the shelf life of past experience is ever shortening and has been estimated recently to range from 3 to 5 years depending on which occupation and on which industry one is looking at. Moreover, it is relatively easy to build skill and experience through training – it is much harder to influence personality. Having the right personalities in a role provides a firm foundation for further development that can push potential contributions even higher.

A South African ROI study involving a sample of broker consultants in a South African financial services group was performed in 2000. It was estimated that the utility gain for the first year of work was R21 335.17 for a broker consultant who stayed with the organisation. It can be seen that the costs incurred in testing are very small if weighed against the production gain per employee per annum. For the total sample of 172 included in this study, the annual savings for the organisation amounted to R3 669 649.20 (SHL, no date).

Conclusion

Since the OPQ's development 24 years ago, various research studies, local as well as international, have supported its psychometric properties. It measures work-related behavioural traits, and can be used to identify candidates with the potential for successful performance in a wide range of areas of work. Detailed information is provided on 32 specific personality characteristics that underpin performance on various competencies. The OPQ32 has a detailed technical manual (Bartram et al., 2006) that was reviewed during development by a panel of independent experts: Professors Barbara Byrne, Ronald Hambleton, Robert Roe and Peter Warr. In addition, there are more recent technical documents and user manuals relating to the OPQ32r (Brown & Bartram, 2009a; SHL, 2009a; 2011; 2012). These manuals can be consulted for more detailed information on the international and South African research performed on the OPQ32.

References

Bartram, D. (2005). The great eight competencies: A criterion-centric approach to validation. *Journal of Applied Psychology, 90(6)*, 1185–1203.

Bartram, D. & Brown, A. (2004). Online testing: Mode of administration and the stability of OPQ32i scores. *International Journal of Selection and Assessment, 12(3)*, 278–284.

Bartram, D. & Brown, A. (2005). *Five Factor Model (Big Five) OPQ32 Report: OPQ32 Technical Manual Supplement.* Thames Ditton, Surrey: SHL Group.

Bartram, D., Brown, A., Fleck, S. Inceoglu, I. & Ward, K. (2006). *OPQ32 Technical Manual.* Thames Ditton, Surrey: SHL Group.

Brown, A. & Bartram, D. (2009a). *Development and Psychometric Properties of OPQ32r: Supplement to the OPQ32 Technical Manual.* Thames Ditton, Surrey: SHL Group.

Brown, A. & Bartram, D. (2009b). *The Occupational Personality Questionnaire Revolution: Applying Item Response Theory to Questionnaire Design and Scoring.* Thames Ditton, Surrey: SHL Group.

Brown, A. & Dowdeswell, K. (2008). Normative-ipsative debate: Old arguments and new debates. Pre-conference workshop at the Annual Society for Industrial and Organisational Psychology of South Africa (SIOPSA) Conference. Pretoria, May 21–23.

Burke, E. (2005). The return on investment from personality testing. *Business Issues Series, 7*, 1–4.

Burke, E., Bartram, D. & Philpott, D. (2009). *OPQ32i International Norm: OPQ32 Technical Manual Supplement.* Thames Ditton, Surrey: SHL Group.

Costa, P. T. & McCrae, R. R. (1992). *Revised NEO Personality Inventory (NEO-PI-R) and NEO Five-Factor Inventory (NEO-FFI) Professional Manual.* Odessa, FL: Psychological Assessment Resources.

Holtzhausen, G. (2004). Mode of administration and the stability of the OPQ32n: Comparing internet (controlled) and paper-and-pencil (supervised) administration. Unpublished Master's thesis, University of Pretoria, Pretoria.

Joubert, T. & Kriek, H. J. (2009). Psychometric comparison of paper-and-pencil and online personality assessments in a selection setting. *SA Journal of Industrial Psychology, 35(1)*, 1–11.

Kotzé, M. & Griessel, L. (2008). The prediction of the academic performance of MBA students by means of specific aptitudes and competencies. *Journal for New Generation Sciences, 6(2)*, 60–79.

Robertson, I. T. & Kinder, A. (1993). Personality and job competencies: The criterion-related validity of some personality variables. *Journal of Occupational and Organizational Psychology, 66*, 225–244.

SHL (1993). *OPQ Concept Model Manual and Users' Guide.* Thames Ditton, Surrey: SHL Group.

SHL (1997). *Customer Contact Styles Questionnaire: Customer Contact Manual and Users' Guide.* Thames Ditton, Surrey: SHL Group.

SHL (1999a). *OPQ32 Manual and Users' Guide.* Thames Ditton, Surrey: SHL Group.

SHL (1999b). *Work Styles Questionnaire: Manual and User's Guide.* Thames Ditton, Surrey: SHL Group.

SHL (2002a). Reliability Study, *Study No. R038, 06 March 2002.* Thames Ditton, Surrey: SHL Group.

SHL (2002b). Validation Study, *Study No. V030, 27 September 2002.* Thames Ditton, Surrey: SHL Group.

SHL (2004). *The Occupational Personality Questionnaire in South Africa: Psychometric Research Perspectives*. Pretoria: SHL Group.

SHL (2008). Development Study, *Study No. D015, November 2008*. Thames Ditton, Surrey: SHL Group.

SHL (2009a). *OPQ32r User Manual*. Thames Ditton, Surrey: SHL Group.

SHL (2009b). Internal research report: Relationships between OPQ32i and OPQ32r, October 2009. Thames Ditton, Surrey: SHL Group.

SHL (2011). *OPQ32r Norm Update Technical Documentation*. Thames Ditton, Surrey, UK: SHL Group.

SHL (2012). *OPQ32r Technical Manual Supplement: OPQ32r International Norm*. Thames Ditton, Surrey: SHL Group.

SHL (no date). *OPQ32: Celebrating Decades of Innovation*. Pretoria: SHL SA.

Visser, D. & Viviers, R. (2010). Construct equivalence of the OPQ32n for black and white people in South Africa. *SA Journal of Industrial Psychology, 36(1)*, 1–11.

21 The Millon Inventories in South Africa

R. Patel and S. Laher

Theodore Millon (1969; 1991; 1994; 1996b; 2010) argues that predominant theories of personality tend to focus primarily on either the intrapsychic, interpersonal, environmental or biological aspects involved in personality development. Instruments, particularly objective, self-report questionnaires, are then developed in relation to these theories to assess personality. However, personality is more than just intrapsychic or interpersonal factors.

Millon attempts to combine the intrapsychic, cognitive and interpersonal spheres in his theory. He also acknowledges that an integrated approach needs to go beyond psychology if it is to be truly holistic (Millon, 1996b). In keeping with this argument, he borrows from evolutionary biology to develop his biopsychosocial evolutionary theory of personality, which underpins a number of instruments developed under the Millon umbrella.

The Millon family of instruments consists of pre-adolescent, adolescent, adult and medical patient inventories. The Millon Pre-Adolescent Clinical Inventory (M-PACI) is a comprehensive clinical tool that is designed to quickly and accurately identify psychological problems in children between the ages of 9 and 12. Unlike other instruments that focus on single clinical areas such as depression or anxiety, the M-PACI provides a synthesis of the child's emerging personality style and clinical syndrome, and can assist with early intervention (Millon, 2010). The Millon Adolescent Personality Inventory (MAPI) is a measure that assesses eight personality style dimensions, expressed concerns and behavioural correlates in normal adolescents aged 13 to 18 years (Millon, 2010). The Millon Adolescent Clinical Inventory (MACI) was developed specifically for use in regard to diagnostic assistance, treatment formulation and outcome measure in the clinical setting, and is used primarily for the evaluation of adolescents with difficulties. The MACI supplements the MAPI in providing a more holistic picture of the adolescent's personality type and clinical difficulties that he or she may be experiencing (Millon, 2010).

The Millon Inventories also include the Millon College Counselling Inventory (MCCI), Millon Behavioural Medicine Diagnostic (MBMD) and Personality Adjective Check List (PACL). The MCCI is an assessment tool that can help address students' concerns and student-specific issues such as depression, stress, anxiety, substance abuse, suicidal ideation, and adjustment and relationship difficulties (Millon, 2010). The MBMD provides medical and health practitioners with an assessment of psychosocial factors that may support or interfere with a chronically ill patient's medical treatment (Millon, 2010). The MBMD is used to identify significant psychiatric problems, as well as to identify personal and social assets that may facilitate a patient's adjustment to his or her physical limitations and lifestyle changes (Millon, 2010). Finally, the PACL is a measure of Millon's eight basic personality types for use in normal adults. The measure is appropriate for use in individuals who are 16 years and older, and is frequently used by psychologists who want to achieve a rapid understanding of their clients' strengths and weaknesses. The PACL is used in relatively higher-functioning individuals (Millon, 2010). The Millon Index of Personality Styles – Revised (MIPS-Revised) and Millon Clinical Multiaxial Inventory – III (MCMI-III) are designed for use on the adult population.

Millon's theory

In a book published more than 40 years ago, Theodore Millon proposed a theoretical grid for the classification of personality (Millon, 1969). Part of the appeal of his proposal was that it grouped together eight different personality prototypes that had long been recognised by clinicians. The scheme leading to the prototypes was eventually revised to consist of three polarities, tendencies that theoretically resulted in the distinguishing characteristics of the different personality prototypes – namely, pain vs pleasure, active vs passive, and self vs other (Millon, 1994; 1996b). The theory influenced the development of the current classification of personality disorders by the American Psychological Association and has led to the creation of four different psychological instruments, of which the MCMI has achieved widespread use with psychiatric patients (Choca, 1998).

According to Millon (1996a, p.13), personality is

> [an] inferred abstraction, a concept or construct, rather than a tangible phenomenon with material existence ... personality may be conceived as a psychic system of structures that parallels that of the body. It is not a potpourri of unrelated traits and miscellaneous behaviors but a tightly knit organisation of stable structures (e.g. internalised memories and self images) and coordinated functions (e.g. unconscious mechanisms and cognitive processes). Given continuity in one's constitutional equipment and a narrow band of experiences for learning behavioral alternatives, this psychic system develops an integrated pattern of characteristics and inclinations that are deeply etched, cannot be easily eradicated, and pervade every facet of their life experience ...

Thus, according to Millon, personality is that abstract concept that consists of an individual's lifelong style of relating, coping, behaving, thinking and feeling.

Based on this, then, one is inclined to conclude that psychopathology is the condition that arises as a result of any internal or external factor that upsets or is incoherent with an individual's lifelong style of relating, coping, behaving, thinking and feeling. Millon (1996a) argues that there is no sharp line that divides normal from pathological behaviour. According to him, they are relative concepts representing arbitrary points on a continuum. Millon's conception of normality and psychopathology is best represented in Figure 21.1.

Figure 21.1 Millon's continuum of personality development

NORMAL PERSONALITY	PSYCHOPATHOLOGICAL PERSONALITY

From Figure 21.1, it becomes clear that normality and psychopathology are opposite ends of a continuum, and it is possible to experience varying degrees of normality and psychopathology. When an individual displays an ability to cope with the environment in a flexible manner, and when his or her typical perceptions and behaviours foster increments in personal satisfaction, then the individual may be said to have a normal or healthy personality. The most common criterion used to determine normality is a statistical one, in which normality is determined by those behaviours that are found most frequently in a social group; and pathology or abnormality, by features that are uncommon in that population. Among diverse criteria used to signify normality are a capacity to function autonomously and competently, a tendency to adjust to one's environment effectively and efficiently, a subjective sense of contentment and satisfaction, and the ability to self-actualise or to fulfil one's potentials. Psychopathology would be noted by deficits among these features. Thus psychopathology reflects the person–environment interaction, and types of psychopathology can be distinguished in terms of the extent to which their determinants derive from personological versus situational forces (Millon, 1996a).

Personality disorders (Axis II)[1] are best conceived as those conditions that are 'activated' primarily by internally embedded structures and pervasive ways of functioning. At the opposite end of the internal–external continuum are the adjustment reactions, which are best construed as specific pathological responses attributable largely to circumscribed environmental precipitants. Between these polar extremes lie the categories of psychopathology that are anchored more or less equally and simultaneously to internal personal attributes and external situational events. These are referred to as clinical syndromes (Axis I)[2] (Millon, 1996a). This is best represented in Figure 21.2.

Figure 21.2 Millon's conceptualisation of the role of personological and situational factors

INTERNAL/ PERSONOLOGICAL FACTORS				EXTERNAL/ SITUATIONAL FACTORS
PERSONALITY DISORDERS	CLINICAL SYNDROMES	NORMAL PERSONALITY	CLINICAL SYNDROMES	ADJUSTMENT DISORDERS

From the discussion thus far it becomes possible to conclude that Millon, unlike some of his predecessors, adopts a holistic view of personality and psychopathology. He regards both personality and psychopathology as being products of the person–environment interaction, and does not subscribe to a wholly intrapsychic or wholly interpersonal approach. Rather, he adopts an integrative theory of personality and psychopathology in which he stresses that 'biological and experiential determinants combine and interact in a reciprocal interplay throughout life ... Etiology in psychopathology may be viewed, then, as a developmental process in which intraorganismic and environmental forces display not only a reciprocity and circularity of influence but an orderly and sequential continuity throughout the life of an individual' (Millon, 1996c, p.59). This forms the basis for Millon's biosocial learning approach towards personality and psychopathology.

In 1990, Millon published *Toward a New Personology: An Evolutionary Model*. In this book he extended his theory to include normal individuals. The MIPS represents an extension of the Millon assessment tools into the measurement of 'normal' individuals. Millon's theory takes evolutionary biology as a point of departure, and then amalgamates concepts from other theorists – Freud, Jung and Leary – as well as some theoretical contributions from the Five-Factor Model. He considers personality to be composed of the nature, the source and the instrumental behaviours that an individual exhibits. Rather than giving primacy either to the 'driving' motivational and emotional roots of personality style (as in Millon's formulation of personality disorders or Freudian theory), or to the overt behavioural expressions of personality (as explicated in the Five-Factor Model, for example), the Millonian approach seeks to conjoin these components by linking them to cognitive functions. In this way, he attempts to integrate the various components of personality into a single coherent whole under the umbrella of evolutionary principles (Millon, 1994).

In accordance with evolutionary psychology, Millon likens the development of an individual's personality to the ontogenetic development of that individual organism's adaptive strategies (Million, 1994; 1996d). Just as an individual organism begins life with a limited subset of its species' genes and the trait potentials they subserve, an individual is also born with a number of potential personality styles. Over time, the salience of these trait potentials – not the proportion of the genes themselves – will become differentially prominent as the organism interacts with its environments. Thus with time, as the individual adapts to his or her environment, different personality styles will become differentially prominent and latent potentialities will be shaped into adaptive and manifest styles of perceiving, feeling, thinking and acting. It is these distinctive modes of adaptation, engendered by the interaction of biological endowment and social experience, that Millon (1991; 1994; 1996d) identifies as 'personality styles'.

In the South African context, we were only able to locate research on the MIPS-Revised and the MCMI-II and MCMI-III. Hence these instruments are focused on in this chapter.

The MIPS

The MIPS-Revised represents an extension of the Millon assessment tools into the measurement of 'normal' individuals. Millon attempts to combine the intrapsychic, cognitive and interpersonal spheres in his theory. However, Millon also acknowledges that an integrated approach needs to go beyond psychology if it is to be truly holistic. In keeping with this argument, he borrows from evolutionary biology to develop his theory. He identifies 24 different characteristics or 12 bipolar traits that can be grouped in numerous different ways to describe an individual's personality style. These 12 bipolar traits are organised into categories such that they represent motivational, cognitive and interpersonal characteristics. Millon's theory thus considers three motivational aims bipolarities, four cognitive modes bipolarities and five interpersonal behaviours bipolarities (see Figure 21.3). These bipolarities are assessed using the MIPS. The MIPS also includes two scales labelled Positive Impression and Negative Impression to measure the test-taking attitude of the examinee. A third Consistency scale establishes the consistency of responses across the questionnaire.

The utility of the MIPS was explored in the South African setting in a sample of 245 university students (Laher, 2001). According to Laher (2001), the descriptive statistics, norms and reliability coefficients obtained in the study were highly satisfactory, as well as comparable to the US norms. Comparable interscale correlations, together with a factor structure that factors into five factors consonant with the Five-Factor Model, were also found. Laher (2001) argued that while the findings of her study lent support to the cross-cultural applicability of the instrument, other evidence from the criterion, content and construct validity explorations indicated that there were differences in the expression of the factors across cultures, and that the factors presented by Millon were not exhaustive. There were other factors which Millon's model, by virtue of being located in a Eurocentric framework, did not take into account. In 2007, Laher published a paper on the Millon approach to personality and demonstrated that whilst the model was theoretically sound, it was not complete. It failed to take into account the environment and, more importantly, cultural differences in its understanding of personality. As such, its utility in a diverse South African culture is debatable (Laher, 2007).

The MCMI-III

The MCMI-III (1997) is a clinical tool, and the primary intent of this assessment inventory is to provide clinical information to professionals about a person's emotional and interpersonal difficulties (Millon, 2010). In the South African context the MCMI-III is employed frequently in both clinical and counselling settings (Foxcroft & Roodt, 2005). It is the only test in the Millon family of instruments that is widely used and researched in South Africa (Foxcroft, Paterson, Le Roux & Herbst, 2004). This instrument is therefore discussed in more detail here, and South African research on the instrument is presented.

Figure 21.3 Diagrammatic representation of Millon's theory of normal personality

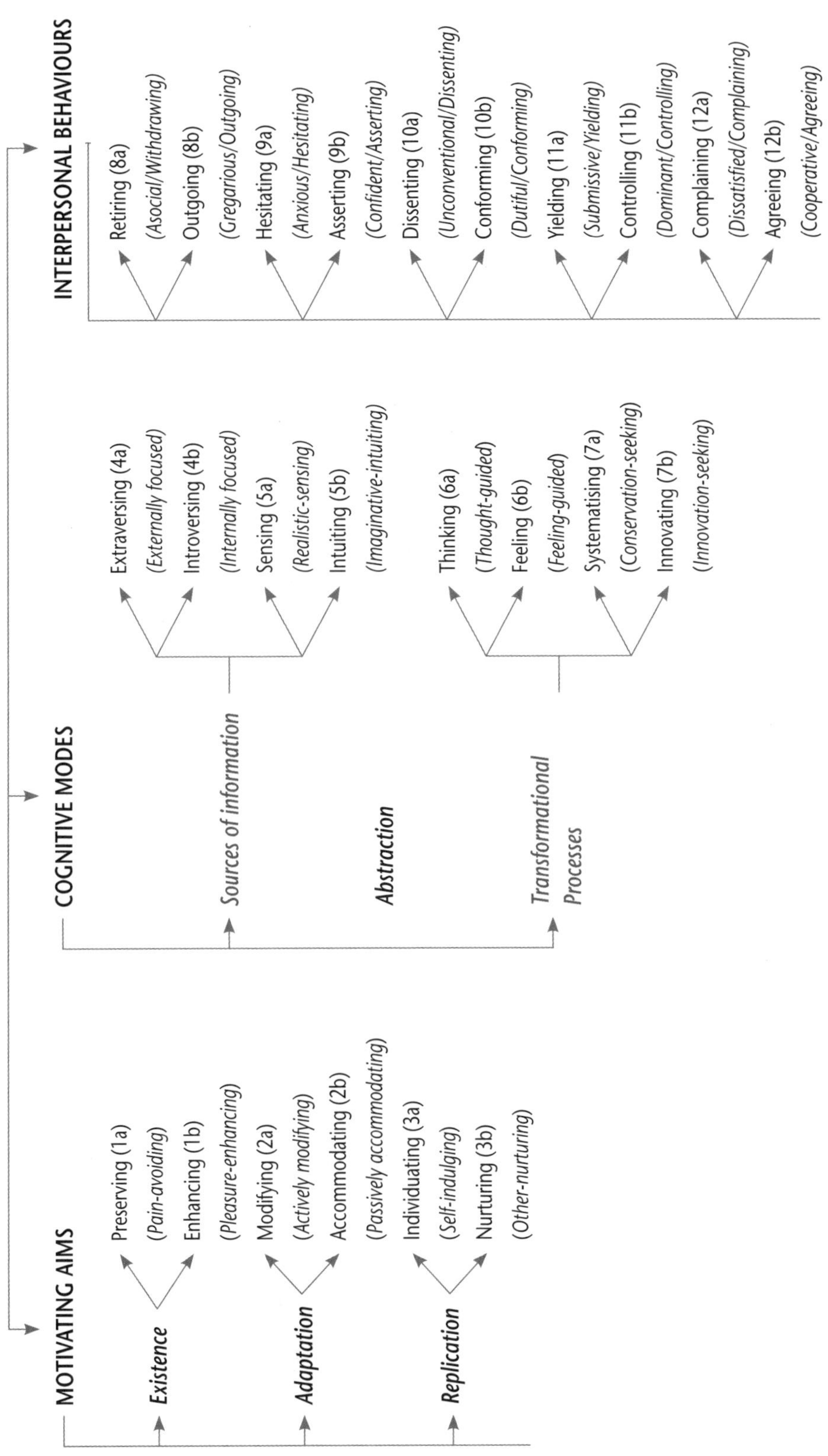

The MCMI-III is a self-report instrument designed to help the clinician assess Axis I disorders (clinical syndromes) and Axis II disorders (personality disorders) based on the DSM-IV-TR (APA, 2004) classification system. Published in 1994, the MCMI-III consists of 175 true-false items, and is appropriate for use on individuals who are 18 years and older and who have at least an eighth-grade reading level. It is used primarily in clinical and counselling settings with individuals who require mental health services for emotional, social or interpersonal difficulties. It can assist in diagnosis, and in developing a treatment plan that takes into account the patient's personality style and coping behaviour. It consists of 11 clinical personality pattern scales, 3 severe personality pathology scales, 7 clinical syndrome scales, 3 severe syndrome scales and 3 modifying indices, as described in Table 21.1.

Table 21.1 Structure of the MCMI-III

Clinical personality patterns	These scales assess the personality of an individual that cuts across the established personality prototypes and that demonstrates a different level of extremeness on any of the given personality patterns.
Schizoid	Individuals who are expressively impassive and interpersonally unengaged. They display a lifelong pattern of social withdrawal, feel uncomfortable with human interaction and are often seen as eccentric, isolated or lonely.
Avoidant	Individuals who are expressively fretful and interpersonally aversive. They are extremely sensitive to rejection that leads to social withdrawal. Although shy they have a strong desire for companionship.
Depressive	Individuals who are expressively disconsolate and interpersonally defenceless. They are characterised by lifelong traits that fall under the pessimistic, anhedonia, self-doubting and chronically unhappy spectrum.
Dependent	Individuals who are expressively incompetent and interpersonally submissive. These individuals subordinate their own needs to those of others. They lack self-confidence and may get others to assume responsibility for major areas of their lives.
Histrionic	Individuals who are expressively dramatic and interpersonally attention-seeking. They are excitable and emotional. They tend to behave in a dramatic and extraverted fashion, and have a high degree of attention-seeking behaviour.
Narcissistic	Individuals who are expressively haughty and interpersonally exploitative. They have a heightened sense of self-importance and feelings of grandiosity. These individuals often feel unique and special.
Antisocial	Individuals who are expressively impulsive and interpersonally irresponsible. They have an inability to conform to social norms of expected adult behaviour. These are individuals who show a reckless disregard for self and others.
Aggressive (sadistic)	Individuals who are expressively reckless, reactive and interpersonally abrasive and coercing. They are strongly opinionated, obstinate and closed-minded and are prone to a hostile mood.

Clinical personality patterns	**These scales assess the personality of an individual that cuts across the established personality prototypes and that demonstrates a different level of extremeness on any of the given personality patterns.**
Compulsive	Individuals who are expressively disciplined and interpersonally respectful. They exhibit unusual compliance with social conventions and can be over-conscientious. They will adhere to rigid hierarchies and can become upset by the unfamiliar.
Passive-Aggressive (Negativistic)	Individuals who are resentful and are characterised by covert obstructionism, procrastination, stubbornness and inefficiency. Such behaviour is the manifestation of passively expressed underlying aggression.
Self-defeating (masochistic)	Individuals who are expressively non-indulgent and interpersonally distant from those who are consistently supportive. They can be simultaneously anxiously apprehensive and, on the other hand, mournful and forlorn.
Severe personality pathology	**These scales determine how functional an individual is. An elevation on this scale represents a dysfunctional personality disorder.**
Schizotypal	Individuals who are peculiar in their mannerisms and are reticent with others. They use magical thinking as a consistent manner of defence and are haphazard and chaotic.
Borderline	Individuals who are dysfunctional, with abrupt shifts in behaviour and interpersonal relationships. These individuals lack an identity consolidation and are characterised by unstable and fluctuating moods that range from euphoria to profound despair.
Paranoid	Individuals who are characterised by long-standing suspiciousness and mistrust of others. They will assign their own feelings of hostility, anger and irritability to others.
Clinical syndromes	**These scales are an extension or distortion of the individual's basic personality pattern. They represent symptoms that can occur within any personality type. They are more transient over time and are psychometrically less stable than the personality traits.**
Anxiety	Relates to an individual's experience of tension, restlessness, possible phobic responses, some physiological symptoms of anxiety and worry.
Somatoform	Relates to complaints of fatigue, pains, aches and strange sensory experiences.
Bipolar-Manic	Degree to which the individual reports elation, overactivity, impulsiveness, flight of ideas and rapid shift in moods.
Dysthymia	Relates to feelings of guilt, dejection, futility, pessimism, problems with concentration and decreased interest in the interpersonal world.
Alcohol dependence	Detects the presence of alcohol use and dependence.
Drug dependence	Detects the presence of substance use and dependence.
Post-Traumatic Stress Disorder	Relates to the painful re-experiencing of a traumatic event, coupled with patterns of avoidance and emotional numbing. Also detects constant hyper-arousal in a person.

continued →

Severe syndromes	**These scales assess more severe symptomatic psychopathology.**
Thought Disorder	Represents symptoms of schizophrenia, schizophreniform disorder or brief reactive psychosis.
Major Depression	Assesses the presence of a profoundly debilitating depressive disorder.
Delusional Disorder	Identifies paranoid individuals with a psychotic level of symptomatic presentation. These individuals are likely to have systemised delusions.
Modifying indices	**These are scales that assess the validity of the MCMI-III profile.**
Desirability Scale	Determines the patient's inclination to be socially attractive.
Debasement Scale	Detects a tendency to devalue oneself by presenting more troublesome emotional problems.
Validity Scale	Includes three bizarre or highly improbable items to see if responses throughout are valid.

Psychometric properties

Millon's normative sample for the MCMI-III consisted of 998 males and females, including patients seen in independent practices, clinics, mental health centres, residential settings and hospitals. Since the norms are based on clinical samples, the instrument is not appropriate for use with nonclinical populations.

An important feature of the MCMI-III is its use of *base rate* scores for norms. Unlike other instruments which calculate norms based on the normal distribution, the MCMI-III uses the clinical prevalence rates in a particular population. Thus there is no assumption that a particular pathology is normally distributed in a population.

Both internal consistency and test-retest reliability are demonstrated in the MCMI-III. Internal consistency for the personality scales ranged from .66 to .90 (N = 398), with alphas exceeding .80 for 20 of the scales. Test-retest reliability coefficients ranged from .82 to .96 (Millon, 1997).

The MCMI-III appears to have good concurrent validity with a wide variety of other personality tests – namely, Beck's Depression Inventory, the General Behaviour Inventory, the Symptom Checklist 90 – Revised and the Minnesota Multiphasic Personality Inventory-2 (MMPI-2), as well as with the MCMI-II (Dyce, O'Connor, Parkins & Janzen, 1997; Millon, 1997). It was also found to correlate well with other tests – namely, the Michigan Alcoholism Screening Test, the Impact of Events Scale and the State-Trait Anxiety Inventory. Similar findings have been reported between the MCMI and the more narrowly bound instruments, including the Profile of Mood States, the General Health Questionnaire and the Interpersonal Checklist (Millon, 1997).

Cultural considerations

The MCMI-III is frequently employed within the South African clinical setting. As such, it is important that its cross-cultural utility be explored within this context in both South African and non-Western cultures.

A Dutch study of 263 inpatient substance abusers looked at establishing cross-cultural equivalence in the MMPI as well as the MCMI-III (Egger, De Mey, Derksen & Van der Staat, 2003). The aim was to establish cross-cultural equivalence across both instruments and per instrument. Egger et al. (2003) found cross-cultural similarities in a component-by-component comparison between the MMPI and the MCMI-III. However, the findings also suggest that the MCMI-III itself showed a limited degree of cross-cultural similarity, leading the researchers to argue that the influence of translation as well as cultural differences cannot be overlooked when using the MCMI-III. On the other hand, a Chinese study that examined the MCMI-III profile of 107 substance abusers at a psychiatric institution in Hong Kong found good predictive validity between the MCMI-III scales and Axis I and Axis II pathologies. This study used the Chinese version of the MCMI-III that had been back-translated into English to account for reduced influence of translation on the outcome of the study (So, 2005).

Benjamin (2006) used the MCMI-II in a study on compliance with chemotherapy in a sample of 134 oncology patients at the Johannesburg General Hospital in South Africa. Significant differences were found between compliant and non-compliant patients on the Disclosure, Debasement, Avoidance, Passive-Aggressive, Self-defeating, Schizotypal, Anxiety, Dysthymia, Alcohol Dependence and Major Depression scales. The most important predictors of non-compliance were the Debasement and Schizotypal scales. Hence these were used to successfully develop a treatment intervention model that improved non-compliance: the Medical Trauma Debriefing Model. One of the features of the MCMI-III is the inclusion of a Post-Traumatic Stress scale. It would be interesting for further research to explore compliance using the model developed, together with the MCMI-III.

As part of a broader South African National Defence Force (SANDF) initiative, Naggan (2001) undertook research in an attempt to screen military personnel and to standardise the MCMI-III for the South African population. This study was conducted on 5 707 members of the SANDF who were based outside South Africa. This sample was representative of race and gender within the military context, and ranged in age from 18 to 65 years. Results found good criterion validity for the Dependent, Schizotypal, Borderline, Paranoid and Compulsive Personality scales, and, to a lesser extent, for the Antisocial and Narcissistic personality scales (Naggan, 2001).

Good criterion and predictive validity was also found in research done by Laher and Rebolo (2010), Tshabalala (2004) and Lloyd (2008). Laher and Rebolo's (2010) study on 23 patients, gender-representative and between the ages of 22 and 68, who had been diagnosed with Bipolar Disorder, showed good predictive outcomes on the Avoidant and Passive-Aggressive scales. A study on a diverse group of 20 African military and humanitarian personnel conducted over a 14-month period found that the Depressive, Narcissistic and Anxiety scales provided good negative indicators on the competency model of civil military officials (Lloyd, 2008). This means that the MCMI-III represented meaningful scales that correlated with the competencies that were required by the members of the civil military, thus demonstrating appropriate criterion validity (Lloyd, 2008). Good predictive outcomes were also found between the personality dynamics of ten male sexual offenders on the clinical syndrome scales as well as on the personality pathology scale (Tshabalala, 2004).

However, despite these findings across the various cross-cultural studies, there are at least four aspects of the MCMI-III that need to be highlighted where culture can affect psychological disorders. The first relates to psychometrics, and considers issues of translation and, more broadly, language proficiency when using tests like the MCMI-III in a South African context. With translation, the first question would be which language the test would be translated into, since South Africa has 11 official languages. Furthermore, research on translation with other personality instruments – for example, the Sixteen Personality Factor Questionnaire (Van Eeden & Mantsha, 2007) and the NEO Personality Inventory (Horn, 2000) – has shown that problems exist with finding equivalent terms, or that there are difficulties with finding the same word in another language. For example, 'blue' and 'green' are expressed by the same word in isiXhosa. Alternatively, the meaning of a word may be different across languages. For example, 'feeling blue' in English means feeling sad, but an equivalent translation in Afrikaans, 'voel blou', means feeling tired. Further issues related to language are those of English proficiency in a country where English is the second language for most of the population. Of the 11 official languages, isiZulu is the most commonly spoken language (23.8 per cent), followed by isiXhosa (17.6 per cent), Afrikaans (13.3 per cent), Sepedi (9.4 per cent), Setswana and English (8.2 per cent), Sesotho (7.9 per cent), Xitsonga (4.4 per cent), Siswati (2.7 per cent), Tshivenda (2.3 per cent), isiNdebele (1.6 per cent) and other languages (0.5 per cent) (Statistics South Africa, 2001). Also related to language is the issue of using translators. Quite often in health-care settings, psychologists rely on nurses and other health professionals to assist with the administration of the MCMI-III, as the psychologist does not speak the language of the patient. This is done on an ad hoc basis, and from experience it is clear that the use of interpreters compromises standardisation and introduces a number of biases into the administration procedure.

Other issues of bias across various groupings also exist. This leads to the second concern, that of equivalence and the use of self-report inventories in cultures other than those in which the instruments were developed and normed. Van de Vijver and Tanzer (1997) argue that it cannot be taken for granted that scores that are obtained in one culture can be compared across cultural groups. Some cultures can be considered similar – for example, the US culture can be seen to be similar to European cultures – but one cannot make the same argument when comparing Western cultures to a country like China (Van de Vijver & Tanzer, 1997). For example, a base rate score on the Narcissistic Personality Disorder may be significantly higher in some cultures that value independence and self-directed behaviour (Rossi, Sloore & Derksen, 2008). Similarly, a study that looked at the differences between US and Korean students differed on 7 of the 11 MCMI-III scales. Korean participants scored significantly higher than their US counterparts on the Dependent scale, reflecting more passive personality orientations, whilst scoring much lower on the Histrionic scale (Gunsalus & Kelly, 2001). The use of base rate scores, whilst useful in the population on which the MCMI-III was normed, is a limitation in all other groups since it cannot be assumed that the prevalence of a particular disorder is the same in every group. As correctly pointed out by a reviewer of this chapter, accurate diagnosis rests upon accurate estimates of base rates. Thus there is a need to develop local base rates, rather than assuming that prevalence rates are comparable in the South African context.

Similar consideration needs to given to demographic variables of race and gender. Scores obtained on the MCMI-III between black and white psychiatric inpatients indicated a difference in predicting psychopathology between the two races (Choca, Stanley, Peterson & Van Denburg, 1990). Lindsay and Widiger (1995) argued that one has to consider that results may be more a prediction of the respondent's gender than of personality dysfunction. In data summarised from six studies, Craig (1999) found that African-Americans consistently scored higher on the Narcissistic, Antisocial, Paranoid, Drug Dependence and Delusional Disorder scales, while Caucasian Americans scored higher on the Dysthymia scale. Furthermore, men scored higher on the Antisocial scale, whilst women scored higher on the Somatoform and Major Depression scales.

Thirdly, the way clients express or explain their problems may differ across cultures (Cheung, 2009; Craig, 2005). For many, mental illness is regarded as a test from God and something that the family and community deal with (Laher & Khan, 2011). Asian individuals tend to somaticise their symptoms more than Western individuals (Cheung, 2009). However, Cheung (2009) alerts one to the bias prevalent in Western models which discuss this tendency to somaticise psychological symptoms as pathological and characteristic of Asian cultures. She reframes it within a different taxonomy of mental illness, where somaticisation is normal and is linked to personality features that emphasise harmony and traditionalism. Cheung (2009, p.46) argues that somaticisation needs to be reconceptualised 'as a metaphor of distress in the cultural context of an illness experience with implications to social relationships, coping and help-seeking behavior'.

Finally, what is considered to be a psychological problem can also differ between cultures (Swartz, 2002). Meyer, Moore and Viljoen (2003) cite the example of schizophrenia, which is commonly misdiagnosed in African individuals. The African belief system advocates communication with ancestors as well as the belief in spiritual illnesses linked to bewitchment. Western practitioners misdiagnose these as paranoid delusions and auditory hallucinations, leading to a misdiagnosis of schizophrenia (Meyer et al., 2003). Ally and Laher (2008) discuss how the conceptualisation of the person and the illness (medical, psychological and spiritual) differ from Western models, which are rooted in Cartesian dualism and fail to take into account a deeper, more essential layer of the person related to the spiritual essence, and how this links to medical and psychological illness.

Both Cheung (2009) and Ally and Laher (2008) argue for the need to move away from the traditional philosophy of Cartesian dualism that underlies current epistemologies of psychopathology, and advocate the consideration of other philosophies. Both studies concur that while current models are useful, and while instruments like the MCMI-III provide useful information, they are limited when used in non-Western contexts. What is also common across both articles is the emphasis on the role of community and context in the understanding, aetiology and treatment of psychological illness, and further research in this regard is warranted.

Conclusion

The MCMI-III is a psychological assessment tool that has been derived from comprehensive theory, and it has been coordinated with the format of the DSM. It enhances diagnostic efficiency by taking the base rates of the disorders that it measures into account. The MCMI-III is also very easy to administer and to interpret, allowing the clinical practitioner to use it as part of a comprehensive assessment strategy (Craig, 1999).

Based on clinical experience, a reviewer for this chapter highlighted the fact that the MCMI-III's brevity and the instrument's correspondence with official diagnostic constructs of the DSM-IV-TR (APA, 2004) mean that it is extremely useful in formulating and communicating diagnoses and treatment plans in a multidisciplinary team setting. It is also useful in looking at the interplay between Axis I and Axis II, as well as the relationship between personality characteristics and clinical syndromes. Furthermore, the MCMI-III has been found to be very useful in that it is quick and simple to administer to patients who are distractible and who tire easily.

On the other hand, responses to the MCMI-III questionnaire are true/false, and this make the test susceptible to acquiescent response sets (Craig, 1999). It also appears to be less effective in assessing individuals with minor personality pathology, and those with very severe dysfunction such as the psychotic disorders (Craig, 1999). There may also be subtypes of different personality disorders, but assessment of these subtypes has not been incorporated into the MCMI-III (Craig, 1999). However, there is a move towards this with the Grossman Facet Subscales (Millon, 2010).

Finally, even though the MCMI-III remains a well-researched instrument, its wide use within the South African clinical and counselling context warrants that a culturally responsive approach must be very seriously considered in its application (Cheung, 2009; Cheung, Van de Vijver & Leong, 2011). Cultural differences can be relative, and may not necessarily describe levels of personality pathology; overlooking the rich diversity inherent in the South African population can mean a misdiagnosis of pathology in individuals (Meyer et al., 2003). Furthermore, ignoring the role of the community and context in the understanding, aetiology and treatment of psychological illness will further limit the use of the MCMI-III (Ally & Laher, 2008; Cheung, 2009). A universal model like the MCMI-III must be applied with caution across cultures.

Notes

1 According to DSM-IV multiaxial diagnosis (APA, 2004).

2 According to DSM-IV multiaxial diagnosis (APA, 2004).

References

Ally, Y. & Laher, S. (2008). South African Muslim faith healers' perceptions of mental illness: Understanding, aetiology and treatment. *Journal of Religion and Health, 47,* 45–56.

APA (American Psychiatric Association) (2004). *Diagnostic and Statistical Manual of Mental Disorders* (4th edition). Washington, DC: American Psychiatric Association.

Benjamin, R. V. N. (2006). Non-compliance with chemotherapy in the oncology patient with a good prognosis. Unpublished PhD dissertation. University of the Witwatersrand, Johannesburg.

Cheung, F. M. (2009). The cultural perspective in personality assessment. In J. N. Butcher (Ed.), *Oxford Handbook of Personality Assessment* (pp. 44–56). London: Oxford University Press.

Cheung, F. M., Van de Vijver, F. J. R. & Leong, F. T. L. (2011). Toward a new approach to the study of personality in culture. *American Psychologist*. Advance online publication. January 24. doi: 10.1037/a0022389.

Choca, J. P. (1998). The Millon Index of Personality Styles. In J. C. Impara & B. S. Plake (Eds), *Thirteenth Mental Measurements Yearbook*. Lincoln, NE: Buros Institute of Mental Measurements.

Choca, J. P, Stanley, L. A., Peterson, C. A. & Van Denburg, E. (1990). Racial bias and the MCMI. *Journal of Personality Assessment, 54*, 479–490.

Craig, R. J. (1999). Overview and current status of the Millon Clinical Multiaxial Inventory. *Journal of Personality Assessment, 72*, 390–406.

Craig, R. J. (2005). *New Directions in Interpreting the MCMI-III*. Hoboken, NJ: John Wiley & Sons.

Dyce, J. A., O'Connor, B. P., Parkins, S. Y. & Janzen, H. L. (1997). Correlational structure of the MCMI-III personality disorder scales and comparison with other data. *Journal of Personality Assessment, 69*, 568–582.

Egger, J., De Mey, H., Derksen, J. & Van der Staat, C. (2003). MMPI-2 and MCMI-III scores among Dutch inpatient substance abusers: Assessing corresponding and cross-cultural equivalence. *Current Psychology: Developmental, Learning, Personality, Social, 22*, 117–124.

Foxcroft, C., Paterson, H., Le Roux, N. & Herbst, D. (2004). *Psychological Assessment in South Africa: A Needs Analysis. The Test Use Patterns and Needs of Psychological Assessment Practitioners*. Pretoria: Human Sciences Research Council.

Foxcroft, C. & Roodt, G. (2005). An *Introduction to Psychological Assessment in the South African Context* (2nd edition). Cape Town: Oxford University Press.

Gunsalus, A. J. C. & Kelly, K. R. (2001). Korean cultural influences on the Millon Clinical Multiaxial Inventory III. *Journal of Mental Health Counseling, 23*, 151–161.

Horn, B. S. (2000). A Xhosa translation of the revised NEO Personality Inventory: A pilot study. Unpublished Master's dissertation. University of Port Elizabeth, Port Elizabeth.

Laher, S. (2001). Exploring the utility of the MIPS in the South African context. Unpublished Master's dissertation. University of the Witwatersrand, Johannesburg.

Laher, S. (2007). Personality reconceptualised: A Millonian approach? *South African Journal of Psychology, 37*, 82–95.

Laher, S. & Khan, S. (2011). Exploring the influence of Islam on the perceptions of mental illness of volunteers in a Johannesburg community-based organization. *Psychology in Developing Societies, 23*, 63–84.

Laher, S. & Rebolo, C. (2010). Personality styles of patients with bipolar disorder: An exploratory study. *South African Journal of Psychology, 40*, 159–164.

Lindsay, K.A. & Widiger, T. (1995). Sex and gender bias in self-report personality disorder inventories: Item analysis of the MCMI-II, MMPI, and PDQ-R. *Journal of Personality Assessment, 65*, 1–20.

Lloyd, G. (2008). An exploratory study for the psychological profile of a civil military coordination officer as a selection tool for training. Unpublished Master's dissertation. University of Stellenbosch, Stellenbosch.

Meyer, W., Moore, C. & Viljoen, H. (2003). *Personology: From Individual to Ecosystem.* Johannesburg: Heinemann.

Millon, T. (1969). *Modern Psychopathology*. Philadelphia, PA: Saunders.

Millon, T. (1990). *Toward a New Personology: An Evolutionary Model.* New York, NY: John Wiley & Sons.

Millon, T. (1991). Normality: What may we learn from evolutionary theory? In D. Offer & M. Sabshin (Eds), *The Diversity of Normal Behaviour* (pp. 356–404). New York, NY: Basic Books.

Millon, T. (1994). *Millon Index of Personality Styles Manual.* Orlando, FL: Psychological Corporation.

Millon, T. (1996a). Personality disorders: Conceptual distinctions and classification issues. In T. Millon (Ed.), *Personality and Psychopathology: Building a Clinical Science* (pp. 11–38). New York, NY: John Wiley & Sons.

Millon, T. (1996b). Contemporary theoretical models. In T. Millon, (Ed.), *Personality and Psychopathology: Building a Clinical Science* (pp. 39–58). New York, NY: John Wiley & Sons.

Millon, T. (1996c). An integrative theory of personality and psychopathology. In T. Millon, (Ed.), *Personality and Psychopathology: Building a Clinical Science* (pp. 59–70). New York, NY: John Wiley & Sons.

Millon, T. (1996d). Foundations of the MIPS scales. In T. Millon, (Ed.), *Personality and Psychopathology: Building a Clinical Science* (pp. 259–294). New York, NY: John Wiley & Sons.

Millon, T. (1997). *MCMI-III Manual* (2nd edition). Minneapolis, MN: National Computer Systems.

Millon, T. (2010). *Institute for Advanced Studies in Personality & Psychopathology.* Retrieved May 24, 2010, from http://www.millon/content/instrumentation.htm.

Naggan, N. (2001). An exploratory study into the relation between Post Traumatic Stress and Axis II personality traits as measured on the MCMI-III in military personnel. Unpublished Master's dissertation. University of Johannesburg, Johannesburg.

Rossi, G. M. P., Sloore, H. V. & Derksen, J. J. L. (2008). The adaptation of the MCMI-III in two non-English speaking countries: State of art of the Dutch language version. In T. Millon & C. Bloom (Eds), *The Millon Inventories: A Practitioner's Guide to Personalized Clinical Assessment* (pp. 360–383). New York, NY: The Guilford Press.

So, H. W. (2005). Substance abuse and psychiatric comorbidity: Millon Clinical Multiaxial Inventory – III profile of Chinese substance abusers. *Hong Kong Journal of Psychiatry, 15*, 89–96.

Statistics South Africa (2001). *Census 2001.* Retrieved May 21, 2010, from http://www.statsa.gov.za/publications/populationstats.asp.

Swartz, L. (2002). *Culture and Mental Health: A Southern African View.* Cape Town: Oxford University Press.

Tshabalala, P. R. (2004). Personality dynamics of sexual offenders. Unpublished Master's dissertation. University of Zululand, KwaDlangezwa.

Van de Vijver, F. J. R. & Tanzer, N. K. (1997). Bias and equivalence in cross-cultural assessments: An overview. *European Review of Applied Psychology, 46*, 263–279.

Van Eeden, R. & Mantsha, T. (2007). Theoretical and methodological considerations in the translation of the 16PF5 into an African language. *South African Journal of Psychology, 37*, 62–81.

22 Assessment and monitoring of symptoms in the treatment of psychological problems

C. Young and D. Edwards

Although the clinical interview is the foundation of assessment for individuals presenting with psychological problems (Edwards & Young, chapter 23, this volume), information from self-report scales provides valuable complementary information. Many self-report scales developed in North America and Britain are used regularly in South Africa with clients from a spectrum of cultural backgrounds. Some have been translated into South African languages, while others may be translated on the spot by the clinician or an assistant during the assessment process. Yet translation of scales, or importing them into cultural contexts different from those in which they were developed and validated, poses a number of problems that may be sufficient to throw doubt on their validity. There has been limited research on this in South Africa, and this chapter will examine the problems involved and the conclusions that can be drawn from existing research with respect to the value in local clinical settings of self-report scales developed overseas.

The role of self-report scales in clinical assessment

Self-report scales can be used in a number of ways during the initial assessment of a case, and as part of the ongoing assessment that continues throughout treatment and even afterwards. Their main applications will be examined in this section.

Determining presence and severity of a clinical problem

A wide variety of specialised scales that tap the specific cognitive, emotional and behavioural aspects of common clinical problems have been used in South Africa, both clinically and in research studies. These include, for example, the Beck Anxiety Inventory (BAI) for anxiety and panic (Beck & Steer, 1993), the Beck Depression Inventory-II (BDI-II) for depression (Beck, Steer & Brown, 1996), and the Post-traumatic Diagnostic Scale (PDS) for post-traumatic stress disorder (PTSD) (Foa, Cashman, Jaycox & Perry, 1997). Scales like these are usually validated in the USA or the UK. On the basis of normative data from these validation studies, cut-off points are determined which act as a guide to clinicians as to whether the symptoms are within the normal range, or whether they point to a mild, moderate or severe degree of clinical concern. While the cut-offs obtained from such normative data are likely to be appropriate in South African contexts where clients are similar socio-economically, educationally and culturally to the normative samples, they may not be valid at all with other groups, especially if the scales are used in translation. This problem will be discussed later in this chapter with specific reference to local research on translations of the BAI, BDI-II and Beck Hopelessness Scale (BHS), and on the application of the Clinical Outcomes in Routine Evaluation – Outcome Measure (CORE-OM) at a university counselling centre.

Using scales as a source of qualitative information

Clinical self-report scales can provide valuable qualitative information, such that their use is not confined to deriving scale scores and interpreting them against normative data. Many self-report scales are checklists. For example, the Adult Psychological Symptoms Checklist (Gilbert, Allan, Nicholls & Olsen, 2005) is a list of common symptoms. Such scales can be used to provide clinicians with information about a range of characteristics or symptoms which might not emerge from a clinical interview. Information from a scale may therefore serve as a useful point for further enquiry. For example, when respondents check the BDI-II item 'I feel guilty much of the time' or the BAI item 'Fear of the worst happening' or the CORE-OM item 'I have been disturbed by unwanted thoughts and feelings', clinicians can ask such questions as 'You checked this item – can you tell me the kinds of things you feel guilty about? ... Can you tell me when you feel this and what it is that you are afraid will happen? ... Can you tell me about the thoughts that have been troubling you?'

Information from self-report scales may also be useful for diagnosis, especially where scales are designed to provide a systematic check of diagnostic criteria for specific disorders. For example, the Symptom Checklist-90 (SCL-90) (Derogatis, 1983) covers a large number of symptoms relevant to the diagnosis of a range of disorders; the BDI-II (Beck et al., 1996) covers the DSM-IV criteria for major depressive disorder; and the PDS (Foa et al., 1997) covers the DSM-IV criteria for PTSD. A diagnosis should never be made solely on the basis of responses to self-report scales, but such scales can help clinicians identify symptoms relevant to specific diagnostic categories and provide information about symptoms that can be followed up by further questioning.

Furthermore, information from self-report scales can contribute towards the ultimate purpose of a clinical assessment, which is to develop a case formulation as a basis for treatment planning (see Edwards and Young, chapter 23, this volume). The kind of detailed information about cognitions, emotions and behaviours that can be provided by carefully chosen self-report scales can make a major contribution here.

Using self-report scales for monitoring response to intervention

Another important role for self-report scales is in monitoring response to treatment. Clinicians should ensure that the measures they choose cover the domains of change that are relevant, since appropriate response to treatment varies with the needs of particular clients. Sometimes the focus is on reduction of psychological symptoms, at other times it needs to be on improving life functioning, while at others, improving well-being is the goal. In many cases changes in all three domains are important (Howard, Lueger, Maling & Martinovich, 1993). By administering the scales at regular intervals throughout the therapy process, clinicians can track progress and, if necessary, adjust their interventions in response to the measurements. For example, if, near the end of therapy, a client's CORE-OM scores suggest improved well-being and symptoms but without any corresponding improvement in life functioning, the therapist might decide to direct future interventions at moving the client towards reclaiming the quality of life that preceded the current distress. Similarly, when there is evidence of problems with well-being, clinicians should consider directing attention to the therapeutic alliance and other efforts to remoralise the client. Scales for monitoring outcome should be carefully chosen to tap the specific symptoms that are causing distress and that led the client to seek treatment. When carefully selected and regularly administered, such scales provide clinicians with ongoing feedback about the effectiveness (or lack of effectiveness) of their intervention strategies. When used for this purpose, there is no need for normative data against which clients' scores are compared; clinicians can simply attend to how the total score or individual item scores change from one measurement to the next. Such feedback has been shown to improve clinical outcomes and speed up response to treatment (Lambert, Whipple, Smart, Vermeersch, Nielsen & Hawkins, 2001).

Assessing clinical significance of change

Where scales are locally validated and normed, clinicians can also determine the extent to which the change in score before and after therapy is clinically meaningful. Assessing clinical significance goes beyond statistical significance, and is concerned with the question of whether the change reflected on outcome measures corresponds with a genuine, practical impact on the life of the client. Various statistical methods have been proposed to measure the clinical significance of change in response to psychotherapy interventions, but classifications based on the different methods are surprisingly similar (Atkins, Bedics, McGlinchey & Beauchaine, 2005). The most widely used method, developed by Jacobson and Truax (1991), requires an outcome measure for which there are appropriate normative data, and two scores, one pre- and one post-intervention. This information allows for the calculation of two indices. The first is *reliable change*, and refers to the minimum size of the difference between pre- and post-intervention scores that can be considered not to be the result of measurement error. Clients can be said to show reliable improvement (or reliable deterioration) if the difference in their outcome measure scores before and after therapy is greater than the reliable change index calculated for that particular measure. The second is *clinical significance*, and is usually thought of as a change in score from above to below the clinical cut-off point. In other words, clinically significant change is obtained when the pre-therapy score is representative of the dysfunctional range of scores and the post-intervention score better representative of the functional range of scores. Therapists should, therefore, aim to achieve change that is both reliable and clinically significant.

The proportions of clients who achieve this can be used as benchmarks to compare different services or to track outcomes within any particular service from one year to the next. In South Africa, however, there are few scales with local norms, and this restricts the use of this approach.

Research evidence

There are three kinds of study which provide evidence for the value of specific self-report scales for clinical assessment in South African settings. In the first, the applicability of a scale in a South African setting is examined systematically in a research programme which investigates the scale's reliability and validity. In some studies, the scale is translated into a local language and the psychometric properties of the translated scale are evaluated. In the second, self-report scales which are of clinical value are used in epidemiological research whose aim is to determine the prevalence of specific kinds of clinical symptoms or clinical problems within various populations. These studies may also use group comparisons to test specific hypotheses about the relationship between different levels of prevalence and various psychological, socio-economic and cultural variables. The studies may provide information about the reliability and validity of the scales, although this may not be the main aim of the research. The third kind of study is the systematic clinical case study which provides an in-depth account of the process of assessment, treatment and outcome evaluation of a clinical case, since such studies often include self-report scales in the data. Examples of each of these kinds of research will be examined in the following sections.

Research on the Beck scales

The first kind of study is illustrated by Steele and Edwards's (2008a; 2008b; Edwards & Steele, 2008) research on developing and evaluating translations into isiXhosa of the BDI-II (Beck et al., 1996), the BAI (Beck & Steer, 1993) and the BHS (Beck & Steer, 1988). First, they showed that the translation process is not straightforward and that it is often more difficult than might be expected to find words and phrases that are equivalent to those in the original version of a scale. Even using the standard procedure of back-translation, they found considerable disagreement among translators about how particular items should be rendered. One contributing factor was that there were different local dialects of isiXhosa, and, in particular, differences between town isiXhosa and 'deep' isiXhosa spoken in traditional rural areas. However, even between towns and cities such as Grahamstown, Port Elizabeth and Cape Town there were differences in idiomatic expression. Another factor was that there was often no clear equivalence between isiXhosa and English words or phrases that referred to psychological or somatic states. As a consequence of these kinds of problems, translations of scales used in social and clinical research have tended to have poorer psychometric characteristics than the originals (Edwards & Leger, 1995; Edwards & Riordan, 1994). In order to resolve these problems, Steele and Edwards (2008a) identified a number of words and phrases that were problematic, consulted dictionary definitions and discussed meanings with informants. Only after considerable detailed work of this kind were translations of the three scales achieved that could be used in clinical settings. These isiXhosa translations are referred to as the XBDI-II, XBAI and XBHS respectively.

Cultural relativists argue that culture shapes the underlying experience of psychological distress to such an extent that depression or anxiety as defined in Western contexts may not be meaningful categories in non-Western cultures. By contrast, a universalist position holds that although culture shapes the meaning given to experience, there are common patterns of experience of distress that are independent of culture. In their validation studies of the isiXhosa versions of the Beck scales, Steele and Edwards found evidence for a universalist position with respect to depression, anxiety and hopelessness. First of all, even though considerable work was needed to find phrases in isiXhosa equivalent to those in the three Beck inventories, the finalised translations were clearly understandable to isiXhosa speakers, did convey meanings with a high degree of equivalence to the original English, and were highly acceptable to isiXhosa-speaking clients and clinicians. Second, the psychometric properties of the translated scales, which were administered to a mixed group of isiXhosa speakers that ranged from students to patients at a psychiatric hospital, were comparable to those obtained with the English versions in the validation studies in the USA (Steele & Edwards, 2008b). Alpha coefficients of .92 (XBAI) and .93 (XBDI-II) and a Kuder-Richardson (KR-20) of .89 (XBHS) are exceptionally high, as it is not uncommon for scales used with other cultural groups to have lower alphas than in the original validation studies, whether in the original language (Muris, Loxton, Neumann, Du Plessis, King & Ollendick, 2006; Taylor & Booyens, 1991) or in translation (Edwards & Leger, 1995; Edwards & Riordan, 1994). Item-total correlations also compared favourably with those from the original validation studies, as did correlations between total scores on each of the three scales. In a study of concurrent validity, groups of patients who had been identified by clinicians as being either depressed, anxious or neither depressed nor anxious completed the scales. As predicted, XBDI scores were markedly higher in the depressed patients than in the group who were neither anxious nor depressed, and XBAI scores were higher in the anxious patients than in the group who were neither anxious nor depressed (Edwards & Steele, 2008).

Research on the CORE-OM

Another example of the first research strategy is Young's (2009) research on CORE-OM developed in Britain. He studied clients at a South African university counselling centre, a setting in which there may be less need for translation of English-language scales because clients have a reasonable fluency in English. The CORE-OM was designed to offer a single instrument that would be used by therapists from a range of therapeutic orientations across research and clinical settings to assess the severity of psychological distress and to measure psychotherapy outcomes (Barkham et al. 1998; Evans et al., 2000). It is based on the phase model of psychotherapy outcomes, in terms of which clients typically first show an improved sense of *well-being*, then a reduction in *symptoms*, followed finally by an increase in *life functioning* (Howard et al., 1993). Whether or not all clients follow this sequence of improvement, all three phases clearly represent important domains of psychotherapy change, and measures that focus predominantly on symptoms might miss the other aspects of clients' lives. The CORE-OM also taps the extent to which clients are at risk of harming themselves or others. This is a fourth domain that is critical to examine in a clinical assessment (see Edwards and Young, chapter 23, this volume). Thus the CORE-OM provides clinicians with a rapid quantification of current well-being, symptom severity, life functioning and risk. In Britain, normative data with clinical cut-offs provide a basis for determining whether a client's score indicates a clinically significant problem.

Young (2009) collected South African data at a university counselling centre where all applicants for services completed the CORE-OM. When these responses were compared with similar data from 11 British university counselling services (Connell, Barkham & Mellor-Clark, 2007), there were no statistical differences between the means of the South African and British data on any of the four domains. Thus, despite the very different contexts, the symptom profiles of South African students and British students seeking counselling were similar. However, within the South African data set, there were interesting differences between black and white clients. Black clients reported significantly greater levels of distress than whites, and had higher risk scores. Furthermore, while the proportions of black and white clients scoring above the clinical cut-off points were similar, black clients were much more likely to score above the cut-off point that indicated severe distress. These results probably reflect real differences between black and white students at a university which is historically white. The inequalities entrenched during the apartheid era have to a large extent persisted, so that black students differ from their white counterparts in having poorer financial resources, social capital and educational preparation (Boughey, 2003; Makgato, 2007; Msila, 2005). Furthermore, historically white campuses are experienced as alienating not only by many black students but also by black lecturers (Gwele, 2002; Makgoba, 1997; Potgieter, 2002). It is hypothesised that these factors are the sources of differences between black and white students with respect to psychological distress. Given the similarity of responses of South African and British students at university counselling centres, the British normative data can be used for evaluating the nature and clinical severity of problems in individual cases. The CORE-OM can therefore offer South African clinicians useful and valid information in contexts where translation into other languages is not needed.

Epidemiological and group comparison research

The work of Muris et al. (2006) provides an example of the second kind of research: an epidemiological study designed to assess the prevalence of psychopathology in specific populations. Black, coloured and white children at primary schools around Stellenbosch in the Western Cape completed the Screen for Child Anxiety and Related Emotional Disorders (SCARED), which 'taps symptoms of generalised anxiety disorder, separation anxiety disorder, social phobia, panic disorder, and school-related phobia' (p.884). The instrument was in English or Afrikaans, whichever was the language of education at the school. Cronbach's alpha for the combined sample was acceptable (.7), but it was lower (around .6) for black and coloured respondents taken separately. However, Muris et al. concluded that 'the SCARED can be used as a screen for DSM-defined anxiety symptoms in South African children and adolescents' (2006, p.893) but that extra caution is needed when using the scale with black and coloured youths. Some of the implications in a clinical situation of this lower level of reliability among the black and coloured sample will be examined later. These kinds of studies often include comparisons between groups that differ with respect to socio-economic status, culture or ethnicity, and may tap a range of variables in order to test hypotheses about the relationship between them. Several epidemiological studies have been conducted on PTSD, although not all of these provide psychometric data on the instruments used (Edwards, 2005).

Systematic case studies

There are many aspects of the science of everyday clinical practice which cannot be investigated by quantitative multivariate methodologies, and this has contributed to an ongoing rift between clinicians and researchers which has been a feature of clinical psychology for several decades. The systematic clinical case study is the research method that is closest to the clinical situation, but this has often been neglected. In a case study, the individual case is the unit of analysis, and qualitative data are used to construct an assessment and case formulation and a treatment narrative. Self-report scales are used in the initial assessment and to monitor the impact of treatment (Dattilio, Edwards & Fishman, 2010). Such studies document the application of self-report scales in practice under a range of South African conditions, and provide evidence for its practical value. Rachman (1958) provides an early example of a South African case study. Apart from the use of a self-report scale before and after treatment, evaluation of progress was largely qualitative, through the therapist regularly questioning the client about specific problems being addressed by the therapy (using sanitary pads, sexual intercourse with her partner, receiving injections in medical settings). By the end of treatment she was no longer experiencing anxiety with respect to any of these, and this was reflected in a large reduction in score on the self-report scale. This study illustrates the principle that when self-report scales are used for monitoring or evaluation of treatment effectiveness, they should be used in conjunction with data from a qualitative enquiry.

On the whole, however, there has been a dearth of such careful clinical case studies locally, although recently several have been published documenting treatment under South African conditions. Two case studies of black students in a group treatment for social phobia demonstrate the usefulness of the BDI-II and BAI in tracking progress, together with specialised scales that monitor thoughts, feelings and behaviours known to be associated with social phobia (Edwards, Henwood & Kannan, 2003; Edwards & Kannan, 2006). Similarly, in a series of case studies of the treatment of PTSD, the BDI-II and BAI have been useful when used in conjunction with specialised measures such as the PDS (Foa et al., 1997) and the Post-traumatic Cognitions Inventory (PTCI) (Foa, Ehlers, Clark, Tolin & Orsillo, 1999). For example, Payne and Edwards (2009) reported the treatment of Zanele, a 15-year-old isiXhosa-speaking township girl, who had been raped and suffered from PTSD and major depressive disorder. Although Zanele was not fluent in English, the English versions of the BDI-II, BAI, PDS and PTCI were employed and there was concordance between changes on these scales and what she reported to the clinician during sessions. On one occasion data from the PTCI alerted the clinician to a particular concern, and further enquiry led the client to disclose that she had contracted a sexually transmitted disease following the rape.

Other South African clinical case studies which provide evidence for the usefulness of specific self-report scales are those of Whitefield-Alexander and Edwards (2009), which employed the Connors Teachers Rating Scale (which is a widely used behaviour checklist), and those of Karpelowsky and Edwards (2005) and Boulind and Edwards (2008), which employed the BDI-II and BAI. The Inventory of Complicated Grief (ICG) (Prigerson et al., 1995) has also proven valuable in systematic case studies which have not yet been published.

These clinical case studies may be more thorough and systematic than much routine clinical practice, but they have the advantage of demonstrating the applicability of self-report scales to a wide range of clients from different cultural backgrounds. In these studies, clinicians track qualitative information by regularly interviewing the client as well as by observing client responses or receiving reports of responses to particular interventions. They therefore have valuable data against which to assess the usefulness of the self-report scales. In fact, one of the criticisms of the various statistical methods of assessing clinical significance is that the concept of clinical significance is not adequately evaluated against multiple external criteria (Kazdin, 1999). Detailed clinical case studies of clients who provide qualitative evidence that they have achieved worthwhile and genuine improvement, and that report pre- and post-therapy scores, can provide useful information to clinicians, especially when there are no local normative data to calculate reliable change indices and clinical cut-off scores.

Use of self-report scales in clinical assessment: basic principles

Taken together, the kinds of research reviewed above provide the basis for some basic guidelines with respect to the usefulness and trustworthiness of self-report scales in clinical assessment. Whether or not a scale has been validated for the kind of population from which specific clients come, it is important to pay attention to whether they understand the task of completing the self-report scale, as well as the content of individual items, especially when giving clients scales in their second language. Lower values of Cronbach's alpha found in Muris et al.'s (2006) black and coloured respondents, as discussed above, point to problems in this area. Another factor to bear in mind is that even with clients who are familiar with the language of the scale, there may be words or phrases in the scale that are unfamiliar. This is illustrated by Edwards and Moldan's (2004) research on the Bulimia Test (BULIT) (Smith & Thelen, 1984), a scale designed to tap eating-disordered thinking and behaviour. The study was conducted with male and female students at the same historically white university as that at which Young obtained his CORE-OM data. In addition to administering the scale to a sample of black and white students, Edwards and Moldan conducted qualitative interviews with some of the respondents. It was found that females generally had a good grasp of the meaning of specialised terms related to eating-disordered thoughts and behaviour, but black and white males were less familiar with this specialised discourse. Several were confused about the meaning of the term 'binge-eating' and some black males completely misunderstood terms such as 'laxatives', 'diuretics' and 'uncontrolled eating', and one did not know the meaning of 'pudding' or 'milk-shake'. There was evidence that

> ... the less respondents understood the items, the less seriously they were likely to take the task of completing the inventory, and the less reliable and valid would be the results. One of the high-scoring black males commented, 'I didn't understand most of the questions and the choices were bad [i.e. the alternatives provided did not apply to me]. I would say that sixty per cent of the stuff I answered was right. The others was [*sic*] because I didn't understand and I was choiceless [*sic*].' (Edwards & Moldan, 2004, p.198)

These findings show what it means to exercise the kind of caution recommended by Muris et al. (2006) when using scales whose psychometric properties for the population from which clients come are either unknown or known to be less robust than in the original validation studies. In quantitative group comparison research, especially with university students, researchers often assume that imported scales will be readily understood. For eating disorders, several self-report scales have been used in South African research that examined samples from different ethnic groups. Edwards, D'Agrela, Geach and Welman (2003) used the Eating Disorders Inventory (EDI) and the BULIT, which has since been replaced by the BULIT-R (Welch, Thomson & Hall, 1993). Wassenaar, Le Grange, Winship and Lachenicht (2000) also used the EDI, while Le Grange, Telch and Tibbs (1998) used the Bulimia Investigatory Test Edinburgh (BITE) and the Eating Attitudes Test (EAT). The EAT was also used by Senekal, Steyn, Mashego and Nel (2001). However, Edwards and Moldan's (2004) research shows the danger of assuming that because students are being educated in English there is no threat to validity from misunderstanding of items, and where scales are used for epidemiological or group comparison purposes there needs to be careful preliminary piloting to ensure that these kinds of problems do not occur (see, for example, Edwards and Leger, 1995).

The same problems are inevitably encountered in clinical settings. They are, of course, likely to be much more serious in clients who are not fluent in the language in which the scale is written, or are educationally disadvantaged. Clinicians should therefore be attentive to the quality of clients' engagement with the material. Where clients do not fully understand the task of completing a self-report scale and/or are not motivated to represent their experience accurately, the information obtained will be untrustworthy, even as a basis for qualitative analysis (Padmanabhanunni, personal communication, 2010). However, because clinical assessment is largely based on a process of qualitative data collection (see

Edwards and Young, chapter 23, this volume) clinicians can still use scales in a second language or in an informal translation, provided that they check for the kinds of problems discussed above and interpret scale scores in the context of other information. Where this is done, self-report scales for which there is no local validation data can be used as valuable sources of qualitative information, as illustrated by several of the clinical case studies cited above.

The validation of self-report scales is less important to the working clinician than it is in a research setting. Validation is important when a scale is used as a means of benchmarking the degree of distress or symptomatology against a normative sample. However, when tracking response to treatment, a comparison is made between the responses of the same client at different times. For such a comparison, reference to a normative sample is not necessary. Bilsbury and Richman (2002) argue that the best way to track therapy progress is to design a personalised scale in consultation with the client which reflects the kinds of changes the client wants to make as a result of treatment. This means that for a self-report scale to be of use clinically in specific South African contexts, it is not necessary for it to have been validated locally in the kind of study carried out by Steele and Edwards for the Beck scales.

Rather, the first step would be to evaluate a scale within a carefully conducted systematic case study, where the contribution of the scale can be evaluated qualitatively in terms of its capacity to elicit clinically useful information and the extent to which clinical progress is reflected in a decline in symptom scores, and/or improved well-being scores and life-functioning scores. Where this kind of evaluation provides evidence for the clinical usefulness of a scale, the scale can then serve a range of valuable functions including, as shown in this chapter, highlighting symptoms that are relevant for diagnosis and case formulation and treatment planning, and providing clinicians with ongoing feedback about the effectiveness of their intervention strategies, which allows therapeutic adjustments that ultimately benefit the client. The authors recommend that researchers use some of the suitable measures to compare different psychotherapies across different South African contexts, in the process of evaluating and adapting therapies to build our local knowledge of what works best for whom. Researchers and clinicians are encouraged to cooperate in writing systematic case studies which document the use of self-report scales in a range of contexts, and in which there is a focus on the qualitative evaluation of their usefulness and trustworthiness in practice. Given the paucity of relevant South African literature, this is a timely and important area of research.

References

Atkins, D. C., Bedics, J. D., McGlinchey, J. B. & Beauchaine, T. P. (2005). Assessing clinical significance: Does it matter which method we use? *Journal of Consulting and Clinical Psychology, 73*, 982–989.

Barkham, M., Evans, C., Margison, F., McGrath, G., Mellor-Clark, J., Milne, D. & Connell, J. (1998). The rationale for developing and implementing core outcome batteries for routine use in service settings and psychotherapy outcome research. *Journal of Mental Health, 7*, 21–35.

Beck, A. T. & Steer, R. A. (1988). *Manual for the Beck Hopelessness Scale*. San Antonio, TX: Psychological Corporation.

Beck, A. T. & Steer, R. A. (1993). *Manual for the Beck Anxiety Inventory*. San Antonio, TX: Psychological Corporation.

Beck, A. T., Steer, R. A. & Brown, G. K. (1996). *Manual for the Beck Depression Inventory-II*. San Antonio, TX: Psychological Corporation.

Bilsbury, C. D. & Richman, A. (2002). A staging approach to measuring patient-centred subjective outcomes. *Acta Psychiatrica Scandinavica (Supplementum no. 414), 106*, 1–40.

Boughey, C. (2003). From equity to efficiency: Access to higher education in South Africa. *Arts and Humanities in Higher Education, 2*, 65–71.

Boulind, M. & Edwards, D. (2008). The assessment and treatment of post-abortion syndrome: A systematic case-study from Southern Africa. *Journal of Psychology in Africa, 18*, 539–548.

Connell, J., Barkham, M. & Mellor-Clark, J. (2007). CORE-OM mental health norms of students attending university counselling services benchmarked against an age-matched primary care sample. *British Journal of Guidance and Counselling, 35*, 41–57.

Dattilio, F. M., Edwards, D. J. A. & Fishman, D. B. (2010). Case studies within a mixed methods paradigm: Towards a resolution of the alienation between researcher and practitioner in psychotherapy research. *Psychotherapy: Theory, Research, Practice & Training, 47*, 427–441.

Derogatis, L. R. (1983). *Administration, Scoring and Procedures Manual–II for the SCL-90-R*. Towson, MD: Clinical Psychometric Research.

Edwards, D. J. A. (2005). Post-traumatic stress disorder as a public health concern in South Africa. *Journal of Psychology in Africa, 15(2)*, 125–134.

Edwards, D. J. A., D'Agrela, A., Geach, M. & Welman, M. (2003). Eating disordered attitudes and behaviours in black and white females at high school and university in South Africa. *Journal of Psychology in Africa, 13(1)*, 16–33.

Edwards, D. J. A., Henwood, J. & Kannan, S. (2003). Cognitive therapy for social phobia: The human face of cognitive science. *Alternation, 10*, 122–150.

Edwards, D. & Kannan, S. (2006). Identifying and targeting idiosyncratic cognitive processes in group therapy for social phobia: The case of Vumile. *Pragmatic Case Studies in Psychotherapy, 2*, 1–30.

Edwards, D. J. A. & Leger, P. (1995). Psychometric properties of the Right Wing Authoritarianism scale in black and white South African students. *International Journal of Psychology, 30*, 47–68.

Edwards, D. J. A. & Moldan, S. (2004). Bulimic pathology in black students in South Africa: Some unexpected findings. *South African Journal of Psychology, 34(2)*, 191–205.

Edwards, D. J. A. & Riordan, S. (1994). Learned resourcefulness in black and white South African university students. *Journal of Social Psychology, 134*, 365–375.

Edwards, D. J. A. & Steele, G. I. (2008). Development and validation of the Xhosa translations of the Beck Inventories: 3. Concurrent and convergent validity. *Journal of Psychology in Africa, 18(2)*, 227–236.

Evans, C., Mellor-Clark, J., Margison, F., Barkham, M., Audin, K., Connell, J. et al. (2000). CORE: Clinical outcomes in routine evaluation. *Journal of Mental Health, 9*, 247–255.

Foa, E., Cashman, L., Jaycox, L. & Perry, K. (1997). The validation of a self-report measure of posttraumatic stress disorder: The Posttraumatic Diagnostic Scale. *Psychological Assessment, 9*, 445–451.

Foa, E. B., Ehlers, A., Clark, D. M., Tolin, D. F. & Orsillo, S. M. (1999). The Posttraumatic Cognitions Inventory (PTCI): Development and validation. *Psychological Assessment, 11*, 303–314.

Gilbert, P., Allan, S., Nicholls, W. & Olsen, K. (2005). The assessment of psychological symptoms of patients referred to community mental health teams: Distress, chronicity and life interference. *Clinical Psychology and Psychotherapy, 12*, 10–27.

Gwele, N. S. (2002). Racial relations in selected faculties in English-language historically white universities in South Africa. *Society in Transformation, 33*, 134–151.

Howard, K. I., Lueger, R. J., Maling, M. S. & Martinovich, Z. (1993). A phase model of psychotherapy outcome: Causal mediation of change. *Journal of Consulting and Clinical Psychology, 61*, 678–685.

Jacobson, N. S. & Truax, P. (1991). Clinical significance: A statistical approach to defining meaningful change in psychotherapy research. *Journal of Consulting and Clinical Psychology, 59*, 12–19.

Karpelowsky, B. & Edwards, D. (2005). Trauma, imagery, and the therapeutic relationship: Langu's story. *Journal of Psychology in Africa, 15*, 185–195.

Kazdin, A. E. (1999). The meanings and measurement of clinical significance. *Journal of Consulting and Clinical Psychology, 67*, 332–339.

Lambert, M. J., Whipple, J., Smart, D., Vermeersch, D., Nielsen, S. & Hawkins, E. (2001). The effects of providing therapists with feedback on patient progress during psychotherapy: Are outcomes enhanced? *Psychotherapy Research, 11*, 49–68.

Le Grange, D., Telch, C. F. & Tibbs, J. (1998). Eating attitudes and behaviors in 1435 South African Caucasian and non-Caucasian college students. *American Journal of Psychiatry, 155(2)*, 250–254.

Makgato, N. (2007). Factors associated with poor performance of learners in mathematics and physical science in secondary schools in Soshanguve, South Africa. *Africa Education Review, 4*, 89–103.

Makgoba, M. W. (1997). *Mokoko. The Makgoba Affair: A Reflection on Transformation.* Johannesburg: Vivlia.

Msila, V. (2005). The education exodus: The flight from township schools. *Africa Education Review, 2*, 173–188.

Muris, P., Loxton, H., Neumann, A., Du Plessis, M., King, N. & Ollendick, T. (2006). DSM-defined anxiety disorders symptoms in South African youths: Their assessment and relationship with perceived parental rearing behaviours. *Behaviour Research and Therapy, 44*, 883–896.

Payne, C. & Edwards, D. J. A. (2009). What services and supports are needed to enable trauma survivors to rebuild their lives? Implications of a systematic case study of cognitive therapy with a township adolescent girl with PTSD following rape. *Child Abuse Research in South Africa, 10*, 27–40.

Potgieter, C. (2002). *Black Academics on the Move: How Black South African Academics Account for Moving Between or Leaving the Academic Profession.* Pretoria: Council for Higher Education Transformation.

Prigerson, H. G., Maciejewski, P. K., Reynolds III, C. F., Bierhals, A. J., Newsom, J. T., Fasiczka, E. et al. (1995). Inventory of Complicated Grief: A scale to measure maladaptive symptoms of loss. *Psychiatry Research, 59*, 65–79.

Rachman, S. (1958). The treatment of anxiety and phobic reactions by systematic desensitization psychotherapy. *Journal of Abnormal and Social Psychology, 58(2)*, 259–263.

Senekal, M., Steyn, N. P., Mashego, T. & Nel, J. H. (2001). Evaluation of body shape, eating disorders and weight management related parameters in black female students of rural and urban origins. *South African Journal of Psychology, 31(1)*, 46–53.

Smith, M. C. & Thelen, M. H. (1984). Development and validation of a test for bulimia. *Journal of Consulting and Clinical Psychology, 52*, 863–872.

Steele, G.I. & Edwards, D. J. A. (2008a). Development and validation of the Xhosa translations of the Beck Inventories: 1. Challenges of the translation process. *Journal of Psychology in Africa, 18*, 207–216.

Steele, G. I. & Edwards, D. J. A. (2008b). Development and validation of the Xhosa translations of the Beck Inventories: 2. Item analysis and internal consistency. *Journal of Psychology in Africa, 18*, 217–226.

Taylor, T. R. & Booyens, J. C. A. (1991). The comparability of scores of blacks and whites on the South African Personality Questionnaire: An exploratory study. *South African Journal of Psychology, 21*, 1–11.

Wassenaar, D., Le Grange, D., Winship, J. & Lachenicht, L. (2000). The prevalence of eating disorder pathology in a cross-ethnic population of female students in South Africa. *European Eating Disorders Review, 8*, 225–236.

Welch, G., Thomson, L. & Hall, A. (1993). The BULIT-R: Its reliability and clinical validity as a screening tool for DSM-III-R bulimia nervosa in a female tertiary education population. *International Journal of Eating Disorders, 14(1)*, 85–105.

Whitefield-Alexander, V. & Edwards, D. J. A. (2009). A case of effective single-session treatment for attention deficit and learning problems in a routine clinical practice: The value of a transdiagnostic approach to case formulation. *Journal of Child and Adolescent Mental Health, 21*, 61–72.

Young, C. (2009). The CORE-OM intake norms of students attending a South African university counselling service: A comparison with UK counselling service data. *British Journal of Guidance and Counselling, 37*, 473–483.

23 Assessment in routine clinical and counselling settings

D. Edwards and C. Young

This chapter examines the principles of psychological assessment applied to clinical and counselling settings where clients typically seek help because they are in emotional distress, experiencing, for example, anxiety, depressed mood or chronic anger. Such problems may be related to a range of other problems such as experiences of trauma, relationship conflicts, social or work difficulties, or excessive attempts at self-control (as in some eating disorders or obsessive-compulsive problems), or to poor impulse control (for example, with respect to aggression, gambling, substance use). The main focus of this chapter is the initial gathering of information in these contexts. This is called an intake assessment.

Figure 23.1 The phases in the process of intake and ongoing assessment

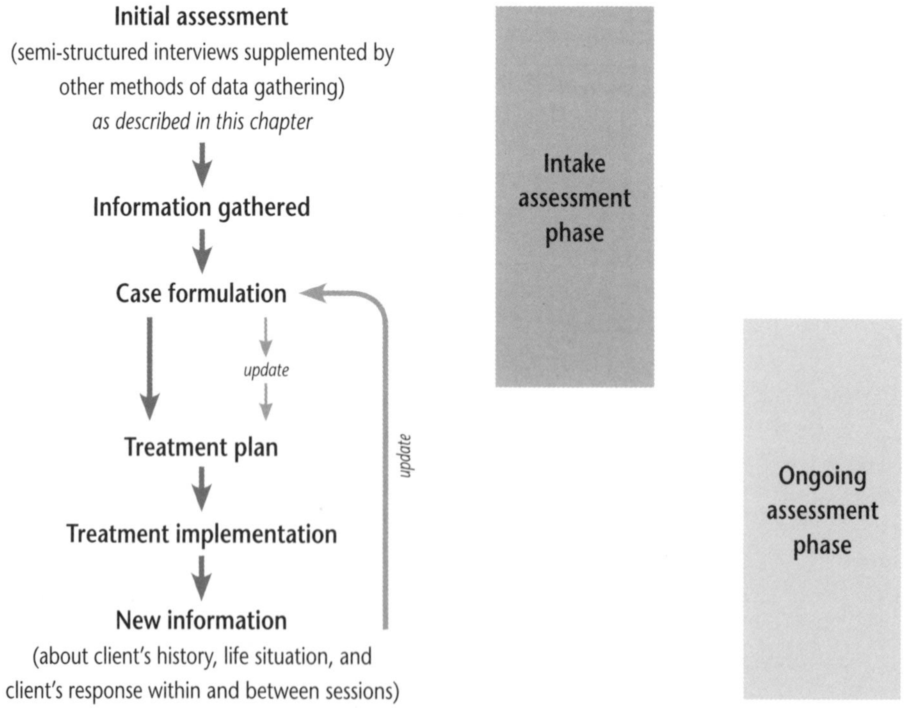

An intake assessment is the first step in a process whose aim is to deliver meaningful help to clients in distress. The second step is to use the information gathered during the assessment to make a case formulation. This incorporates a psychological understanding of clients' problems that can serve as the basis for the third step, the making of a treatment plan. Since the implementation of a treatment plan usually requires at least a few further sessions (and sometimes a large number), it is only worth embarking on the assessment process where it can be expected that a client seeking help can attend a series of sessions on a regular basis. A clinical assessment of this sort does not end once the intake is completed. Once treatment is implemented, new information is gained and the clinician engages in an ongoing assessment process that may lead to modifying the case formulation, and, in turn, the treatment plan, as illustrated in Figure 23.1.

A flexible and pragmatic qualitative investigation

The general principles of assessment, case formulation and treatment planning have a long history within clinical and counselling psychology in Europe and North America (for example, Freeman, Pretzer, Fleming & Simon, 2004; Kuyken, Padesky & Dudley, 2008; Mace, 1995), and have been regularly applied in South Africa since clinical and counselling psychologists began to develop a professional identity here in the 1970s and even before then (for example, Rachman, 1958). This chapter examines the application of clinical assessment under South African conditions based on case examples and published case studies, and discusses the problems and challenges that practitioners face due to time constraints, shortage of resources or cultural and contextual factors.

Unlike most other chapters in this volume, this one does not describe a rigidly structured assessment technique with quantified results and normative data. This is because a clinical assessment is a pragmatic investigation that is largely a process of qualitative evaluation based on the same principles as phenomenological-hermeneutic research (see Kvale, 1996). The phenomenological aspect is that the main interest is the lived experience of clients – their everyday thoughts, beliefs and attitudes (conscious or unconscious), emotions, body sensations and behaviour within the contexts of their everyday lives. The hermeneutic aspect is that clinicians draw on existing clinical knowledge and theory to guide their questioning and to interpret the information obtained. In formulating the case, clinicians need to ensure that they do not arbitrarily impose an interpretation from theory that is not supported by the information obtained from the client. The problems of many clients can be satisfactorily understood in terms of existing clinical theory, but, where they cannot, the case could be written up and published as a means of extending and refining existing theory (Dattilio, Edwards & Fishman, 2010; Edwards, Dattilio & Bromley, 2004).

A semi-structured interview is the main method of gathering information. Clinicians need to facilitate a balance between encouraging clients to express themselves in their own words and obtaining the specific kinds of information that will enable them to provide meaningful help. They also need to be responsive to the personal characteristics of the clients being assessed, the particular details of their lives, and the socio-economic and cultural contexts in which they live. Some of the information that clinicians ask about will be sensitive and likely to evoke distressing emotions in the client. For this reason, clinicians will not only be covering a list of important questions, but will be putting their client at ease, offering hope, building trust, and laying a relational foundation for any future work together if a course of treatment is indicated (Tantam, 1995).

In order to obtain the information that will be needed for a meaningful formulation of the case, other individuals may need to be interviewed. In assessing children, parents or caregivers are interviewed to provide background information. Such interviews also enable the clinician to assess the degree of support within the family, which may be essential if treatment is to be effective (Leibowitz-Levy, 2005; McDermott, 2005). Interviews with parents/caregivers and teachers are often central in the assessment of children's scholastic problems (see, for example, Whitefield-Alexander & Edwards, 2009). In assessing Tumeleng, a boy with severe conduct problems, Smith (2006) also interviewed the boy's father and sister, as well as two members of the school staff who knew him well. In addition to the interview, clinicians may draw on several other methods of gathering information that will contribute to an understanding of clients' problems.

Another method of data collection is to ask clients to observe their own behaviour and report back to the clinician at the next session. The clinician or an assistant may even observe the client's behaviour in a natural setting: observations of children's behaviour in the classroom may be valuable in the assessment of scholastic or behavioural problems. In assessing children, clinicians can obtain valuable information about factors related to their problems by observing the mother playing with her child in a clinic playroom, or by observing the child's spontaneous play or drawings. Self-report scales may be used to measure a range of responses, including those associated with depression, anxiety and post-traumatic stress (this aspect is elaborated by Young and Edwards in chapter 22 of this volume). For children, parents may complete a parenting scale that taps their style of parenting and administering discipline (Smith, 2006), and parents or teachers may complete behaviour checklists (Mashalaba & Edwards, 2005; Whitefield-Alexander & Edwards, 2009).

Much useful information is also available from clients' nonverbal behaviour: the volume, speed and intensity of their speech; their posture and gestures; their clothing; and their punctuality. As important as what clients say may be 'what they're not saying', and clinicians may use this to probe for 'information that might be out of their current awareness' (Padesky, 1996). Projective tests can also help to access aspects that clients cannot verbalise. Although these can be formally scored if appropriate norms are available, they can also be interpreted using standard methods of qualitative research and linking themes with other material obtained during the assessment. This is illustrated by McDermott's (2005) case study of 11-year-old Nosipho, where the Draw-A-Person Test provided valuable information about her identity as a black child, and the game of making a 'life road' became an instrument not only for ongoing assessment but also for treatment. Killian, Van der Riet, O'Neill, Hough and Zondi (2008) also provide evidence for the value of these methods in providing information about children's experience. Their study of children's agency under conditions of extreme adversity used focus groups in which a range of methods drawn from clinical practice were used, including making a 'life road' and other projective techniques. Material obtained in this way can largely be interpreted qualitatively, in conjunction with other information and further questioning of the client. Quantitative analysis of projective drawings can be misleading, though: in an earlier study of preschool children exposed to township violence, Magwaza, Killian, Petersen and Pillay (1993) found that the most severely traumatised children showed *less* trauma content in their drawings.

Areas to be covered in a clinical assessment

The aim of the assessment is to obtain enough information to form the basis for a case formulation, management recommendation and treatment. This means that clinicians are not just going through a checklist of information to be obtained, but are asking questions with specific goals in mind. The kinds of information that need to be gathered during a psychological assessment in order to inform such a final recommendation are summarised in Table 23.1 (note that not all of the items in the table are elaborated below).

Table 23.1 Kinds of information to be gathered in a clinical assessment

Presenting problems	The specific concerns that led the client to seek treatment: behavioural (relationship conflict or abuse, substance misuse, eating disorders, compulsive behaviours, sexual difficulties); emotions and mood (anxiety, depression, anger). Other prominent current psychological problems that emerge from the assessment interviews.
History, time course and impact of presenting problems	Onset, time course and severity of each problem or symptom. Impact on the client's everyday life (social and occupational functioning).
Case history	A summary of the main events of the client's life from birth to the present. Needs to include information about family, peer relationships, education and occupation, major life changes or traumatic events, medical problems, sexual orientation and history.
Screening	Check for problems that client may avoid disclosing such as substance use or abusive behaviour. Be alert for problems related to factors which cannot be addressed by psychological treatment: for example, headaches may be caused by a brain tumour, memory difficulties may be the result of brain injury following a motor vehicle accident, dizzy spells may be due to epilepsy.
Risk assessment	An assessment of whether the client is at risk of harming self (suicide, self-mutilation) or others (assault, murder, drunken driving).

continued →

Contextual factors	Factors likely to have a bearing on delivery of an intervention. These include social support (family, community), neighbourhood (safety, resources, services), cultural aspects (religious or cultural beliefs of client and family), current employment and financial stability.
Vulnerabilities	Developmental vulnerabilities (see predisposing factors in Table 23.2). Current vulnerabilities (lack of social support, unsafe or abusive environment, financial problems, etc.).
Strengths	Factors that may help clients to address their problems (motivation, social support, personality strengths).

Presenting problems, course and severity

Initially, the most important focus is the presenting problem or problems that led the client to seek help. While the clinician may begin with open-ended questions to facilitate clients' sharing their problems in their own words, this is followed up by more focused questions based on the clinician's knowledge of the kind of problem the client is presenting, and the kinds of psychological and behavioural processes that might be associated with it. For example, where a client is presenting with low mood, lack of motivation and fatigue, clinicians will ask questions to establish whether this fits the picture of a clinical depression, and, if so, what particular symptoms are present. It is also important to establish how severe the client's symptoms are, and the degree of their negative impact on the client's everyday life (Gilbert, Allan, Nicholls & Olsen, 2005). Information about the time course of the problem is also important. For example, is this the first experience of depressed mood or has the client been depressed like this for years? Does the client regularly experience episodes of depressed mood following events such as disappointments or relationship conflicts? The therapist should pay attention to any events that might have precipitated the current problem. For example, a client who has coped with a sense of failure by putting great effort into his work finds himself depressed after being retrenched from his job (see discussion of precipitating factors below). Where there are several problems, it is important to establish the time course of each: for example, a client may have a history of social anxiety going back to early high school days, but may only have experienced significant depression at the age of 25.

Case history

Taking a case history means surveying the course of a client's whole life, including the circumstances of his or her birth, his or her family relationships, relocations (moving house, moving towns), his or her progress at school, his or her peer relationships at different phases, traumatic events (family deaths, experiences of abuse, crime and violence), his or her intimate (including sexual) relationships, birth of children and work history. It is particularly important to gather information about life events that might render an individual vulnerable to psychological difficulties. Stressful conditions that increase vulnerability to psychological problems include many events that have the potential to disrupt family stability and the security of the child's attachment to caretakers. An example would be living in a family where parents are neglectful, emotionally unstable or unpredictable, verbally or physically abusive, in chronic conflict, abusing alcohol or drugs, or suffering from other serious mental health problems such as depression or psychotic disorders. Clinicians should also be alert for information about such events as chronic disabling illness of a parent, the death of a parent or sibling, a sudden shift in caretaking arrangements (for example, a child who has been cared for by the mother is suddenly left with a grandmother), or breakdown in the relationship between parents (including separation and divorce). The relationship between these kinds of events and psychological problems is well established by research both internationally (Agrawal, Gunderson, Holmes & Lyons-Ruth, 2004; Chapman, Dube & Anda, 2007; Edwards, Holden, Anda & Felitti, 2003) and locally (Seedat, Stein, Jackson, Heeringa, Williams & Myer, 2009).

Screening and risk assessment

Questions should not be confined to what clients talk about spontaneously. Clients and those concerned about them are often unaware of what causes their problems, or of the connection between different problems. Tumeleng's violent behaviour at school followed on his being sent away to boarding school in another country and being severely bullied (Smith, 2006). A student who became so depressed that she could not study did not realise that the main factor behind this was an abortion she had had a few months earlier (Boulind & Edwards, 2008). Alcohol abuse and dependence often lead to depressed mood and severe anxiety states, but clients may report the depression and anxiety without reporting the substance problem and without understanding that they are connected. For this reason, investigation of the presenting problems should include the use of screening questions that probe substance abuse, self-harm and other impulse-control symptoms that clients might not readily admit. Symptom checklists or checklists based on DSM or *International Classification of Mental and Behavioural Disorders* (ICD) diagnostic criteria can be a valuable means of ensuring that important information is not missed (Young & Edwards, chapter 22, this volume).

A risk assessment needs to be carried out early in the assessment to ascertain whether clients are a danger either to themselves (for example, by attempting suicide) or to others (for example, by assaulting or even killing someone). Research shows that suicidal ideation is associated most strongly with affective disorders, followed by substance abuse (especially alcohol) and schizophrenia, and, while suicidal thoughts are common, actual suicide is rare, so suicidal ideation is not necessarily indicative of high suicide risk (Davies, Naik & Lee, 2001). The sensitivity and specificity of the known risk factors is low, which means that there is no sure way of predicting whether clients will attempt suicide (Powell, Geddes, Deeks, Goldacre & Hawton, 2000). However, there is significant risk associated with having made previous suicide attempts, as well as with hopelessness. Client impulsiveness and aggressiveness are also causes for concern. In these kinds of cases, clinicians should use direct questioning about the nature of suicidal thoughts, the strength of the client's intent and whether the client has firm plans using a specific method. Where there is clear intent, clinicians should ask about access to lethal methods (for example, whether clients have been collecting medications on which to overdose, or own a gun) since there is a greater risk when means are available (Hawton & Van Heeringen, 2009). The same general approach would hold in cases where clients actively threaten to assault or kill someone. Clinicians must also be alert for clients who may be at risk of being harmed by others (for example, a child who is being sexually or physically assaulted by a family member).

Where clinicians establish that there is significant risk, they are ethically required to take action. Where a child is being abused, this may need to be reported to authorities. In the case of suicidal ideation, for less severe cases clinicians can consider using anti-suicide contracts, but their effectiveness has not been clearly established (Lee & Bartlett, 2005). Where there is more severe intent, it may be important to alert family members, and interventions might include the removal of firearms and/or lethal medication and voluntary or, in extreme cases, involuntary hospital admission. The appropriate course of action will depend on local mental health resources and should preferably be discussed with a supervisor or colleague (Allan, 2008). In the long term, the only sure way of decreasing suicide risk is to treat the client's mental disorder (Cavanagh, Carson, Sharpe & Lawrie, 2003), and therefore suicide management strategies that risk alienating clients from mental health services should be used sparingly. Bantjes and Van Ommen (2008) have developed a Suicide Risk Assessment Interview Schedule which provides a detailed checklist of risk factors to be probed in the course of a semi-structured interview. They illustrate its application using two case examples of students who sought assistance at a South African university counselling service, and discuss principles for making appropriate management decisions that are no more intensive than necessary, and most likely to preserve the therapeutic relationship.

A final aspect of screening is to be attentive to problems or symptoms that are not caused by psychological factors. For example, a client suffering from infectious mononucleosis (glandular fever) may experience loss of energy and motivation (Candy, Chalder, Cleare, Wessely & Hotopf, 2004); a client who has suffered a recent concussion may experience headaches, dizziness or concentration difficulties related to bruising of the brain (Lovell et al., 2006; Shuttleworth-Edwards, Whitefield-Alexander & Radloff, chapter 30, this volume); and a client in the early stages of AIDS may develop a number of cognitive impairments (Joska, Fincham, Stein, Paul & Seedat, 2010).

Contextual factors, vulnerabilities and strengths

Clients' psychological difficulties are embedded in their everyday lives, so they cannot be understood without information about their families, friendships and intimate relationships, work setting, financial means, access to medical care, and the kind of home and neighbourhood they live in (with respect to such factors as overcrowding and exposure to crime). For example, at a South African university counselling centre, black students seeking counselling were more distressed than their white counterparts, possibly because of issues such as racism, financial strain, trauma, poor academic preparation and a lack of social support (Young, 2009). Trauma, too, is a common feature of South African society (Edwards,

2005), and individual treatment of members of communities affected by chronic violence may have limited impact unless support structures are also built within the affected community (Higson-Smith & Killian, 2000). In addition, poverty – with its associated poor living conditions and poor nutrition – makes a significant contribution to poor mental health. Failure to take into account such contextual factors that might cause, shape or aggravate psychological disorders will in all likelihood result in a poor response to treatment.

An evaluation of clients' strengths provides an important counterpoint to the identification of factors in the case history that might confer vulnerability (as discussed above). Some individuals show remarkable resilience in the face of adversity, and remain optimistic in the face of very difficult life circumstances. The inclusion of the client's strengths may result in a case conceptualisation that is more acceptable to the client, which can promote therapist/client collaboration (Kuyken et al., 2008). In such cases, therapy can focus on enhancing strengths as well as alleviating problems, which can enhance the prevention of relapse (Brewin, 2006).

Assessment and intervention: managing priorities

Clinicians must exercise judgement with respect to how they manage the gathering of all this information. To cover all the areas in Table 23.1 comprehensively could take several hours. Meanwhile, the client may have urgent concerns that are not being addressed. One way to overcome this is to schedule two to three hours at a time. Breaks can be included for the client to rest, and for the clinician to reflect on the information obtained and plan the focus for the next part of the interview. Where clients are in crisis, the clinician may need to intervene immediately to calm intense emotions or reduce suicide risk. In such cases the clinician may have to move between conducting the assessment and a crisis-intervention approach (Dattilio & Freeman, 2007).

Because of time constraints the clinician may choose to obtain only a limited history, and build up a fuller history as details emerge in the course of treatment. This allows for problems that might respond to brief structured interventions to be addressed more rapidly. Where clinicians elect to do this, it is particularly important to view the process of assessment as ongoing so that, as they build up a fuller picture over the course of a few sessions, they can reformulate the case and renegotiate with the client about what is likely to be involved in treatment (see Figure 23.1).

The disadvantage of skipping aspects of the assessment process is that information vital for case formulation may be missed, resulting in inappropriate interventions being offered. This could waste time and undermine the clinician's credibility. Another reason for not plunging into treatment prematurely is that psychotherapy or counselling may not be appropriate for all clients who are assessed, and it is one aim of the assessment to determine whether a psychological intervention is appropriate at all. Furthermore, a systematic assessment means that the clinician may open up areas of experience that the client might otherwise avoid, and this can benefit the client. If very traumatic experiences are touched on that clients are too distressed to go into detail about (such as childhood sexual abuse), the clinician can at least note their significance and consider their possible contribution to current problems. For some clients the assessment process itself can result in some improvement, as measured by the sorts of measures used to evaluate therapy outcomes (Young, 2006a). This is because having had the opportunity to discuss their problems with a sympathetic therapist, and having felt understood, they may subsequently put insights gained from this process into action to improve their lives (Young, 2006b).

Case formulation

Throughout the assessment process, information is gathered in such a way as to serve as a basis for the steps set out in Table 23.2: making a diagnosis, developing a case formulation, making recommendations for management and devising a treatment plan.

A provisional diagnosis is made by using the diagnostic criteria in, for example, the ICD-10 (World Health Organization, 1992) or DSM-IV (APA, 2000), and systematically checking to see if the client meets them.

Table 23.2 Case formulation, management recommendation and treatment plan

Diagnosis (ICD-10; DSM-IV)		A formal diagnosis based on the criteria set out in the ICD-10 and/or DSM-IV.
Case formulation	Predisposing factors	Factors in the client's history that render him/her vulnerable to particular kinds of psychological problems: insecure or disturbed attachment in infancy and childhood, traumatic events (deaths in family, violence, etc.), ongoing adversity (family conflict, neglect, abuse, poverty).
	Precipitating factors	Was there a critical event which seems to have caused or exacerbated the current difficulties?
	Maintaining factors	Aspects of the client's current thinking and behaviour which are keeping the problem going.
Management recommendations		Should the client be referred for further specialist assessment (for example, by a psychiatrist or neurologist)? Does the client need crisis intervention? Does the client need to be hospitalised? Can the client be helped with a course of psychotherapy or counselling?
Treatment plan		This should address the presenting problems based on the factors that are currently maintaining them. Interventions need to be selected according to the evidence base in the clinical research literature and adapted to suit the contextual features of clients' lives, and taking into account their vulnerabilities and strengths.

A case formulation, also called a case conceptualisation, describes and explains the client's distress. It incorporates clinical hypotheses about the factors underlying the development and the maintenance of the problem (Kuyken et al., 2008; Persons, 2006). Although there may be differences in how this is done within different approaches to psychotherapy, case formulation is central to most approaches to psychotherapy (Eells, 2007; Mace, 1995) and formulations from different approaches can be remarkably similar (Persons, Curtis & Silberschatz, 1991). This chapter summarises the basic principles, based on an analysis of predisposing, precipitating and maintaining factors, using examples set out in Table 23.3. However, case formulation is a complex process to which many clinicians pay inadequate attention (Eells, Lombart, Kendjelic, Turner & Lucas, 2005), and a full treatment is beyond the scope of this chapter.

Table 23.3 Contrasting treatment plans for three cases of women with major depressive disorder

Client	Context and formulation	Treatment focus
Sindi	Ongoing marital discord. Husband regularly criticises and belittles her and sometimes physically assaults her. She is feeling chronically helpless and hopeless. She was raised in a home where such abuse was routine and watched her mother being treated in the same way.	Educate her about the relationship between abuse and depression, and about women's rights. Help her stand up to and confront her husband or take steps to leave him. Increase her social support. Discuss possible legal action.
Bulelwa	Unresolved bereavement – started when her 6-month-old baby died of a severe infection a few months ago. She is unable to talk about this without bursting into tears.	Help her accept the loss using bereavement therapy.
Nomvuyo	As a child her father expected her to perform at a high level, and often implied that she was incompetent. She was recently promoted but has been having panic attacks related to the extra responsibilities she has to undertake. The panic attacks are interfering with her work performance, and she fears that her superiors can see how poorly she is doing and will fire her. She feels increasingly out of control and helpless about solving the problem.	Address her anxiety about being evaluated. Train her in anxiety management techniques and panic control. Help her get an accurate appraisal of her ability to meet her responsibilities, and use a problem-solving approach to mastering the new challenges in her work.

Predisposing factors are those that have rendered clients vulnerable to their current problems. For example, a client's depression may be directly related to an unstable family situation in the first few months or years of life, the death of a parent, or a sexual molestation that occurred in early childhood. A client whose mother died when she was an infant and who was sent from one caretaker to another over the following ten years would be vulnerable to intense feelings of abandonment, and the resulting insecurity could predispose her to intense anxiety and difficulties in current intimate relationships. The meaning such events had for the client will need to be explored to provide a basis for understanding how these may have conferred vulnerability. The experience of emotional and physical abuse as routine while growing up may result in learned helplessness (as with Sindi in Table 23.3). Parental criticism may impart beliefs about the self such as 'I'm incompetent' (as with Nomvuyo in Table 23.3). Many clients are unaware of the link between past distressing events and current psychological functioning, and it is the task of the clinician, in developing the case formulation, to put forward credible hypotheses about this. In developing contexts such as South Africa, where poverty, crime and illness are not uncommon, it is particularly important to consider the impact of the accumulation of stressful life events and adversity both in conferring vulnerability and in the development of resilience (Turner & Butler, 2003).

Precipitating factors are those that set off a particular problem. In the examples in Table 23.3, the death of Bulelwa's baby and Nomvuyo's promotion are precipitating factors, as they are associated with the onset of symptoms. In the case of Sindi there may be no precipitating factor. Having been raised in an abusive family from which she progressed into an abusive marriage, she may have been depressed for so long that no clear onset can be identified.

Maintaining factors are those that keep the problem going. It is important to recognise that what may have caused a problem might be very different from what maintains it, and that both may need to be addressed in therapy. A depressed person withdraws socially and feels lonely, which exacerbates the depression. A woman in an abusive relationship (like Sindi in Table 23.3) may believe that if she perseveres, her partner will change, or may simply believe that this is what happens to women. A bereaved person who is too distressed to talk about the loss (like Bulelwa in Table 23.3) is unable to grieve and let go. Individuals experiencing panic attacks (like Nomvuyo in Table 23.3) may feel less and less able to cope, and even believe that they have a chronic incurable illness, and this demotivates them from trying to address their problems.

The management recommendation and treatment plan

The case formulation is the basis for a management recommendation. Since not all symptoms have a psychological basis, some clients may need to be referred to a medical practitioner or specialist to rule out any serious undiagnosed medical condition. Persistent headaches, for example, could be related to chronic anxiety or suppressed anger, but they can also be caused by a brain tumour or another underlying neurological disorder. Similarly, where clients report episodes of loss of consciousness, a referral for investigation of a possible diagnosis of epilepsy should be made. Some clients' problems may be too severe for outpatient psychotherapy or counselling, and the outcome of the assessment may be a referral to a psychiatrist or a recommendation for hospitalisation or referral to a specialised substance abuse unit.

For many cases, however, the outcome of the assessment is a recommendation for a course of psychotherapy or counselling, and the case formulation will provide the basis for the treatment plan. This step is illustrated by the three cases described in Table 23.3 of women suffering from major depressive disorder. Presenting the formulation and treatment plan is an important step which, if done well, can motivate the client and give them hope. If you imagine yourself presenting the treatment plan to each of these three women, you will be able to understand why Ahmed and Westra (2009) found that where clinicians can provide clients with a clear understanding of the cause of their distress and a rationale for the treatment plan, clients are more likely to be motivated to engage with treatment.

Currently there is a debate about the extent to which psychological treatments can be defined and manualised. A closely manualised treatment would be one that follows the same fixed protocol across a set number of sessions for any client. While such manuals work for less complicated procedures such as systematic desensitisation, most treatments are more complex, and treatment manuals emphasise general principles for planning treatment based on theory rather than prescribing the details session by session. This kind of flexible manualisation is widely recommended in cognitive behaviour therapy approaches stemming from the work of Beck (Westbrook, Kennerley & Kirk, 2007), and found in the treatment of post-traumatic stress disorder (PTSD) (Ehlers & Clark, 2000) and borderline personality disorder (Giesen-Bloo et al., 2006). It is also an increasing characteristic of psychodynamic approaches (Cabaniss, Cherry, Douglas & Schwartz, 2010; Leichsenring et al., 2009).

In these approaches, clinicians do an initial assessment of the kind described in this chapter, followed by an ongoing assessment based on new information that emerges from treatment sessions, clients' response to treatment, and clients' behaviour and experience between sessions. On this basis the case formulation is regularly refined and updated (see Figure 23.1). Such ongoing assessment is a feature of Edwards's (2009) model for working with South African clients with PTSD or complex trauma, which allows clinicians to be responsive to the needs of each client on a session-by-session basis.

Assessment for psychotherapy in practice in South Africa

In multicultural societies the principles of assessment need to be flexibly adapted to working with clients from different backgrounds and in different settings. Since a clinical assessment is a form of qualitative investigation that is responsive to the individual characteristics of each client, sensitivity to culture and context is an essential feature of the process. Even where clinicians are from a similar cultural background to their clients, there may be differences in perspective related to such factors as family traditions, school experience, political loyalties and religious affiliation. The more clinicians understand these kinds of contextual factors, the more they can draw on resources within the client's environment. Donald and Hlongwane (1989) show how clinicians working with black African children intervened with psychotherapy to address some aspects of their problems, but addressed other aspects by encouraging families to work with African healers.

Eagle (2004) describes cases of African clients with PTSD where, in order to plan treatment, the clinician needed to understand how traditional African beliefs impacted on the way trauma was experienced. Religious syncretism, whereby people follow Christian belief systems and simultaneously hold traditional cultural beliefs and practise cultural rituals that are often in contradiction to their Christian belief system, is not uncommon (Leclerc-Madlala, Simbayi & Cloete, 2009). The clinician, therefore, should explore how clients understand their problems and the cultural context in which these problems have developed. A woman who believes that a particular religious practice offers her protection from witchcraft might present with anxiety if something happens to prevent her from carrying out her practice, or if her faith in the practice is undermined.

The process of assessment described here has not been the focus of much formal research (Tantam, 1995). Despite this, it forms the basis of treatment planning in the majority of scientific evaluations of psychological interventions – for example, in randomised controlled trials. It is also fundamental to conducting systematic case studies (Dattilio et al., 2010). The applicability to South African contexts of the kind of assessment described in this chapter has been documented in several case studies which describe the treatment of a range of clinical problems. These include several cases of PTSD: in a male student who had had to identify his brother who had been killed in a road accident and badly burned (Karpelowsky & Edwards, 2005); in a schoolgirl whose policeman father had treated her and her mother abusively and whose mother had died of AIDS (McDermott, 2005); in a schoolgirl who had twice been raped near her township home (Payne & Edwards, 2009); and in a female student who developed depression and PTSD following an abortion (Boulind & Edwards, 2008). Other clinical problems addressed in published case studies include childhood Attention Deficit/Hyperactivity Disorder (Whitefield-Alexander & Edwards, 2009), childhood conduct disorder (Mashalaba & Edwards, 2005; Smith, 2006) and social anxiety disorder (Edwards, Henwood & Kannan, 2003; Edwards & Kannan, 2006). There is thus a clear body of evidence that the principles set out in this chapter are appropriate for a diverse range of clinical contexts in South Africa.

References

Agrawal, H. R., Gunderson, J., Holmes, B. M. & Lyons-Ruth, K. (2004). Attachment studies with borderline patients: A review. *Harvard Review of Psychiatry, 12(2)*, 94–104.

Ahmed, M. & Westra, H. A. (2009). Impact of a treatment rationale on expectancy and engagement in cognitive behavioral therapy for social anxiety. *Cognitive Therapy and Research, 33*, 314–322.

Allan, A. (2008). *Law and Ethics in Psychology: An International Perspective*. Somerset West: Inter-Ed Publishers.

APA (American Psychiatric Association) (2000). *Diagnostic and Statistical Manual of Mental Disorders IV-TR*. Washington, DC: American Psychiatric Press.

Bantjes, J. & Van Ommen, C. (2008). The development and utilisation of a suicide risk assessment interview schedule. *South African Journal of Psychology, 38*, 391–411.

Boulind, M. & Edwards, D. (2008). The assessment and treatment of post-abortion syndrome: A systematic case-study from Southern Africa. *Journal of Psychology in Africa, 18*, 539–548.

Brewin, C. R. (2006). Understanding cognitive behaviour therapy: A retrieval competition account. *Behaviour Research and Therapy, 44*, 765–784.

Cabaniss, D. L., Cherry, S., Douglas, C. J. & Schwartz, A. R. (2010). *Psychodynamic Psychotherapy: A Clinical Manual*. New York, NY: Wiley.

Candy, B., Chalder, T., Cleare, A., Wessely, S. & Hotopf, M. (2004). A randomised controlled trial of a psycho-educational intervention to aid recovery in infectious mononucleosis. *Journal of Psychosomatic Research, 57(1)*, 89–94.

Cavanagh, J. T. O., Carson, A. J., Sharpe, M. & Lawrie, S. M. (2003). Psychological autopsy studies of suicide: A systematic review. *Psychological Medicine, 33*, 395–405.

Chapman, D. P., Dube, S. R. & Anda, R. F. (2007). Adverse childhood events as risk factors for negative mental health outcomes. *Psychiatric Annals, 37(5)*, 359–364.

Dattilio, F. M., Edwards, D. J. A. & Fishman, D. B. (2010). Case studies within a mixed methods paradigm: Towards a resolution of the alienation between researcher and practitioner in psychotherapy research. *Psychotherapy: Theory, Research, Practice & Training, 47*, 427–441.

Dattilio, F. M. & Freeman, A. (2007). *Cognitive-Behavioral Strategies in Crisis Intervention* (3rd edition). New York, NY: The Guilford Press.

Davies, S., Naik, P. C. & Lee, A. S. (2001). Depression, suicide, and the national service framework. *British Medical Journal, 322*, 1500–1501.

Donald, D. R. & Hlongwane, M. M. (1989). Issues in the integration of traditional African healing and Western counselling in school psychological practice: Three case studies. *School Psychology International, 10*, 243–249.

Eagle, G. T. (2004). Therapy at the cultural interface: Implications of African cosmology for traumatic stress intervention. *Psychology in Society, 30*, 1–22.

Edwards, D. J. A. (2005). Post-traumatic stress disorder as a public health concern in South Africa. *Journal of Psychology in Africa, 15(2)*, 125–134.

Edwards, D. J. A. (2009). Responsive treatment of posttraumatic stress disorder: An integrative model grounded in case-based research in South Africa. *Journal of Psychology in Africa, 19(2)*, 189–198.

Edwards, D. J. A., Dattilio, F. & Bromley, D. B. (2004). Developing evidence-based practice: The role of case-based research. *Professional Psychology: Research and Practice, 35*, 589–597.

Edwards, D. J. A., Henwood, J. & Kannan, S. (2003). Cognitive therapy for social phobia: The human face of cognitive science. *Alternation, 10*, 122–150.

Edwards, D. & Kannan, S. (2006). Identifying and targeting idiosyncratic cognitive processes in group therapy for social phobia: The case of Vumile. *Pragmatic Case Studies in Psychotherapy, 2*, module 2, 1–30.

Edwards, V. J., Holden, G. W., Anda, R. F. & Felitti, V. J. (2003). Experiencing multiple forms of childhood maltreatment and adult mental health: Results from the Adverse Childhood Experiences (ACE) study. *American Journal of Psychiatry, 160(8)*, 1453–1460.

Eells, T. D. (Ed.) (2007). *Handbook of Psychotherapy Case Formulation* (2nd edition). New York, NY: The Guilford Press.

Eells, T. D., Lombart, K. G., Kendjelic, E. M., Turner, L. C. & Lucas, C. P. (2005). The quality of psychotherapy case formulations: A comparison of expert, experienced, and novice cognitive-behavioral and psychodynamic therapists. *Journal of Consulting and Clinical Psychology, 73*, 579–589.

Ehlers, A. & Clark, D. M. (2000). A cognitive model of posttraumatic stress disorder. *Behaviour Research and Therapy, 38*, 319–345.

Freeman, A., Pretzer, J., Fleming, B. & Simon, K. M. (2004). *Clinical Applications of Cognitive Therapy* (2nd edition). New York, NY: Kluwer Academic/Plenum.

Giesen-Bloo, J., Van Dyck, R., Spinhoven, P., Van Tilburg, W., Dirksen, C., Van Asselt, T. et al. (2006). Outpatient psychotherapy for borderline personality disorder: Randomized trial of schema-focused therapy vs. transference-focused psychotherapy. *Archives of General Psychiatry, 63*, 649–658.

Gilbert, P., Allan, S., Nicholls, W. & Olsen, K. (2005). The assessment of psychological symptoms of patients referred to community mental health teams: Distress, chronicity and life interference. *Clinical Psychology and Psychotherapy, 12*, 10–27.

Hawton, K. & Van Heeringen, K. (2009). Suicide. *The Lancet, 373*, 1372–1381.

Higson-Smith, C. & Killian, B. (2000). Caring for children in fragmented communities. In D. Donald, A. Dawes & J. Louw (Eds), *Addressing Childhood Adversity* (pp. 202–224). Cape Town: David Philip.

Joska, J., Fincham, D., Stein, D., Paul, R. & Seedat, S. (2010). Clinical correlates of HIV-associated neurocognitive disorders in South Africa. *AIDS and Behavior, 14*, 371–378.

Karpelowsky, B. & Edwards, D. (2005). Trauma, imagery, and the therapeutic relationship: Langu's story. *Journal of Psychology in Africa, 15*, 185–195.

Killian, B., Van der Riet, M., O'Neill, V., Hough, A. & Zondi, V. (2008). Children's loss of agency under extreme adversity. *Journal of Psychology in Africa, 18*, 403–412.

Kuyken, W., Padesky, C. A. & Dudley, R. (2008). The science and practice of case conceptualization. *Behavioural and Cognitive Psychotherapy, 36*, 757–768.

Kvale, S. (1996). *Interviews: An Introduction to Qualitative Research Interviewing*. Thousand Oaks, CA: Sage.

Leclerc-Madlala, S., Simbayi, L.B. & Cloete, A. (2009). The sociocultural aspects of HIV/AIDS in South Africa. In P. Rohleder, L. Swartz, S. C. Kalichman & L. C. Simbayi (Eds), *HIV/AIDS in South Africa 25 Years On* (pp. 13–25). New York, NY: Springer Verlag.

Lee, J. B. & Bartlett, M. L. (2005). Suicide prevention: Critical elements for managing suicidal clients and counselor liability without the use of a no-suicide contract. *Death Studies, 29*, 847–865.

Leibowitz-Levy, S. (2005). The role of brief term interventions with South African child trauma survivors. *Journal of Psychology in Africa, 15*, 155–163.

Leichsenring, F., Salzer, S., Jaeger, U., Kächele, H., Kreische, R., Leweke, F. et al. (2009). Short-term psychodynamic psychotherapy and cognitive-behavioral therapy in generalized anxiety disorder: A randomized, controlled trial. *American Journal of Psychiatry, 166*, 875–881.

Lovell, M. R., Iverson, G. L., Collins, M. W., Podell, K., Johnston K. M., Pardini D. et al. (2006). Measurement of symptoms following sports-related concussion: Reliability and normative data for the Post-Concussion Symptom Scale. *Applied Neuropsychology, 13(3)*, 166–175.

Mace, C. (Ed.) (1995). *The Art and Science of Assessment in Psychotherapy*. London: Routledge.

Magwaza, A. S., Killian, B. J., Petersen, I. & Pillay, Y. (1993). The effects of chronic violence on preschool children living in South African townships. *Child Abuse and Neglect, 17*, 795–803.

Mashalaba, E. & Edwards, D. (2005). A successful cognitive-behavioural intervention that failed: A case study of adolescent conduct disorder at a school for the disadvantaged. *Journal of Child and Adolescent Mental Health, 17*, 69–78.

McDermott, R. (2005). The great arch of unimagined bridges: Integrative play therapy with an abused child. *Journal of Psychology in Africa, 15*, 165–175.

Padesky, C. A. (1996). *Guided Discovery: Using Socratic Dialogue.* Video recording. Newport Beach, CA: Center for Cognitive Therapy.

Payne, C. & Edwards, D. J. A. (2009). What services and supports are needed to enable trauma survivors to rebuild their lives? Implications of a systematic case study of cognitive therapy with a township adolescent girl with PTSD following rape. *Child Abuse Research in South Africa, 10,* 27–40.

Persons, J. B. (2006). Case formulation-driven psychotherapy. *Clinical Psychology: Science and Practice, 13(2),* 167–170.

Persons, J. B., Curtis, J. T. & Silberschatz, G. (1991). Psychodynamic and cognitive-behavioral formulations of a single case. *Psychotherapy, 28(4),* 608–617.

Powell, J., Geddes, J., Deeks, J., Goldacre, M. & Hawton, K. (2000). Suicide in psychiatric hospital in-patients: Risk factors and their predictive power. *British Journal of Psychiatry, 176,* 266–272.

Rachman, S. (1958). The treatment of anxiety and phobic reactions by systematic desensitization psychotherapy. *Journal of Abnormal and Social Psychology, 58(2),* 259–263.

Seedat, S., Stein, D. J., Jackson, P. B., Heeringa, S. G., Williams, D. R. & Myer, L. (2009). Life stress and mental disorders in the South African stress and health study. *South African Medical Journal, 99,* 375–382.

Smith, I. (2006). A cognitive-behavioural treatment programme for conduct disorder: The case of Tumeleng. *Journal of Psychology in Africa, 16,* 231–241.

Tantam, D. (1995). Why assess? In C. Mace (Ed.), *The Art and Science of Assessment in Psychotherapy* (pp. 8–25). London: Routledge.

Turner, H. A. & Butler, M. J. (2003). Direct and indirect effects of childhood adversity on depressive symptoms in young adults. *Journal of Youth and Adolescence, 32,* 89–103.

Westbrook, D., Kennerley, H. & Kirk, J. (2007). *An Introduction to Cognitive Behaviour Therapy: Skills and Applications.* London: Sage.

Whitefield-Alexander, V. & Edwards, D. J. A. (2009). A case of effective single-session treatment for attention deficit and learning problems in a routine clinical practice: The value of a transdiagnostic approach to case formulation. *Journal of Child and Adolescent Mental Health, 21,* 61–72.

World Health Organization (1992). *International Classification of Mental and Behavioural Disorders ICD-10.* Geneva: World Health Organization.

Young, C. S. (2006a). What happens when people wait for therapy? Assessing the clinical significance of the changes observed over the waiting period for clients referred to a primary care psychology service. *Primary Care Mental Health, 4,* 113–119.

Young, C. S. (2006b). The personal experiences and views of waiting for cognitive therapy in the NHS: A qualitative account. *Counselling Psychology Review, 21,* 19–26.

Young, C. S. (2009). The CORE-OM intake norms of students attending a South African university counselling service: A comparison with UK counselling service data. *British Journal of Guidance and Counselling, 37,* 473–483.

24 Projective assessment of adults and children in South Africa

K. Bain, Z. Amod and R. Gericke

This chapter provides an introduction to the theoretical concepts that underlie projective assessment and includes a brief history of projective testing. The current debates in the literature that surround projective assessment are outlined, and the limitations of projective tests are discussed in relation to research conducted into the reliability and validity of various projective tests. The criticisms levelled against these tests are balanced against arguments for their clinical utility. The prevalence of this form of testing in clinical practice, internationally and in South Africa, is briefly discussed, as is the use of this form of testing in adult and child populations. The use of these tests in forensic settings is also briefly addressed; however, research into the cross-cultural validity of this form of testing is a central focus of the chapter. Common problems relating to the cross-cultural use of these Westernised assessment measures are also outlined. A discussion of the fact that clinical practice often precedes research regarding adaptations in the use of tests is included, and clinical illustrations of adapted interpretations accounting for socio-economic and cultural variations are described. The necessity for socio-cultural awareness in mental health practitioners in relation to this form of testing is highlighted.

The scope of projective assessment

Projective assessment refers to the measurement of personality traits or characteristics, using instruments in which the stimulus is a task or activity that is vague or ambiguous. These tests allow for a less restricted response from the person being assessed than the limited choice of responses usually associated with objective personality measures, such as 'yes', 'no', 'sometimes' or a Likert scale. Typically, when using projective assessments, a task such as responding to an image, telling a story about a picture, completing an unfinished sentence or drawing a picture is presented to a person who is then required to generate a response, with minimal external guidance or constraints imposed on the nature of that response. The assumption that underlies these tests is that when a person is called upon to generate a response in the face of ambiguity, the person projects elements of her personal characteristics into her response (Meyer & Kurtz,

2006). Most of these tests are premised largely on psychoanalytic theories of personality. Due to the unstructured nature of the tasks presented, most often the subject matter being assessed is unclear to examinees, which requires them to draw upon their own internal representations, schemas or internal working models in order to make sense of the stimulus. Thus, the responses constructed by the examinee can often reveal important psychological characteristics that can be measured and interpreted by the psychologist. Rather than being used for diagnostic purposes, projective tests are used to generate hypotheses about how examinees view themselves, others and the world. Projective tests should not be used in isolation, but rather as part of an assessment battery or group of tests, as projective test results are most usefully understood within the context of a person's history and their other test responses, rather than through blind interpretation. It is important to note that according to the South African Health Professions Act No. 56 of 1974, any tests or measures that assess psychological constructs must be used, interpreted and controlled by psychologists. According to the Health Professions Council of South Africa (HPCSA), the administration of a projective test constitutes a 'psychological act', and due to the fact that these tests assess personality functioning, it is possible that a projective test could 'in terms of its content or responses required, result in either embarrassment or anxiety to the test-taker' (HPCSA, 2005, p.1); hence personality and diagnostic measures, in particular projective tests, are allowed to be used only by registered psychologists.

Most Master's courses in clinical, counselling and educational psychology teach the use of projective assessment measures, with various universities placing emphasis on different tests, such as the Rorschach Inkblot Technique, the Thematic Apperception Test (TAT) and projective drawings. Most courses cover the administration, scoring and interpretation of these tests; the theoretical foundations upon which they are based; the clinical uses; and the diagnostic and prognostic indicators of the tests. Students are usually also expected to learn how factors such as anxiety, organicity, personality traits, culture and socio-economic status affect the measurement and interpretations of projective test results.

The history of projective testing

The first recorded projective techniques were based on word association, which was used by Galton and Freud in the late 19th century (Rook, 2006). Projective techniques were then developed for use in clinical psychology in the early 20th century, primarily for the purpose of personality assessment. However, other uses for these techniques were soon discovered. During the 1940s, they were adapted from their clinical settings for use in market research to determine buyer attitudes and opinions (Smith, 1954); however, this adaptation of clinical personality tests for use in market research was controversial and a number of reservations were voiced about the fact that these tests attempt to tap into areas of the psyche that people might rather leave concealed (Bellenger, Bernhardt & Goldstucker, 1976).

Reliable interpretation of projective test data was found to be problematic, and as the validity of projective tests began to be questioned their use declined sharply after the 1950s. The focus remained on the weaknesses of projective tests for decades, and it was only in the 1980s that they appear to have been 'rediscovered' (Catterall & Ibbottson, 2000). Projective assessments are now widely used in clinical practice, both internationally and in South Africa (Foxcroft, Paterson, Le Roux & Herbst, 2004; Piotrowski, Keller & Ogawa, 1993), and as improved statistical methods have developed, controversy regarding the utility and validity of projective testing has continued. The debates surrounding these measures revolve around the relevance of their psychoanalytic theoretical underpinnings and the sufficiency of empirical support (Erickson, Lilienfeld & Vitacco, 2007), in addition to concerns about cultural fairness (Foxcroft et al., 2004). According to Moletsane (2004), in terms of apartheid policies in South Africa psychological tests were designed according to racial groups, with very few then being appropriate for use with all South Africans. An example of a racially and culturally specific test developed during this time is the TAT-Z, designed for use with Zulu people. The limited number of tests normed for all racial and cultural groups in post-apartheid South Africa then led to the practice of psychologists using measures, amongst these projective tests, normed only on US or European samples, and then applying caution to the interpretation of results. Moletsane (2004, p.10) states that, due to the fact that 'very few empirical studies have been undertaken into test bias, the testers are left with very little certainty about the validity and cultural appropriateness of the measures they use'. However, despite continuing debate about them in the academic community, the practitioner community continues to find projective techniques useful (Foxcroft et al., 2004; Pruitt, Smith, Thelen & Lubin, 1985).

Theoretical concepts underlying projective testing

The basic assumption underlying these measures is that when a person is presented with a number of ambiguous stimuli and is invited to respond to such stimuli, projection occurs and aspects of the examinee's own characteristics and needs appear in the responses to the ambiguous stimuli (Anastasi & Urbina, 2007). The concept of projection was originally based on Freud's theory of projection, wherein he proposed that there are parts of ourselves we can't accept or tolerate, thus, we 'project' those repressed thoughts and feelings onto other people and things. Projective tests are

> based on the well-recognised fact that when someone attempts to interpret a complex social situation he is apt to tell as much about himself as he is about the phenomenon on which his attention is focused. At such times, the person is off his guard, since he believes he is merely explaining objective occurrences. To one with 'double hearing', however, he is exposing certain inner forces and arrangements, wishes, fears and traces of past experiences. (Morgan & Murray, 1935, p.390)

However, as psychoanalytic theory has developed, Freud's initial conception of projection as a defence mechanism has been broadened, and currently projective tests are thought to elicit both repressions, in the Freudian sense, that the examinee would consciously deny or disavow, and more everyday projections that are also often symbolically important, such as beliefs, feelings or action tendencies (Wagner, 2008). People are constantly projecting aspects of themselves onto the outer world, usually without awareness, and so when presented with an unstructured task, a person similarly projects his or her personality onto the content and structure of the response. According to Wagner (2008) it is the unstructured nature of projective tests which allows for an infinite variety of responses that can sometimes reveal insights into examinees' psychodynamics, and can also detect deviancy through responses that contradict reality (Wagner, 2008). An example of a response on the Incomplete Sentence Blank (ISB) that reveals elements of an examinee's psychodynamics is: '*A father* always knows what is right and gets angry if you do wrong.' An example on the ISB that depicts deviancy is: '*I suffer* because they put devices in my ears at night to give me orders.' Wagner (2008) also considers ambiguity an important aspect of projective tests and states that a moderate amount of ambiguity is best, with highly structured or unstructured stimuli not lending themselves well to projections. Tests with recognisable, yet ambiguous, pictures seem to elicit the most meaningful projective responses.

Empirical evidence for the concept of projection

In 1989, McClelland, Koestner and Weinberger published an important review that has been extremely influential in the past three decades as it linked the controversial concept of projection to the learning and memory literatures. This field proposes a distinction between 'explicit' and 'implicit' memory. While explicit memory involves the conscious retrieval of information, such as names or childhood memories, implicit memory refers to memory that is only observable in behaviour, but that cannot be consciously brought to mind (Schacter, 1992). A great deal of research has been done on implicit memory and a number of different types of implicit memories have been identified, such as procedural memory – for example, driving a car – or associative memory, which refers to the formation of associations that guide mental processes outside of conscious awareness (Westen, 1999) – for example, priming by advertisements. In their review, McClelland et al. (1989) suggest that while most objective measures tend to assess 'explicit' needs – in other words, self-attributed needs and motives that a person acknowledges as being characteristic of his or her day-to-day functioning and experience – projective tests tend to assess 'implicit' needs, which are the needs and motivations that influence a person's behaviour automatically, usually without her awareness that her behaviour is influenced by these motives (Bornstein, 2002). McClelland et al. (1989, pp.698–699) state that 'conscious goal-setting is analogous to episodic recall: It involves a voluntary act. And implicit motives are more like semantic memory: They automatically influence behavior without conscious effort.' Hence, behaviour or responses that are thought out and conscious reflect explicit memory, while behaviour and responses that are more spontaneous or unconscious reflect implicit memory (Weinberger & McClelland, 1990). Explaining why results on objective and projective measures of the same construct often differ, McClelland et al. (1989) noted that the explicit memory used to answer questions regarding the self and relationships on objective (self-report) measures tends to be filtered through analytic thought, and so reflects conscious constructions of the self and others. In contrast, the implicit memory used to respond to more unstructured stimuli is 'more often built on early, prelinguistic affective experiences, whereas self-attributed motives are more often built on explicit teaching by parents and others as to what values or goals it is important for a child to pursue' (McClelland et al., 1989, pp.698–699). Hence, responses that elicit implicit memory tend to 'provide a more direct readout of motivational and emotional experiences than do self reports' (p.698). According to Bornstein (2002, p.50), when comparing explicit and implicit achievement strivings Weinberger and McClelland (1990) found that projective measures, such as the TAT, were a particularly effective predictor of 'spontaneous achievement-related behaviour across a variety of situations and settings, whereas questionnaire measures of self-attributed achievement needs show greater predictive validity in situations where the person's attention is focused on the achievement-related aspects of his or her actions'. Bornstein (2002) also found that by combining implicit (projective) and self-attributed (objective) dependency test scores, the overall accuracy of behavioural prediction was increased as the results managed to encompass both spontaneous and goal-directed dependent behaviour in different contexts and settings. Thus, the differences between results on objective and projective measures can be clinically useful. If both types of measures are used it appears that a more complete picture regarding the examinee's personality structure and interpersonal style might be gained, allowing clinicians to make more accurate situation-specific predictions regarding an individual's behaviour.

Connotations of the word 'projective'

Since Freud (1920/1959) first wrote about the 'projection' of unwanted aspects of the self, tests that aim to gather information regarding these aspects of the self or personality have been called projective tests. For decades personality tests have been classified by psychologists as being either *objective* or *projective*. These terms have become entrenched in academic literature and psychological discourse; however, debate has recently begun around whether these terms are in fact accurate. According to Meyer and Kurtz (2006, p.223), '[i]n the interest of advancing the science of personality assessment, we believe it is time to end this historical practice and retire these terms from our formal lexicon and general discourse describing the methods of personality assessment'.

Meyer and Kurtz (2006) argue that the terms 'objective' and 'projective' are misleading and carry unfair connotations. Certain researchers and clinicians feel that the fact that the term 'objective' implies accuracy and a lack of bias has contributed to 'projective' tests being regarded as inferior forms of assessment. Meyer and Kurtz (2006) state that it is important to remember that although 'objective assessments' rely considerably less on the judgement of assessors to interpret the examinee's response (as the response is usually one of a limited choice of responses and scored according to a pre-existing key), the judgement of the examinee is still a factor that needs to be taken into account. These tests rely on the examinee's ability to negotiate the ambiguity inherent in the test items, to evaluate herself, and to decide whether a characteristic describes her personality, and on her judgement regarding how honestly she should convey this information in her response. Meyer and Kurtz (2006, p.223) state that

> if the kind of self-report scales that are classified as objective actually were 'objective' in a meaningful sense of that word, then there would not be such a huge literature examining the various response styles and biases that affect scores derived from these instruments. In fact, the literature addressing the topic of response styles, malingering, and test bias in these measures appears larger than the literature on any other focused issue concerning their validity or application.

Meyer and Kurtz (2006) suggest that these forms of assessment should rather be called 'self-report' measures and that projective tests could be described by the term 'performance-based' tests.

Current use of projective assessments with children and adults

Many psychology graduate programmes include coverage of projective assessments or techniques (Cohen & Swerdlik, 2004), and according to Foxcroft et al. (2004) the most commonly used projective tests in psychiatric hospitals, psychotherapy centres, community clinics and private practice in South Africa are the Children's Apperception Test (CAT) (Bellak & Abrahams, 1997; Murray, 1943), the Draw-A-Person Test (DAP) (Goodenough, 1926; Harris, 1963), the Rorschach (Exner, 1993; Rorschach, 1942) and the TAT (Bellak & Abrahams, 1997; Murray, 1943). Other frequently used projective tests include the Rotter Incomplete Sentence Test (RISB) (Rotter, Lah & Rafferty, 1992), the Kinetic Family Drawing (KFD) (Burns & Kaufman, 1972) and the House-Tree-Person Test (HTP) (Buck, 1985; Goodenough, 1926; Harris, 1963). While the Rorschach and the TAT are used with adult populations, the CAT and DAP are used with children. The RISB is used in both populations; however, it is important to note that the RISB was originally developed and validated as a measure of adult psychosocial functioning (Weis, Toolis & Cerankosky, 2008), and that the use of the RISB with clinic-referred children and adolescents may be problematic due to the fact that although there are three versions of the RISB (one for adolescents, one for university students and one for adults), the scoring manual and normative data refer only to university students (Weis et al., 2008). When the test was originally developed, Rotter et al. (1992, p.59) stated that if used on populations other than university students, practitioners should 'exercise caution' during interpretation.

The clinical use of projective tests in South Africa tends to be for the purposes of screening for socio-emotional problems, to corroborate diagnoses, to obtain information about clients' personalities and to identify themes that may be addressed in treatment. The forensic use of projective assessments internationally and in South Africa, however, is more contentious, especially in the area of family court proceedings. While sometimes still used in forensic assessments, the reliability and validity of projective assessments have been questioned in numerous articles in both social science and law journals (Eaton, 2004; Emery, Otto & O'Donohue, 2006; Erickson, 2003; Erickson et al., 2007; Tippins, 2005; Tippins & Wittmann, 2005). It is acknowledged that psychologists provide a valuable service in legal proceedings, providing insight into the behaviours of those standing accused and their fitness to stand trial or their ability to distinguish between right and wrong, and through offering opinions in custody cases fraught with complex emotional issues. However, while contention and doubt exist as to the reliability and validity of projective assessments, caution is recommended with regard to the use of projective tests in forensic assessments. In the USA the Daubert ruling applies in all federal courts and most state courts, and holds that the judge is required to evaluate the substance of the expert testimony, closely scrutinising the expert's method and qualifications before permitting the jury to hear it (Hoyt & Aalberts, 1997). Due to a lack of scientific evidence of reliability and validity, projective tests do not meet the Daubert requirements. In South Africa, the classification, possession, control and use of psychological tests and other devices used for assessing individuals is strictly controlled by two sets of legislation. The one set is that which includes the Constitution of the Republic of South Africa (Act No. 108 of 1996), the Labour Relations Act No. 66 of 1995 and the Employment Equity Act No. 55 of 1998. These Acts deal with matters of individuals' rights, both generally and in the workplace. The second set of legislation is contained in the Health Professions Act, in which the scope of the profession of psychology and the responsibilities and functions of psychologists are addressed within the context of health care in the country (Mauer, 2000). With regard to psychological assessment in the workplace, Section 8 of the Employment Equity Act states: 'Psychological testing and other similar assessments of an employee are prohibited unless the test or assessment being used – (a) has been scientifically shown to be valid and reliable; (b) can be applied fairly to all employees; (c) is not biased against any employee or group' (Mauer, 2000, p.5). Projective tests do not meet these criteria; therefore it is not permitted to use them within a nonclinical setting.

Interpreting projective assessments

When analysing and interpreting projective data, there are two broad approaches. The first is a more objective approach and entails using a specific scoring technique or a scoring blank. The second approach is more subjective, and consists of either a content analysis or a more interpretive approach based on a theoretical framework, which is most often psychoanalytic. Sometimes a combination of a content analysis and an interpretive approach is used. With regard to objective scoring techniques, the most widely used scoring system for the Rorschach is the Exner (1993) system of scoring. For information on the scoring and interpretation of the TAT and projective drawings, see chapters 25 and 26 in this volume respectively. In relation to the more subjective methods of interpretation, content analysis is a well-documented method and entails an examination of the content of examinees' responses in order to identify recurring themes. It is important to note, however, that the subjective interpretation of responses to projective stimuli is regarded as problematic in terms of reliability and validity (Wiederman, 1999). According to Dawes (1994), the information received about a client beforehand and the beliefs that this information creates about the client in the clinician's mind – for example, that the client is dependent – can bias a scorer's subjective interpretation. Holding certain beliefs about a particular examinee can influence the scorer to pay more attention to responses that fit with these beliefs, and pay less attention to responses that don't (Dawes, 1994). While subjective interpretation of responses on projective measures by experienced clinicians can lead to important insights into examinees' functioning, the general use of clinical judgement rather than norms and statistics to interpret projective tests seems to have led to a belief that projective assessments are deficient and unreliable, as results can be different each time a test is given to the same person, or depending on who interprets the protocol. However, many practitioners continue to rely on projective testing. Hence, for research purposes especially, it is important for users of projective measures to use objective scoring techniques in order to achieve adequate reliability and validity.

With regard to the interpretation of projective assessments used with children, it is essential to be sensitive to developmental trends and to be aware of what would constitute an age-appropriate response or performance. For example, when using the DAP or Kinetic Family Drawings (KFDs), it is important to bear in mind the child's age and current level of development when interpreting drawings. According to Vinter (1999) developmental trends, although highly sensitive to context, appear to emerge in drawing, whether it is the 'what' or the 'how' of drawing that is considered. It is also important to consider cultural influences when interpreting children's drawings. See chapter 26 for more specific information with regard to children's developmental age and cultural influences on drawing styles.

The benefits of using projective techniques

Projective techniques are versatile and are used within a wide range of applications, such as assessment, research and psychotherapy. Once respondents adjust to the initial surprise or embarrassment at what they are required to do, projective techniques can be more fun for respondents than cognitive assessments or self-report questionnaires, and are even sometimes used in order to establish therapeutic rapport with clients (Anastasi & Urbina, 2007). Projective tests can access feelings, perceptions and attitudes that might be more difficult to access using more direct questioning techniques, and can also be a rich source of new ideas for researchers (Catterall & Ibbotson, 2000; Oppenheim, 1992). While long questionnaires with little variety in response format can bore and demotivate respondents, projective techniques tend to generate respondent curiosity because they are intriguing (Catterall & Ibbotson, 2000). Cramer (2004) states that the value of storytelling has been rediscovered in psychology due to dissatisfaction with self-report questionnaires on psychological functioning. Projective techniques have been found to be particularly useful in accessing children's and adolescents' perceptions of their reality, as these groups can rarely be engaged in conversation regarding their intrapsychic conflicts. Sunderland (2004) states that children's views and feelings find more complete representation through storytelling than through direct statement. Children tend to find more creative and spontaneous ways to communicate their feelings and their conflicts, and telling stories or drawing are often more effective methods of accessing these feelings (Brandell, 2000).

The disadvantages of projective tests

Some projective tests are used less often today because administration and scoring is time-intensive, and because the reliability and validity of these assessments is considered controversial. Projection plates of various kinds have been researched in more than a thousand psychological studies (Cramer, 2004), and while there have been a number of studies detailing the reliable use of these assessments (Costantino, Colon-Malgady, Malgady & Perez, 1991; Harris, 1963; Meyer, 2001; Riethmiller & Handler, 1997; Spangler, 1992; Weiner, 2005; Westen, 1991), there have also been a number of studies demonstrating the numerous pitfalls associated with projective testing, such as their sensitivity to context, the manner of administration and cross-cultural influences (Gregory, 2000; Grieve, 2003; Kaufman & Kaufman, 2001). Queries as to the cross-cultural applicability of projective tests are of particular relevance in South Africa; this issue will be discussed in more detail later in this chapter. Studies noting the variability of interpretations through lack of a uniform interpretation system have also been conducted (Ball, Archer & Imhof, 1994; Groth-Marnat, 2003; Hunsley, Lee & Wood, 2003; Jenkins, 2008; Rossini & Moretti, 1997; Teglasi, 2001). The Rorschach Inkblot Test, in particular, has been criticised for its lack of norms for subscales of the test. Despite the fact that global meta-analyses, which are mathematical combinations of all Rorschach test scores for a particular individual, show the Rorschach test to have a validity that may approach that of the Minnesota Multiphasic Personality Inventory-2 (MMPI-2) (Hiller, Rosenthal, Bornstein, Berry & Brunell-Neuleib, 1999), several studies have found that due to this lack of norms for individual subscales, results gained on specific test scales can lead psychologists to overestimate examinees' psychopathology (Shaffer, Erdberg & Haroian, 1999; Wood, Nezworski, Lilienfeld & Garb, 2003). Human figure drawings have also been criticised for their lack of norms, poor inter-rater reliability and failure to detect general psychopathology (Hunsley et al., 2003; Kahill, 1984; Lally, 2001; Riethmiller & Handler, 1997; Scribner & Handler, 1987).

The influence of socio-economic status and culture

In 1956, Rothney and Heimann documented the fact that Wedemeyer had achieved atypical and meagre Rorschach reports from 136 navy enlisted men of average intelligence, and that this was attributed to the fact that the examiner was female. Rothney and Heimann (1956) also described a study conducted by

Robin, Nelson and Clark, which found that the content of Rorschach responses is in part a function of current perceptual experience (the physical setting prior to which or in which testing occurs). Robin et al. (in Rothney & Heimann, 1956) compared the responses on the Rorschach of a group of US examinees who waited prior to testing in a room displaying either anatomical and medical photographs, or 'sexy' pictures, or in a room with bare walls. The study found that sexually related responses increased to an almost significant level for the first two groups, when compared to the third group who sat in a room with bare walls. Ehrenreich (1990) also found that socio-economic status can influence responses on the TAT. Differences were found between the responses of individuals from middle and lower socio-economic circumstances with regard to patterns of dependency and locus of control, with a lower socio-economic status being associated with more dependency and a more external locus of control. These kinds of findings have highlighted the need to take into account the culture and socio-economic status of examinees and the context in which testing takes place.

According to Bornstein (2002) it is important to conceptualise psychological assessment as a dynamic interpersonal process, in which assessment results are interpreted within the context in which they were obtained. This context includes the physical setting; the interpersonal milieu within which testing occurred; the language, and current and past cultural and socio-economic status of the examinee; and the wider societal environment. This statement is particularly relevant for South Africa, with its multilingual and multicultural population and history of apartheid. According to Foxcroft (2002, p.5), '[p]sychological testing was brought to Africa in the colonial era, and is not something that is indigenous to Africa and its peoples'. Hence Moletsane (2004) has voiced uncertainty about the use of measures developed internationally, and the validity and reliability of decisions about individuals that are based on these techniques. This is especially pertinent with regard to the projective tests commonly used in South Africa, the majority of which were developed internationally. The fact that tests are used on people who did not form a part of the norm group is problematic and renders the results questionable. The limited empirical certainty about the extent to which tests used in South Africa are culturally applicable and valid, and the lack of local research regarding test bias, have been recognised by the South African Professional Board for Psychology (Matthews & Bouwer, 2009), and for the past few years the Board has been encouraging psychologists to research the cultural bias associated with psychological tests and make the necessary adaptations (HPCSA, 2005).

Some research on the use of projective tests with African populations within South Africa has begun – for example, Matthews and Bouwer's (2009) study on the use of the TAT with South African adolescents. This study addressed a pitfall of the TAT when used cross-culturally with South African adolescents, in that 'psychologists presenting projection plates to adolescent clients in South Africa frequently obtain little more than one-liners from standard procedures, raising doubts about viability and reliability of the technique' (Matthews and Bouwers, 2009, p.231). Matthews and Bouwers developed a revised method of questioning and probing, called dynamic assessment (DA), that did not compromise the projective value of responses. The results of this study suggested that the use of DA with South African adolescents appeared to access deeper and broader projections in the form of richer stories. Moletsane and Eloff's (2006) study on the use of the Rorschach with black learners in South Africa also involved adjusting procedures used when administering the Rorschach Comprehensive System (RCS) to young South African learners. The study found that when standard procedures for conducting the RCS were used, half of the participants failed to provide the number of responses required for interpretation in terms of the Rorschach system. The adjustments made to the administration procedure considered possible inhibiting factors, and the response rates of participants increased significantly.

Other South African studies have not focused on adaptation of tests, but rather on examining the use of certain projective tests as is with a South African population. Makunga and Shange's (2009) study on whether projective drawings can provide a reliable method of exploring the worlds of black bereaved children in KwaZulu-Natal found that the emotional indicators on Human Figure Drawings (HFDs) reflected symptoms that are generally known as characterising bereaved individuals. According to Makunga and Shange (2009, p.27), results showed statistically significant differences between the two groups on four indicators in HFDs (big figure; teeth; monster/grotesque; hands cut off) and on two indicators in the Self Portraits (slanting figure and hands cut off). The KFDs and the children's Own Choice Drawings could not statistically differentiate the two groups, but were found to be useful with regard to gaining insight into the family dynamics of those in the bereaved group. Douglas's (2010) study into the use of KFDs with regard to attachment classifications with children in care in Johannesburg found that the KFD can be a helpful tool in the classification of children's attachment patterns, and can provide insight into children's current emotional functioning. Douglas's (2010) study aimed to examine the convergent validity between the KFD and a storytelling/narrative task and their associated scoring systems, in an effort to extend the research on measures of attachment employed during middle childhood, specifically within a South African context. According to Douglas (2010, p.25), '[t]he kinetic family drawing was scored using both the Kaplan and Main (1986) system and the Family Drawing Global Rating Scale (FDGRS) (Fury, Carlson & Sroufe, 1997); and the story telling/narrative task was scored using the Attachment Story Completion Task (ASCT) modified by Granot & Mayseless (2001)'. The study found that the Kaplan and Main scoring system requires a workshop and/or revision to improve inter-rater reliability and validity of the attachment-based measure, and that improved inter-rater reliability and validity can be achieved through the combined use of the Kaplan and Main scoring system and the FDGRS to assess children's family drawings. The attachment classifications that resulted from the combined classification from the Kaplan and Main scoring system and the FDGRS were shown to be highly significant to those yielded from the ASCT when using the Fisher's Exact Test ($p \leq 0.0001$). While this study is currently being prepared for publication, most South African studies have been conducted for either honours or Master's research dissertations and have not found their way into mainstream publications. However, it is hoped that future research in South Africa will focus on expanding this area of study and that publication will be encouraged.

Despite the fact that significant differences in the way that people from different cultural groups and groups of varying social status process information cognitively and emotionally have been documented on instruments such as the Rorschach (Krall et al., 1983), the TAT (Ehrenreich, 1990) and the DAP (Koppitz, 1968), research investigating cross-cultural differences on projective tests is relatively scarce, and the use of these tools internationally, without any standardised modification, continues (Anastasi & Urbina, 2007). In addition, most cross-cultural research appears to have occurred with groups of varying cultures outside of South Africa. A number of methodological weaknesses have also been found in these cross-cultural studies, where the effects of variables such as educational level, IQ, language and socio-economic status have not been taken into account, making it difficult to determine whether the differences found among varying cultural groups are due to real personality differences or to bias in the way the test is constructed (Van de Vijver & Tanzer, 2004).

Bias due to culture and language that occurs during the use of projective tests takes many forms. It includes administration bias, where language differences create communication problems with regard to instructions (Van de Vijver & Tanzer, 2004). Bias in cross-cultural testing situations may also arise from ethnocentric interpretations, where the examiner does not understand an aspect of an examinee's culture and the influence that this may have on her perception and interpretation of a particular projective stimulus (Banks, Ge & Baker, 1991). A common example of this within an African context relates to the issue of fertility. According to Dyer (2007), parenthood motives in African countries differ from those of parents in Western countries. In African countries 'children secure conjugal ties, offer social security, assist with labour, confer social status, secure rights of property and inheritance, provide continuity through re-incarnation and maintaining the family lineage, and satisfy emotional needs' (Dyer, 2007, p.69). Hence the meaning of desiring a baby could be interpreted very differently, depending on cultural attributions.

Tester effects are another potential source of administration bias, in that the mere presence of a person from a different culture can have a significant effect on respondents' behaviour (Singer & Presser, 1989). This is particularly pertinent in South Africa, given the country's history of racial tension. When conducting testing this needs to be carefully considered as, according to Foxcroft, Roodt and Abrahams (2001), the relationship between the examiner and the person being examined represents a power relationship in which the examiner holds most of the power; thus the client can be considered to be in a vulnerable position. Also, Van de Vijver and Tanzer (2004) state that projective techniques, questionnaires and interviews are the most likely to be affected by phenomena such as social desirability with regard to response styles, where examinees may censor their responses in order to appear socially acceptable to the examiner. In South Africa, with our history of racial tension, tester effects are particularly relevant, and it is likely that examinees will express more positive attitudes than they may normally do towards a particular cultural group if the examiner is from that group (Reese, Danielson, Shoemaker, Chang & Hsu, 1986). In this regard, the impact of meta-stereotypes also needs to be taken into account.

Meta-stereotypes can be defined as 'the stereotypes that members of a group believe that members of an out-group hold of them' (Finchilescu, 2005, p.465). Thus, how an examinee perceives the tester is thinking about the examinee may also influence the examinee's behaviour.

Another difficulty facing the users of projective measures in South Africa is acculturation (Van de Vijver & Tanzer, 2004), which refers to the degree to which an individual begins to adopt the cultural characteristics of a new culture, usually the dominant culture in her place of residence. The effects of acculturation have been examined in populations internationally and it has been found that while recent immigrants to a country tend to display similar emotional patterns to their culture of origin, second- and third-generation or other highly acculturated individuals tend to display the characteristics of the new culture within which they are living (Liem, Lim & Lien, 2000). In South Africa, increasing urbanisation and Westernisation have resulted in many individuals adopting norms and beliefs of a variety of cultures, making it difficult for examiners to know which cultural context to use when interpreting results.

Ethical issues to consider before using projective tests in the South African context

Ethical testing practices are highlighted in the International Guidelines for Test Use developed by the International Test Commission (ITC, 2001). According to these guidelines, ethical assessment practices require that the examiner 'use tests appropriately, professionally, and in an ethical manner, paying due regard for the needs and rights of those involved in the testing process, and the broader context in which the testing takes place' (2000, p.6). However, according to Foxcroft et al.'s (2004) survey, clinicians using projective tests within the South African context have expressed concern regarding 'the adequacy of the training that practitioners receive in projective tests and also the cultural appropriateness of some projective tests' (p.134). Hence, the need to pay due regard to the broader social and cultural context is especially significant within the South African context, where sensitivity to examinees' cultural backgrounds and values is required during all phases of assessment – namely, test selection, administration, interpretation and reporting phases of the testing process (Foxcroft, 2002).

As postmodernism has developed and emphasised the possibility of multiple truths, objectivity in assessment has been questioned. Given this paradigmatic shift, Bornstein (2002, p.60) has suggested that the heuristic value of test data can be increased 'if the dynamics of the testing situation are scrutinized (or even manipulated) instead of being statistically controlled (or worse, ignored)'. In other words, it is essential to acknowledge that testing cannot be absolutely objective, and for results to reflect as closely as possible the examinee's reality, examiners need to acknowledge and take into account the effects of the examinee's and examiner's subjectivities, the effects of culture and language and the effects of the broader context of testing. Foxcroft (2002) states that examiners should never presume to know how best to assess or interpret aspects of human functioning without first having knowledge of the lived world of the examinee. This implies adopting an emic approach to testing, which is one in which thought and behaviour are examined using criteria that are related to a specific culture, as opposed to using criteria that are presumed to be universal, which is representative of an etic approach (Foxcroft, 2002).

Using projective assessments within the South African context

There are a number of ways in which practitioners can approach projective testing that may improve the ethical respectfulness and methodological soundness of results. The first of these is to be aware of the limitations of tests with regard to their cross-cultural use. According to Moletsane (2004), cross-cultural assessment is difficult to conduct and requires special reflection to ensure appropriate interpretation. Next, it is important to ensure that when testing, the practitioner has a thorough knowledge of the client's current and previous social and cultural context. This can be done through immersing oneself in the examinee's world (Foxcroft, 2002). According to Foxcroft (2002, p.13), '[t]he learning that I have gained ... is that being well prepared and being sensitive to the test-taker's community and cultural background lies at the very heart of following ethical testing practices in multicultural contexts, in Africa and elsewhere in the world'. This immersion can be accomplished through visiting the examinee's broader environment – for example, their village, township, workplace, hospital or shelter – or through asking about it. Ivey, Ivey and Simek-Morgan (1997) recommend using community and family genograms in order to gain greater understanding of the cultural factors involved in individual and family development within particular families and cultures. According to Van de Vijver and Tanzer (2004), the use of informants with a good knowledge of the local culture and language helps to deal with both construct and method bias in cross-cultural assessment. It is also important for the examiners to be well trained in the administration and interpretation of tests in order to decrease method bias (Van de Vijver & Tanzer, 2004), and to be very familiar with the specific test intended for use and with common patterns of tester–testee interactions, as then any differences in interaction that occur can be examined and taken into account.

Another important way to approach projective testing in a more ethical and methodologically sound manner is to be aware of the influence of the examiner. It can be helpful to acknowledge that a difference in culture and language may make it more difficult for an examinee to understand instructions or express himself clearly. Establishing a strong rapport before attempting projective testing can also minimise tester effects, as examinees may then feel free to clarify aspects that they do not understand or feel that the examiner does not understand. The use of interpreters should also be handled with thought and sensitivity. Despite extensive training, interpreters are often still faced with difficulties in fully capturing expressions and meanings across languages (Foxcroft, 2002).

Conclusion

Projective assessment in South Africa remains controversial and yet clinically popular, as it invites dynamic expression of thoughts, feelings and conflicts, acknowledging the complexity of individual psychology. In this chapter the points have been highlighted that projective tests seem to be most effectively conducted within a battery of other tests, such as intelligence and self-report or objective personality measures, and that results are best interpreted within the particular individual's context. While it is hoped that future research in South Africa will focus on the cross-cultural applicability of these tests, in order to use the tests in the most ethical manner possible, it is recommended that awareness of the influences of culture, history and context are foremost in practitioners' minds when deciding to use or administer a projective test, or interpret the results.

References

Anastasi, A. & Urbina, S. (2007). *Psychological Testing* (7th edition). Delhi: Pearson Education & Dorling Kindersley (India).

Ball, J. D., Archer, R. P. & Imhof, E. A. (1994). Time requirements of psychological testing: A survey of practitioners. *Journal of Personality Assessment, 63*, 239–249.

Banks, S. P., Ge, G. & Baker, J. (1991). Intercultural encounters and miscommunication. In N. Coupland, H. Giles & J. M. Wiemann (Eds), *Miscommunication and Problematic Talk* (pp. 103–120). Newbury Park, CA: Sage.

Bellak, L. & Abrams, D. M. (1997). *The TAT, the CAT and the SAT in Clinical Use* (6th edition). Boston, MA: Allyn and Bacon.

Bellenger, D. N., Bernhardt, K. L. & Goldstucker, J. L. (1976). *Qualitative Marketing Research.* Chicago, IL: American Marketing Association.

Bornstein, R. F. (2002). A process dissociation approach to objective–projective test score interrelationships. *Journal of Personality Assessment, 78(1)*, 47–68.

Brandell, J. R. (2000). *Of Mice and Metaphors.* New York, NY: Basic Books.

Buck, J. (1985). *The House-Tree-Person Technique: Revised Manual.* Los Angeles, CA: Western Psychological Services.

Burns, R. C. & Kaufman, S. H. (1972). *Action, Styles and Symbols in Kinetic Family Drawings (KFD): An Interpretive Manual.* New York, NY: Brunner/Mazel.

Catterall, M. & Ibbotson, P. (2000). Using projective techniques in education research. *British Educational Research Journal, 26(2)*, 245–256.

Cohen, R. J. & Swerdlik, M. E. (2004). *Psychological Testing and Assessment* (6th edition). New York, NY: McGraw-Hill.

Costantino, G., Colon-Malgady, G., Malgady, R. G. & Perez, A. (1991). Assessment of attention deficit disorder using a thematic apperception technique. *Journal of Personality Assessment, 57*, 87–95.

Cramer, P. (2004). *Storytelling, Narrative, and the Thematic Apperception Test.* New York, NY: The Guilford Press.

Dawes, R. M. (1994). *House of Cards: Psychology and Psychotherapy Built on Myth.* New York, NY: Free Press.

Douglas, D. (2010). Representations of attachment in the kinetic family drawings of children in care: A pilot study. Unpublished honours mini-dissertation. University of the Witwatersrand, Johannesburg.

Dyer, S. J. (2007). The value of children in African countries – insights from studies on infertility. *Journal of Psychosomatic Obstetrics & Gynecology, 28(2)*, 69–77.

Eaton, L. (2004). For arbiters in custody battles, wide power and little scrutiny. *New York Times*, May 23. Retrieved May, 2010, from http://www.nytimes.com.

Ehrenreich, J. H. (1990). Effect of social class of subjects on normative responses to TAT cards. *Journal of Clinical Psychology, 46(4)*, 467–471.

Emery, R. E., Otto, R. K. & O'Donohue, W. T. (2006). A critical assessment of child custody evaluations: Limited science and a flawed system. *Psychological Science in the Public Interest, 6*, 1–29.

Erickson, S. (2003). Psychological testimony on trial: Questions arise about the validity of popular testing methods. *New York State Bar Journal, 75(6)*, 19–26.

Erickson, S. K., Lilienfeld, S. O. & Vitacco, M. J. (2007). A critical examination of the suitability and limitations of psychological tests in family court. *Family Court Review, 45(2)*, 157–174.

Exner, J. E. (1993). *The Rorschach: A Comprehensive System. Volume 1: Basic Foundations*. New York, NY: John Wiley & Sons.

Finchilescu, G. (2005). Meta-stereotypes may hinder inter-racial contact. *South African Journal of Psychology, 35*, 460–472.

Foxcroft, C. D. (2002). Ethical issues related to psychological testing in Africa: What I have learned (so far). In W. J. Lonner, D. L. Dinnel, S. A. Hayes & D. N. Sattler (Eds), *Online Readings in Psychology and Culture* (Unit 5, Chapter 4). Center for Cross-cultural Research, Western Washington University, Bellingham, Washington, USA. Retrieved July 20, 2010, from http://www.wwu.edu/~culture.

Foxcroft, C., Paterson, H., Le Roux, N. & Herbst, D. (2004). *Psychological Assessment in South Africa: A Needs Analysis. The Test Use Patterns and Needs of Psychological Assessment Practitioners*. Pretoria: Human Sciences Research Council.

Foxcroft, C. D., Roodt, G. & Abrahams, F. (2001). The practice of psychological assessment: Controlling the use of measures, competing values, and ethical practice standards. In C. D. Foxcroft & G. Roodt (Eds), *An Introduction to Psychological Assessment in the South African Context* (pp. 93–105). Cape Town: Oxford University Press.

Freud, S. (1920/1959). *Beyond the Pleasure Principle*. New York, NY: Norton.

Goodenough, F. (1926). *Measurement of Intelligence by Drawings*. New York, NY: Harcourt, Brace & World.

Gregory, R. J. (2000). *Psychological Testing* (3rd edition). Boston, MA: Allyn and Bacon.

Grieve, K. W. (2003). Factors affecting assessment results. In C. Foxcroft & G. Roodt (Eds), *An Introduction to Psychological Assessment in the South African Context* (pp. 224–241). Cape Town: Oxford University Press.

Groth-Marnat, G. (2003). *Handbook of Psychological Assessment* (4th edition). Hoboken, NJ: John Wiley & Sons.

Harris, D. B. (1963). *Children's Drawings as Measures of Intellectual Maturity*. New York, NY: Harcourt, Brace & World.

Hiller, J. B., Rosenthal, R., Bornstein, R. F., Berry, D. T. R. & Brunell-Neulieb, S. (1999). A comparative meta-analysis of Rorschach and MMPI validity. *Psychological Assessment, 11*, 278–296.

Hoyt, R.W. & Aalberts, R. J. (1997). New requirement for the appraisal expert witness. *Appraisal Journal, 65(4)*, 342–350.

HPCSA (Health Professions Council of South Africa) (2005). *Form 208. Policy on the Classification of Psychometric Measuring Devices, Instruments, Methods and Techniques.* Pretoria: Health Professions Council of South Africa.

Hunsley, J., Lee, C. M. & Wood, J. M. (2003). Controversial and questionable assessment techniques. In S. O. Lilienfeld, J. M. Lohr & S. J. Lynn (Eds), *Science and Pseudoscience in Contemporary Clinical Psychology* (pp. 39–76). New York, NY: The Guilford Press.

ITC (International Test Commission) (2000). International guidelines for test use. Retrieved 16 July 2010, from http://www.intestcom.org.

Ivey, A. E., Ivey, M. B. & Simek-Morgan, L. (1997). *Counselling and Psychotherapy: A Multicultural Perspective* (4th edition). Boston, MA: Allyn and Bacon.

Jenkins, S. R. (2008). *A Handbook of Clinical Scoring Systems for Thematic Apperceptive Techniques*. New York, NY: Lawrence Erlbaum Associates.

Kahill, S. (1984). Human figure drawing in adults: An update of the empirical evidence, 1967–1982. *Canadian Psychology, 25*, 269–292.

Kaufman, A. S. & Kaufman, N. L. (2001). Series Preface. In H. Teglasi, *Essentials of TAT and Other Storytelling Techniques Assessment* (pp. vii–viii). New York, NY: John Wiley & Sons.

Koppitz, E. M. (1968). *Psychological Evaluation of Children's Human Figure Drawing*. New York, NY: Grune & Stratton.

Krall, V., Sachs, H., Lazar, B., Rayson, B., Growe, G., Novar, L. & O'Connell, L. (1983). Rorschach norms for inner-city children. *Journal of Personality Assessment, 47*, 155–157.

Lally, S. J. (2001). Should human figure drawings be admitted into court? *Journal of Personality Assessment, 76*, 135–149.

Liem, R., Lim, B. A. & Lien, J. H. (2000). Acculturation and emotion among Asian Americans. *Cultural Diversity and Mental Health, 61*, 13–31.

Makunga, N. V. & Shange, L. O. (2009). Drawings as a method of evaluation and communication with bereaved children. *Inkanyiso, Journal of Human and Social Sciences, 1(1)*, 27–33.

Matthews, L. & Bouwer, C. (2009). Enhancing adolescents' responses to projection plates through a dynamic assessment technique of questioning. *South African Journal of Psychology, 39(2)*, 231–241.

Mauer, K. F. (2000). *Psychological Test Use In South Africa.* Retrieved February 8, 2011, from http://www.pai.org.za/Psychological%20test%20use%20in%20South%20Africa.pdf.

McClelland, D. C., Koestner, R. & Weinberger, J. (1989). How do self-attributed and implicit motives differ? *Psychological Review, 96*, 690–702.

Meyer, G. J. (2001). Evidence to correct misperceptions about Rorschach norms. *Clinical Psychology: Science and Practice, 8*, 389–396.

Meyer, G. J. & Kurtz, J. E. (2006). Advancing personality assessment terminology: Time to retire 'objective' and 'projective' as personality test descriptors. *Journal of Personality Assessment, 87*, 223–225.

Moletsane, M. K. (2004). The efficacy of the Rorschach amongst black learners in South Africa. Unpublished PhD dissertation. University of Pretoria, Pretoria.

Moletsane, M. K. & Eloff, I. (2006). The adjustment of Rorschach Comprehensive System procedures for South African learners. *South African Journal of Psychology, 36(4)*, 880–902.

Morgan, C. D. & Murray, H. A. (1935). A method for investigating fantasies: The Thematic Apperception Test. *Archives of Neurological Psychiatry, 34*, 289–306.

Murray, H. A. (1943). *Thematic Apperception Test Manual*. Cambridge, MA: Harvard University Press.

Oppenheim, A. N. (1992). *Questionnaire Design and Attitude Measurement*. London: Pinter Publishers.

Piotrowski, C., Keller, J. W. & Ogawa, T. (1993). Projective techniques: An international perspective. *Psychological Reports, 72*, 179–182.

Pruitt, J. A., Smith, M. C., Thelen, M. H. & Lubin, B. (1985). Attitudes of academic clinical psychologists toward projective techniques: 1963–1983. *Professional Psychology: Research and Practice, 16*, 781–788.

Reese, S. D., Danielson, W. A., Shoemaker, P. J., Chang, T. & Hsu, H.-L. (1986). Ethnicity-of-interviewer effects among Mexican-Americans and Anglos. *Public Opinion Quarterly, 50*, 563–572.

Riethmiller, R. J. & Handler, L. (1997). The great figure drawing controversy: The integration of research and clinical practice. *Journal of Personality Assessment, 69*, 488–496.

Rook, D. W. (2006). Let's pretend: Projective methods reconsidered. In R. W. Belk (Ed.), *Handbook of Qualitative Research Methods in Marketing* (pp. 143–155). Northampton, MA: Edward Elgar Publishing.

Rorschach, H. (1942). *Psychodiagnostics* (5th edition). Berne: Verlag Hans Huber.

Rossini, E. & Moretti, R. (1997). Thematic Apperception Test (TAT) interpretation: Practice recommendations from a survey of clinical psychology doctoral programs accredited by the American Psychological Association. *Professional Psychology: Research and Practice, 28*, 393–398.

Rothney, J. W. M. & Heimann, R. A. (1956). Development and applications of projective technics. *Review of Educational Research, 26(1)*, 56–71.

Rotter, J. B., Lah, M. I. & Rafferty, J. E. (1992). *Rotter Incomplete Sentences Blank: Manual* (2nd edition). San Antonio, TX: Psychological Corporation.

Schacter, D. L. (1992). Understanding implicit memory: A cognitive neuroscience approach. *American Psychologist, 47*, 559–569.

Scribner, C. M. & Handler, L. (1987). The interpreter's personality in Draw-A-Person interpretation: A study of interpersonal style. *Journal of Personality Assessment, 51*, 112–122.

Shaffer, T. W., Erdberg, P. & Haroian, J. (1999). Current nonpatient data for the Rorschach, WAIS-R, and MMPI-2. *Journal of Personality Assessment, 73*, 305–316.

Singer, E. & Presser, S. (1989). The interviewer. In E. Singer & S. Presser (Eds), *Survey Research Methods* (pp. 245–246). Chicago, IL: University of Chicago Press.

Smith, G. H. (1954). *Motivation Research in Advertising and Marketing*. New York, NY: McGraw-Hill.

Spangler, W. D. (1992). Validity of questionnaire and TAT measures of need for achievement: Two meta-analyses. *Psychological Bulletin, 112*, 140–154.

Sunderland, M. (2004). *Using Story Telling as a Therapeutic Tool with Children*. Oxon: Speechmark Publishing.

Teglasi, H. (2001). *Essentials of TAT and Other Storytelling Techniques Assessment*. New York, NY: John Wiley & Sons.

Tippins, T. M. (2005). Custody evaluations, part XI: 'Daubert' and the rise of empiricism. *New York Law Journal*, March, 3–12.

Tippins, T. M. & Wittmann, J. P. (2005). Empirical and ethical problems with custody recommendations: A call for clinical humility and judicial vigilance. *Family Court Review, 43*, 193–218.

Van de Vijver, F. & Tanzer, N. K. (2004). Bias and equivalence in cross-cultural assessment: An overview. *European Review of Applied Psychology, 54*, 119–135.

Vinter, A. (1999). How meaning modifies drawing behavior in children. *Child Development, 70(1)*, 33–49.

Wagner, E. E. (2008). Beyond 'objective' and 'projective': A logical system for classifying psychological tests. Comment on Meyer and Kurtz (2006). *Journal of Personality Assessment, 90(4)*, 402–405.

Weinberger, J. & McClelland, D. C. (1990). Cognitive versus traditional motivational models: Irreconcilable or complementary? In R. Sorrentino & E. T. Higgins (Eds), *Handbook of Motivation and Cognition* (pp. 562–597). New York, NY: Academic.

Weiner, I. B. (2005). Some observations of the reliability of the Rorschach inkblot method. *Psychological Assessment, 8*, 206–213.

Weis, R., Toolis, E. E. & Cerankosky, B. E. (2008). Construct validity of the Rotter Incomplete Sentences Blank with clinic-referred and nonreferred adolescents. *Journal of Personality Assessment, 90(6)*, 564–573.

Westen, D. (1991). Clinical assessment of object relations using the TAT. *Journal of Personality Assessment, 56*, 56–74.

Westen, D. (1999). The scientific status of unconscious processes: Is Freud really dead? *Journal of the American Psychoanalytic Association, 47(4)*, 1061–1106.

Wiederman, M. W. (1999). A classroom demonstration of potential biases in the subjective interpretation of projective tests. *Teaching of Psychology, 26(1)*, 37–39.

Wood, J. M., Nezworski, M. T., Lilienfeld, S. & Garb, H. (2003). *What's Wrong with the Rorschach? Science Confronts the Controversial Inkblot Test*. San Francisco, CA: Jossey-Bass.

25 The use of the Children's Apperception Test and Thematic Apperception Test in South Africa

R. Gericke, K. Bain and Z. Amod

This chapter explores the practice and cross-cultural application of two thematic projective techniques, the Children's Apperception Test (CAT) and the Thematic Apperception Test (TAT). A brief introduction to, and definition of, thematic storytelling techniques is followed by discussions on reliability and validity, test administration and clinical application. The chapter has a strong focus on clinical application within a South African context and provides guidelines for clinicians. The focus on case material also allows the utility of these tests to be illustrated in depth.

The development of apperception testing

The origin of projective testing was Herman Rorschach's (1924a; 1924b) accidental discovery that people automatically and unconsciously project their own hidden desires, fears, wishes, feelings, conflicts and attitudes onto unstructured stimuli. As with individual interpretations given to a work of art, so we canvas our experiences, perceptions and reflections from an internal palette. He termed this process 'apperception' (Rorschach, 1924b, p.359). The concept 'projection', however, developed from Freud's (1938) theory of the unconscious and of the consequent use of projection as a defence. Freud conceived of the unconscious as a repository of instincts, wishes and fantasies deemed unacceptable to consciousness, thereby becoming the object of repression, hidden from conscious awareness. These unacceptable feelings and impulses are projected outside the self so that, for example, a group of people are experienced in a certain way that is more telling of the subject than of the other. To quote Freud, 'experience shows that we understand very well how to interpret in other people ... the same acts which we refuse to acknowledge as being mental in ourselves' (1955, p.171). Projective assessments are therefore administered to describe a person's subjective experience of him- or herself, and relationships with others and the world, often in response to queries about the psychological underpinnings of reported emotional and/or behavioural problems, or to assist with diagnosing emotional disturbances.

Morgan and Murray (1935) also referred to the process as 'apperception' and described a technique for investigating fantasies in their introduction to the TAT. Subsequent to this initial introduction, the TAT has seen numerous revisions, inclusion of scoring systems and development of an apperception test specifically tailored for use with children (Bellak, 1944; 1954; 1971; 1975; 1986; 1993; Bellak & Abrams, 1997; Bellak & Bellak, 1949; 1965).

The TAT

The TAT comprises 31 ambiguous pictures portraying everyday life situations. Clinicians typically administer 10 to 12 cards in a session. The ambiguity allows the participant to reveal him- or herself, as a direct relationship between perception and personality is assumed to hold. Bellak and Abrams (1997) recommend administering a standard battery comprising cards 1, 2, 3BM, 4, 6BM, 7BM, 11, 12M and 13MF to males, and 1, 2, 3BM, 4, 6GF, 7GF, 9GF, 11 and 13MF to females, which can then be added to. The batteries recommended for children are: 1, 3BM, 7GF, 8BM, 12BM, 13B, 14 and 17BM; and for adolescents, 1, 2, 5, 7GF, 12F, 12M, 15, 17BM, 18BM and 18GF (Obrzut & Boliek, 1986). To decide on the battery, one should consider the reasons for referral and the participant's history. For example, if assessing an adolescent who complains of an over-involved mother, one may want to include card 5, which facilitates narratives of an intrusive mother. Card 13B evokes rich clinical material from children, adolescents and adults. Card 14 is often a useful prognostic indicator for success of engagement with a therapeutic process. The stimuli provided by the recommended cards and Bellak's scoring categories are presented in Tables 25.1 and 25.2. No objective scoring system has, however, been developed (Dana, 1982). When interpreting responses, one should consider the stimulus pull of the cards and whether the pull to a particular story is strong, such as with cards 4 and 13MF.

The original instruction given to children by Murray was as follows:

> This is a story-telling test. I have some pictures here that I am going to show you, and for each picture I want you to make up a story. Tell me what has happened before and what is happening now. Say what the people are feeling and thinking and how it will come out. You can make up any kind of story you please. (1943, p.4)

Spreen and Strauss (1998) recommend a similar instruction for low-functioning or low-education adults, more clearly asking participants to state how the story will end. The instruction is elaborated for adolescents and higher-functioning adults to invite more fantasy projection. They begin the instruction as follows:

> We have here a test to study fantasy. I will show you some pictures, and for each picture I want you to make up as dramatic a story as you can. Please look at the picture and tell me what happens in the picture at the moment – what the people in the picture are thinking, feeling, planning to do. Please make a complete story, inventing how it came to this situation, what happened before, how it developed further, and how it came out in the end. (pp.652–653)

Missing story elements are queried once the participant has completed their story.

Table 25.1 Popular TAT cards and their abbreviated stimulus pull

1	Relationship with parental figures
	Achievement or mastery drives
	Body or self-image
	Obsessive preoccupations
2	Family relations
	Autonomy versus compliance with the conservative
	Oedipal issues
	Sexuality
	Compulsive tendencies
	Role of the sexes
3BM	Aggression (inwardly or outwardly directed) or defended against
	Depression
	Suicidality
	Latent homosexuality
4	Male-female relationships
	Sexuality
	Triangular jealousy
	Minority groups
5	Watchful/*intrusive** mother
	Masturbation guilt
	Voyeuristic material
	Fear of attack
	Rescue fantasies
6BM	Mother-son relationships
6GF	*The role of females*
	Relationship of females to the father
7BM	Father-son relationship
7GF	Mother-daughter relationship
8BM	Aggression
	Ambition or mastery
9GF	Sibling rivalry
	Mother-daughter hostility
	Paranoia
11	Infantile or primitive fears
	Oral aggression
12M	Relationship of a younger man to an older man
	Homosexual fears

continued →

13B	Stories of childhood
	Abandonment
	Loneliness
13MF	Sexual conflict in both men and women
	Economic deprivation
	Oral deprivation
	Obsessive-compulsive tendencies
14	Suicidal tendencies
	Depression
	Fears in relation to darkness
	Sexual identification
	Prognostic indicator
17BM	Oedipal fears
	Homosexual feelings
	Competitiveness
	Body image

Source: Bellak and Abrams (1997).

Note: * Italics indicates stimulus pull; added by the authors.

Table 25.2 Bellak's ten scoring categories for the TAT and CAT

The main theme	This can be on both a conscious, descriptive level as well as an unconscious, interpretative level.
The main hero	The character who is mostly spoken about and whose feelings are described, usually the closest to the participant in age and sex. Secondary figures may express unconscious attitudes. Adequacy of the hero to accomplish tasks is often an indication of ego strength.
Main needs and drives of the hero	Does the hero experience needs as being gratified or frustrated? Are expressed needs fantasy needs prohibited from expression due to cultural sanctions or reality-based behaviours – for example, aggression or sexual activity versus autonomy strivings? The first three variables provide a description of the unconscious structure and needs of the subject.
Conception of the environment	Examples are: hostile, demanding, violent, supportive or caring.
Social relationships	The attitude of the hero towards parental figures, peers, and so forth.
Significant conflicts (between drives and superego)	What is the nature of these conflicts and what defences are employed against them?
Nature of anxieties and defences employed	Examples are: denial, intellectualisation, identification, projection, passive-aggression, acting out, displacement, splitting, regression, somatisation, withdrawal, omnipotence, humour, identification, affiliation and repression.

Main defences against conflicts and fears	The defensive structure may account for observed behaviours or reasons for referral.
Adequacy of superego	Indicated by 'punishment' for 'crimes' committed – severity of the superego is indicated by the relationship between type of punishment and severity of offence.
Integration of ego	The extent to which the demands of the id, reality and superego are integrated. Coping ability is indicated by how well the hero is able to deal with problems. Attempts by the storyteller to distance self from the story reveal a weak ego that is not able to deal with the emotional stimuli of the story.

Source: Bellak and Abrams (1997).

The CAT

Children and adolescents are often unable to say what is troubling them, or unable to verbalise their feelings (Smith & Handler, 2007), whilst parents and teachers are also often unable to articulate the complex psychological processes under investigation (Kelly, 2007). The CAT is available in three forms – a human form and two animal forms – as preferred identification figures for children. The animal form is often preferred for the younger child. The CAT is usually administered to children aged 3 to 10 or 11 for cognitively lower-functioning children, while the TAT is administered to adolescents and adults. While this is a rule of thumb, the decision as to which test to administer needs to be informed by clinical judgement as the TAT can be administered to children as young as six (Kelly, 2007). Although the pictures are felt by some to be inappropriate for young children (Cashel, Killilea & Dollinger, 2007), for others the TAT is the preferred apperception test for children (Cramer, 1996; Teglasi, 1993). The CAT consists of ten black-and-white picture cards administered in sequential order (Table 25.3).

For both the TAT and the CAT, one card at a time must be revealed by laying it down on a desk in front of the subject of the test. The instruction is: 'I am going to show you some pictures and I want you to tell me a story about what you think is happening in the picture.' The assessor should explain to the child that this is not a test of their abilities, and provide encouragement and prompts throughout the process of the test. When the child has completed the story, the assessor should ask 'Who is your favourite person?' and 'How is that person feeling?' If necessary, the assessor should provide prompts such as *sad, cross, scared, happy* or *worried*. It is useful to ask whom the child likes the most in the picture, as the protagonist is not as clear in the CAT as in the TAT. As with the TAT, the responses should be transcribed verbatim. Once the test has been completed, the assessor can return to stories and question elements of them as necessary.

Table 25.3 CAT cards and their abbreviated stimulus pull

1	Relationship with mother figure
	Oral gratification
	Sibling rivalry
2	Family conflict / anger and how it is resolved
	Relationship with anger and aggression
	Parent identified with
	Discipline
	Castration fears
3	Relationship with father figure
	Vulnerability
4	Sibling rivalry
	Place in the family
	Origin of babies
	Relation to mother
	Independence
5	Oedipal issues
6	*Feelings of rejection*
	Jealousy
	Masturbation
7	Fears of aggression and how it is dealt with / Is it inwardly or outwardly directed?
	Hostility
8	How are children viewed in the family?
9	Abandonment issues
	Fear of attack
10	Toilet training issues
	How are children disciplined? Superego functioning
	Masturbation
	Regression

Source: Bellak and Bellak (1949).

Note: Italics indicates stimulus pull; added by the authors.

Assessing object relations

The Social Cognition and Object Relations Scale – Revised (SCOR-R) is an interpretative paradigm analysing TAT stories according to six dimensions that are then quantitatively scored (Kelly, 2007). In object relations theory 'objects' refer to an infant's experiences of caregivers or parts of caregivers that are internalised, initially as concrete objects due to the fact that infants experience their world in a concrete way (Rustin, Rustin & Shuttleworth, 1989). These early experiences with caregivers form internal representations of expected interpersonal ways of relating. Object relations can be assessed interpretively or by applying a psychometrically validated scale of object relations, the SCOR-R. An interpretive approach would focus on the relationships between the subject and primary figures (peers, love objects, parental figures, authority figures, siblings, sexual partners) described in the stories. The assessor would be interested in who is perceived to be doing what to whom in these interactions. The SCOR-R has been validated for use on adults and children from age six (Kelly, 2007). The six dimensions of this scale are Complexities of Representations of Self and Other, Emotional Investment in Values and Moral Standards, Understanding of Social Causality, Capacity for Investment in Relationships, Affect Tone of Relationship Paradigms, and Dominant Interpersonal Concerns (for example, nurturance, autonomy and mastery) (Kelly, 2007).

Scoring manuals available from Hilsenroth, Stein and Pinsker (2004), Westen (2002) and Westen, Lohr, Silk, Kerber and Goodrich (1985) are easy to understand and apply to clinical settings. The data obtained are rich and multidimensional, and the measure is validated by the theoretical underpinnings by which it is informed (including object relations theory and developmental psychology). Convergent validity between the Rorschach and TAT scales of object relations has been shown (Ackerman, Hilsenroth, Clemence, Weatherill & Fowler, 2001). The administration of 10 to 12 cards is needed to obtain internal consistency (Hibbard, Mitchell & Porcerelli, 2001).

Reliability and validity statistics

While projective tests have not reported good validity and reliability results (Entwisle, 1972; Klinger, 1966), a meta-analytic study of 66 psychological and medical tests produced reliability and validity results for the TAT interchangeable with those for other tests (Meyer, 2004). These tests included the Minnesota Multiphasic Personality Inventory, Rorschach, Wechsler Adult Intelligence Scale, Magnetic Resonance Imaging and Creatinine Clearance Test Results and Kidney Function Test. Inter-rater reliability was between .80 and .86 (for the Defence Mechanism Manual, the SCOR-R and Personal Problem Solving Scale), test-retest stability .45, and validity .22 for Achievement Motivation and Spontaneous Achievement Behaviour. Validity coefficients vary depending on the criterion under investigation. Implicit motives usually assessed are Achievement, Affiliation and Power. TAT validity has been shown to be strongly influenced by instructions given, as variations in this influence the results obtained (Allan, 1988).

Other reports of test-retest stability are around .30 (Entwisle, 1972). Test-retest reliability is, however, felt to be adversely affected by the expectation that a different story be produced at retest (Winter & Stewart, 1977) and by situational variables, such as fatigue, test anxiety, hunger and so forth (Moretti & Rossini, 2004), as with intellectual assessments (Snyderman & Rothman, 1987). Apperceptive tests reveal the participant's current psychological status; however, interpretative skill is required to discern temporary behaviours from more enduring central motives and needs (Moretti & Rossini, 2004). When training students, it is important to evaluate inter-scorer reliability for agreement on central constructs (construct validity) (Dana, 1999). This is useful in helping students think about what the central motives are and how to report on these. Problems with low internal consistency can be corrected by increasing the number of cards administered (Tuerlinckx, De Boeck & Lens, 2002).

Tuerlinckx et al. (2002) reject the application of a classical psychometric approach to the TAT. It is important to bear in mind that the TAT is not a diagnostic instrument (Spreen & Strauss, 1998); its strength is its 'ability to elicit the content and dynamics of interpersonal relationships and the psychodynamic patterns' (Bellak, 1975, pp.66–67).

Applicability and utility of the instruments in the South African context

The CAT and TAT are consistently selected as favoured tests across professional registrations, with the TAT being the test most favoured by clinical psychologists in South Africa (Foxcroft, Paterson, Le Roux & Herbst, 2004). Table 25.4 lists the popularity of the tests according to professional registration. The TAT and CAT are widely taught as the preferred apperception tests at local training institutions and internship sites. Given this, the cross-cultural implications of using these tests need to be addressed (Bellak & Abrams, 1997; Hofer & Chasiotis, 2004).

Table 25.4 The use of the TAT and CAT in South Africa, by registration category

Clinical Psychology	Educational Psychology	Research Psychology	Counselling Psychology
1. TAT (Murray)	4. CAT	5. TAT (Murray)	8. TAT (Murray)
6. CAT	8. TAT (Murray)		
	10. CAT-H		

Source: Foxcroft, Paterson, Le Roux and Herbst (2004).

Despite the tests' popularity, 13 per cent of clinicians have indicated a need for culturally unbiased tests (Foxcroft et al., 2004). The prediction of behaviour on the basis of fantasy is questioned in cross-cultural applications (Bellak & Abrams, 1997). As apperceptive or cultural norms form the backdrop against which comparisons are made, it is critical to possess a thorough knowledge of cultural groups within South Africa. An African TAT was developed in 1953 (De Ridder, 1961; Lee, 1953a; 1953b), but this version has not been utilised or further researched. Dana (1999, p.188), whose work in cross-cultural application spans over 30 years, states that 'culturally recognizable pictures, scoring variables germane to the culture, availability of normative data, and culturally specific interpretation procedures for these TAT applications' are needed. In agreement with Murstein (1965), Hofer and Chasiotis (2004) do not believe it necessary to show African persons to African participants in order to assess meaningful data or obtain validity, although content production has been found to increase if the racial characteristics of the stimuli match those of the subjects (Bailey & Green, 1977; Duzant, 2005). Empirical research has not proven increased identification, better assessment results or test utility (Aronow, Weiss & Reznikoff, 2001). The strength of the projective hypothesis may also be illustrated when participants are asked to respond to vague stimuli with no knowledge of their inherent cultural norms with which to mask responses. Responses from children or adults in the African population where unknown animals are replaced with familiar animals are considered acceptable – for example, calling the tiger a lion. The Human Sciences Research Council (HSRC) adapted the CAT for South Africans and published the Beginners Children's Apperception Test – Supplement (CAT-S) (Foxcroft et al., 2004), but this test is no longer in production.

The utility of thematic apperception methods in cross-cultural studies is supported (Holtzman, 1980) and has been used in research with persons of ethnic diversity internationally (Mussan & Naylor, 1954; Rousseau, Corin, Morrison & Stolk, 1986) and nationally (Arzul, 2005; Pond, 1987; Roper, 2007; Spuy, 1972; Straker & Jacobson, 1981; Tshabalala, 2004). However, a number of methodological concerns relating to method and item bias have been raised by Hofer and Chasiotis (2004), among others. Given the cultural diversity of the South African population and the lack of apperception tests standardised for this population, the recommendations suggested by Hofer and Chasiotis can be addressed as follows:

- Elicit themes through the use of thematic content analysis and not a predefined scoring category with possible cultural biases.
- During analysis maintain awareness of participants' cultural background and practices. Avoid imposing Westernised views of what constitutes a healthy family, so that, for example, it is understood that for economic reasons a child may be raised by a grandmother, aunt or other family member and not the biological mother (Van IJzendoorn, Bakermans-Kranenberg & Sagi-Swartz, 2006).
- Maintain awareness that the stimulus pull of the picture cards, or the strength thereof, may differ across cultural groups due to differences in value orientations (Hofer & Chasiotis, 2004; Hofer, Chasiotis, Friedlmeier, Busch & Campos, 2005; Pang & Schultheiss, 2005). Use verbal cues to clarify motives being ascribed to characters.
- Provide clear and detailed instructions.
- As far as possible, allow participants to narrate stories in their vernacular.

There is a dire lack in the assessment of implicit motives in non-Western populations and the development of culture-independent sets of picture stimuli. Few researchers have studied implicit motives across cultures using the TAT (Hofer & Chasiotis, 2003; 2004; Hofer et al., 2005; McClelland & Winter, 1969). Hofer et al. (2005) used differential item functioning to identify differences in the stimulus pull of cards, using a comparison between populations from Cameroon, Germany and Costa Rica. They found that implicit motives (for Power, Affiliation and Achievement) are understood to be universal needs not bound to a culture-specific test. However, interestingly, they found that within the Cameroonian sample 'an individual's achievement-related behavior seems also to be motivated by affiliation-intimacy-oriented strivings (e.g., concern for others, wish to be part of group, love of other people)' (Hofer et al., 2005, p.697). This confirmed that the distinction between achievement and affiliation motives appears to be less clear among individuals from cultures with an interdependent self-construal (Hofer et al., 2005). The culturally sensitive TAT-type measurement Tell Me a Story Test (Constantino, Malgady & Rogler, 1988) can be used with children aged between 5 and 18. Unfortunately, norm data are only available for US minority groups from low socio-economic urban districts.

Interpretation procedure

Analysis is dependent on the interpreters' knowledge of psychodynamic theory and participants' social and cultural environments (De Ridder, 1961). In administering an apperception test, the following steps are recommended:

- Read the personal history and reason for referral to provide a contextual framework.
- Take note of the subject's social and cultural environment.
- Read the entire protocol to derive a sense of the mood and prevailing themes.
- Analyse each story thematically.
- Consider each story in relation to the rest of the protocol to extract dominant relationship themes, clarify the meaning of each response in a larger context, obtain support for hypotheses generated and distinguish fantasy wishes from behaviour.
- Integrate all the information to provide a coherent, meaningful interpretation.
- Write the report in a way that is accessible to the reader and use age-appropriate language.

The clinician is interested in the emergence of repetitive themes in apperceptive tests that then provide substantiation for interpretative hypotheses made. Corroboration is also attained by repetition of themes across emotional assessment measures. In clinical work it is important not to interpret the CAT or TAT protocols in isolation, but to consider the responses with reference to personal history so that actual behaviours can be separated from compensatory fantasy material. For example, a self-sufficient child may express fantasised wishes of regressing to dependence on the mother. Whilst caution is voiced in interpreting the responses of borderline and lower-functioning individuals (Cashel et al., 2007), their responses have been found to be psychodynamically useful as understood within the constraints of their cognitive functioning.

Whilst there are no right or wrong responses to projective tests, respondents, especially children, can become anxious about the open-ended nature of the assessment and respond with a defensive 'I don't know' (Smith & Handler, 2007). Thus, it is important for the assessor to provide a safe 'holding environment' (Smith & Handler, 2007; Winnicott, 1965) to facilitate the verbalisation of projections. A defensive response remains psychodynamically meaningful, as it may point to a deep-seated anxiety being projected onto the stimulus material that feels too threatening to be engaged with, even through displacement. Whilst children, adolescents and adults referred for psychological assessments present with an array of emotional, social and behavioural problems and therefore can be considered vulnerable (Smith & Handler, 2007), the anxiety provoked by the testing situation often enables deep-seated anxieties and fantasies to surface, as well as the defences typically employed to combat these anxieties. Cramer (1982, 1996) developed a measure to assess for three defence mechanisms from responses to the TAT and CAT: namely, denial, projection and identification. While it is very important to establish rapport and provide a holding relationship, clinicians are also very interested in accessing the underlying anxieties, phobias, fears and fantasies that can help them understand the psychological underpinnings of the reasons for referral. The following is an example of how a deep anxiety is expressed in the testing situation:

> The rabbit is sleeping in his bed and it's in the night and the stars is sleeping, the moon, the sun and the door is wide open, wide, wide open. The door and the windows is open and the curtains is open and the frame is falling. The whole house is breaking. Here's the boogy man. The boogy man is going to eat him up. (CAT-9, 6-year-old, 2005)

This extremely anxious young boy decompensates when he feels abandoned (everyone is sleeping) and experiences that he has no ego boundaries or defences to provide protection (the whole house is breaking). It is also possible that his boundaries (physical and/or psychological) have not been respected so that he easily feels invaded.

Clinical use

In this section clinical material from children, adolescents and adults of different cultural groups within South Africa is discussed. The rich material obtained supports the applicability of the CAT and TAT for children from diverse cultural backgrounds.

Children

Traumatised child

> The lion is sitting in a castle. The mouse is looking out. The mouse tickled the king and the king felt happy. Mouse, oh so happy! Gardener felt sadness because the lion had badness first but the gardener took the badness of the lion and the lion took the gardener's happiness. (CAT-3, 6-year-old, 2003)

The spoiling of the good is told in the story of this girl whose father had committed suicide three months previously. What was once good in the relationship between the lion and mouse (representative of the father and child) was spoilt when an act of violence robbed the gardener, or child, of her happy feelings. This child assumed responsibility for the emotional well-being of the king whom she would 'tickle' to make happy and her happiness (the mouse's) was contingent on the king's happiness.

Nurturance needs

Ruan was referred for a very poor appetite and fussiness with food.[1]

> Once upon a time, a mother lives in a poor house (mother is emotionally depleted). She wondered about the money because the husband did not work (father is experienced as not being able to support his family). Mother picked four bowls of porridge. The father came home and said, 'I have money'. Both went shopping and got all the food. They ate till the pot was empty. The next morning they woke up and the children were starving. There was one porridge for each child. Lizzy said she is not sharing with Biv and Chip. When daddy comes home there was nothing to eat only bowls. I like Chip the most. I am Chip. (CAT-1, 8-year-old, 2009)

Ruan does not feel emotionally secure, as in his experience needs are not reliably and consistently met. There are not enough resources in the family to meet everyone's needs, so there is rivalry for the limited resources. He may also experience his parents as emotionally unstable, not dependable. His attachment status is insecure.

> Once upon a time, there was a father and a child, the father was too lazy. When he comes from work, the boy wanted to play with dad at the park, boy likes racing with his bike at the park (he wishes to spend more time with his father). Father said no when the boy wants to ride, you can walk how far you want and you can cry all you want. Mum said yes when the boy asked mom (mom is more emotionally available to him) but father does not want to send the boy anywhere, because his chair is too comfortable. The boy and his brother hide dad's chair (angry with father for being passive). Father was too cross and the children were laughing from inside the cupboard (his relationship with his father evokes hostile feelings in him). Father opened the cupboard, he looked everywhere and saw the chair handle. Boy was watching the father every minute and every movement the baby also moved. Father did not like it at all. (CAT-3)

Father is experienced as a withholding and strict figure, who is unresponsive to his son's feelings, needs and distress.

Neglected child

Timmy is an 8-year-old boy who has been living in a children's home following removal from an abusive mother.

> They pull rope. *(What happens?)* The rope goes snap. Flies that baby, flies the mother on top of him. Splash! *(Who do you like the most?)* Baby. *(How is the baby feeling?)* Happy. *(What is making him feel happy?)* He is playing with his mother. (CAT-2, 2004)

Timmy misses his mother terribly and would rather have bad experiences with her than none at all, although he needs protection from her, as her instability hurts him.

> The rabbit went to sleep then a big ghost came. *(What happened?)* The ghost didn't kill him. *(Who do you like the most?)* Ghost, he's happy, he's got his own baby. *(Who?)* The rabbit. (CAT-9)

He wishes he could hold onto someone who would never leave him. This need is so intense he is at risk of attaching himself to people who could harm him.

Family conflict

> One, two babies are pulling on the right. One bear is pulling on the left. They are thinking 'why are we doing this on the outside because on the inside they are feeling sad.' Coz they don't know why they are doing this, pulling the rope. (CAT-2, 8-year-old, 2005)

The child is aware that although his family are fighting with each other they are actually feeling sad but are not able to express this.

Pathology

Below are responses indicating avoidant attachment and genesis of a narcissistic construction.

> Oh, a king? Lion. There was a lion and he didn't have any friends. Everyone just gave him stuff but they never received stuff from him but then one day he gave stuff to them. *(Feeling?)* Sad. (CAT-3, 8-year-old, 2006)

> Once there was a baby bear and he lost his mom and didn't have anywhere to go, only a cold cave that was dark. Nobody, only himself in it. He felt sad. (CAT-6)

> Once upon a time there was a tiger and a baboon. The tiger was trying to attack the baboon – but climbed the tree. Then one day he was climbing the tree and the tiger ate it so he wasn't feeling hungry anymore but the baboon was dead so what could he feel (smiles). (CAT-7)

His father is felt to be preoccupied with his own needs and therefore struggles to be emotionally involved with his son. He feels that he has been trying to meet his father's needs to win his favour (card 3). Emotionally starved, he is desperate for emotional warmth from his mother (6) and generosity from his father (3), but experiences that he has been abandoned to look after himself (6). Most worrying is the child's experience of emotional deadness and denial of his feelings (7).

The responses below indicate suicide risk.

> The boy is looking at the gun. *(What will happen?)* The boy is going to pick up the gun and use it. (TAT-1, 10-year-old, 2006)

> The boy is all alone. *(Feeling?)* Very, very sad. (TAT-13B)
>
> The man is standing by the window where it is very dark. *(Why?)* He is looking out. *(Will anything happen?)* Maybe he wants to jump out. *(Feeling?)* Angry. (TAT-14)
>
> The old man is trying to touch the lady's face. *(How come?)* Maybe he wants to kill her. (TAT-12M)

Michael presented as a raging child (cards 1, 12M) who feels unloved, alone and rejected (13B). This, together with his impulsivity, makes him a suicide risk (1, 13B and 14).

The next excerpts are from 6-year-old Chris, who was diagnosed with pseudo-autism following a psychological and psychiatric assessment. He had lost both his parents two-and-a-half years previously after witnessing his father shoot his mother and then himself. He has been placed with foster-parents but his foster-mother reports not liking him.

> The birds are climbing inside, eating in the nest, on the table ... *(Happen?)* Going to die. Going to die. *(Favourite?)* Middle one. *(Feeling?)* Sad. (CAT-1, 2006)
>
> They breaking the house down and the floors. They breaking ... *(Who?)* Fire ambulance. *(Why is there an ambulance?)* Coz there's an accident. (CAT-5)
>
> The puppy's making him cute and big. *(Who is he with?)* The daddy. *(Why?)* Keeping the baby puppy cute and safe. He's cute, he's cute, he's cute. He tries to keep the puppy safe. *(Favourite?)* The baby. *(How is he feeling?)* Happy. *(Why?)* Coz his daddy's keeping him safe. (CAT-10)
>
> He's going to die again. (CAT-6)

Chris's stories indicate that he is a very traumatised boy who continually re-experiences the traumatic death and loss of his parents. He perceives his family of origin as transient, characterised by violence and as abandoning him. Thus the world is a dangerous and unsafe place where adults can't protect him (1, 5, 6). Potential nurturing female figures evoke anxiety in him (1). However, there does appear to be a tenuous attachment to his foster-father (10). He fears he could easily be harmed, damaged and annihilated by the adults in his world. An insecure boy who lacks resilience and ego strength, he is unable to cope with the demands of life (1, 5, 6).

Adolescents

Superego functioning

> The child is in a dark room, he becomes very scared and he jumps out the window. *(What happens?)* Then he runs away. *(How does he feel then?)* Very unhappy because he found out he wasn't supposed to run away. (TAT-14, 12-year-old, 2005)

This teenager tries very hard to do what is right and expected of him, but experiences that people are not aware of how bad he is feeling and therefore of what prompts his behaviour.

HIV/AIDS orphan

> I think the lady is begging the man to stay. Before the scene, they were happily married, but all of a sudden the man wants to leave her for the military. After the scene, if the poor guy likes the girl he will stay. When asked why does she want him to stay – the lady thinks he is going to go forever so she doesn't want to lose him. (TAT-4, 15-year-old, 2010, mild intellectual disability)
>
> The lady is sneaking in the office and the husband caught her. Before the scene, maybe the lady suspected that the husband is keeping a secret. After, the lady confronts the man that he is keeping a secret, which turns out to be an affair. (6GF)

Relationships between men and women are not perceived to be open and honest. Women can't necessarily trust men. This understanding may impact on her ability to form and trust in future relationships (6GF), especially as she expects to be abandoned (4).

Mastery

> Boy forced to do instrument. Looks stressed. He does not look interested. Before he wanted to do something else but was pushed to do it. In the future he will end up quitting. (TAT-1, 17-year-old, 2010)

Sibusiso is feeling pressured to perform in areas in which he cannot manage and is at risk of disinvesting. He feels others place expectations on him instead of helping him to develop his own interests.

Adults

> Oh that looks sad. Or someone is very tired or very 'moedeloos' [discouraged]. The person, no the person is not tired. It's both, 'moedeloos' and completely depressed and probably not the motivation to keep on living. *(What is this?* Points to gun) Flower! Where would the flower have come from? That's what I'd like to know … maybe it was a cemetery. I don't know. (TAT-3BM, 45-year-old, 2000, admitted to an inpatient facility)
>
> Oh goodness, it looks as if someone, it's also completely dark, the room. Everything that is light is coming in through the window. So that person is looking out the dark to the light. I wonder if it is emotionally like that for him, if he experiences it like that in him. That he is looking to the future when it will be light again. *(What will he do?)* I don't know. It looks like he wants to jump out the window? But it looks like he, he still wants to go on because his hands are stretched out, otherwise a person

> gives everything up if you don't have hope. Or he wants to jump out the window, I don't know but I think his attitude would be different. The picture is unclear to say further ... (TAT-14)

This adult is very depressed and struggling to find the inner resources to motivate herself (3BM). Although she has ideated about suicide, and probably still does (3BM, 14), she is striving towards a better future and would work well therapeutically (14). She struggles to know what she is feeling and how to reach a better emotional place (14). While her aggression is fiercely defended against, it is not successfully repressed (cemetery) (3BM), indicating a weak ego and continued risk of possible suicidal behaviour.

Socio-cultural variables

The fear of loss to violence is reflected in the TAT and CAT story fragments below:

1) 'Long ago people are feeling sad.'
2) 'Long ago they didn't have to go ... transport ... and no homes.'
3) 'Long ago no friends.'
4) 'Long ago children had babies and they were cross.'
5) 'Long ago ... no friend ... drunk.'
6) 'Long ago ... no homes ... no food.'
7) 'Now people are dying and crying.' (TAT, 10-year-old boy, 2004)

This young boy had lost family and friends to HIV/AIDS. The frequently expressed fear of abandonment by many South African children suggests a fragmentation of society's capacity to contain, protect and provide for families in a way that allows children to subjectively experience support.

> Once there was one boy, one auntie, one mother, one father – four monkeys. Then they went to the pool. Baby one did drown. The auntie went and also got drowned. Only the mother and father left. Then they were walking across the road. Then one taxi skipped the robot. Then they were all dead. (CAT-8, 7-year-old girl, 2003)

> Once there was a little boy. He sat by a door. Robbers came and shot him dead. The robbers lived happily after. (TAT-13B, 10-year-old boy, educational assessment, 2003)

Our society is felt to be an unsafe, angry place in which justice is not served. This anger is also felt to destroy the good, as illustrated in the story about the robbers above. The fear of crime as well as threats to the physical integrity of self and others cannot simply be reduced to internal fears in the face of reality-based external factors. The expressed fears were also not primary to specific psychiatric disorders, but are specific to South African society. The fear of being knocked down by a taxi that has skipped the traffic lights is also a South African experience. These world views of extreme vulnerability are, however, expressed by children in countries at war, such as Israeli and Palestinian children (Laufer & Solomon, 2006).

The samples used in this section to illustrate the various themes have come from the lower socio-economic strata, and there are more stressors and fewer resources available in this group. However, a substantially large portion of South African society falls within this group; between 10 and 15 million South Africans live in extreme poverty (Statistics South Africa, 2010).

Conclusion

As has been illustrated in this chapter, through projection, access to the internal world is gained using a means that is less threatening than being subjected to interviews or self-report questionnaires. More research, however, is needed into the cross-cultural application of the CAT, TAT and other apperception tests in the South African context. Specifically, this research could explore how cultural expectations of normative behaviour may influence the content of stories, representations of attachment figures where there is not one primary attachment figure, and, in our multilingual society, the influence of narrating stories in a second or third language, or using a translator, on the richness of data obtained.

Note

1 Pseudonyms are used in this discussion.

References

Ackerman, S. J., Hilsenroth, M. J., Clemence, A. J., Weatherill, R. & Fowler, J. C. (2001). Convergent validity of Rorschach and TAT scales of object relations. *Journal of Personality Assessment, 77(2)*, 295–306.

Allan, L. (1988). Instructional set and Thematic Apperception Test validity. *Journal of Personality Assessment, 52(2)*, 309–321.

Aronow, E., Weiss, K. A. & Reznikoff, M. (2001). *A Practical Guide to the Thematic Apperception Test*. London: Routledge.

Arzul, J. P. (2005). An investigation into the object relational patterns of violent male juvenile offenders. Unpublished Master's dissertation. University of the Western Cape, Cape Town.

Bailey, B. E. & Green, J. (1977). Black Thematic Apperception Test stimulus material. *Journal of Personality Assessment, 41(1)*, 25–30.

Bellak, L. (1944). The concept of projection: An experimental investigation and study of the concept. *Psychiatry, 7*, 353–370.

Bellak, L. (1954). *The Thematic Apperception Test and the Children's Apperception Test in Clinical Use*. New York, NY: Grune & Stratton.

Bellak, L. (1971). *The Thematic Apperception Test and the Children's Apperception Test in Clinical Use* (2nd edition). New York, NY: Grune & Stratton.

Bellak, L. (1975). *The Thematic Apperception Test and the Children's Apperception Test in Clinical Use* (3rd edition). New York, NY: Grune & Stratton.

Bellak, L. (1986). *The Thematic Apperception Test and the Children's Apperception Test in Clinical Use* (4th edition). Boston, MA: Allyn & Bacon.

Bellak, L. (1993). *The Thematic Apperception Test and the Children's Apperception Test in Clinical Use* (5th edition). Boston, MA: Allyn & Bacon.

Bellak, L. & Abrams, D. M. (1997). *The Thematic Apperception Test and the Children's Apperception Test and the Senior Apperception Technique in Clinical Use* (6th edition). Boston, MA: Allyn & Bacon.

Bellak, L. & Bellak, S. (1949). *The Children's Apperception Test*. Larchmont, NY: C.P.S.

Bellak, L. & Bellak, S. (1965). *The C.A.T.-H-A Human Modification*. Larchmont, NY: C.P.S.

Cashel, M. L., Killilea, B. & Dollinger, S. J. (2007). Interpretation of storytelling. In S. R. Smith & L. Handler (Eds), *The Clinical Assessment of Children and Adolescents* (pp. 185–206). Mahwah, NJ: Lawrence Erlbaum Associates.

Constantino, G., Malgady, R. & Rogler, L. (1988). *TEMAS (Tell-Me-A-Story) Manual*. Los Angeles, CA: Western Psychological Services.

Cramer, P. (1982). Defense mechanism manual. Unpublished dissertation. Williams College, Williamstown, Massachussetts.

Cramer, P. (1996). *Storytelling, Narrative, and the Thematic Apperception Test*. New York, NY: The Guilford Press.

Dana, R. H. (1982). *Picture Story Cards Sioux/Plains Indians*. Fayetteville, AR: University of Arkansas.

Dana, R. H. (1999). Cross-cultural–multicultural use of the Thematic Apperception Test. In L. Geiser & M. I. Stein (Eds), *Evocative Images: The Thematic Apperception Test and the Art of Projection* (pp.177–190). Washington, DC: American Psychological Association.

De Ridder, J. C. (1961). *The Personality of the Urban African in South Africa: A Thematic Apperception Test Study*. New York, NY: The Humanities Press.

Duzant, R. (2005). Differences of emotional tone and story length of African Americans respondents when administered the Contemporized Themes Concerning Blacks Test versus the Thematic Apperception Test. Unpublished manuscript. Chicago School of Professional Psychology, Chicago.

Entwisle, D. R. (1972). To dispel fantasies about fantasy-based measures of achievement motivation. *Psychological Bulletin, 77*, 377–391.

Foxcroft, C., Paterson, H., Le Roux, N. & Herbst, D. (2004). *Psychological Assessment in South Africa: A Needs Analysis. The Test Use Patterns and Needs of Psychological Assessment Practitioners*. Pretoria: Human Sciences Research Council.

Freud, S. (1938). *An Outline of Psychoanalysis*, translated by James Strachey. New York, NY: Norton.

Freud, S. (1955). *On Metapsychology: The Theory of Psychoanalysis*, translated by James Strachey. London: Penguin Books.

Hibbard, S., Mitchell, D. & Porcerelli, J. (2001). Internal consistency of the object relations and social cognition scales for the Thematic Apperception Test. *Journal of Personality Assessment, 77(3)*, 408–419.

Hilsenroth, M., Stein, M. & Pinsker, J. (2004). Social cognition and object relations scale-global rating method (SCORS-G): Training manual. Unpublished manuscript. Derner Institute of Advanced Psychological Studies, Adelphi University, Long Island.

Hofer, J. & Chasiotis, A. (2003). Congruence of life goals and implicit motives as predictors of life satisfaction: Cross-cultural implications of a study of Zambian male adolescents. *Motivation and Emotion, 27*, 251–272.

Hofer, J. & Chasiotis, A. (2004). Methodological considerations of applying a TAT-type picture-story test in cross-cultural research. *Journal of Cross-Cultural Psychology, 35,* 224–241.

Hofer, J., Chasiotis, A., Friedlmeier, W., Busch, H. & Campos, D. (2005). The measurement of implicit motives in three cultures: Power and affiliation in Cameroon, Costa Rica and Germany. *Journal of Cross-Cultural Psychology, 36(6),* 689–716.

Holtzman, W. H. (1980). Projective techniques. In H. C. Triandis & R. W. Brislin (Eds), *Handbook of Cross-cultural Psychology* Volume 2 (pp. 245–278). Boston, MA: Allyn & Bacon.

Kelly, F. D. (2007). The clinical application of the social cognition and object relations scale with children and adolescents. In S. R. Smith & L. Handler (Eds), *The Clinical Assessment of Children and Adolescents* (pp. 169–184). Mahwah, NJ: Lawrence Erlbaum Associates.

Klinger, E. (1966). Fantasy need achievement as a motivational construct. *Psychological Bulletin, 66,* 291–308.

Laufer, A. & Solomon, Z. (2006). Posttraumatic symptoms and posttraumatic growth among Israeli youth exposed to terror incidents. *Journal of Social and Clinical Psychology, 25(4),* 429–447.

Lee, S. G. (1953a). Manual of a thematic apperception test for African subjects. Unpublished manuscript. Pietermaritzburg.

Lee, S. G. (1953b). Manual of a thematic apperception test for African subjects: Set of 22 pictures. Unpublished manuscript. University of Natal, Pietermaritzburg.

McClelland, D. C. & Winter, D. G. (1969). *Motivating Economic Achievement.* New York, NY: Free Press.

Meyer, G. J. (2004). The reliability and validity of the Rorschach and Thematic Apperception Test (TAT) compared to other psychological and medical procedures: An analysis of systematically gathered evidence. In M. Hilsenroth & D. Segal, D. (Eds), *Comprehensive Handbook of Psychological Assessment* (pp. 315–342). Hoboken, NJ: John Wiley & Sons.

Morgan, C. D. & Murray, H. M. (1935). A method for investigating fantasies: The Thematic Apperception Test. *Archives of Neurology and Psychiatry, 34,* 289–306.

Moretti, R. J. & Rossini, E. D. (2004). The Thematic Apperception Test. In M. Hersen, M. J. Hilsenroth & D. L. Segal (Eds), *Comprehensive Handbook of Psychological Assessment: Personality Assessment* (pp. 356–371). Hoboken, NJ: John Wiley & Sons.

Murray, H. A. (1943). *Thematic Apperception Test Manual.* Cambridge, MA: Harvard University Press.

Murstein, B. I. (1965). *Projective Techniques.* New York, NY: Basic Books.

Mussan, P. H. & Naylor, H. K. (1954). The relationships between overt and fantasy aggression. *Journal of Abnormal and Social Psychology, 49(2),* 235–240.

Obrzut, J. E. & Boliek, C. A. (1986). Lateralization characteristics in learning disabled children. *Journal of Learning Disabilities, 19,* 308–314.

Pang, J. S. & Schultheiss, O. C. (2005). Assessing implicit motives in U.S. college students: Effects of picture type and position, gender and ethnicity, and cross-cultural comparisons. *Journal of Personality Assessment, 85(3),* 280–294.

Pond, T. S. (1987). A psychodynamic approach to the adolescent unmarried mother. Unpublished Master's dissertation. University of Pretoria, Pretoria.

Roper, M. (2007). *Integrated Youth Offender Project Three-Year Evaluation Report 2004–2006.* Centre for the Study of Violence and Reconciliation, Johannesburg.

Rorschach, H. (1924a). The application of the interpretation of form to psychoanalysis. *Journal of Nervous & Mental Disease, 60(3)*, 225–248.

Rorschach, H. (1924b). The application of the interpretation of form to psychoanalysis. *Journal of Nervous & Mental Disease, 60(4)*, 359–379.

Rousseau, C., Corin, G., Morrison, E. & Stolk, Y. (1986). Conflict armé et trauma: Une étude clinique chez des enfants réfugiés latinamericains. *Revue Canadien de Psychiatrie, 34*, 376–385.

Rustin, M., Rustin, M. & Shuttleworth, J. (1989). Psychoanalytic theory and infant development. In L. Miller (Ed.), *Closely Observed Infants* (pp. 22–51). London: Duckworth.

Smith, S. R. & Handler, L. (2007). The clinical practice of child and adolescent assessment. In S. R. Smith & L. Handler (Eds), *The Clinical Assessment of Children and Adolescents* (pp. 1–18). Mahwah, NJ: Lawrence Erlbaum Associates.

Snyderman, M. & Rothman. S. (1987). Survey of expert opinion on intelligence and aptitude. *Testing American Psychologist, 42(2)*, 137–144.

Spreen, O. & Strauss, E. (1998). *A Compendium of Neuropsychological Tests: Administration, Norms, and Commentary* (2nd edition). New York, NY: Oxford University Press.

Spuy, H. I. J. (1972). The influence of alcohol on the mood of the alcoholic. *British Journal of Addiction to Alcohol & Other Drugs, 67(4)*, 255–265.

Statistics South Africa (2010). *Work Programme 2010/11*. Pretoria: Statistics South Africa.

Straker, G. & Jacobson, R. S. (1981). Aggression, emotional maladjustment, and empathy in the abused child. *Developmental Psychology, 17(6)*, 762–765.

Teglasi, H. (1993). *Clinical Use of Story Telling: Emphasizing the TAT with Children and Adolescents*. Boston, MA: Allyn & Bacon.

Tshabalala, P. R. (2004). Personality dynamics of sexual offenders. Unpublished Master's dissertation. University of Zululand, KwaDlangezwa.

Tuerlinckx, F., De Boeck, P. & Lens, W. (2002). Measuring needs with the Thematic Apperception Test: A psychometric study. *Journal of Personality and Social Psychology, 82(3)*, 448–461.

Van IJzendoorn, M. H., Bakermans-Kranenberg, M. J. & Sagi-Swartz, A. (2006). Attachment across diverse sociocultural contexts: The limits of universality. In K. H. Rubin & O. B. Chung (Eds), *Parenting Beliefs, Behaviors, and Parent-Child Relations: A Cross-cultural Perspective* (pp. 107–142). New York, NY: Psychology Press.

Westen, D. (2002). *Current Rating Summary Sheet*. Department of Psychology, Emory University.

Westen, D., Lohr, N., Silk, K., Kerber, K. & Goodrich, S. (1985). *Social Cognition and Object Relations Scale (SCORS): Manual for Coding TAT Data*. Department of Psychology, University of Michigan, Ann Arbor.

Winnicott, D. W. (1965). The theory of the parent-infant relationship. In D. W. Winnicott, *The Maturational Process and the Facilitating Environment* (pp. 37–55). New York, NY: International Universities Press.

Winter, D. G. & Stewart, A. J. (1977). Power motive reliability as a function of retest instructions. *Journal of Consulting and Clinical Psychology, 45*, 436–440.

26 Projective assessment using the Draw-A-Person Test and Kinetic Family Drawing in South Africa

Z. Amod, R. Gericke and K. Bain

Interest in human figure drawings and their evaluation dates back to the 18th century. Drawings are considered to serve as projective techniques, as they present individuals with an unstructured and ambiguous situation, inviting them to make meaning of these tasks by drawing on their own life experiences. This allows for the exploration of a rich tapestry of material which depicts their inner world, emotions, perceptions, personality, needs and interpretation of reality (Zubin, Eron & Schumer, 1965) which may not be possible through direct communication (Machover, 1949/1980). The use of projective techniques is based on the assumption that the individual is driven by psychological forces blocked from consciousness. Unconscious conflicts are revealed by the projection of the individual's characteristic modes of response, thought processes, impulses, needs and anxieties onto the unstructured projective task. Projection is commonly regarded as the general tendency to externalise aspects of the self (Rabin, 1981).

According to Machover (1949/1980), the human figure drawing can be understood to be the way the individual projects his inner reality of past experience and current moods, tensions and concerns by the symbolism of his body image. This inner reality is the self-concept. The psychoanalytic view holds that there are both conscious and unconscious aspects of the self, and it is the unconscious expression of conflicts, body image, self and the environment as well as sexual identity which is projected in drawings (Furth, 1988; Hammer, 1997; Koppitz, 1968). Kanchan, Khan, Singh, Jahan and Sengar (2010) point out that projection of the self should not be defined in narrow terms, as it includes not only the individual's actual self but also the ideal self and the feared self. The theoretical concepts that underlie projective assessment are discussed more fully in chapter 24 of this volume.

Despite the ongoing controversy surrounding projective drawing tests (Matto & Naglieri, 2005; Roback, 1968; Swensen, 1968; Williams, Fall, Eaves & Woods-Groves, 2006), human figure drawings remain among the most widely used psychological tests by clinicians (Camara, Nathan & Puente, 2000). The Draw-A-Person (DAP) Test is rated among the top 10 to 15 most frequently used projective tests abroad (Hojnoski, Morrison, Brown & Matthews, 2006; Yama, 1990) and a similar rating is given for the popularity of the DAP and the Kinetic Family Drawing (KFD) amongst South African practitioners (Foxcroft, Paterson, Le Roux & Herbst, 2004).

In this chapter, an introductory overview of the DAP and the KFD will be given. Reference will be made to various texts and manuals which provide guidelines for the analysis and interpretation of these tests. Cross-cultural issues will be focused upon, using a few case examples. While projective drawing tests are extensively utilised by practitioners in South Africa, there is a paucity of locally published literature and research in this field. Some of the pioneering studies that have been conducted in this country will be discussed, and suggestions will be offered with regard to the future use of the DAP and KFD tests within our local context.

The DAP

The foundation of projective drawing tests lies in the work of Goodenough (1926), who developed the Draw-A-Man (DAM) Test and examined its relationship to the intellectual development of children aged 5–10 years. She foresaw further development and use of children's drawing to study personality variables. Others such as Buck (1948; 1966), Machover (1949/1980), Hammer (1953), Harris (1963) and Koppitz (1968) expanded on the knowledge of projective drawing tests. The use of the DAP has been extended to work with adults. It can, for instance, be used for clinical diagnosis, to assess personality dynamics and emotional adjustment, for the study of self-perception and body image, and to assess change over a course of therapy (Hammer, 1981; 1997).

The DAM test was later refined by Harris (1963) to include the drawing of a woman and of the self. He developed the Goodenough Harris scoring system for the Draw-A-Human Test for the age range 3 to 15 years. This scoring system is widely used to assess cognitive maturity (Fabry & Bertinetti, 1990). According to Salvia and Ysseldyke (1985), the scores on human figure drawing tests tend to correlate positively with other intelligence measures, with correlations ranging from .05 to .92. However, studies conducted over the years have not been consistently able to support the utilisation of the human figure drawing as a measure of intelligence, as compared to other assessment instruments such as the Wechsler Intelligence Scales and Raven's Progressive Matrices, although they do appear to have a relationship with Piagetian measures (Fernandes, 2000).

Machover's (1949/1980) seminal work on the DAP served as the foundation for literature relating to the interpretation of the human figure drawing as a measure of the projected self. Her work, which emerged from psychoanalytical theory, outlined general guidelines for the identification of particular characteristics or signs that were associated with specific intrapersonal and interpersonal conflicts. For example, meaning was ascribed to shading or scribbling (suggestive of preoccupation and anxiety), size (diminished or exaggerated view of self) and pressure (suggestive of inward or outward direction of impulse). Over the past half-century an extensive body of work has been conducted to further explore and develop Machover's original work. While many case studies have shown the clinical usefulness of Machover's hypotheses (Maloney & Glasser, 1982), other studies have yielded negative or mixed results (Daoud & Breik, 2009; Kahill,

1984; Roback, 1968; Swensen, 1968). Thomas and Jolley (1998) argue that there is a limitation in using Machover's approach to interpretation with children, as her scheme was largely aimed at adolescents and adults.

With the emphasis placed by researchers on the need for objective methods in the interpretation of human figure drawings, Koppitz (1968) developed a standardised scoring system using 30 emotional indicators to detect the evidence of distress in the drawings of children aged 5 to 12 years. Koppitz (1968) controlled for developmental changes in children, and presented data which showed large differences between the total number of specific signs (emotional indicators) for disturbed and normal populations. The Koppitz approach reflected a shift from looking at individual specific characteristics in analysing drawings, as postulated by Machover (1949/1980), to the use of a global or holistic approach whereby a number of specific indicators are counted to assess psychological disturbance (Dans-Lopez & Terroja, 2010). The utility of the Koppitz scoring system has received support both overseas and in South Africa, particularly in studies describing emotional manifestations in children's drawings (Daglioglu, Calisandemir, Alemdar & Bencik Kangal, 2010; Groves & Fried, 1991; Rudenberg, Jansen & Fridjhon, 1998; 2001; Williams, 2000). However, several research studies have challenged the diagnostic validity of Koppitz's system of emotional indicators when subjected to empirical evaluation (Snyder & Gaston, 1970; Tharinger & Stark, 1990). A suggestion was made in a South African study (March, 2004) that there is a need for revision and refinement of some of the Koppitz indicators.

Two further quantitative scoring systems that use the sum of specific indicators on the DAP to obtain a profile of functioning are those developed by Naglieri, McNeish and Bardos (1991), who devised the Draw-A-Person Screening Procedure for Emotional Disturbance (DAP-SPED) for use with children, and the Human Figure Drawing Test (HFDT) designed for adults by Mitchell, Trent and McArthur (1993). The DAP-SPED is a screening instrument rather than a diagnostic tool, which assists in identifying children and adolescents between the ages of 6 and 17 years who may have emotional and behavioural problems that require further evaluation. Lev-Wiesel and Witztum (2006) consider the DAP-SPED as the most psychometrically advanced figure assessment measure, as its discriminant validity and reliability evidence were found to be strong. On the other hand, the HFDT scoring and interpretation system evaluates psychopathology and cognitive impairments in adults. A recent research study (Dans-Lopez & Tarroja, 2010) demonstrated the usefulness of both the DAP-SPED and the HFDT scoring systems, especially when using large sample sizes. High inter-rater reliability was shown in this study, which was conducted with Filipino adults. A further study conducted in India by Kanchan et al. (2010) found the HFDT to be a useful tool when used with other sources of collateral information to compare the cognitive and personality patterns of male and female schizophrenic patients.

The most recently developed scoring system, the Draw-A-Person Intellectual Ability Test for Children, Adolescents and Adults (DAP: IQ), has been developed by Reynolds and Hickman (2004). This requires the testee to draw a single human figure of him- or herself, which is analysed using a standardised and objective scoring system consisting of 23 criteria. Reynolds and Hickman (2004) provide evidence for item consistency and inter-scorer reliability. In their study conducted with college students, Williams et al. (2006) reported similar reliability coefficients.

Reliability and validity

While many clinicians attest to the usefulness of projective drawing tests, their reliability, and particularly their validity, are extremely difficult to document. The popularity of human figure drawings 'lies in how interpretation is validated by further tests, rather than how research confirms interpretations' (Dans-Lopez & Tarroja, 2010, p.17). Test-retest reliability of the DAP ranges from fair to good (Handler, 1996), with only a few studies reporting test-retest reliabilities below .80 (Kahill, 1984). An earlier review of empirical studies reflected inter-rater reliability as being generally high, with $r > 0.80$ for both specific and global indicators (Kahill, 1984). On the other hand, there is limited validity evidence for human figure drawings (Ter Laak, De Goede & Van Rijswijk, 2005; Roback, 1968; Swensen, 1968; Thomas & Jolley, 1998; Yama, 1990). While some of Machover's (1949/1980) hypotheses have not found empirical support, others have yielded inconsistent results (Kahill, 1984).

Administration, scoring and interpretation

The instruction given for the DAP is for the testee to 'draw a picture of a person' on an A4 drawing page. If a cartoon or stick figure is drawn, a request is made for the drawing of a complete person. The testee is then asked to draw a picture of the opposite sex (Machover, 1949/1980). However, Koppitz (1968) suggested that a child be asked to make only one drawing of a person, because she believed that the second drawing did not often provide additional information. A variation of the DAP test instruction, used by many clinicians to economise on time, is to instruct the testee to 'draw a person, any person, but not a stick figure'.

Once the drawing is completed, many psychologists ask for details such as the age of the figure that is drawn and the activity that she or he is engaged in. Questions such as whom the person drawn likes the most and the least could also be asked, which could give an indication of attachment-related issues. The testee's responses and verbalisations assist in obtaining a further understanding of the drawing. Particularly when assessing culturally diverse individuals, drawings should be used as stimuli for discussion which could allow them to elaborate on the meaning of their drawings.

The Goodenough Harris scoring system provides an indication of nonverbal cognitive ability. Guidelines for the interpretation of emotional functioning on the DAP are provided by Machover (1949/1980), Handler (1996) and Ogdon (2001). Quantitative scoring systems such as those developed by Koppitz (1968) for children or the HFDT for adults, more qualitative approaches such as Machover's technique or Ogdon's approach, or a combination of these systems could be used to analyse the DAP. The purpose of the assessment should determine the approach that is chosen. In the quantitative approach, individual emotional indicators are classified into categories of global functioning. For example, in the Koppitz (1968) scoring system, two or more of the following indicators need to be present to categorise the drawing in the insecure/inadequate category: a slanting figure, a tiny head, hands that are cut off, a monster or grotesque figure, and an omission of the arms, legs and feet.

Within the qualitative approach, the overall quality of the drawing is analysed and hypotheses are formulated based on a configuration of signs. The interpreter could start by analysing the global feeling elicited by the drawing; for instance, does the figure appear sad, happy or tense? Cues are observed from the size, posture or facial expression of the figure. Graphomotor signs that are interpreted include erasing responses, placement of the drawing on the page, pressure factors and the size of the drawing. Hypotheses are based on the presence of other signs in the drawing, such as detailing of the figure and symmetry, as well as distortions and omission of body parts (Ogdon, 2001). The artistic quality of the drawing, such as the more-or-less accurate rendering of body parts and sufficiency of details, is considered to be an important factor in reflecting the degree of psychopathology (Handler, 1996). Drawing of the same gender as the client is considered normative (Daoud & Breik, 2009; Machover, 1949/1980). Guidelines on the characteristics of a 'typical' adult DAP drawing, which is about 15–17 cm in size on an A4 page, are given in Ogdon (2001). Discussion related to the drawing, once the testee has completed it, offers further insight into his or her functioning.

Some general considerations when interpreting human figure drawings are:

- Signs/indicators in drawings should not be interpreted in isolation but within a holistic context, taking into consideration and integrating all sources of data. This may include other formal and informal assessment procedures, clinical observations, behaviour rating scales, background history, clinical interview data and information from significant others such as parents and teachers.
- While human figure drawings are considered to represent the drawer's self-perception and body image, situational and temporary changes in attitude and mood are also expressed. Clinical experience is needed to differentiate between 'durable characteristics' in drawings and 'transient' ones (Ogdon, 2001, p.72).
- The individual's culture and social context need to be considered to better understand projective drawing test results and to make tentative inferences. For example, children's drawings are influenced by the attitudes towards art in a particular social context. A reluctance to draw or shyness of drawing may be found in individuals for whom drawing is not a commonplace activity, or for whom pencil and paper are not readily available.
- Chronological age is an important factor to consider in drawing performance, and the clinician needs to be aware of the developmental stages of children when interpreting drawings. Except for severe handicapping conditions, children follow expected and progressive changes in their drawing (Malchiodi, 1998). Very young children produce scribbles, and as they mature and develop cognitively their drawings represent shapes and forms and then complex human figure drawings (Golomb, 2004). Kellogg (1969),

Di Leo (1973) and Golomb (2004) provide an understanding of children's drawings from a developmental perspective. Knowing what is expected for a particular age group helps the clinician to understand and interpret what may be unusual in a drawing.
- Gender differences are evident in drawings. The content and style of drawings by males and females would, in many instances, be influenced by societal, cultural and gender socialisation variables. Studies by Koppitz (1968), and more recently by others such as Cherney, Seiwert, Dickey and Flichtbeil (2006) and Oluremi (2010), showed that girls reflected more details such as body parts and clothing in their drawings than boys. This variation needs to be considered when scoring and interpreting drawings.
- Individual differences in fine motor skills can confound the outcome of drawing tests (Pianta & McCoy, 1997).
- As drawing tests are screening devices to be used with other sources of information, hypotheses and interpretations made need to be tentative.

While the more quantitative scoring system could improve the reliability of the drawing test measure, it can be reductionist by not considering the drawing outcome holistically. On the other hand, qualitative approaches to analysis face the risk of subjectivity in interpretation. The clinician needs to be well skilled and self-aware, taking cognisance of the fact that personal emotions can impact upon the interpretations that are made.

Uses and limitations

The DAP is widely applicable, as it is a nonverbal assessment tool which is inexpensive and quick to administer. It provides an estimate of current nonverbal cognitive functioning on a screening level which is less influenced by cultural and language differences. Many case studies appear in the literature that attest to the usefulness of the projective drawing technique in a range of clinical situations.

Issues related to reliability and validity present as the major limitations of projective drawing tests. The compounding difficulty is that most of the evidence reported on projective drawings is in the form of clinical case studies and subjective data, rather than controlled experimental research. Projective drawing tests are not registered with the Health Professions Council of South Africa (HPCSA) as psychological tests, and local research is needed to support their widespread use in this country.

Research using projective drawings to make inferences about internal psychological states has been criticised in the literature. A further criticism is that when making interpretations the negative aspects of drawings which emphasise deficiency and pathology are mainly focused upon.

Test variations

A well-known projective drawing test that can be used for adults and children is Buck's (1948; 1966) House-Tree-Person (HTP) Test. Quantitative and qualitative scoring criteria have been designed for this test, which provides a measure of self-perception and conscious and unconscious associations regarding home and the environment. Some other DAP test variations that have been developed are the 'Draw-A-Person in the rain' modification, which attempts to assess self-concept in the face of environmental stress (Hammer, 1981), and more recently the 'Draw a mother and child' technique (Gilliespie, 1994; 1997). The latter test is thought to be a useful way to understand issues of early development from an object relations perspective.

The KFD

Burns and Kaufman (1970; 1972) published an introduction to the use of the KFD as a tool for assessing family dynamics and the development of the self within the family. Burns (1982) subsequently focused on the application and research related to the KFD, with some new guidelines for interpretation. The KFD involves a kinetic factor by asking the child to draw his or her family doing something. This allows one to gain a sense of the child's perceptions of family interactions, subsystems within the family, and whether any conflict or difficulties exist in the family. The KFD is also useful in understanding changes in family dynamics over time, as well as the adjustment issues related to changes in the composition of the family. Some examples of these changes include loss and bereavement in a family, the addition of a new sibling, a reconstituted family, or where a child has been removed from parental care.

Reliability and validity

After a comprehensive review of literature and research, Handler and Habenicht (1994) concluded that the KFD scales can be scored with a high degree of inter-rater reliability. The median percentages of inter-rater agreement in the studies that they reviewed were between 87 per cent and 95 per cent. Test-retest reliability was variable, which Handler and Habenicht interpreted as being related to the day-to-day variability in children's moods and feelings. Validity results were mixed, as Handler and Habenicht noted that researchers had in most cases modified the original scoring system devised by Burns and Kaufman (1970; 1972), making it difficult to draw comparisons between studies.

Administration, scoring and interpretation

The KFD is an individually administered test. The test instruction is 'Draw a picture of everyone in your family, including you, doing something. Try to draw whole people, not cartoons or stick people. Remember to make everyone doing something – some kind of action' (Burns & Kaufman, 1970, pp.19–20). If the testee asks whom to include in the picture, a non-directive answer is given indicating that it could be whomever his or her family is, so as not to impose any direction. Once the drawing is completed, it is discussed with the testee.

The general considerations for the interpretation of human figure drawings listed earlier in this chapter also apply to the KFD. Although some of the factors in the initial KFD scoring system proposed by Burns and Kaufman (1970; 1972) were taken from work done mainly by Machover (1949/1980) on the DAP, they also added other unique variables. Burns' (1982) scoring method uses a cluster of categories consisting of actions, styles and symbols to interpret family drawings. Distances, barriers and positions of family members are also analysed, as well as the physical characteristics of the figures that are drawn. Physical characteristics comprise the inclusion of essential body parts, the sizes of the figures and facial expression, among others. In the category of distances, barriers and positions, some of the factors that are analysed are the distances between family members, the direction faced by each figure, and the barriers placed between family members. Action, as defined by Burns and Kaufman (1970), refers to the content or theme of the drawing (for example, the type of activity depicted for each family member). Style refers to the manner of arranging the family figures on the page. Burns (1982) indicated several style variables that may suggest psychopathology or emotional disturbance, such as the underlining of the entire drawing (characteristic of family instability) and compartmentalisation (suggestive of an attempt to isolate the self).

In more recent years, some work on the interpretation of children's family drawings from the perspective of attachment theory has been published (Fihrer & McMahon, 2009; Fury, Carlson & Stroufe, 1997; Grossman & Grossman, 1991; Kaplan & Main, 1986). Kaplan and Main classified children's family drawings using four dimensions – secure, avoidant, ambivalent and disorganised/disorientated. Based on their research using Kaplan and Main's classification system, and teacher ratings of classroom socio-emotional and behaviour functioning (controlling for the variables of age, ethnic status, intelligence and fine motor skills), Pianta, Longmaid and Ferguson (1999) concluded that this coding system may be more valuable than the informal and hypothesis-generating approaches that are used to interpret family drawings.

Studies reported by Fury et al. (1997) and Madigan, Ladd and Goldberg (2003) also support the Kaplan and Main (1986) scoring system for family drawings, although like Solomon and George (2008), they caution that further reliability and validity data are needed. In a recent South African exploratory study conducted by Douglas (2010), it was suggested that the Kaplan and Main scoring system provided insight into the attachment patterns of the sample used in her study. However, she suggested that this scoring system requires a conferencing workshop and/or modifications to improve inter-rater reliability and validity.

Uses and limitations

The KFD offers a tool to understand family dynamics, as well as a change in family dynamics, and like the DAP is simple to administer. It can be used where other techniques may be limited by factors such as language barriers, cultural issues and communication difficulties. Burns and Kaufman (1970) and Burns (1982) provide ample case examples which illustrate the potential use and value of the KFD projective technique.

Drawings can, in many instances, serve as a powerful medium of communication where an individual is not able to verbalise his or her thoughts and emotions. For example, in his KFD, a 13-year-old boy drew himself and his mother pouring buckets of water over a hut that was aflame. His two siblings were walking away from this scene. When his history was probed, the social worker reported that this young boy was six years old when the informal settlement where he stayed with his mother and two brothers had burnt down. He was placed in a children's home and was separated from his siblings. The boy had last seen his mother two years prior to the occasion when he drew the family picture. He reportedly had not ever spoken to anyone at the children's home about his traumatic history. Not only was the boy able to represent his past experience in his KFD, but he was also able to express his unresolved feelings about not being able to 'save' his home and keep his family together.

In the studies reviewed by Handler and Habenicht (1994), cultural variations in family drawings were identified. In South Africa, grandparents and extended family members have a significant role to play in the day-to-day upbringing of children in many communities. In the writers' clinical experience, this experience is often depicted in children's family drawings. Research is needed to explore the KFD's cross-cultural application and validity in South Africa.

Test variations

Prout and Phillips (1974) developed the Kinetic School Drawing (KSD) for school-going children and teenagers. This test requires the child to draw a picture of him- or herself, a teacher and one or more classmates. The KSD picture assesses the child's attitude towards people at school and his or her functioning within the school environment. Knoff and Prout (1985) subsequently integrated the KFD and KSD into a system called the Kinetic Drawing System (KDS), which assesses socio-emotional differences across home and school. Their test manual summarises the relevant literature and research for the KFD and the KSD.

Cross-cultural issues with specific reference to the South African context

Chapter 24 of this volume presents a discussion of cultural and language bias issues in relation to projective testing. There has been an assumption that a human figure drawing test may serve as a useful trans-cultural measure, transcending language. However, the significant cross-cultural effects in terms of race, ethnicity, socio-economic status, societal values and norms, and religion have also been recognised in the literature (La Voy, Pedersen, Reitz, Brauch, Luxenberg & Nofsinger, 2001; Malchiodi, 1998; Rübeling, Schwarzer, Keller & Lenk, 2011).

In South Africa, there is an ongoing debate regarding the adaptation of existing international tests and the development of new culturally appropriate assessment tools (Foxcroft, 2002; Paterson & Uys, 2005). Helms (1992) and Nell (2000) have argued that tests are primarily Eurocentric in nature, developed by white psychologists who have been socialised both interpersonally and professionally in a Eurocentric environment. Foxcroft (2002) believes that the adaptation or development of culturally relevant tests and norms is paramount to enhancing the practice of psychological testing in South Africa. On the other hand, Shuttleworth-Jordan (1996) believes that due to many different cultural groups being at different stages of Westernisation, internationally recognised and well-researched tests could be used in South Africa.

There are many instances where there would be a universal understanding in the interpretation of a human figure drawing. However, an overarching factor is that when using and interpreting projective drawing tests on samples other than those for whom they have been normed, extreme caution and sensitivity is needed. Inapplicable norms should not be used at all, in some instances. Members from all cultural groups should be involved in the development of appropriate assessment measures for the South African context.

Some case examples are presented below. Although caution needs to be applied in relation to overgeneralisation, the case examples A–G in Figures 26.1 and 26.2 reflect the likelihood that there would be a similar universal meaning for practitioners, without too much cross-cultural variation. On the other hand,

Figure 26.1 Drawing test case examples

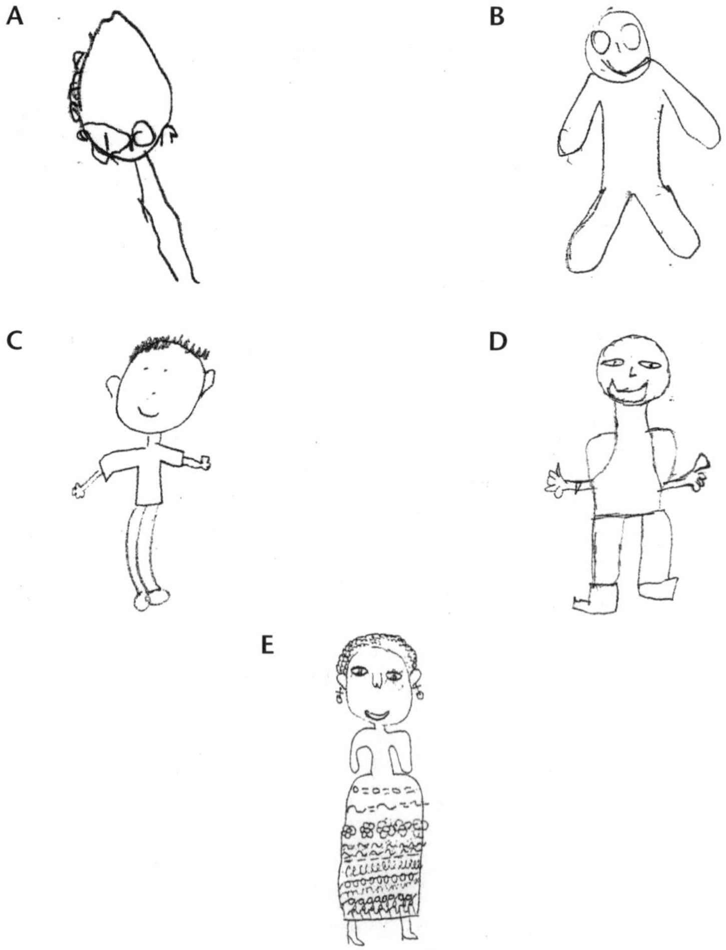

case example G in Figure 26.2 raises some cross-cultural issues. As drawing test findings are always interpreted in context to gain a holistic understanding of the testee, individual drawings are used here only for illustrative purposes.

The DAP picture A (7 cm in size) was drawn by a 9-year-old Down's Syndrome boy. Developmental delay is indicated on the drawing (Stage 111 human form, ages 4 to 7 years: rudimentary, tadpole-like figure; see Harris, 1963; Malchiodi, 1998).

An 8-year-old boy drew picture B (6 cm in size), which suggests emotional immaturity in terms of form and detail, and the figure drawn appears much younger than the subject (he said the boy in the picture was himself). His Wechsler Intelligence Scale for Children – Revised Fourth Edition (WISC-IV) Verbal and Performance Scale scores were average, except for a scaled score of 4 (significantly below average) on the Comprehension subtest, which was suggestive of a limitation with social reasoning. His Goodenough Harris score on the DAP placed him at a 6-year-old level. Reports by his teacher also confirmed emotional immaturity and a socialisation difficulty at school.

A 20-year-old male attending a drug outpatient clinic drew DAP picture C (6 cm in size), doing 'nothing'. He had a history of separation anxiety as a child and was subsequently diagnosed with depression. The DAP suggests lowered self-esteem, inadequacy and possible depressive tendencies (unusually small drawing placed at the bottom of the page, lack of detail; see Ogdon, 2001).

DAP picture D (8 cm in size) was placed on the top left-hand corner of the page by a 21-year-old psychiatric patient. He had been diagnosed with autism as a child. The figure drawn suggests a distortion of body image, possible emotional instability and interpersonal awkwardness. The open mouth may indicate unmet emotional needs (see Ogdon, 2001). The testee did not make any eye contact during the assessment and appeared to be distant and detached, suggesting an interpersonal relationship difficulty.

In DAP picture E, a girl aged 13 years drew a picture of herself 'posing for a photograph'. While her ethnic identity was reflected in her DAP, not all individuals necessarily show their cultural identity in their drawings. The testee's attention to detail with hair, ears and dress could be reflective of a typical adolescent wish to appear physically attractive, and of a concern about how she is perceived by others. However, the attention to detail may indicate anxiety about her physical appearance (Machover, 1949/1980).

The KFD picture F (photo-reduced) in Figure 26.2 was drawn by a girl aged 8 years, whose parents had just separated. She drew herself as the last figure on the right-hand side, jumping up and down. Her mother was next to her, carrying her baby sibling, and next to the mother was her sister, playing with dolls. Her father was playing soccer (the ball could symbolise outwardly directed energy/conflict; see Burns and Kaufman, 1972). The child's father had unexpectedly moved out of home and the KFD reflects her perceptions of the family dynamics in a potent way. Two dolls (a barrier (Burns and Kaufman, 1972)) separate the child, her mother and siblings on the one side of the drawing and her father on the other side. Insecurity (ground line, no feet except for father (Burns & Kaufman, 1972)) and anxiety (shading of figures (Machover, 1949/1980; Burns & Kaufman, 1972)) are also suggested and the mother appears to be anxious (shaded eyes (Machover, 1949/1980)).

Figure 26.2 Further drawing test case examples

F

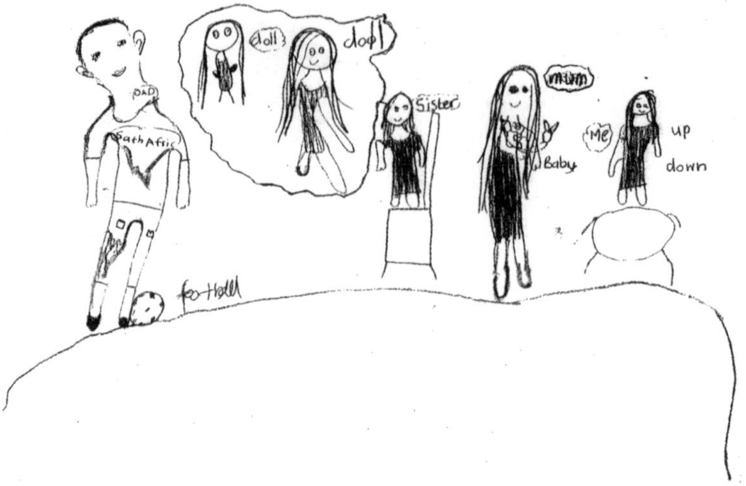

G

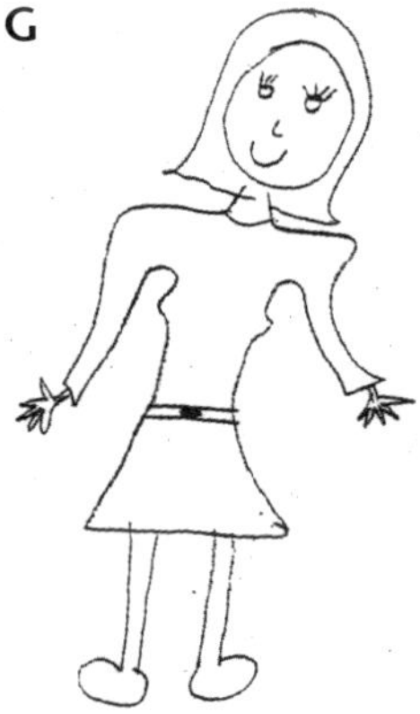

DAP figure G was drawn by a 14-year-old Muslim girl. Muslim children are not encouraged to draw human figures, particularly the pupils of the eyes, for religious reasons. After drawing the picture, the girl commented that she was not comfortable about drawing the eyes. Had a clinician not been aware of this, empty eyes would have been interpreted to indicate intrusive, self-absorbed tendencies, or a communication difficulty (Ogdon, 2001). There may also be occasions where Muslim children might refuse to comply when asked to draw a person, which, if not understood, could be interpreted as a lack of cooperation or negativity. The form and content of their drawings may also be underdeveloped, although this aspect needs to be researched.

In many South African communities, children are raised within extended families and also by substitute caregivers. This may result in cultural variation in relation to the KFD. For example, many clinicians have experienced the situation where children are not sure whom they need to include in their KFD. Some children find it difficult to complete the KFD as there are too many people to draw, or they would say that there is limited space available on the page.

A sample of South African research

In this section a sample of some of the research conducted in relation to projective drawing tests in South Africa is presented. These studies will be discussed in terms of their implications for further research.

Richter, Griesel and Wortley (1989) compared human figure drawings of 415 black children with figures of people drawn by children in 1938 and 1950. While children from 5 to 8 years of age showed no change in performance over the 50-year time span, there was a significant improvement in the Goodenough (1926) scores obtained by the older children tested in 1988, in comparison with the historical samples. According to the researchers, whilst the improvement of the social milieu of black people in South African could have been associated with these changes, no significant relationships between DAM scores and socio-economic status could be demonstrated for the older children in the 1988 sample. Richter et al. (1989) concluded that the DAM test appears to have some validity as a general cognitive measure amongst local black children between the ages of five and eight years, but that it seems to be unsuitable for children over eight years of age, because from this age onwards it underestimates abilities considerably. Since this study is dated, these assertions should be explored in relation to more recent research.

More recently, Piek (2007) conducted a study that compared the DAP using the Goodenough Harris scoring system with the Junior South African Individual Scales (JSAIS). A non-probability sample consisting of 66 white, black and coloured preschool children was used in this study. While the results cannot be generalised to the broader population, the significant correlation between the DAP and the Performance IQ on the JSAIS seemed to confirm Richter et al.'s (1989) findings, suggesting that the DAP could be used effectively within a South African context.

Rudenberg et al. (1998) used the DAP test and drawings of the street or area that children live in, as well as a behaviour checklist completed by teachers, to study the effect of violence on a sample of black and white children, aged 8–12 years. A rating and scoring system was used based on Koppitz's (1968) emotional indicators, although some additional items were added based on research conducted by others, such as Buck (1948). Two trained independent raters analysed the drawings, and Cohen's kappa was used to select only drawings with significant inter-rater agreement. Rudenberg et al. concluded that the use of the DAP together with a drawing of the street or area where a child lives correlated significantly with teacher ratings, although use of the DAP alone did not show this correlation. Their results also suggested that the DAP tapped the child's inner world rather than overt behaviour, indicating the need to obtain multiple sources of information before making definite predictions based on the DAP.

In a related study, Rudenberg et al. (2001) compared the drawings of the subjects in their South African study to drawings of subjects in West Belfast (Northern Ireland). Their findings showed cross-national differences in levels of stress and emotional indicators using the Koppitz (1968) scoring system. The researchers concluded that the analysis of children's drawings is an appropriate method of evaluating children's levels of stress and emotional adjustment.

Davidow (1999) conducted a qualitative exploratory study using two groups consisting of 30 children each, with black and white latency-phase children. A comparison was made between the two groups in their projective drawing styles using Buck's (1948; 1966) HTP test. Three independent, qualified raters were used and no substantial differences were found in the two groups' drawing styles. Davidow tentatively concluded that drawing styles are not culture-bound and that drawing tests can be usefully applied in the South African setting, although further research is needed in this area.

A pilot study conducted by Suttner (2000) examined the inter- and intra-rater reliability of scores and diagnoses by two clinicians from a clinical sample of 104 Bender Visual Motor Gestalt Test and DAP test protocols. The age range of the subjects was 8–12 years. The Koppitz (1968) scoring system was successfully used in this study, showing no significant inter-rater or intra-rater differences in the scoring of the DAP. These findings need to be validated in South Africa by further large-scale studies.

Williams (2000) explored the level and types of distress found in the drawings of female latency-age children exposed to different forms of violence within a township setting. The Koppitz (1968) scoring system was also used in this study, which supported the use of the DAP as a screening device when assessing distress as a result of trauma in children.

Emotional indicators using the Koppitz (1968) scoring system of the DAP were analysed by March (2004) in a study of children who were victims of or witnesses to crime and violence. No statistically significant differences were found in the presence of individual emotional indicators between the two experimental groups (children who were victims of crime and violence and those who were witnesses to crime and violence) and the control group (children who had never been exposed to crime and violence). All the drawings included more emotional indicators than a normal population predicted by Koppitz. In this study, stress signs, based on the research of Buck (1948) and Machover (1949/1980), were also used and no significant difference was established between the experimental and control groups. The researcher suggested that, as South Africa is a violent society, one could expect that most children would include emotional indicators in their drawings. The lack of a statistically significant difference between the groups could thus reflect this, as well as cross-cultural differences or issues related to sampling.

Makunga and Shange (2009) used four projective drawings which included the DAP and the KFD to study bereavement in young children. A statistically significant difference was found between the experimental group (recently bereaved children) and the control group (children who had never suffered any bereavement) in relation to drawn features which reflected emotional distress (such as teeth, monster/grotesque figures and hands cut off). The KFDs did not differentiate between the two groups, although the researchers stated that they added insight regarding the family dynamics of the children.

In summary, there is evidently a dearth of published research in relation to projective drawing tests in South Africa. The studies that have been conducted at tertiary training institutions tend to be limited in scope in terms of sample size and representativeness. Most of the studies described used Koppitz's (1968) quantitative scoring system, which appears to lend itself to research application. More recently developed scoring systems such as the DAP: IQ (Reynolds & Hickman, 2004) have not been explored in South African research, and data on the KFD are almost nonexistent. The documentation of well-designed studies that explore the cultural appropriateness of projective drawing tests will contribute to the optimal use and application of these tests within the multicultural South African context.

Conclusion

According to Thomas and Jolley (1998, p.135), '[t]here continues to be a gulf between clinical practice and the requirements of psychological science', and there is therefore an urgent need in South Africa to integrate the available rich clinical material with research, in order to develop an indigenous body of knowledge on projective drawing tests. This is crucial to justify the ongoing local use of these tests, to ensure that a high level of professional and ethical responsibility is maintained, to enhance initial and ongoing professional training, and also to contribute to international developments in the field of projective testing.

References

Buck, J. (1948). *The House-Tree-Person Technique.* Los Angeles, CA: Western Psychological Services.

Buck, J. (1966). *The House-Tree-Person Technique: Revised Manual.* Los Angeles, CA: Western Psychological Services.

Burns, R. C. (1982). *Self-Growth in Families: Kinetic Family Drawings (KFD) Research and Application.* New York, NY: Brunner/Mazel.

Burns, R. & Kaufman, S. (1970). *Kinetic Family Drawings (KFD): An Introduction to Understanding Children through Kinetic Drawings.* New York, NY: Brunner/Mazel.

Burns, R. C. & Kaufman, S. H. (1972). *Actions, Styles and Symbols in Kinetic Family Drawings (KFD): An Interpretive Manual.* New York, NY: Brunner/Mazel.

Camara, W. J., Nathan, J. S. & Puente, A. E. (2000). Psychological test usage: Implications in professional psychology. *Professional Psychology: Research and Practice, 31,* 141–154.

Cherney, I. D., Seiwert, C. S., Dickey, T. M. & Flichtbeil, J. D. (2006). Children's drawings: A mirror to their minds. *Educational Psychology, 26(1),* 127–142.

Daglioglu, H. E., Calisandemir, F., Alemdar, M. & Bencik Kangal, S. (2010). Examination of human figure drawings by gifted and normally developed children at preschool period. *Elementary Education Online, 9(1),* 31-43. Retrieved January 15, 2011, from http://ilkogretim.online.org.tr.

Dans-Lopez, G. & Terroja, M. C. H. (2010). Exploring human figure drawings as an assessment tool for departing OFW domestic helpers and caregivers. *Philippine Journal of Counselling Psychology, 12(1),* 13–38.

Daoud, F. S. & Breik, W. D. (2009). Relationship between family structure variables and sexual identification as measured by the Draw-A-Person Test. *Social Behaviour and Personality, 37(4)*, 545–553.

Davidow, M. (1999). A comparison of the styles of projective drawings of black and white school children. Unpublished Master's research report. University of the Witwatersrand, Johannesburg.

DiLeo, J. (1973). *Children's Drawings as Diagnostic Aids*. New York, NY: Brunner/Mazel.

Douglas, D. (2010). Representations of attachment during middle childhood in a sample of children in care in South Africa as determined by two attachment measures. Unpublished Master's research report. University of the Witwatersrand, Johannesburg.

Fabry, J. J. & Bertinetti, J. F. (1990). A construct validation study of the Human Figure Drawing Test. *Perceptual and Motor Skills, 70(2)*, 465–466.

Fernandes, F. S. (2000). Relationships of the Piagetian cognitive development to human figure drawing. *Child Study Journal, 30(4)*, 225–232.

Fihrer, I. & McMahon, C. (2009). Maternal state of mind regarding attachment, maternal depression and children's family drawings in the early school years. *Attachment and Human Development, 11(6)*, 537–556.

Foxcroft, C. D. (2002). Ethical issues related to psychological testing in Africa: What I have learned (so far). In W. J. Lonner, D. L. Dinnel, S. A. Hayes & D. N. Sattler (Eds), *Online Readings in Psychology and Culture* (Unit 5, Chapter 4). Center for Cross-cultural Research, Western Washington University, Bellinghan, Washington. Retrieved January 30, 2011, from http://www.wwu.edu/~culture.

Foxcroft, C., Paterson, H., Le Roux, N. & Herbst, D. (2004). *Psychological Assessment in South Africa: A Needs Analysis. The Test Use Patterns and Needs of Psychological Assessment Practitioners*. Pretoria: Human Sciences Research Council.

Furth, G. M. (1988). *The Secret World of Drawings: Healing through Art*. Boston, MA: Sigo Press.

Fury, G. S., Carlson, E. A. & Stroufe, L.A. (1997). Children's representations of attachment relationships in family drawings. *Child Development, 68*, 1154–1164.

Gilliespie, J. (1994). *The Projective Use of Mother-and-Child Drawings: A Manual for Clinicians*. New York, NY: Brunner/Mazel.

Gilliespie, J. (1997). Projective mother-and-child drawings. In E. Hammer (Ed.), *Advances in Projective Drawing Interpretation* (pp. 137–151). Springfield, IL: Charles C. Thomas.

Golomb, C. (2004). *The Child's Creation of a Pictorial World*. Mahwah, NJ: Lawrence Erlbaum Associates.

Goodenough, F. (1926). *Measurement of Intelligence by Drawings*. New York, NY: Harcourt, Brace & World.

Grossman, K. E. & Grossman, K. (1991). Attachment quality as an organizer of emotional and behavioral responses in a longitudinal perspective. In C. M. Parkes, J. Stevenson-Hinde & P. Marris (Eds), *Attachment across the Life Cycle* (pp. 93–114). London: Tavistock/Routledge.

Groves, J. R. & Fried, P. A. (1991). Developmental items on children's human figure drawings: A replication and extension of Koppitz to younger children. *Journal of Clinical Psychology, 41(1)*, 140–148.

Hammer, E. F. (1953). Frustration-aggression hypothesis extended to socio-racial areas: Comparison of Negro and white children's H-T-Ps. *Psychiatric Quarterly, 27*, 597–607.

Hammer, E. F. (1981). Projective drawings. In A. I. Rabin (Ed.), *Assessment with Projective Techniques* (pp. 151–185). New York, NY: Springer Publishing Company.

Hammer, E. F. (1997). *Advances in Projective Drawing Interpretation*. Springfield, IL: Charles C. Thomas.

Handler, L. (1996). The clinical use of drawings. In C. S. Newmark (Ed.), *Major Psychological Assessment Instruments* (pp. 165–216). Newton, MA: Allyn & Bacon.

Handler, L. & Habenicht, D. (1994). The Kinetic Family Drawing technique: A review of the literature. *Journal of Personality Assessment, 62(3)*, 440–464.

Harris, D. (1963). *Children's Drawings as Measures of Intellectual Maturity*. New York, NY: Harcourt, Brace & World.

Helms, J. E. (1992). Why is there no study of cultural equivalence in standardized cognitive ability testing? *American Psychologist, 47(9)*, 1083–1101.

Hojnoski, R. L., Morrison, R., Brown, W. & Matthews, W. J. (2006). Projective test use among school psychologists. *Journal of Psychoeducational Assessment, 24(2)*, 145–159.

Kahill, S. (1984). Human figure drawing in adults: An update of the empirical evidence, 1967–1982. *Canadian Psychology, 25*, 269–292.

Kanchan, A., Khan, N. A., Singh, A. R., Jahan, M. & Sengar, K. S. (2010). Personality pattern of male and female schizophrenics on human figure drawing test. *SIS Journal of Projective Psychology and Mental Health, 17(1)*, 63–68.

Kaplan, N. & Main, M. (1986). Instructions for the classification of children's family drawings in terms of representation of attachment. Unpublished manuscript. University of California, Berkeley.

Kellogg, R. (1969). *Analyzing Children's Art*. Palo Alto, CA: Mayfield.

Knoff, H. M. & Prout, H. T. (1985). *Kinetic School Drawing System for Family and School: A Handbook*. Los Angeles, CA: Western Psychological Services.

Koppitz, E. M. (1968). *Psychological Evaluation of Children's Human Figure Drawings*. New York, NY: Grune & Stratton.

La Voy, S. K., Pedersen, W. C., Reitz, J. M., Brauch, A. A., Luxenberg, T. M. & Nofsinger, C. C. (2001). Children's drawings: A cross-cultural analysis from Japan and the United States. *School Psychology International, 22*, 53–63.

Lev-Wiesel, R. & Witztum, E. (2006). Child molesters vs rapists as reflected in their self-figure drawings: A pilot study. *Journal of Child Sexual Abuse, 15(1)*, 105–117.

Machover, K. (1949/1980). *Personality Projection in the Drawing of the Human Figure*. Springfield, IL: Charles C. Thomas.

Madigan, S., Ladd, M. & Goldberg, S. (2003). A picture is worth a thousand words: Children's representations of family as indicators of early attachment. *Attachment & Human Development, 5(1)*, 19–37.

Makunga, N. V. & Shange, L. O. (2009). Drawings as a method of evaluation and communication with bereaved children. *Inkanyiso, Journal of Humanities and Social Sciences, 1(1)*, 27–33.

Malchiodi, C. A. (1998). *Understanding Children's Drawings*. New York, NY: The Guilford Press.

Maloney, M. P. & Glasser, A. (1982). An evaluation of the clinical utility of the Draw-A-Person Test. *Journal of Clinical Psychology, 38*, 183–190.

March, C. (2004). Emotional indicators in human figure drawings of children who have been victims of or witness to crime and violence. Unpublished Master's research report. University of the Witwatersrand, Johannesburg.

Matto, H. C. & Naglieri, J. A. (2005). Race and ethnic differences and human figure drawings: Clinical utility of the DAP-SPED. *Journal of Clinical Child and Adolescent Psychology, 34(4)*, 706–711.

Mitchell, J., Trent, R. & McArthur, R. (1993). *Human Figure Drawing Test (HFDT): An Illustrated Handbook for Clinical Interpretation and Standardized Assessment of Cognitive Impairment.* Los Angeles, CA: Western Psychological Services.

Naglieri, J., McNeish, T. & Bardos, A. (1991). *Draw-A-Person: Screening Procedure for Emotional Disturbance (DAP:SPED) Examiner's Manual.* Austin, TX: Pro-Ed.

Nell, V. (2000). *Cross-cultural Neuropsychological Assessment: Theory and Practice.* London & Mahwah, NJ: Lawrence Erlbaum Associates.

Ogdon, D. P. (2001). *Psychodiagnostics and Personality Assessment: A Handbook.* Los Angeles, CA: Western Psychological Services.

Oluremi, A. M. (2010). Gender and preferred content in children's drawing among selected primary school children in Zaria Metropolis, Kaduna State. *Gender and Behaviour, 8(2)*, 3168–3198.

Paterson, H. & Uys, K. (2005). Critical issues in psychological test use in the South African workplace. *South African Journal of Industrial Psychology, 31(3)*, 12–22.

Pianta, R. C., Longmaid, K. & Ferguson, J. E. (1999). Attachment-based classification of children's family drawings: Psychometric properties and relations with children's adjustment in kindergarten. *Journal of Clinical Child Psychology, 28(2)*, 244–255.

Pianta, R. C. & McCoy, S. (1997). The first day of school: The predictive utility of an early school screening program. *Journal of Applied Developmental Psychology, 18*, 1–22.

Piek, J. (2007). The construct validity of the Goodenough-Harris Drawing Test as a screen for intellectual functioning in a group of preschool children. Unpublished Master's research report. University of Stellenbosch, Stellenbosch.

Prout, H. T. & Phillips, P. D. (1974). A clinical note: The Kinetic School Drawing. *Psychology in the Schools, 11(3)*, 303–306.

Rabin, A. (1981). *Assessment with Projective Techniques: A Concise Introduction.* New York, NY: Springer Publishing Co.

Reynolds, C. R. & Hickman, J. A. (2004). *Draw-A-Person Intellectual Ability Test for Children, Adolescents and Adults: Examiner's Manual.* Austin, TX: Pro-Ed.

Richter, L. M., Griesel, R. D. & Wortley, M. E. (1989). The Draw-A-Man test: A 50-year perspective on drawings done by black South African children. *South African Journal of Psychology, 19(10)*, 1–5.

Roback, H. (1968). Human figure drawings: Their utility in the psychologist's armamentarium for personality assessment. *Psychological Bulletin, 70(1)*, 1–19.

Rübeling, H., Schwarzer, S., Keller, H. & Lenk, M. (2011). Young children's nonfigurative drawings of themselves and their families in two different cultures. *Journal of Cognitive Education and Psychology, 10(1)*, 63–76.

Rudenberg, S. L., Jansen, P. & Fridjhon, P. (1998). The effect of exposure during an ongoing climate of violence on children's self-perceptions, as reflected in drawings. *South African Journal of Psychology, 28(2)*, 107–115.

Rudenberg, S. L., Jansen, P. & Fridjhon, P. (2001). Living and coping with violence: A cross-national analysis of children's drawings using structured rating indices. *Childhood, 8*, 31–55.

Salvia, J. & Ysseldyke, J. (1985). *Assessment in Special and Remedial Education*. Boston, MA: Houghton Mifflin.

Shuttleworth-Jordan, A. B. (1996). On not reinventing the wheel: A clinical perspective on culturally relevant test usage in South Africa. *South African Journal of Psychology, 26(2)*, 96–102.

Snyder, R. T. & Gaston, D. S. (1970). The figure drawing of the first-grade child: Item analysis and comparison with Koppitz norms. *Journal of Clinical Psychology, 26*, 377–383.

Solomon, J. & George, C. (2008). The measurement of attachment, security and relevant constructs in infancy and childhood. In J. Cassidy & P. R. Shaver (Eds), *Handbook of Attachment: Theory Research and Clinical Applications* (2nd edition, pp. 383–418). New York, NY: The Guilford Press.

Suttner, V. (2000). Inter- and intra-rater reliability of the scoring and analysis of the Bender Gestalt and human figure drawing protocols in a clinical setting. Unpublished Master's research report. University of the Witwatersrand, Johannesburg.

Swensen, E. (1968). Empirical evaluations of human figure drawings. *Psychological Bulletin, 70(1)*, 20–44.

Ter Laak, J., De Goede, M., Aleva, A. & Van Rijswijk, P. (2005). The Draw-A-Person Test: An indicator of children's cognitive and socio-emotional adaptation? *Journal of Genetic Psychology, 166(1)*, 77–93.

Tharinger, D. J. & Stark, K. (1990). A qualitative versus quantitative approach to evaluating the Draw-A-Person and Kinetic Family Drawing: A study of mood- and anxiety-disorder children. *Psychological Assessment: A Journal of Consulting and Clinical Psychology, 2*, 365–375.

Thomas, G. V. & Jolley, R. P. (1998). Drawing conclusions: A re-examination of empirical and conceptual bases for psychological evaluation of children from their drawings. *British Journal of Clinical Psychology, 37*, 127–139.

Williams, J. A. (2000). An analysis of the drawings of sexually abused, traumatized and a non-clinical population of girls. Unpublished Master's research report. University of the Witwatersrand, Johannesburg.

Williams, T. O., Fall, A., Eaves, R. C. & Woods-Groves, S. (2006). The reliability of scores for the Draw-A-Person intellectual ability test for children, adolescents and adults. *Journal of Psychoeducational Assessment, 24(2)*, 137–144.

Yama, M. F. (1990). The usefulness of human figure drawings as an index of overall adjustment. *Journal of Personality Assessment, 54(1 & 2)*, 78–86.

Zubin, J., Eron, L. D. & Schumer, F. (1965). *An Experimental Approach to Projective Techniques*. New York, NY: John Wiley & Sons.

27 The Rorschach in South Africa

M. Brink

Psychologists worldwide have used the Rorschach Inkblot Method ever since Hermann Rorschach first published his research in 1921 (Rorschach, 1921/1942). The clinician presents a standard set of ten cards with inkblots and asks the client to indicate what she or he sees on each card, where it is seen and what characteristics of the blot make it look the way it does. Clients' responses suggest how people perceive and think about their world, solve problems, make decisions, manage stress and view themselves and others. The Rorschach has been accurately described as a perceptual, an associational, an interpersonal and a sequential task. Taken together, these features enable the Rorschach user to come to a remarkably comprehensive interpretation of personality processes and structures (Weiner, 2000).

Those in South Africa who use the Rorschach as more than a mere projective technique currently use the Exner Comprehensive System, into which all of the empirically defensible features of other, earlier approaches have been merged. Exner's work represents a major attempt, mostly successful, at integrating some of the most meaningful contributions of earlier interpretation systems – for example, those of Rorschach himself, Piotrowski, Rapaport, Beck, Hertz and Klopfer. Research regarding the Exner Comprehensive System is still ongoing, also in South Africa.

The Rorschach as a personality test

The main aim of the Rorschach is not to achieve a specific psychiatric diagnosis, but to enhance understanding of the interactive, dynamic personality processes and characteristics of a unique individual (Exner, 2003; Meloy, 2005).

The Exner Comprehensive System enables the Rorschach user to come to well-validated conclusions about personality features such as capacity for control and coping with stress, affective functioning, interpersonal perception, self-perception and cognitive processes. The latter include the use of cognitive defences, rationality of thinking, accuracy of perception and problem-solving style. Because it measures personality processes, the data gathered can contribute to identifying conditions that are defined by personality characteristics (Weiner, 2000). Specific diagnostic indices have been developed, but have to be applied with caution, taking into consideration contextual information and the results of other personality tests. These indices include a Suicide Index, a Depression Index, a Perceptual-Thinking Index (picking up on irrational thinking and perceptual distortions often associated with psychosis or organic brain syndromes), a Coping Deficit Index (sensitive to features associated with personality disorders), a Hypervigilance Index and an Obsessive Style Index.

One of the major advantages of the Rorschach is that it provides a full picture of total personality structure and functioning, including both assets and liabilities. As such, it has proven to be most useful in detecting the presence of inner resources, prognosis with various types of psychotherapy and potential for improvement or healing if pathology exists (Janson & Stattin, 2003; Weiner, 1998).

When using the Exner Comprehensive System, the sheer comprehensiveness and detail of the scoring and statistical data may give the impression that qualitative aspects are not given sufficient cognisance. Actually this is not the case. Exner himself emphasises repeatedly that both quantitative and qualitative features have to be carefully considered and used in a complementary way when interpreting a protocol (2003; Exner, Weiner & PAR Staff, 2008). This view is confirmed by other researchers (Ritzler, 2001; Weiner, 2000). Exner (2003; 2005) also emphasises that while acknowledgement of the projective process enhances the usefulness of the Rorschach, structural features should not be neglected. Since personality traits are enduring characteristics, these may not be directly linked to projection. What may happen is that a strong trait may give rise to rich projective material which has to be taken into account with the structural data. He regards the structural data as the 'hard data' of the Rorschach which will generally be the most meaningful in forming hypotheses about personality structure and functioning. When interpretive hypotheses regarding one 'cluster' (for example, affect or self-perception) prove to be too general, too narrow, or misleading, one needs to first consider qualitative data before proceeding to a following cluster (Exner, 2003).

Even when adhering to the Exner comprehensive approach, it may still be useful to base one's understanding of the data on earlier theoretical foundations of the Rorshach as explicated by Piotrowski (Daly, 2005) and Klopfer (Klopfer, Ainsworth, Klopfer & Holt, 1954).

In the world of Western psychology, the Rorschach is presently used more widely and has generated more published research than any other personality measure, with the exception of the Minnesota Multiphasic Personality Inventory (MMPI) (Meyer & Archer, 2001). In contrast, its usage in South Africa has diminished over the past decade. This could be due to the phasing out (retirement and death) of experts, a minimal follow-up of young scholars, a gradual decrease in interest in 'projectives', the increasing use of tests and questionnaires whose results are more easily quantified and interpreted via the use of computer programs, and the increasing preference for cognitive therapy. Due to the serious paucity of research in South Africa, this chapter will include references to overseas publications, insofar as these are relevant to working with the Rorschach in South Africa.

Psychometric properties of the Rorschach: nomothetic and idiographic approaches

The utility of the Rorschach, as indicated by an increasing body of research, is confirmed in an article in the *South African Rorschach Journal* (Mattlar, 2005). Over time the quality, integrity and strength of the Rorschach have continued to evolve. In an extensive study, Weiner (2001) concluded that the Rorschach exemplifies all of the sound principles of a scientific test.

Reliability studies have indicated that inter-rater reliability is excellent: namely, between .85 and .97, which is as good as that of the MMPI (Meyer & Archer, 2001; Meyer, Hilsenroth, Baxter, Exner, Fowler & Piers, 2002).

Research concerning the validity of the Rorschach has shown that the test is conceptually valid when used in the manner for which it was designed and intended (Brink, 2005; Weiner, 2001). Validity data were found to be comparable to those of the MMPI.

Users of the Rorschach are nevertheless cautioned to take note of research that indicates that certain Rorschach indicators, especially those which are regarded as being related to affective functioning, have been proven to be invalid when used in isolation, and therefore suggests that an idiographic approach to the data should not be dismissed (Aronow & Rodriguez-Srednicki, 2004).

In response to the need to accommodate the Rorschach to cultural differences, multiple normative research contributions from 15 countries have recently been published (Shaffer, Erdberg & Meyer, 2007) and updated (Meyer, Viglione, Mihura, Erard & Erdberg, 2012). These international norms are now being used by some researchers and clinicians inside and outside the USA. This approach to challenging normative data across international boundaries is a continuous process, and will hopefully be extended to cultural groups within South Africa.

The abovementioned research shows that the Rorschach lends itself well to a nomothetic approach to psychological assessment. It also allows for idiographic and meaning-oriented approaches, which are absent from purely objective measures such as the MMPI. An important development in the Rorschach in recent years is the shift to more fully incorporating both nomothetic and idiographic interpretation approaches. Information from both the Structural Summary – that is, the formal, nomothetic data – and from content analysis contributes to a fuller understanding of an individual's psychological functioning. This is in line with the research format suggested by De Vos (2007). The newly revised approach to the Rorschach, 'The Rorschach performance assessment system' (Meyer et al., 2012), repeatedly emphasises the importance of holistic interpretation, including both the new norms and idiographic information.

Exner (2003) encourages the reading and understanding of specific responses – for example, those that include pairs, movement, cooperation and aggression – as well as responses that reflect poor reality testing.

The following examples from adult clients illustrate the importance of taking cognisance of nomothetic as well as idiographic aspects of a protocol:

1. Card 1, a response to the whole blot: *Two evil witches in dark black robes, dancing around a victim bound to a pole. The victim is already dead.*

Versus: *Two fairies performing some intricate dance around a magical treasure chest. They are wearing dark robes. So beautiful and delicate.*

Both responses will receive a $M_aFC'+$ as determinants (active human movement and achromatic colour) and a (H) for contents (fantasy human figures), but considering them qualitatively suggests a very different meaning regarding each response.

2. Card 3, a response to D1, an area which often evokes a human response: *Two waiters carrying a large bowl of soup to a table. They are dressed in fancy black uniforms. It must be a rather posh restaurant.*
   Versus: *Two ugly goblins mixing a poisonous potion. Their bodies are painted black.*

Both qualify for an active human movement and an achromatic colour determinant M_aFC', but again the contents should be taken into account, as it should be for any pair and movement response.

3. Card 7, a response to D1: *A young lady admiring herself in a mirror. She is dressed like a queen. Very beautiful indeed.*
   Versus: *Card 8, a response to D1: An animal climbing up a steep mountain. One can see his reflection in the water beneath him.*

While the reflection in both cases will be given an Fr as determinant, the quality of the possible narcissism in the two responses is clearly very different.

4. Card 10, a response to D11: *Two tiny ants playing football.*
   Versus: *a response to the same location: Two insects attacking a nuclear bomb.*

Both earn a Special Score – namely, FABCOM – for the content, which refers to an impossible combination of percepts, but where the first one suggests playfulness, perhaps immaturity or even creativity, the second one could be indicative of irrational thinking.

Each of the above examples should, of course, be considered within the context of the whole protocol, both nomothetically and idiosyncratically.

For those interested in analysing the Rorschach from a psychoanalytic and psychodynamic perspective, the work by Leichtman (2000) will be of great relevance. The more recent work of Berant and Mikulincer (2005), which focuses on implicit processes inherent in attachment systems functioning, adds to this dimension of understanding the Rorschach. Bornstein (2007) also questions a purely nomothetic approach which does not allow for an understanding of the projective aspects of the test.

The responsible Rorschach user accepts that one group of determinants or 'cluster' of nomothetic information should never be interpreted in isolation from other structural data, content, form quality or psychodynamic content analysis (Gacono, 2001, p.64).

Raskin (2001) discusses ways in which constructivism complements and adds to existing Rorschach methodologies. A constructivist therapist sees the Rorschach as a test of meaning construction. Contextual and relationship factors do contribute to Rorschach responses and have to be taken into consideration. This is why it is risky to rely too heavily on computerised reports based exclusively on nomothetic data.

Determining the reliability and the validity of the Rorschach regarding different variables and different populations should be seen as an ongoing endeavour for those wanting to implement the Rorschach in a scientifically acceptable manner (Liebman, Porcerelli & Abel, 2005; Meyer, 2000a; 2000b).

The Rorschach as part of a test battery

Assessment is a process that integrates the results of several carefully selected tests with relevant facts from a subject's history, as well as observation, in order to form an accurate, in-depth understanding of an individual (Weiner, 2004). The rationale for using a combination of tests includes the argument that no one test is so broad in its scope as to test everything; and, since various tests overlap to some extent, there is a possibility of cross-validating information derived from any single test (Exner, 2003, p.38). The Rorschach is helpful in providing information about the cognitive, affective, social perceptive and self-perceptive characteristics, as well as the coping mechanisms, of individuals that would probably not be identified through structural interviews or self-report tests and inventories (Hartman, 2003).

Exner (2003) suggests that in contemporary assessment which targets a reasonably full picture of a person, three tests might best be considered as forming the nucleus of the assessment procedure: one of the Wechsler Intelligence Scales, the Rorschach and the MMPI. Each is empirically well founded, and each provides rich information from which a well-trained practitioner can generate many important and meaningful hypotheses concerning an individual.

The Rorschach can thus form a meaningful adjunct to a well-selected battery of tests where the understanding of an individual is important, be it for clinical, counselling, forensic or research purposes. It is currently used in South Africa in all of these settings, and knowledge of the advantages of using this test can be of considerable benefit to a practitioner working in any of these areas.

Criticisms of the Rorschach

Many of the criticisms aimed at the Rorschach, both in South Africa and overseas, are marked by a sort of naïveté, bias or lack of understanding. Most critics focus on findings derived from one or a single combination of determinants, ignoring supportive nomothetic and idiographic data.

A recent criticism by Wood, Nezworski, Lilienfeld and Garb (2003) in *What's Wrong with the Rorschach?* clearly advocates a certain biased point of view rather than a balanced look at the Rorschach (Meloy, 2005). Meloy illustrates how this book makes use of distortion of the existing literature and deliberate exaggerations, refers to unpublished and inaccessible sources, and neglects to mention the importance of interpreting certain indicators within the context of the entire protocol.

Critics of the Rorschach, such as Wood et al. (2003) and Lilienfeld (2001), tend to recognise only a few variables as tenable, and neglect to look at the total picture that arises from all of the information gained (Aronow & Rodriques-Srednicki, 2004, p.30). Responsible users of the Rorschach understand that a specific finding should never be interpreted in isolation from other structural data and psychodynamic analysis of the content (Gacono, 2001; Meloy, 2005, p.345). This is why the Rorschach is such a complex instrument but also such a satisfying one, giving a full picture of personality with all of its strengths and its difficulties. Weiner (2000; 2001) addresses the many criticisms of the Rorschach and convincingly emphasises its usefulness and reliability.

Research on the Rorschach in South Africa

The challenges inherent in doing research in the social sciences in South Africa are addressed in the work of Strydom (2007). A number of articles published in South Africa empirically document the wide clinical and research use of the Rorschach (Aronstam, Daws & Swanepoel, 2006/2007; Daws & Aronstam, 2005; Odendaal, 2011).

In South Africa, as overseas, Rorschach findings are used to facilitate decision-making in the field of career counselling, personnel selection and promotion, and professional fitness or competence (Meloy, Acklin, Gacono, Murray & Peterson, 1997). Most of this South African work is, unfortunately, not available in published form. It has often been the focus of advanced discussion groups for professionals who have mastered the basics of Rorschach scoring and interpretation (Brink, 2002; 2010). In addition, the Rorschach has been implemented in several studies to assess subjects' readiness and dynamic capacity for various forms of psychotherapy (Nygren, 2004).

Meloy, as senior editor of the book *Contemporary Rorschach Interpretation* (Meloy et al., 1997), comments favourably on the use of this test for forensic purposes. Almost 200 legal citations were found in which the Rorschach was discussed by the courts in substantive, if not foundational, terms. Many of these articles have arisen from forensic cases, and illustrate the depth and range of Rorschach data in contributing to the resolution of legal questions. Issues such as the psychological 'fit' between each parent and a child, the suitability of persons as parents or adoptive parents, and criminal responsibility were often addressed. Again, published work is scarce, but forensic psychologists such as Dr Visser (Pretoria), Ms Van Niekerk (Secunda), Ms Bothma (Johannesburg) and Ms MacNab (Johannesburg) are known and respected for their inclusion of Rorschach findings in their work. De Ruyter and Veen (2004) mention in the *South African Rorschach Journal* that there is much room for research in forensic psychological assessment in the South African context. Those who are interested in the use of the Rorschach for forensic purposes will find the earlier work by Gacono (2001) and the more recent comprehensive work edited by Gacono, Evans, Gacono and Kaser-Boyd (2008) of great interest and relevance.

Finally, the Rorschach has been used extensively in research regarding a wide variety of subjects. Some of this research, particularly that done in South Africa, will be discussed below.

As the Rorschach involves culture-free stimuli, it is an ideal instrument for exploring cross-cultural differences. Various authors have concluded that it can be regarded as a universally applicable and cross-culturally relevant instrument. Some of the methodological issues in cross-cultural and multicultural research have been addressed by authors such as Allen and Dana (2004).

In South Africa appropriate guidelines and norms have not been developed, although some important efforts have been made in this direction. Cultural influences on the administration process, response coding and the impact of language have been explored, at least to some extent. Some of the published studies by Aronstam and Macklin (2004) and Moletsane and Eloff (2006) are important in this regard. Various ongoing and completed doctoral studies, in which the Rorschach is used as a measuring instrument, are also promising in terms of the future use of this test in the South African context.

Aronstam and Macklin (2004) point out that while the Rorschach has definite cross-cultural application value, there remains concern about its culture-fairness and bias regarding both the normative data and the qualitative interpretation of the data. Clients are often rooted in strong traditional beliefs and values that need to be approached from an unbiased stance. Aronstam (Aronstam & Macklin 2004) reports on the development of a method of self-interpretation of the Rorschach, wherein the subjects contribute directly to the final interpretation of their own protocols. He presents vignettes from two case studies to illustrate the rationale and method, and how the data generated complement and enhance more traditional Rorschach interpretation.

Moletsane and Eloff (2006) have developed an adapted procedure for the administration of the Rorschach to young South African learners. They took into consideration the earlier research by Hartman (2001), who compared the effect of different instructions on Rorschach performance. In the adjustment the researchers took into account the language and some social factors that may inhibit participants from giving sufficient responses. Explanations were given at least twice, and participants were encouraged to ask questions if they were still uncertain about what was expected from them. Participants were allowed to mix languages, since it was found that none of them was able to keep to their home language when giving responses. They were allowed to respond in any language with which they felt comfortable, and were not penalised for this. In cases where participants had difficulty in providing answers in any of the languages they commonly used, they were encouraged to explain the image further or even to draw what they saw. Inquiry was conducted immediately after each card was responded to, and not in the conventional manner after all ten cards had been administered. Participants were given a choice regarding seating arrangements:

face-to-face, side-by-side or catty-corner seating (examiner and client sitting at an angle of 90 degrees). A significant increase in response rate was found as a result of the flexibility of this administration procedure, which made for more valid, interpretable protocols. Subjects consistently produced 14 or more responses, which was not the case when the conventional instructions were given, in which case nomothetic interpretation is not regarded as viable. This study supports the position that excessive dependence on standardised assessment procedures can limit the value of such assessments. Standardised instruments may have to be modified, adjusted or corrected for use with diverse populations. The examiner should demonstrate appropriate flexibility and professional discretion when doing assessments cross-culturally.

The study by Odendaal (2011) contributes to the research of Theron (2004) and Theron, Cameron, Lau, Didkowsky and Mabitsela (2009) concerning resilience among youth in South Africa. Veeren and Morgan (2009) specifically address the role of South African culture in the development of resilience. Adhering to the guidelines proposed by Moletsane and Eloff (2006) regarding language usage and administration procedure, Odendaal (2011) assessed protective processes that enable adolescents at risk. Her interpretation of the Rorschach data relies on an integration of structural and content data analysis to describe how individual and culturally informed habits, traits and styles are constructed and reflected. Her aims were both to conduct a culturally sensitive interpretation of the Rorschach to identify latent schema associated with resilience in black South African adolescents, and to provide guidelines for a culturally fair interpretation of the Rorschach to identify latent resources which nurture black adolescent resilience. The relevance of psychodynamic and constructivist approaches to Rorschach interpretation regarding the experience of adolescence as a black South African was explored. As such, the Rorschach was implemented effectively as a culturally sensitive and fair instrument (Odendaal, 2011).

In 2002 Dr Aronstam and colleagues established the South African Rorschach Discussion Group. This group has international connections and provides a forum for all interested Rorschach clinicians and researchers. It invites presentations from young researchers so that they can share their research findings. Dr Aronstam, a senior lecturer in the Department of Psychology at the University of Pretoria, started the *South African Rorschach Journal* in 2004. Various important and interesting research articles have been published which use both nomothetic and idiographic approaches.

Several studies have focused on various areas of psychopathology, indicating how Rorschach data could enhance our understanding of these conditions.

Aronstam and Macklin (2004) published a study on the development of diagnostic criteria for Borderline Personality Disorder, based on Rorschach data. In a separate study by Daws, Du Preez and Aronstam (2004), the Perceptual Thinking Index of the Rorschach was evaluated within a psychotic and nonpsychotic South African population. They indicated the importance of using this index with a definite consideration of the traditional belief systems and values of different cultural groups in South Africa. In another study Smuts and Aronstam (2004) explored aetiological and prognostic considerations for Trichotilomania.

Aronstam, Daws and Pearce (2006) explored the manifestation of anorexia nervosa within a South African sample. Aronstam, Daws and Swanepoel (2006/2007) also published a study investigating schizoid character organisation and the anorexic patient. In a similar vein, Aronstam (2008) published articles on the relevance of the Rorschach in exploring anxiety and Burning Mouth Syndrome (Daws & Aronstam, 2005). In her completed but unpublished Master's dissertation, Smit (2010) reported on her research regarding Rorschach indicators of self-harm amongst South African adolescents. Another study of particular value within the current climate of South Africa, which is characterised by an unusually high crime rate, was that of E'Silva and Aronstam (2006/2007), which focused on the impact of multiple traumas on victims by exploring impaired perceptual thinking, as evidenced on the Rorschach, amongst victims of repetitive armed robbery at the workplace. A solid basis for this study can be found in the work of Luxemberg and Levin (2004), who explored the use of the Rorschach in the diagnosis and treatment of trauma.

Unfortunately research on the Rorschach in South Africa is limited, possibly due to the limited training currently available. Universities and other training institutions which place more emphasis on 'objective' measurement and on cognitive-behavioural therapies are, because of their theoretical and ideological bias, uninterested in pursuing this training with their students. These students are often exposed to negative attitudes and opinions regarding the Rorschach, despite the fact that numerous well-devised studies have shown many criticisms to be inaccurate (Odendaal, 2011).

The training of novices requires a substantial commitment and, of course, expert knowledge from the trainer. It is time-consuming, and each student will initially need much individual guidance with scoring as well as with interpretation. Personality theory, developmental theory and knowledge of psychopathology form the backdrop to understanding Rorschach results and to the writing of meaningful reports.

It takes a minimum of regular (weekly) sessions for a period of six months for a student to grasp the basics of coding, interpretation and report-writing. Further exposure to the literature and a variety of case studies, in addition to supervised work related to their own work in this field, is necessary before the psychologist will feel confident about regularly using the Rorschach as part of an assessment battery. Consequently, many higher education institutions are unable to devote time and/or expertise to offering this training.[1]

Conclusion

The tendency today is to incorporate both idiographic and nomothetic approaches when using the Rorschach. In the South African context, research may be more meaningful following a conceptual rather than a strictly nomothetic approach, as the norms provided by Exner are not standardised for the South African population as such. The interpretation of content in Rorschach protocols, in addition to taking some cognisance of nomothetic data, seems to be the most acceptable route.

The value of the Rorschach, as part of a test battery aimed at a better understanding of the individual, should not be underestimated. It can contribute substantially to establishing a diagnosis, considering a prognosis and planning appropriate treatment. It has also been shown to be most valuable in other contexts, such as career planning and forensic work.

Rorschach results provide us with exceptionally rich information that cannot be gained from any other measurement of the individual personality in a manner that is not dependent solely on self-report. Thus it would be unfortunate if training and research on this instrument were to be abandoned, since it has been proven to be a valuable and unique instrument. As Aronstam (2004) indicates, it may well be that the optimal way of using the Rorschach in the 21st century (and in South Africa) has yet to be devised. This is an exciting challenge for clinicians facing multiple dilemmas inherent in working within a multicultural society.

Note

1 Dr Aronstam, editor of the *South African Rorschach Journal*, is well known for the training he provides to students and other interested professionals in Pretoria. Dr Visser, of the University of South Africa, provides intensive Rorschach training at a Master's level in clinical psychology. She uses the Rorschach regularly in her own forensic work. Similar training is offered at the University of the North-West, in the Department of Clinical Psychology. In Johannesburg, Dr Brink offers a basic Rorschach course, as well as an advanced discussion group to registered psychologists.

References

Allen, A. & Dana, R. H. (2004). Methodological issues in cross-cultural and multicultural Rorschach research. *Journal of Personality Assessment, 83(2)*, 189–206.

Aronow, E. & Rodriguez-Srednicki, O. (2004). The relationship of Rorschach determinants to affective functioning: Implications for Rorschach usage. *South African Rorschach Journal, 1(1)*, 26–32.

Aronstam, M. (2004). Rorschach self-interpretation: Towards a culture-fair understanding of Rorschach content data. *South African Rorschach Journal, 1(1)*, 33–46.

Aronstam, M. (2008). Harry Stack Sullivan's *not-me* anxiety and the Rorschach Inkblot Test: Can the two meet? *South African Rorschach Journal, 4(1)*, 26–52.

Aronstam, M., Daws, L. & Pearce, A. (2006). An exploration of anorexia nervosa within a South African sample: A Rorschach study. *South African Rorschach Journal, 3(3)*, 29–41.

Aronstam, M., Daws, L. & Swanepoel, N. (2006/2007). Schizoid character organization and the anorexic patient. *South African Rorschach Journal, 3(2)*, 34–48.

Aronstam, M. & Macklin, D. (2004). The development of diagnostic criteria for the Borderline Personality Disorder. *South African Rorschach Journal, 1(2)*, 46–64.

Berant, E. & Mikulincer, M. (2005). Rorschach correlates of self-reported attachment dimensions: Dynamic manifestations of hyperactivating and deactivating strategies. *Journal of Personality Assessment, 84(1)*, 70–81.

Bornstein, R. F. (2007). Might the Rorschach be a projective test after all? Social projection of an undesirable trait alters Rorschach oral dependency scores. *Journal of Personality Assessment, 88(3)*, 354–367.

Brink, M. (2002). Notes on Rorschach interpretation. Unpublished course notes. Johannesburg.

Brink, M. (2005). Scientific basis for using the Rorschach: Research, reliability and validity: A meta-study. Unpublished course notes. Johannesburg.

Brink, M. (2010). Revised notes on Rorschach interpretation. Unpublished course notes for the Advanced Discussion Group. Johannesburg.

Daly, W. C. (2005). Theoretical foundations of Rorschach by Piotrowski. *Education, 125(4)*, 669–673.

Daws, L. & Aronstam, M. (2005). Burning Mouth Syndrome (Part 1): A Rorschach case study. *South African Rorschach Journal, 2(1)*, 53–70.

Daws, L., Du Preez, I. & Aronstam, M. (2004). The Schizophrenic and Perceptual Thinking Index within a psychotic and non-psychotic population in South Africa. *South African Rorschach Journal, 1(2)*, 65–91.

De Ruyter, C. & Veen, V. (2004). Forensic psychological assessment: The case of an arsonist. *South African Rorschach Journal, 1(2)*, 23.

De Vos, A. S. (2007). Combined quantitative and qualitative approach. In A. S. De Vos, C. B. Fouche & C. S. L. Delport (Eds), *Research at Grass Roots for the Social Sciences and Human Service Professions* (pp. 357–355). Pretoria: Van Schaik.

E'Silva, J. & Aronstam, M. (2006/2007). Multiple traumas: The Rorschach and impaired thinking amongst victims of repetitive armed robbery at the workplace. *South African Rorschach Journal, 3(2)*, 34–48.

Exner, J. E., Jr (2003). *The Rorschach: A Comprehensive System. Volume 1: Basic Foundations and Principles of Interpretation* (4th edition). Hoboken, NJ: John Wiley & Sons.

Exner, J. E., Jr (2005). *The Rorschach: A Comprehensive System. Volume 2: Advanced Interpretation* (3rd edition). Hoboken, NJ: John Wiley & Sons.

Exner, J. E., Jr, Weiner, I. B. & PAR Staff (2008). *Rorschach Interpretation Assistance Program: Version 5*. Lutz, FL: Psychological Assessment Resources.

Gacono, C. B. (Ed.) (2001). *The Clinical and Forensic Assessment of Psychopathy: A Practitioner's Guide*. Mahwah, NJ: Lawrence Erlbaum Associates.

Gacono, C. B., Evans, B. F., Gacono, L. A. & Kaser-Boyd, N. (Eds) (2008). *The Handbook of Forensic Rorschach Assessment*. New York, NY: Routledge Taylor & Francis Group.

Hartman, E. (2001). Rorschach administration: A comparison of the effect of two instructions. *Journal of Personality Assessment, 76(3)*, 461–471.

Hartman, E. (2003). Depression and vulnerability as assessed by the Rorschach method. *Journal of Personality Assessment, 81(3)*, 242–255.

Janson, H. & Stattin, H. (2003). Prediction of adolescent and adult delinquency from childhood Rorschach ratings. *Journal of Personality Assessment, 81(1)*, 51–63.

Klopfer, B., Ainsworth, M. D., Klopfer, G. & Holt, R. R. (1954). *Developments in the Rorschach Technique: Technique and Theory*. New York, NY: Harcourt, Brace & World.

Leichtman, M. (2000). Psychoanalytic perspectives on the Rorschach. Book review. *Bulletin of the Menninger Clinic, 64(3)*, 432–434.

Liebman, S. J., Porcerelli, J. & Abel, S. C. (2005). Reliability and validity of Rorschach aggression variables with a sample of adjudicated adolescents. *Journal of Personality Assessment, 85(1)*, 33–39.

Lilienfeld, S. O. (2001). The Rorschach test is scientifically questionable. *Harvard Mental Health Letter, 18(6)*, 5–6.

Luxemberg, T. & Levin, P. (2004). The role of the Rorschach in the assessment and treatment of trauma. In J. P. Wilson & T. M. Keane (Eds), *Assessing Psychological Trauma and PTSD* (2nd edition, pp. 231–239). New York, NY: The Guilford Press.

Mattlar, C. (2005). The utility of the Rorschach Comprehensive System: An increasing body of supportive research. *South African Rorschach Journal, 2(1)*, 3–31.

Meloy, J. R. (2005). Some reflections on *'What's wrong with the Rorschach?'*. *Journal of Personality Assessment, 85(3)*, 344–346.

Meloy, J. R., Acklin, M. W., Gacono, C. B., Murray, J. F. & Peterson, C. A. (Eds) (1997). *Contemporary Rorschach Interpretation*. London: Lawrence Erlbaum Associates.

Meyer, G. J. (2000a). Incremental validity of the Rorschach prognostic rating scale over the MMPI ego strength scale. *Journal of Personality Assessment, 74(3)*, 356–370.

Meyer, G. J. (Ed.) (2000b). The utility of the Rorschach for clinical assessment. *Psychological Assessment (Special section), 12*, 235–302.

Meyer, G. J. & Archer, R. (2001). The hard science of Rorschach research: What do we know and where do we go? *Psychological Assessment, 13*, 486–502.

Meyer, G. J., Hilsenroth, M. J., Baxter, M. J., Exner, J. E., Fowler, J. C. & Piers, C. C. (2002). An examination of interrater reliability for scoring the Rorschach Comprehensive System in eight data sets. *Journal of Personality Assessment, 78*, 219–274.

Meyer, G. J., Viglione, D. J., Mihura, J. L., Erard, R. E. & Erdberg, P. (2012). *The R-Pas System: Administration, Coding, Interpretation, and Technical Manual* (pp. 317–374). Retrieved May 28, 2012, from www.r-pas.org.

Moletsane, M. & Eloff, I. (2006). The adjustment of Rorschach Comprehensive System procedures for South African learners. *South African Journal of Psychology, 36(4)*, 880–902.

Nygren, M. (2004). Rorschach Comprehensive System variables in relation to assessing dynamic capacity and ego strength for psychodynamic psychotherapy. *Journal of Personality Assessment, 83(3)*, 277–292.

Odendaal, I. E. (2011). Rorschach indicators of resilience in adolescents. Unpublished PhD dissertation. University of the North-West, Vanderbijlpark.

Raskin, J. D. (2001). Constructivism and the projective assessment of meaning in Rorschach administration. *Journal of Personality Assessment, 77(1)*, 139–161.

Ritzler, B. A. (2001). Multicultural usage of the Rorschach. In L. A. Suzuki, J. G. Pontrotto & P. J. Meller (Eds), *Handbook of Multicultural Assessment: Clinical, Psychological, and Educational Applications* (pp. 237–252). San Francisco, CA: Jossey-Bassey.

Rorschach, H. (1921/1942). *Psychodiagnostics*. New York, NY: Grune & Stratton.

Shaffer, T. W., Erdberg, P. & Meyer, G. J. (2007). An international reference sample for the Rorschach. *Journal of Personality Assessment, 89(51)*, 139–161.

Smit, M. (2010). Self-harm amongst adolescent girls in Afrikaans schools: An explorative Rorschach investigation. Unpublished Master's dissertation. University of Johannesburg, Johannesburg.

Smuts, S. & Aronstam, M. (2004). Aetiological and prognostic considerations for Trichotilomania. *South African Rorschach Journal, 1(1)*, 47–66.

Strydom, H. (2007). Ethical aspects of research in the social sciences and human service professions. In A. S. De Vos, H. Strydom, C. B. Fouche & C. S. L. Delport (Eds), *Research at Grass Roots for the Social Sciences and Human Service Professions* (pp. 239–261). Pretoria: Van Schaik.

Theron, L. C. (2004). The role of personal protective factors in anchoring psychological resilience in adolescents with learning difficulties. *South African Journal of Education, 24(4)*, 317–321.

Theron, L. C., Cameron, A., Lau, C., Didkowsky, N. & Mabitsela, M. (2009). A day in the lives of four resilient youth: An investigation of the cultural roots of resilience. Paper presented at the 14th South African Psychology Conference, Cape Town, August 11–14.

Veeren, V. & Morgan, T. (2009). Examining the role of culture in the development of resilience for youth at risk in contested societies of South Africa and Northern Ireland. *Youth & Policy, 102*, 53–66.

Weiner, I. B. (1998). *Principles of Rorschach Interpretation*. London: Lawrence Erlbaum Associates.

Weiner, I. B. (2000). Making Rorschach interpretation as good as it can be. *Journal of Personality Assessment, 74(2)*, 164–174.

Weiner, I. B. (2001). Advancing the science of psychological assessment: The Rorschach Inkblot Method as exemplar. *Journal of Psychological Assessment, 13(4)*, 423–433.

Weiner, I. B. (2004). The future of Rorschach assessment. *South African Rorschach Journal, 1(1)*, 3–11.

Wood, J., Nezworski, M. T., Lilienfeld, S. & Garb, H. (2003). *What's Wrong with the Rorschach?* San Francisco: Jossey-Bass.

Section Three

Assessment approaches and methodologies

28 Ethical perspectives in assessment

N. Coetzee

The etymological basis of the word *ethics* is the Greek word *ethos*, which, when it is translated into English, means a set of moral principles (Pharos, 2010). According to Leach and Oakland (2007), the first official document ever to express the need for imposing rules that would govern professional behaviour was the Code of Hammurabi (circa 1795–1750 BCE). Their research revealed that the Hippocratic Oath (circa 400 BCE) was the first known example of a professionally generated code of ethics. In 1958, the American Psychological Association (APA) established the first ethical code for psychologists (Leach & Oakland, 2007). Since then, many countries have developed ethical codes addressing issues associated with psychological practice and psychological assessment. South Africa is one of many countries that have produced an ethical code largely influenced by the 2002 APA code (Leach & Oakland, 2007). The South African code is published under the heading 'Rules of Conduct Pertaining Specifically to Psychology' by the Professional Board for Psychology, which falls under the auspices of the Health Professions Council of South Africa (HPCSA) (HPCSA, 2010a).

Louw (1997a) perceives the existence of a South African code as evidence of the intention of local psychologists to adhere to professional standards of practice. He notes that such a code is a defining characteristic of the discipline and serves as proof that psychology in South Africa deserves its scientific status. Since the Professional Board for Psychology falls under the auspices of the HPCSA, clients are legally protected against any possible harm and control is exerted over the conduct of assessment practitioners. Despite an ongoing debate over the feasibility of these institutions in South Africa (AfricaRights, 2007a; 2007b), it should be noted that international commentators advocate the existence of statutory control no matter what the type or form (Hall, Howerton & Bolin, 2005; ITC, 2001; Leach & Oakland, 2007).

In South Africa there are various forms of legislation that contribute to psychological assessment in some form. In addition to the Rules of Conduct Pertaining Specifically to Psychology, and the relevant legislation, one will note that the International Test Commission's (ITC) International Guidelines for Test Use (Version 2000) (ITC, 2001) and the Code of Practice for Psychological and Other Similar Assessment in the Workplace, published by the Society for Industrial and Organisational Psychology of South Africa (SIOPSA) in association with People Assessment in Industry (PAI) (SIOPSA, 2006), are the other two most often cited and used documents for understanding and discussing ethical issues relating to psychological assessment in South Africa. It is the author's contention that these separate documents need to be brought together in a single document, thus making the ethical code more accessible to students and professionals in the field.

Allan (2008) and Bricklin (2001) have noted, however, that being ethical does not only involve behaviour that constitutes avoiding harm, but also involves thorough knowledge of legislation pertaining to psychological assessment. Bricklin (2001, p.202) proposes that psychological assessment practitioners should develop an 'ethical consciousness'. Such a consciousness would be evident amongst those practitioners who have a sufficient understanding of the relevant ethical codes and standards of conduct. In addition, such practitioners would display proper knowledge of the legislation pertaining to psychological assessment. To be ethical when doing psychological assessment thus means demonstrating a thorough understanding not only of the legislation governing assessment practices, but also of the relevant codes and standards of conduct. This chapter will demonstrate this approach, using the model in Figure 28.1, where it is proposed that a thorough understanding of ethical issues in South Africa involves the joint consideration of three areas – namely, a code of conduct, a specification of standard practices, and sufficient knowledge of legislation. Each of these is discussed hereunder.

Figure 28.1 The three main components of an ethical code

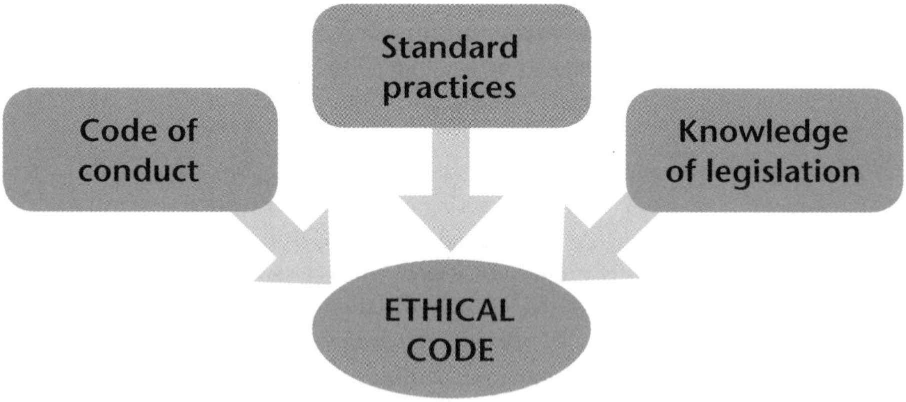

A code of conduct

For the purposes of this chapter, conduct is defined as the behaviour practitioners display whilst doing psychological assessment. In order to establish a code of conduct that is representative of the field of psychology, a thematic analysis was conducted on the Ethical Principles of Psychologists and Code of Conduct of the APA (2002), the Professional Board for Psychology's Rules of Conduct (HPCSA, 2010a) and policy documents from the HPCSA (HPCSA, 2010c; 2010d). These documents were included in the analysis because all of them provide guidance on how practitioners should behave when conducting psychological assessment. The analysis revealed several dominant themes, related to the following topics:

- the boundaries of competence;
- avoiding harm;
- informed consent;
- confidentiality; and
- the fair use of assessment.

Boundaries of competence

In South Africa, the Health Professions Act No. 56 of 1974 specifies the boundaries of competence for those who conduct psychological assessment. According to this Act, two sorts of individuals are allowed to do psychological assessment. The first category is registered psychologists. The main impetus of the Act is the notion that registered psychologists are individuals who have undergone rigorous professional training that qualifies them to psychologically assess intellectual or cognitive ability or functioning, aptitude, interest, personality make-up or personality functioning (HPCSA, 2010a; 2010b; 2010c; 2010d). Having knowledge and understanding of only those instruments one is trained in directly impacts on the boundaries of competence. Psychologists are thus bound to make use only of those forms of assessment for which they have received appropriate training and in which they have gained sufficient experience (Louw, 1997b; Murphy & Davidshofer, 2005).

The second category of individuals who are allowed by the Health Professions Act to conduct psychological assessment includes psychometrists and professionals from other health professions, such as speech and occupational therapists (HPCSA, 2010b). At the time of writing this chapter, changes had been proposed to the Labour Relations Act No. 66 of 1995, amongst which was an amendment that only psychologists and psychometrists may administer and score psychological tests. This was highly contested and, at the time of writing, the legislation had not been passed.

There are a number of conditions that need to be met before individuals commence an assessment (HPCSA, 2010b):

- The measure must be categorised by the Psychometrics Committee of the Professional Board for Psychology as a measurement instrument that may be administered by a psychologist, psychometrist or other professional (but see the comment above about proposed changes to legislation).
- The assessment administrator must comply with the restrictions placed on him or her by his or her category of registration with the HPCSA. A psychometrist, for example, may administer, score and do a preliminary interpretation of assessment results but is not allowed to report on such results.
- The assessment administrator must seek the mentoring of a psychologist if specialist input is needed to enhance the assessment process and further understanding of the results it yielded.
- The assessment administrator must have received appropriate training, and achieved the minimum competencies required to use the assessment measure.

Based on the above, it thus appears that an ethical assessment practitioner would be someone who is aware of their level of competence and will not operate outside their professional limits. Such an individual would rely on his or her training and quality of experience to display ethical behaviour when conducting a psychological assessment. Acknowledging and adhering to these requirements is the first step in the development of an ethical consciousness.

Avoiding harm

Within the context of psychological assessment, avoiding harm implies that the practitioner will take reasonable steps to avoid or minimise any form of harm to individuals during the assessment process (APA, 2002; HPCSA, 2010a). One example of a situation where harm could occur as the result of psychological assessment is in the workplace. Here, the results of an assessment process often impact on the job aspirations of some individuals. Such results are used to determine, for example, which candidate is accepted for a position and who is rejected, who will be promoted and who not. The individual who was not selected for a highly sought-after position or promotion could deem the rejection a failure, and some harm has thus occurred. This form of harm could, however, be minimised by providing professional feedback to the unsuccessful applicant that would enable him or her not to internalise the failure but to consider other career opportunities.

Another way of avoiding harm is by being sensitive to any needs the individual undergoing the assessment, or other relevant parties (for example, parents of children), may have. In some instances, these needs might include basic physical and psychological needs. In other situations, it will be expected of the assessment practitioner to accommodate individuals with more specific needs. Examples of such needs are being visually impaired, physically disabled, hard of hearing, not speaking the same language as the assessment practitioner, having a different cultural background, being unfamiliar with psychological assessment, and so on.

The most important aspect of avoiding harm involves being sensitive to the information obtained during assessment procedures. Psychological assessment often gives practitioners an in-depth look into aspects of an individual's life which are deemed private. Practitioners will gain insight into the personalities and lives of individuals, and must be sensitive yet professional when dealing with clients. When dealing with the latter, practitioners must display respect and unconditional acceptance (Allan, 2008; HPCSA, 2010a). Since it is one of the obligations of an ethical assessment practitioner to protect the individuals they are assessing, and because they find themselves in positions where they are privy to sensitive information, the aspects of informed consent and confidentiality become even more important in the ethical make-up and ultimately the ethical consciousness of the assessment practitioner.

Informed consent

Informed consent is the practice of obtaining, in writing, consent from an individual, the parent of a child or the legal guardian or representative of any person incapable of providing consent, to participate in psychological assessment. The consent form should contain the following information (HPCSA, 2010a):

- all relevant details of the individual being assessed;
- the nature of the assessment procedure and a list of the assessment measures to be used; and
- any limits that might be imposed when conducting the assessment, such as the individual refusing to be assessed, limits to confidentiality, or any potential harmful effects inherent in the assessment procedure.

It is important to note that individuals have the right to ask questions about the assessment procedure before giving their consent. When an individual (or the representative of the individual) refuses to consent to participating in the assessment, he or she must be informed in a respectful and professional manner of the consequences of such a refusal (Foxcroft, Roodt & Abrahams, 2009; Moerdyk, 2009). Written consent is not necessary in some instances. These are (HPCSA, 2010a):

- when the assessment is a legal requirement (for example, during custody battles, the Family Advocate's office will require both parents to undergo psychological assessment);
- when informed consent is implied because the assessment is conducted as a routine activity (for example, when applying to become an airline pilot, psychological assessment will form part of the selection procedures); or
- if the purpose of the assessment is to evaluate an individual's ability to make decisions or to determine mental incapacity.

Although it is not a prerequisite to obtain informed consent from individuals with questionable capacity, or from individuals who have been instructed by a court to undergo psychological assessment, the practitioner displaying ethical behaviour will still inform the concerned individual about the nature and purpose of the proposed assessment. This must be done in a language that is reasonably comprehensible to the individual (HPCSA, 2010a).

In a multilingual society such as South Africa, assessment practitioners will sometimes need to acquire the services of an interpreter. In such instances, the individual who will undergo the assessment must consent to the use of the interpreter. The practitioner, however, will still be held responsible for the safekeeping of confidential information arising from the assessment. It is also the practitioner's ethical duty to note the use of an interpreter in any report written subsequent to the assessment, thus making others aware of the limitation that the use of an interpreter may have posed on the procedure (HPCSA, 2010a).

In addition to what is prescribed by the HPCSA on the issue, the author is of the opinion that an ethically conscious practitioner should employ an interpreter who is either registered in one of the categories acknowledged by the Professional Board for Psychology, or has intimate knowledge of the fields of psychology and psychological assessment. This will ensure that the interpreter will understand the importance of keeping obtained information confidential. Such an interpreter will also realise that he or she is under an ethical obligation to interpret exactly what has been said by the assessed individual. In the unlikely event that an assessment practitioner cannot find a suitable interpreter, it will be his or her responsibility to train an individual in the matters of correct interpretation and confidentiality. It is also recommended that the assessment practitioner enter into a contractual agreement with any interpreter used, in order to ensure ethical conduct.

Records of informed consent, contractual agreements, the assessment process and the results it has yielded must be stored and maintained by the practitioner for a minimum period of five years (Allan, 2008). In doing so, the practitioner will not only comply with the legal requirements pertaining to record-keeping, but will also be able to facilitate any inquiry or subsequent professional interventions (HPCSA, 2010a).

Confidentiality

According to the Professional Board for Psychology's Rules of Conduct (HPCSA, 2010a) and the APA's Code of Ethics (2002), practitioners must safeguard all confidential information obtained during the course of psychological assessment procedures. This includes information obtained about the individual being assessed, such as biographical information, information obtained from significant others (for example, family, colleagues and peers) and the results of the assessment(s) conducted. Practitioners must, at the onset of the assessment process and before assent is obtained, discuss the issue of confidentiality with the individual or group of individuals who will be assessed. During this discussion, the practitioner must inform the person or group of persons involved of the measures that will be taken to guarantee confidentiality. Such a person or group of persons must also be informed of the limitations that exist with regard to confidentiality (Allan, 2008; APA, 2002; HPCSA, 2010a). One example of such a limitation is where an individual is legally incapable of making decisions on his or her own behalf (for example, a child, or a person suffering from severe brain damage). The parent(s), legal guardian or legal representative of such a person will then be informed about the outcome of the assessment process. Another example of a limitation on confidentiality is when an exceptional circumstance occurs. When the assessment practitioner learns that a client is abusing a child or poses a clear danger to other persons, he or she must inform the authorities (Allan, 2008). If practitioners are confronted with what they believe to be an exceptional circumstance, but doubt whether alerting the authorities would be the ethical thing to do, they should approach the Professional Board for Psychology or the HPCSA for legal guidance. Yet another example is an instance where the assessment practitioner is ordered by court or some other legal imperative to release the information (HPCSA, 2010a).

Apart from the limitations on confidentiality that exist, assessment practitioners may release confidential information when given the proper authorisation by a client, a parent of a minor, or the legal guardian or legal representative of an incapable person (HPCSA, 2010a). A practitioner needs to be aware of these issues relating to confidentiality, as this is the requirement of the HPCSA Code of Conduct. However the ethically conscious practitioner does not relate to this simply because it is stated in an official document, but rather because he or she feels the moral obligation to adopt the correct approach within the context.

Fair use of assessment

Practitioners must ensure that they only use assessment procedures which are deemed appropriate for the aim of the assessment process (APA, 2002; Foxcroft et al., 2009; ITC, 2001; Kaplan & Saccuzzo, 2009). Neuropsychological assessment measures, for example, cannot be administered on a learner seeking assistance in making the correct subject choices. They may only be utilised if initial assessment procedures indicate neurological fallouts and further investigation is warranted. Practitioners should further make certain that they only make use of assessment measures that are valid and reliable (APA, 2002; Foxcroft et al., 2009; ITC, 2001; Moerdyk, 2009; SIOPSA, 2006). This implies that practitioners will be aware of the limitations of the measures and techniques they use as part of the assessment (Moerdyk, 2009).

An important point coinciding with this is that practitioners must know if the assessment measures and techniques they intend to use are appropriate for individuals from the target population being assessed (APA, 2002; Moerdyk, 2009). In a multicultural society such as South Africa, practitioners might sometimes find themselves in a position where they are dealing with individuals who have not been assessed before or who are illiterate. Assessing these individuals using psychological tests, for example, will constitute the unfair use of assessment. South African practitioners therefore need to be flexible in ensuring the ethical and fair use of assessment. This means that when practitioners find themselves in a situation dealing with individuals who are not familiar with assessment practices or who are illiterate, they should be able to replace one form of assessment with a suitable alternative. For example, a practitioner is approached by an individual who experiences some emotional problems. In order to get to know the person, the practitioner wants to learn more about the specific personality traits displayed by the individual. The individual, however, is illiterate and cannot complete any personality questionnaire. The practitioner then makes use of other forms of assessment, such as behavioural observations, clinical interviews and interviewing significant others (such as family, colleagues and elders) in the community to learn more about the personality of the client (Foxcroft, 2002).

The fair use of assessment forms the foundation of the ethical code of conduct that guides the work of psychological assessment practitioners. Even if a practitioner has been able to gain the trust of an individual, has obtained his or her informed consent and has professionally conducted the assessment, making use of techniques that are unfamiliar to the individual who is being assessed, or which are not appropriate for the purposes of the particular assessment process, will have a negative impact on the assessed person. This must be avoided at all costs, especially in South Africa where not all sectors of society are familiar with psychological assessment practices. Individuals who are assessed must experience the process as helpful, and must be guided to use the knowledge gained to their advantage. Such practices will help to ensure that psychological assessment will become known as a 'helpful' practice instead of becoming known as a 'hurtful' practice.

Standard practices

In the previous section, the behaviour that ethical assessment practitioners will display was discussed. As stated at the start of the chapter, however, these behaviours form only one part of the ethics involved in psychological assessment. The second part consists of specific standards that assessment practitioners should adhere to when conducting assessment. These standards will be discussed next.

Preparing for the assessment

Before the commencement of any assessment process, the practitioner needs to do the following (ITC, 2001; Moerdyk, 2009; SIOPSA, 2006):

- Ensure that, if psychological testing forms part of the process, all the materials as specified by the instructor's manual are readily available. These materials must be in good condition and should contain no marks or notes which are not specified by the manual.
- Make certain that the assessment venue is well illuminated and ventilated, as well as free of any form of disturbances. If the venue is not located at the practitioner's office, arrangements for a facility must be made well in advance. Assessment venues must be accessible and individuals being assessed should be informed beforehand of the location of the venue. When assessing large groups, the venue must be large enough to comfortably accommodate the group.
- Make sure that anyone assisting the practitioner is qualified and competent in the use of the assessment techniques employed.
- Make appropriate arrangements for assessing those with specific needs.
- Anticipate any problems that might occur and counteract them through thorough preparation. A simplistic example is to ensure that a pencil sharpener is at hand to sharpen pencils, when pencil-and-paper testing forms part of the assessment.
- Upon arrival of the individual(s) being assessed, remove any distractions such as cellular phones.

Conducting the assessment

During the assessment, the practitioner must (Foxcroft et al., 2009; ITC, 2001; Moerdyk, 2009; SIOPSA, 2006):

- establish rapport and deal with any possible anxieties that are displayed;
- use a calm and clear tone of voice when providing instructions;
- if psychological tests are used, read instructions from the manual and make certain that the individual(s) being assessed understand(s) them;
- maintain the interest and cooperation of the individual(s);
- in instances where time restrictions are allocated to certain forms of the assessment procedure, adhere to these restrictions;
- observe and record all behaviour which will enhance understanding when the results are interpreted (examples of such behaviour are response times, continuous nervous or anxious fidgeting, non-committal responses, and so on);
- not leave the individual(s) being assessed unsupervised; and

- make certain that when assessment materials such as psychological tests have been used, all such material is accounted for at the end of the assessment.

Securing the information

Once the assessment process has been completed, the practitioner must make sure that all information obtained and the assessment materials that were used (for example, psychological tests) are stored in a safe and secure place (Allan, 2008; ITC, 2001; Moerdyk, 2009; SIOPSA, 2006).

Analysing and interpreting the results

The following guidelines should be adhered to during the analysis and interpretation of assessment results, in order to ensure ethical practice:

- If, during the assessment process, any standardised procedures were used (for example, norm-based psychological tests or structured interviews), the practitioner should follow the prescribed rules for scoring as indicated in the manuals of such measures (ITC, 2001).
- Practitioners must ensure, when analysing results where some subjective interpretation of the information is needed (for example, scoring projective techniques, or unstructured or semi-structured interviews), that they have taken the necessary steps to limit the effects of their own bias. One possible way to deal with this is to submit the material to another qualified individual for scoring (Moerdyk, 2009). Inter-rater reliability is then established to determine the amount of bias that might have occurred.
- All the information obtained during the assessment process should be utilised when making a decision about the individual – whether it concerns appointing the person, institutionalising him or her, making a clinical diagnosis, and so on. It is recommended that the results of the various forms of assessment are correlated with one another to determine the accuracy of the practitioner's judgement (ITC, 2001; Murphy & Davidshofer, 2005).
- Results must be interpreted within the context of the assessment process, and any problems that might have occurred during its duration (such as power failure, or an individual assessed not feeling well) should be taken into account (ITC, 2001).
- Cognisance must be taken of the limitations of the assessment measures or any other factors, such as cultural or language differences, that might affect the outcome of the assessment (ITC, 2001).
- Practitioners must consider the impact that prior experience of assessment processes or the assessment measures used could have on the current situation (ITC, 2001).

Reporting the results

When reporting the results of the assessment process, it is important for the practitioner to consider the following (ITC, 2001; Moerdyk, 2009; SIOPSA, 2006):

- Identify all stakeholders who may legitimately receive the results. If the assessment process was, for example, the consequence of the individual's own request (for example, to assist with subject choices or career planning, or to deal with emotional problems), a report of the results will be given directly to him or her. In other instances, such as the industrial and organisational context, the party who pays for the assessment process is the one who receives the report. It should be noted, however, that the individual being assessed in such an instance has the right to feedback, and arrangements should thus be made if he or she wants access to the information.

- Reports, whether in oral or written form, should be clear and easy to understand and thus must be free from technical jargon. Derogatory comments, negative labels or any other forms of language that could have a destructive impact on the individual must be avoided.
- Practitioners should report only those results that relate to the reasons for the use of the assessment, and must avoid overgeneralisation of results to other aspects of the individual's life that were not dealt with during the assessment process.
- The individual assessed must be given an idea of how the results will impact on his or her future decision-making. Even in organisations and industries where assessment is used (for example, for selection purposes), the outcome (albeit negative) could advantage the individual if reported in a constructive manner. For example, John is a certified chartered accountant who applied for a position with an accounting firm that only deals with big conglomerates in the private sector. John did not get the position, because during the assessment it was discovered that he is not a team player. As a result of the assessment, John realises he will fare better in situations where he works on his own and deals with few individuals at a time. He now knows that he should rather seek employment with firms that deal with small and individually owned businesses. The assessment process has thus assisted John to get to know himself better and to make more informed decisions when looking for a job.
- Any report (oral or written) should contain a clear summary of the results and recommendations that the individual should consider when making any decisions. It is imperative that all forms of report always be presented in a constructive and supportive manner.

Knowledge of legislation

The third element necessary for inclusion in an ethical code is knowledge and understanding of all forms of legislation related to psychological assessment practices. This section will thus deal with the legislation, or acts of law, which assessment practitioners need to consider when conducting psychological assessment.

The Health Professions Act (No. 56 of 1974)

The Health Professions Act applies to all forms of psychological assessment. This Act was thoroughly discussed earlier in this chapter, in the section on 'Boundaries of competence', and will not be pursued further. Practitioners are urged, in the interests of developing an ethical consciousness, to obtain the entire Act from the HPCSA's website and read through it.

The Bill of Rights as contained in the Constitution of the Republic of South Africa (Act No. 108 of 1996)

In addition to the Health Professions Act, assessment practitioners operating in the discipline of psychology need to avail themselves of the contents of the Constitution of the Republic of South Africa. The Constitution is the supreme law of the Republic and hence must be upheld by its citizenry (Mauer, 2000). The Constitution contains the Bill of Rights, which forms the cornerstone of the South African democracy. It protects the rights of people living in South Africa and affirms the democratic rights of human dignity, equality and freedom. Practitioners should pay special attention to Section 9 of the Bill (Mauer, 2000), which deals with Equality and Human Dignity, and states the following:

9.1 Everyone is equal before the law and has the right to equal protection and benefit of the law;

9.2 Equality includes the full and equal enjoyment of all rights and freedom. To promote the achievement of equality, legislative and other measures designed to protect or advance persons, or categories of persons, disadvantaged by unfair discrimination may be taken;

9.3 The state may not unfairly discriminate directly or indirectly against anyone on one or more grounds, including race, gender, sex, pregnancy, marital status, ethnic or social origin, colour, sexual orientation, age, disability, religion, conscience, belief, culture, language and birth;

9.4 No person may unfairly discriminate directly or indirectly against anyone on one or more grounds in terms of subsection (3);

9.5 Discrimination on one or more of the grounds listed in subsection (3) is unfair unless it is established that the discrimination is fair.

The implication Section 9 holds for psychological assessment is clear: any individual being assessed must be respected and treated with dignity, irrespective of their background or biographical features. It is important to note that this section allows for 'fair' discrimination. Few assessment practitioners realise that when using appropriate assessment measures under the right circumstances, assessment presents them with the ideal tool to discriminate in a fair manner. Assessment, and especially the results it yields, helps practitioners to discern ('discriminate') who is the best candidate for the position, who has a personality disorder, which subjects would be most suitable for a Grade 10 learner to take, and so on.

Another subsection of the Bill of Rights which aptly applies to the context of psychological assessment is noted under Section 14(4) (Mauer, 2000). This particular subsection deals with the disclosure of information and states that:

> Everyone has the right to privacy, which includes the right not to have:
> 14.4 the privacy of their communications infringed.

Section 14(4) reminds practitioners how important it is to abide by the rules of confidentiality. They should not, however, let Section 14(4) confuse them and remember that within the boundaries of psychological assessment, limits to confidentiality exist. These must be discussed and explained to the individual who is about to undergo psychological assessment.

The Children's Act (No. 38 of 2005)

Conducting psychological assessment of children is complicated. First of all, children cannot provide consent to undergo psychological assessment; this consent must be obtained from parents or legal guardians (APA, 2002; HPCSA, 2010a). Secondly, not all forms of assessment may be used on children. Practitioners working with children should use assessment measures especially developed for them. In addition, specific attention needs to be focused on inherent factors at the time the child is assessed (APA, 2002; HPCSA, 2010a; Murphy & Davidshofer, 2005). Examples of such factors are age, grade level, level of emotional development and level of cognitive functioning. It is for these reasons that children are perceived as individuals with specific needs and, as was pointed out in the section above on 'Avoiding harm', practitioners should be attentive to these needs when conducting psychological assessment. It is also important to note that Section 10 of the Children's Act specifies:

> Every child that is of such age, maturity and stage of development as to be able to participate in any matter concerning that child has the right to participate in an appropriate way and views expressed by the child must be given due consideration.

Within the context of assessment, this means that practitioners should always have the child's best interest at heart. If, for example, the practitioner does not deem a particular form of assessment to be in the child's best interest but the parents insist that it must be done, the practitioner could refuse to conduct such an assessment based on what the Act specifies. It should further be noted that, according to the Act, children have the right to be informed about the purpose and nature of the assessment. Should the child have any questions or express concern with the assessment procedure, these issues need to be dealt with immediately in an appropriate way. Unfortunately the Act is vague on what practitioners should do in a situation where parents have given consent for a child to undergo psychological assessment but the child refuses to cooperate. Given the fact that the Act is still relatively new, no form of precedent has yet been established and practitioners need to urge the Professional Board for Psychology to provide guidance on this matter.

The Labour Relations Act (No. 66 of 1995)

The Labour Relations Act applies mainly to those practitioners who conduct psychological assessment in industrial and organisational settings. As is the case with all legislation introduced after 1994, the Constitution of the Republic of South Africa also forms the foundation of the Labour Relations Act (Juta, 2009a; Mauer, 2000). The main aim of this Act is to advance economic development, social justice and the democratisation of the workplace (Juta, 2009a; Mauer, 2000). The purpose of the Act is thus to ensure equality and human dignity in the workplace (Juta, 2009a). Although this Act is mostly associated with workplace assessment practices, it should rather be perceived by all psychological assessment practitioners as a reminder of how important legislation is in establishing an ethical code and, ultimately, an ethical consciousness.

With regard to workplace assessment practices, Section 16(5) of the Act provides rather specific guidelines on the disclosure of information obtained in the workplace (Juta, 2009a). According to Section 16(5):

An employer is not required to disclose information:

(a) that is legally privileged;
(b) that the employer cannot disclose without contravening a prohibition imposed on the employer by any law or order of any conduct;
(c) that is confidential and, if disclosed, may cause substantial harm to an employee or employer; or
(d) that is private personal information relating to an employee, unless that employee consents to the disclosure of that information.

This section of the Act thus coincides with what is dictated by the Ethical Principles of Psychologists and Code of Conduct of the APA (2002) and the Professional Board for Psychology's Rules of Conduct Section 16(5) (HPCSA, 2010a) with regard to keeping information confidential. Although informed consent in general is deemed not necessary when it is implied (for example, for selection purposes), it seems that the Act requires that some form of consent be obtained when sensitive or personal information is dealt with in the industrial or organisational context. The implications of this for psychological assessment practices still need to be determined, since no other legal regulation or precedent relating to the issue has thus far been established.

The Employment Equity Act (No. 55 of 1998)

The purpose of the Employment Equity Act is to achieve equity in the workplace (Juta, 2009b). According to the Act, this is achieved by:

(a) Promoting equal opportunity and fair treatment in employment through the elimination of unfair discrimination; and
(b) Implementing affirmative action measures to redress the disadvantages in employment experienced by designated groups, in order to ensure their equitable representation in all occupational categories and levels in the workforce.

Chapter 2 of the Act deals with unfair discrimination (Mauer, 2000). According to Section 8 of this chapter, the use of psychological testing and other similar assessments of employees is prohibited unless the measure (Juta, 2009b; Mauer, 2000):

(a) Has been scientifically shown to be valid and reliable;
(b) Can be applied fairly to all employees; and
(c) Is not biased against any employee or group.

Section 8 provides assessment practitioners with specific guidelines on what is deemed the fair use of assessment in industrial and organisational contexts (Juta, 2009b; Mauer, 2000). Practitioners specialising in industrial and organisational assessment practices thus need to be aware of these specifications so as to ensure that no misconduct takes place when assessing individuals in the workplace.

Conclusion

In order to develop an ethical consciousness, psychological assessment practitioners need to be exposed to all documents pertaining to ethical issues in psychology and psychological assessment. Thus it makes sense to explore an ethical code in terms of three main areas of focus: namely, (1) a code of conduct; (2) adherence to standard practices when assessment is conducted; and (3) a thorough knowledge and understanding of legislation related to psychological assessment practices. This chapter has aimed to bring together this information in one discussion.

Practitioners should be forewarned that no one issue is ever more important than the others. Treating them unequally will have an adverse impact on the development of an ethical consciousness, which could result in the practitioner behaving unethically whilst doing psychological assessment. At this stage many people will start to wonder if it is possible to teach an ethical code to practitioners, so that they can develop an ethical consciousness. According to Velasquez, Andre, Shanks, Meyer and Meyer (1987), the answer is an unequivocal 'yes'. These authors note that moral development is a continuous process which does not end at any specific stage of human development. This therefore implies that student practitioners can be trained in how to act ethically when performing psychological assessment. Practitioners who are already working in the field of psychological assessment will not have an excuse, either. Being ethical also means taking personal responsibility for what one is doing (Allan, 2008), and such individuals will therefore have to avail themselves of new and current trends in assessment practices. In the end, everyone will realise that continuous professional development is just another way of ensuring that one maintains an ethical consciousness.

References

AfricaRights (2007a). *The South African People vs Professional Board for Psychology.* Retrieved November 22, 2007, from http://africarights.wordpress.com/2007/11/22/the-south-african-people-vs-professional-board-of-psychology/.

AfricaRights (2007b). *Psychological Suppression under Fire.* Retrieved December 12, 2007, from http://africarights.wordpress.com/2007/11/12/psychological-suppression-under-fire-/.

Allan, A. (2008). *Law and Ethics in Psychology: An International Perspective.* Somerset West: Inter-Ed Publishers.

APA (American Psychological Association) (2002). *Ethical Principles of Psychologists and Code of Conduct.* Retrieved April 12, 2010, from http://www.apa.org/ethics/code2002.html.

Bricklin, P. (2001). Being ethical: More than obeying the law and avoiding harm. *Journal of Personality Assessment, 77(2)*, 195–202.

Foxcroft, C. D. (2002). Ethical issues related to psychological testing in Africa: What I have learned (so far). In W. J. Lonner, D. L. Dinnel, S. A. Hayes & D. N. Sattler (Eds), *Online Readings in Psychology and Culture* (Unit 5, Chapter 4). Retrieved April 20, 2010, from http://www.ac.wwu.edu/~culture/foxcroft.htm.

Foxcroft, C., Roodt, G. & Abrahams, F. (2009). The practice of psychological assessment: Controlling the use of measures, competing values, and ethical practice standards.

In C. Foxcroft & G. Roodt (Eds), *Introduction to Psychological Assessment* (3rd edition, pp. 94–105). Cape Town: Oxford University Press.

Hall, J. D., Howerton, L. D. & Bolin, A. U. (2005). The use of testing technicians: Critical issues for professional psychology. *International Journal of Testing, 5(4),* 357–375.

HPCSA (Health Professions Council of South Africa) (2010a). *Professional Board for Psychology: Rules of Conduct Pertaining Specifically to Psychology.* Retrieved April 12, 2010, from http://www.psyssa.co./HPCSA%20ethical%20Code%20of%20Professional%20Condcut.pdf.

HPCSA (2010b). *The Professional Board for Psychology: Policy on the Classification of Psychometric Measuring Devices, Instruments, Methods and Techniques.* Retrieved April 12, 2010, from http://www.hpcsa.co.za/downloads/psycho_policy/form_208.pdf.

HPCSA (2010c). *The Professional Board for Psychology: Training and Examination Guidelines for Psychometrists.* Retrieved April 12, 2010, from http://www.hpcsa.co.za/downloads/psycho_policy/form_94.pdf.

HPCSA (2010d). *The Professional Board for Psychology: Generic Examination Guidelines for Psychologists, Registered Counsellors and Psychometrists.* Retrieved April 12, 2010, from http://www.hpcsa.co.za/downloads/psycho_policy/form_255.pdf.

ITC (International Test Commission) (2001). International guidelines for test use. *International Journal of Testing, 1(2),* 93–114.

Juta (2009a). *Labour Relations Act: Act 66 of 1995* (13th edition). Cape Town: Juta & Co.

Juta (2009b). *Employment Equity Act: Act 55 of 1998* (12th edition). Cape Town: Juta & Co.

Kaplan, R. M. & Saccuzzo, D. P. (2009). *Psychological Testing: Principles, Applications and Issues* (7th edition). Belmont, CA: Wadsworth Cengage Learning.

Leach, M. M. & Oakland, T. (2007). Ethics standards impacting test development and use: A review of 31 ethics codes impacting practices in 35 countries. *International Journal of Testing, 7(1),* 71–88.

Louw, J. (1997a). Regulating professional conduct Part I: Codes of ethics of national psychology associations in South Africa. *South African Journal of Psychology, 27(3),* 183–188.

Louw, J. (1997b). Regulating professional conduct Part II: The Professional Board for Psychology in South Africa. *South African Journal of Psychology, 27(3),* 189–195.

Mauer, K. F. (2000). *Psychological Test Use in South Africa.* Retrieved April 22, 2010, from http://www.pai.org.za/Psychological%20test%20use%20South%20Africa.pdf.

Moerdyk, A. (2009). *The Principles and Practice of Psychological Assessment* (1st edition). Pretoria: Van Schaik.

Murphy, K. R. & Davidshofer, C. O. (2005). *Psychological Testing: Principles and Applications* (6th edition). Upper Saddle River, NJ: Pearson Education International.

Pharos (2010). *English-Afrikaans Dictionary.* Cape Town: NB Publishers.

SIOPSA (Society for Industrial & Organisational Psychology of South Africa) (2006). *Code of Practice for Psychological and Other Similar Assessment in the Workplace.* Retrieved April 12, 2010, from http://www.pai.org/code%20of%20practice.pdf.

Velasquez, M., Andre, C., Shanks, T., Meyer, S. J. & Meyer, M. J. (1987). *Can Ethics Be Taught?* Retrieved April 13, 2010, from http://www.scu.edu/ethics/practicing/decision/canethicsbetaught.html.

29 Using computerised and internet-based testing in South Africa

N. Tredoux

Test users need to be aware of the complexities involved in the use of computerised tests in South Africa. Firstly, it is important to understand that not all computerised tests are the same, and that they differ greatly in their sophistication. This has implications for the professional decisions we make regarding the use of particular tests. This chapter begins with a discussion of the different ways in which computerised testing can be understood. We shall also review the historical background of computerised testing in this country with regard to both the technical aspects and the regulatory framework of psychological tests, in order to help users make informed decisions regarding the use of computerised tests.

What does 'computerised testing' mean?

Not all 'computerised' tests rely on computer technology to the same degree, or were designed and programmed for implementation on computers with the same level of skill and sophistication. Several aspects of testing can be computerised, such as the administration of the test, scoring and norming, and the generation of narrative reports or data summaries. Sometimes, for a particular test, not all these aspects are implemented to the same degree of sophistication, or at all. Test administration systems also vary in how they employ computer technology. If a test is delivered 'online', for instance, it means that the program that controls the test administration is located on a server somewhere on the internet, and not on the computer used for administration. Online, or internet-based, administration creates the possibility of administering a test in an unsupervised way, at the respondent's convenience. However, it is quite possible to administer an online test with some degree of control, provided that the necessary technology is in place and is properly utilised.

Scoring and norming

The simplest form of computerisation in psychometrics is the use of computer software to score multiple-choice tests that have been administered using pencil and paper. Data input can be manual, using a spreadsheet or similar software, or even software especially written for the test in question. It can also be mechanised, or purely electronic. Early forms of mechanised data acquisition involved special cards, with the respondent punching a hole in the card to indicate his or her answer. Optical mark readers have been the predominant technology for mechanical input of test responses for the past few decades. These machines require the test to be answered on specially printed answer sheets. These sheets can sometimes be difficult to read and complete, which can interfere with the reliability of the measures. They also sometimes require the use of a special pencil, and errors in answering are difficult to correct. The scoring key is also fed into the computer, either as a separate data file or coded into the scoring software. The same applies to norm data. The software then scores the responses, relates the raw scores to the norms and can print out raw and normed scores. Often this is done in the form of a profile.

The advantage of computerised or computer-assisted scoring lies in the reduction of errors, and in the considerable time-saving that can be achieved. It is especially valuable for questionnaires that measure multiple dimensions. The following types of scoring and norming errors that occur with pencil-and-paper scoring are eliminated:

- using the wrong scoring mask;
- skewed orientation and/or misalignment of the scoring mask;
- miscounting of item endorsements;
- errors in transcribing scores;
- errors in looking up standard scores in norm tables; and
- incorrect positioning of scores on profile sheets.

Even when computers are used to score tests, errors can still occur, and users should be aware of the following sources of error that can occur with the use of computer technology:

- When doing manual response capturing, the capturer can get out of step in typing in the responses, and end up typing the wrong response against a particular question.
- Whether using optical mark readers or manual capturing, the wrong test for a particular answer key can be chosen in the software.
- Errors can also occur when specifying the norm groups in the software.
- Errors in capturing biographical details or creating new database records for respondents can result in inaccurate reporting and corrupted data.
- Answer sheets that are designed for optical mark readers are typically more difficult to complete, and respondents can make errors that can cause their protocols to be unscorable or inaccurate. Test users need to be vigilant for this during test administration.

Computer-generated reports

Computers can make a more sophisticated and potentially valuable contribution to the assessment process by generating a narrative report from normed scores.

The quality and style of such computer-generated narrative reports vary widely depending on the system used and the particular reporting program. The best of them are difficult to distinguish from reports written by expert psychologists, and are even able to integrate results from different tests. The most elementary computer-generated reports do little more than give a description of the constructs that have been measured, with the level of score the respondent attained. The use and interpretation of computer-generated reports is discussed in more detail later in this chapter.

Test administration

Computers can be programmed to present test instructions, examples and test items. In most cases this is done by means of text displayed on the computer monitor. Sometimes voice recording or synthesised speech can be used. Highly sophisticated test administration systems can handle a multitude of response formats, and some can adapt the items to the respondent's level of ability while the test is being administered. The more interactive and sophisticated the computerised test administration system, the more expensive it is to develop. It must be recognised that computerised tests force respondents into a more structured manner of answering compared to pencil-and-paper tests where, for instance, it is much easier to refer back to earlier answers, or use certain answering and checking strategies (Bugbee & Bernt, 1990). Not all candidates react equally positively to computerised test administration (Moe & Johnson, 1988), and there may be systematic differences between population groups in terms of how they experience being tested on a computer (Legg & Buhr, 1992).

The speed of technological progress

Computers decrease in size and price and improve in speed, storage capacity and visual display capability at an astonishing rate. The resolution and flicker of computer screens used to be a concern from an ergonomic point of view, but with the quality of computer displays available at the time of writing, those concerns appear to have become irrelevant. Rapid advances continue in terms of technologies such as voice synthesis and recognition, text and handwriting recognition, as well as the processing and analysis of text. Future testing systems will not need to be limited to the scoring of multiple-choice responses, or even need to receive responses through mouse-clicks, touch screens or keyboards. Open-ended questions, written responses, gestures and spoken responses can all be processed by computers already, even if these capabilities have not yet been incorporated into psychological testing systems. These advances could mean that with sufficient ingenuity and investment, the computer literacy of respondents as a limiting factor for psychological testing could be almost eliminated. Rapid technological advances also mean that test developers and even test users need to be proactive in staying technologically aware, in order to evaluate the significance and implications for psychometrics of new developments.

The pervasiveness of computer technology

Computer technology used to be limited to organisations such as universities, government departments, research institutes and large corporations. When computers were rare and expensive, they were also relatively primitive. Now many individuals have computers of their own. People who do not have access to their own computer can use public computers that can be found in schools, libraries, community centres and internet cafés. Domestic appliances, motor cars and cellphones contain processors that would, in the past, have been considered relatively powerful in terms of computing capability. Cell phones, electronic game consoles, music players and other electronic devices can have internet access. These devices can be highly portable and compact. This means that one cannot assume that when a test is delivered over the internet, it will be completed in an office or quiet home environment, on a computer with a screen of a certain size. This has implications for the standardisation of test conditions when internet-based test administration is used.

Unequal access to computer technology

Even though computer technology is becoming very widespread and inexpensive, it is still mostly available only to fairly affluent people, in relatively urbanised environments (Technology Access Foundation, 2010). The very poor, and people in rural areas, have probably not been exposed to computer technology to the same degree as affluent urban populations, if indeed they have had any exposure to computers at all (Sutton, 1991). Some people have an aversion to computers that may prevent them from becoming comfortable with them, even if they have the opportunity to accustom themselves (Brosnan, 1998). Even with efforts to familiarise respondents with the devices to be used for testing, the fact that some may have had access to similar devices before and others not creates an inequality which raises concern in terms of bias and fairness. It is important that assessment practitioners be observant when testing respondents on computers. They should be alert for respondents who show obvious signs of discomfort with the medium of administration, and watch out for people who struggle with the mouse, keyboard or whatever means is used to enter the test responses. It is helpful to have a nonthreatening computer-based exercise to introduce respondents to the computer. Good rapport and handling of questions during the instructions and early phase of testing are very important. If necessary, an alternative means of assessment should be used if respondents remain very uncomfortable with the computer. Of course, it is very difficult to deal with these issues if the test is administered without supervision.

Computerised testing in South Africa

To understand the current controversy surrounding computerised testing in South Africa, it is important to be aware of the historical background: South Africa's innovative leadership in computerised testing experienced a setback when concerns were raised about the fairness of psychometric testing. The regulation of psychometric tests, whether pencil-and-paper-based or computerised, is still in dispute.

Early computer-based developments

During the late 1970s and early 1980s, researchers at the National Institute for Personnel Research (NIPR) did pioneering work in computerised testing. A computer-based system to administer tests of intellectual ability was developed on a Varian minicomputer. Subsequently, an extremely ambitious system was written to administer a wide range of psychological tests over a wide area network using touch screens. This testing system adapted the Control Data 'Plato' system (Plato Learning, 2010), which was designed for education and training, for psychological testing. It had many groundbreaking features, such as the ability to recover from system interruptions or power failures, resuming where the respondent had left off with all test response data intact.

The NIPR Plato-based testing system allowed the psychologist who controlled it to set up batteries of tests for administration in other cities. Respondents would not necessarily complete the tests under professional supervision, because at the time psychologists were allowed to delegate any psychological action to an unregistered person, provided these actions were supervised (Department of Health, 1977). The Plato-based testing system included its own training module for familiarising respondents with the computer, and all respondents completed this. Respondents who could not answer the example items correctly after a number of attempts were not allowed to complete the rest of the tests. The test responses were routed across a wide area network and processed centrally on a mainframe computer. The system included programs for calculating norms and reliabilities. The Plato-based testing system was implemented at some universities, some state-owned enterprises and the NIPR's own assessment services. Most of the tests programmed for this system were conversions of existing pencil-and-paper tests. There were, however, some instruments developed specifically to take advantage of the computer system's interactive capabilities. Among these were a simulation exercise called 'Maze' designed to assess managerial decision-making (Tredoux, 1985), and a comprehension test that involved the reordering of sentence segments.

These early developments took place during the apartheid era. At this time, different race groups did not compete for the same jobs. The profession of psychology was also relatively young in South Africa, and there was no official, enforceable code of ethical conduct for psychology practitioners. Most of the respondents who were tested on the system were white; therefore cross-cultural studies were not undertaken on data collected on this system. It was not expected that any of the respondents would be computer-literate, and therefore group differences in computer literacy were not considered a factor that might potentially make the tests unfair.

Sanctions and the move to microcomputers

As a result of political and economic sanctions, Control Data, the company that supplied the Plato system and the hardware on which it ran, withdrew from South Africa. Eventually it was no longer feasible to maintain the Plato-based testing system and it fell into disuse. Soon afterwards, microcomputers became available, despite continuing sanctions. In the mid-1980s the NIPR, by then part of the Human Sciences Research Council (HSRC), developed a comprehensive microcomputer-based testing system called PsiTest. Another system, called Siegmund, was also developed at the HSRC. Both these systems were used fairly widely. The PsiTest system had optional enhancements for managing testing sessions, utilising the capabilities of microcomputer networks. A simulator-type system to test vehicle drivers was also developed at the NIPR, using an Apple computer. A clerical office work simulation for assessment was developed on the Microsoft Windows platform. The HSRC also did research on, and acted as a supplier for, the Austrian-developed Vienna Testing System, which specialised largely in computerised psychomotor testing (Schuhfried Gmbh, 2010).

The HSRC's microcomputer-based testing systems brought computer-based testing within reach of psychologists in private practice, as well as larger organisations. The systems were sold only to psychologists, and since the internet was not yet functional the tests were always administered under supervision, even if the supervision was not done by a registered person. A registered psychologist was always professionally responsible for the testing session.

Backlash against testing

During the 1980s, psychometric testing in South Africa became subject to increasingly strong criticism. The HSRC was the statutory organisation responsible for research and development in psychometric technology and was ill-prepared to answer the criticisms that it had not paid sufficient attention to bias and fairness (Taylor, 1987). Insufficient cross-cultural research had been done on the HSRC tests. This was partly due to the fact that the HSRC had developed separate tests for different race groups, and partly due to the historical situation that black and white applicants had not been competing for the same positions, and hence had not been tested on the same tests, leading to a lack of comparative data. Around this time, people (including psychologists) were turning against psychological testing, questioning its fairness and even its legality (Taylor & Radford, 1986), which inhibited further data collection. The HSRC started paying explicit attention to the bias and fairness of the tests that it was supplying (Owen, 1989a; 1989b). The South African Personality Questionnaire, in particular, was examined for cultural bias and found wanting (Taylor & Boeyens, 1991). Amid political unrest and eventual changes in government, state-funded research and development in psychometrics were curtailed. Early drafts of the Employment Equity Act banned psychometric testing for employment purposes (Employment Equity Bill No. 60, 1998). When the final version of this Act, the Employment Equity Act No. 55 of 1998, was eventually promulgated, allowing psychometric testing subject to the tests meeting technical psychometric and fairness requirements, many experts in psychometrics had already left the country or joined the private sector.

Computerised testing becomes highly commercialised

Even before the HSRC reduced its involvement in psychometrics and computerised testing in the early 1990s, some publishers in the private sector had already entered the field of computerised testing. One of the early South African initiatives was a report-writing system for the Sixteen Personality Factor Questionnaire (16PF), developed by Professor Dan Steyn. The computerised testing systems that had been supported by the HSRC, such as the Vienna System and the HSRC computer-administered testing system (CAT), were taken over by private sector organisations.

Drs Dawie Minnaar and Pieter Erasmus developed the Potential Index Battery (PIB), which later evolved to become 'Speex'. This set of tests, each measuring a single dimension, gained widespread acceptance in industry. It featured computerised administration and scoring, and the ability to calculate norms from data that had been collected. Also active in the South African market was Thomas International Ltd with the Personal Profile Assessment (PPA), which produced a comprehensive narrative report from a short ipsative questionnaire (Thomas International, 2010).

The Discus system featured a very similar questionnaire to the PPA, also with computer-generated reporting targeting the same dimensions (Axiom Software, no date). Jopie van Rooyen and Partners acquired the South African distribution rights for a large number of tests and questionnaires. Several of these, notably the 16PF and Myers-Briggs Type Indicator (MBTI), soon featured computer-generated reports available through bureau scoring (JvR Group, 2010). M&M Initiatives (2010) developed the Learning Potential Computerised Adaptive Test (LPCAT), based on item response theory. Dr Terry Taylor formed a company called Aprolab and entered the market with two learning potential measures, Transfer, Automatisation and Memory (TRAM) and (Conceptual) Ability, Processing of Information, and Learning (APIL), that featured computer-assisted reporting although they were originally administered using pencil and paper (Aprolab, 2010). Maretha Prinsloo of Cognadev developed the Cognitive Process Profile (CPP), a computer-administered measure of thinking style and potential (Cognadev, 2010).

Saville and Holdsworth Limited (SHL) entered South Africa in the mid-1990s with a suite of computerised products that encompassed job analysis, personality and ability testing. Dr Kobus Neethling developed a range of instruments measuring thinking styles and preferences (Neethling Brain Instruments, 2010). The Neethling brain profiles were, however, never classified as psychological tests. Psytech International products, also including a range of personality and ability tests with narrative reports, were introduced to South Africa in 1994. Since 1998, access to the Psytech tests and testing software has been restricted to registered professionals (Psytech South Africa, 2010).

The PIB, Discus, SHL, Neethling and Thomas International products were sold for use by people who had been trained by the publisher, and who were not necessarily registered psychologists or psychometrists. Some of the publishers – notably, Neethling, SHL and Thomas International – accredited unregistered users to use their instruments independently of the Health Professions Council of South Africa (HPCSA) registration system, in line with their organisations' international practices (Neethling Brain Instruments, 2010; SHL South Africa, no date; Thomas International, 2010). Within approximately a decade, computerised testing in South Africa had changed from a largely state-funded and controlled activity to a highly competitive, highly commercialised industry. There was and still is a lack of consistency between different providers in the restriction of access to computer-delivered psychological tests.

The advent of internet-delivered testing

In the mid-1990s access to the internet started becoming widespread in South Africa. Very soon, numerous local and international tests became available to anyone with internet access. Some of these were from reputable publishers, but several tests that were clearly psychological in nature were made available by people who had no intention of having the tests evaluated or classified, or of limiting access only to people registered with the HPCSA to use tests. Several of these tests were accessible on a 'pay per use' basis, whereby any person could pay an amount via credit card and then was given access to the test and the report. The website hosting the test and processing the transaction could be anywhere in the world, thus bypassing regulations in countries that regulate testing strictly. However, even with websites that are clearly South African and that fail to abide by the South African rules regarding psychological tests, the Professional Board for Psychology has not been successful in exercising control. Where the websites are run by unregistered people, the Board is not able to prosecute and needs to refer the matter to the National Prosecuting Authority. This has not yet resulted in any successful prosecutions.

Considering the scale on which unregistered persons use psychological tests via the internet, there have been remarkably few complaints to the Professional Board. The reason could be that respondents are not aware of their rights, or that, as job applicants, they feel too disempowered to take action. Even more remarkable is that psychology professionals have lodged so few professional conduct complaints with the HPCSA about psychologists allowing unregistered persons to access tests via the internet, although the author has been the recipient of numerous informal complaints.

The International Test Commission (ITC) has formulated guidelines for the use of computerised and internet-based testing (ITC, 2005). These guidelines outline the responsibilities of various stakeholders in the testing process and distinguish between different modes of administration, ranging from managed mode (administration in a special facility with a supervisor present) to open mode (unsupervised self-administration open to any person). Between these extremes is controlled mode administration, where the identity of the respondent is verified and other technologies are employed to prevent cheating, but the administration still essentially proceeds unsupervised. The Professional Board for Psychology has not accepted the ITC guidelines for unchanged application in South Africa. A limited version of these guidelines was published, allowing only managed mode, but the HPCSA eventually withdrew it after legal action by test publishers (ATP vs HPCSA, Pretoria High Court, Case No. 4218/07).

Critical evaluation of the advantages of computer-administered testing

Facilitation of research

Well-designed computerised testing systems will store the test responses in a database that is accessible for research, or will have options that enable users to export the data to a format that is compatible with data analysis programs. To protect confidentiality of the respondents, it should be possible to make the data anonymous. Errors of scoring and transcribing data can be eliminated if the test is administered directly on the computer. If a test is in development, items can be trialled on computerised testing systems without the cost of printing pencil-and-paper materials that will need to be discarded afterwards. New, updated versions of tests and norms can be made available quickly and inexpensively over the internet, rather than requiring users to purchase new printed copies. These are enormous advantages for test developers, and also make it more feasible to do the psychometric and cross-cultural research that is required in South Africa for compliance with the Employment Equity Act. Hence, well-designed computerised testing systems can also help to protect the rights of respondents by ensuring that up-to-date norms and item sets are used.

Monitoring of usage

From the point of view of test distributors and developers, the fact that computer systems can count the number of times a particular test is used, and by whom it is used, is an important benefit. Pencil-and-paper tests are very vulnerable to copyright violations which cost test developers a lot of money, thus inhibiting further research and development. Computerised test administration makes it much easier for test developers to ensure that they profit from their efforts.

Standardisation of administration

Insofar as test administration consists of presenting instructions and test items to the respondent, timing the responses and scoring them, computers can do that very well. The computer is dispassionate and objective. It treats everybody in exactly the same way. But is this all that test administration should be in a society where there are numerous obstacles to fair administration in terms of culture, language and computer literacy? Is it professionally justifiable in South Africa to allow respondents to complete tests unsupervised over the internet? An examination of the ethical code and defined competencies regarding test administration, as specified by the Professional Board for Psychology, suggests that this is not the case.

The competencies that a psychology professional should master with regard to test administration include more than the accurate conveying of instructions and test items, timing and scoring. These competencies are spelled out with particular reference to psychometrists, although they apply to other categories of professionals who administer tests as well (Professional Board for Psychology, 2006). Among other things, the psychometrist is supposed to ensure that the environment in which testing takes place is conducive to testing. The psychometrist should observe the respondents to consider whether they are in a fit state to be tested. There should be a process of building rapport, obtaining informed consent for testing and observation of behaviour during testing. The psychometrist should evaluate whether all the respondents understand the instructions fully, and give special attention when necessary. The psychometrist should also make sure that the respondents do not cheat, obtain help during testing or remove test materials from the test room. The psychometrist should consider whether the use of an interpreter may be required. In a computerised test room, the psychometrist should consider, by observation, whether all the respondents are coping with the computer interface, and whether an alternative mode of testing would not be more appropriate. The psychometrist should also deal with the eventuality of a power failure or equipment malfunction and its effect on the respondents. Much of this professional administration process is aimed at protecting the right of the respondent to be treated fairly. Test administration according to the standards specified by the HPCSA is not just the mechanical process of reading instructions, timing and scoring. Rather it is a professionally compassionate, interactive process of observation and adaptation of the testing process when necessary, to ensure that respondents are tested fairly and not merely uniformly.

The ethical code for psychologists, now incorporated into the Health Professions Act No. 56 of 1974 as a regulation (Department of Health, 2006), warns psychologists to limit their findings appropriately when there has been any deviation from standard testing practice. They are even warned to limit their conclusions when group test administration rather than individual test administration has been done. They are also instructed to limit their conclusions when using any computer-mediated processes. The ethical code further specifically states that psychological assessment must take place in the context of a defined professional relationship. It is difficult to see how this requirement could be met with unsupervised test administration. In many cases there is no personal contact between the person responsible for the assessment project and the respondent completing an unsupervised internet-based test. Respondents usually simply get an email with a link on which they click to bring up the test. The person in charge of the testing process also usually has no control over the time of day when the test is completed, whether testing conditions are adequate and whether some respondents receive help during testing.

It is thus clear that when tests are administered unsupervised over the internet, the rights of the respondents are not as protected as when the tests are administered under the supervision of a psychologist or psychometrist. Some candidates, particularly those with lower levels of literacy and computer experience, may be more disadvantaged than others. Supervised computerised test administration can, however, have considerable advantages – provided it is properly managed. Systems are becoming available for supervising test administration sessions remotely through web cameras and using instant messaging facilities (Psytech International Limited, 2010). Other verification systems, mainly aimed at controlling cheating, involve doing a verification test under supervised conditions after screening applicants based on an unsupervised test (SHL Group, no date).

Technical considerations

In choosing and implementing computerised tests, psychologists and psychometrists should bear a number of factors in mind. These are discussed below.

System stability

If the computer system is unstable due to hardware or software factors, it is not suitable for testing. The computer should meet the minimum system requirements for the testing software. Security systems on the network or computer, such as antivirus software and firewalls, should not obstruct the functioning of the testing software. The system should also be free of viruses and malware that can slow down performance. Any necessary modules that are needed to display item content, such as special software to display video and animation, sound and video drivers, and so forth, should be installed and up to date. If an internet connection is required, it should be up and running, and the connection speed should be adequate. This is particularly important if the nature of the test administration is highly interactive. It may be necessary to take special precautions to ensure that the testing session will not be interrupted by a power failure. It should be part of the preparation for the testing session to ensure that everything works as it should. If anything on the system has changed since it was last used for testing – such as the updating of the operating system or reconfiguration of the firewall – this is particularly important.

Well-designed testing systems should be able to resume with data intact after an unforeseen termination, and to display test items correctly even when the line speed is slow. However, not all testing systems are capable of doing this. The test administrator should be aware of the risks and vulnerabilities of the particular systems that are being used.

Connection speed

Some assessment systems, particularly those that involve video, require a very fast internet connection. Well-designed assessment systems will download the necessary information before commencing the test. However, in areas where the connection is slow, this can take a lot longer than expected and may interfere with the scheduled start of the testing session.

Systems that allow test administration to be observed remotely through web cameras are particularly vulnerable to slow internet connections. Hopefully this situation will improve as South Africa's connectivity infrastructure is upgraded. In deciding to use systems that rely on fast internet connections, professionals must consider their environment. If testing will take place in rural areas and will connect to the internet through cellular modems, it is necessary to verify whether connectivity will be available in the area and whether it will be possible to connect at full speed. Some internet services are affected by bad weather. If the connection will be slow, extra preparation time may be required to download the items.

Purchasers should bear in mind that systems developed in other countries, where internet speeds are much faster, may never have been tested with bandwidth as limited as we have in South Africa. Poorly designed internet-based assessment systems will simply fail, slowing down or halting during testing if the connection becomes too slow. They may even lose information. If the program is not written to take account of variations in line speed, it could result in inaccurate timing of tests. This is not conducive to standardised testing procedure, and psychology professionals should verify that this will not happen before committing to using such a system.

Security considerations

Computer-based and internet-delivered tests need to be programmed with a greater awareness of security than normal applications. Aspects that should be considered include access control, security of item content and scoring keys, and security of results. These will now be discussed in more detail.

Access control

As with pencil-and-paper test materials, access to computerised testing systems should be limited to authorised users. Many systems are password-protected. Users should know how to change their passwords, and not use a password that is easily guessed or used by a lot of other people. Some systems permit several levels of access. Some individuals may, for instance, be able to set up test batteries, customise reports and change norms, whereas others would only be allowed to perform limited administrative functions such as data capturing on the system. Professional users should be aware that when they share their password or give another person access to a computerised testing system, they are potentially delegating actions that may be reserved for the profession of psychology. The ethical code specifies that such actions should only be delegated to persons who are competent and appropriately trained to perform them.

Security of item content and scoring keys

It is important to pay attention to the computer file formats in which test items and scoring keys are stored on the computer. Item text and graphics should be encrypted so that they cannot be accessed by unauthorised people using a word processor or graphics program. Internet-delivered tests are particularly vulnerable in this regard. Some internet-delivered tests leave files containing the test items behind in the internet cache, or temporary file folder. These files can then be accessed and saved or printed after the test has been completed. This is a serious breach of security and can compromise the integrity of the test and the assessment process. Test users should be aware of this and make sure that they do not use systems that 'leak' confidential information in this way.

There is a possibility that respondents may deliberately try to copy items while doing tests. This risk is much greater when tests are administered unsupervised and respondents may be completing the test in their own homes or offices. Securely designed testing systems do not allow respondents to make screen copies or printouts while the test is in progress. Many internet-based tests can be copied by screen-capturing or printing the items, and practitioners should avoid tests that have this security vulnerability. Even if the 'print screen' key is disabled, some people may try to photograph the items. As a precaution, it is better not to allow respondents to have cell phones accessible while they do computerised tests, since many cell phones incorporate cameras.

Security of results

When obtaining informed consent for testing, the limits to confidentiality must be clarified (Department of Health, 2006). In so doing, the respondent agrees to the persons, other than the psychologist or psychometrist, who may have access to his or her test results and the report based on them. The psychologist then has a fiduciary duty to respect these limits and to make sure that nobody else accesses this confidential information. Psychology professionals in South Africa are also obliged to store psychological assessment results securely for five years. Password-protected databases can be a great help in this regard. Databases should, however, be backed up regularly. Backups should be done onto a different physical device than the one where the original records are stored. Removable media are a good solution. Backup copies should be stored securely, again preferably in a different location to the original data.

Computer-generated reports are usually produced as word-processor documents. Security violations can easily occur when these are saved to hard drives or sent through email, or when printouts are distributed within organisations. It is the responsibility of the psychologist or psychometrist to ensure that unauthorised people do not see psychological reports. The identities of the people who are permitted to see the reports should be clarified when obtaining written informed consent from the respondent before testing. Report documents should preferably also be password-protected. Recipients of the reports should be warned not to have printouts lying around in accessible places, such as in in-trays or on desks. All reports should be clearly marked 'confidential'.

Human–computer interface considerations

When a respondent is completing a psychological test using a computer, he or she should not be struggling to deal with the apparatus rather than attending to the test content. The interface elements – keyboard, mouse and screen – should not 'get in the way' of the test items. This is more difficult to achieve for people who have had little experience with computers. However, it is also important to make sure that the equipment being used is of a sufficient quality that it does not in itself place the respondent at a disadvantage.

Display quality

The image on the computer screen should be crisp, clear, stable and not distorted. If the equipment is relatively new, this should not be a problem. However, older screens can develop problems that may interfere with test administration. If the screen is of different dimensions than the screen for which the item material was programmed, items can appear distorted if the program was not written to compensate for this. If groups of people are tested at the same time, they should be tested on equipment of comparable quality to avoid creating an unfair situation.

Keyboard familiarity

Some respondents have not had the opportunity to learn keyboard skills. This can be the case with people from economically deprived backgrounds, but also with older respondents who may hold senior executive or professional positions, and do not personally use computers at work because they have support staff who do it for them. Well-designed computerised tests should not demand an inappropriate level of computer skill from the respondent, relative to the construct being measured and the purpose of measurement.

Pointing devices and touch screens

In most computerised tests, respondents indicate their choice of answer with a pointing device. Pointing devices come in many types, the computer mouse being the most common. However, light-pens, trackballs, joysticks, touch-sensitive screens and touch pads are also used. Usually, the test program does not distinguish between different types of pointing device. It is up to the test administrator to see that the respondents are comfortable using the particular pointing device. In the author's experience, the most acceptable, inexpensive and reliable pointing device is the ordinary computer mouse, preferably the optical type. The touch pads and little mini-joysticks found on some laptop computers are difficult to use for people who are not used to them and they are best avoided for testing purposes.

Technological literacy

Psychology professionals who use computerised testing should consider their own technological literacy as well as the technological literacy of the respondents. If the test administrator is not able to cope with the technical demands of the assessment system, the assessment process may be discredited and could place the respondents at a disadvantage. In considering the appropriateness of computerised testing for a given group of respondents, the psychologist or psychometrist should verify that there isn't a subgroup who is significantly more technologically sophisticated than the rest. It is differences in technological literacy between people who are being assessed for the same purpose that create unfairness, rather than the overall technological sophistication of the group. This is especially true if lack of technological literacy will affect test performance, and if technological literacy is not in itself relevant to the construct being assessed.

Advancing the state of the art

Even when discussing the limitations of computerised testing systems, one must be aware of the fact that this is a field of technology that has the potential for very rapid development. With the technology becoming available, it is possible to create testing systems that are interactive, responsive to individual needs and secure. However, implementing the new advances will require a commitment from developers. Users also have to be discerning, since many of the systems available today are based on outdated technology.

Item content

Multimedia item content in computerised testing is not new, but it is becoming easier and less expensive to implement. The potential this offers is not only in making tests more attractive and exciting, but also in accommodating people who are visually impaired. Tests can now be made more interactive, in the sense that the testing system responds to the person who is completing the test and adapts the testing process accordingly. The task set for the respondent can also be made more meaningful than merely choosing an answer from a number of options. The CPP is an example of how the interaction with the computer can be used to externalise mental processes.

Processing of responses

To be truly interactive, a testing system needs to process responses while the respondent is completing the items, and not only afterwards. Computerised testing systems can be programmed to take account of response latencies (the time lag between the presentation of the item and the response), the number of errors made and the number of corrections. Computers can monitor and assess learning that takes place during the testing process. With voice recognition, handwriting recognition and sophisticated text-processing capabilities, computers can be programmed to assess the quality of a person's thinking as well as tally the number of errors made.

Supporting advances in psychometrics

With the capabilities mentioned above, computerised testing systems are essential for implementation of tests that go beyond classical psychometrics. With the limitations of classical psychometrics becoming increasingly apparent, it is essential for test developers to embrace new technologies – for instance, tests based on item response theory. Test users must likewise remain up to date with new approaches to psychometrics.

Adaptive tests

Using item response theory and related sophisticated algorithms, it is no longer necessary for all respondents doing a particular test to complete the same set of items in the same sequence. Testing systems can adapt the difficulty level of the items to the candidate and thus test them more accurately and economically. This approach also makes it much easier to protect the integrity of the test, because such tests are much more difficult to copy.

Advanced reporting

Users of computerised tests have come to expect narrative computer-generated reports, and in many cases are prepared to pay extra for the convenience. High-quality computer-generated narrative reports can appear so credible that the test user could even be tempted to overlook the psychometric limitations of psychological tests and take them at face value.

Computerised narrative reports are not inherently difficult to produce. They can make use of artificial intelligence, but this is not necessary for a good report. Computer-generated reports essentially need to consider all the different possible score combinations and generate text for them. They do require a great deal of work, since text needs to be generated for very large numbers of score permutations. This requires not only programming expertise, but also conscientious application and cooperation from insightful psychologists with expertise in the tests. There are specialised software systems available that assist in the customisation and automation of computer-generated reports. An example is the GeneSys system from Psytech International (Agnew, 2003). It is even possible for a knowledgeable user to program a narrative report using spreadsheet software or word-processing software and a database. This is, however, beyond the competence of most psychology professionals, and they rely on the test vendors to provide them with the reporting technology.

Simple reports that merely report on the scores for a single test are the most common. However, with sufficient effort, expertise and investment, it is possible for computer-generated reports to move beyond reporting into the realm of interpretation. Reports can also be developed that integrate results from a whole battery of tests. Advanced reports can evaluate a person's test scores within a specified context. For instance, the report can compare different score combinations against the desired profile for a given position, which can be very useful when using tests for selection. The report-writing program can calculate how well a respondent can be expected to perform on specific work-related competencies or in a specific role, and give an explanation of what can be expected from the person, and which of his or her core characteristics give rise to this expectation. Advanced computer-generated reports can guide a manager in overcoming a respondent's development needs and maximising his or her potential strengths. A very useful type of report is one that generates a follow-up interview schedule that enables the professional to probe or clarify certain measured characteristics. This can act as a means of collecting additional information, and also help to verify or clarify the findings from psychometric tests. Reports such as these enable test users to acquire the ability to use a test in a sophisticated manner very quickly. What used to take years of experience, training and supervision can now be made possible very quickly with the help of a computer.

In some cases, the report-writing program does calculations on scores before interpreting them. These calculations could be estimations of certain dimensions that were not directly measured by the test. They are often called 'derived scores'. The formulae used to do these calculations are sometimes based on empirical research and sometimes on expert opinion. Both of these sources of information contribute to raising the cost of producing the report program.

It is expected that, due to the cost of refining and customising computer-generated reports, the majority of reports will probably continue to be somewhat generic, rather than adapted to a respondent's individual circumstances and the requirements of a particular role. It is usually necessary for a professional to do some editing and contextualising to take account of the respondent's individual circumstances and the specific context in which the assessment is done. Even sophisticated reports are usually developed for the international market, and it is often necessary for test users to edit the reports to incorporate the South African social, cultural and language considerations afterwards.

Professional control

The issue of professional control over computerised testing in South Africa has been controversial. The Professional Board for Psychology accepted a policy on computerised testing which was largely based on the policy published by the ITC. The South African policy, however, did not allow unsupervised testing and placed an age restriction of 18 on clients who could be serviced through computerised means. Test publishers opposed the policy and forced the Board to withdraw it. The policy has been put before the Board several times and has been accepted unanimously on each occasion. Meanwhile, the Health Professions Act was amended, and regulations allowing unregistered persons to perform psychological acts were repealed (Regulation R993, Health Professions Act, September 14, 2008). Moreover, testing for employment was added to the actions reserved for the profession of psychologist. Thus, in terms of the legal and ethical regulation of testing, the situation is now more strictly controlled than when the South African policy on computerised and internet-delivered testing (HPCSA, 2006) was first accepted. Whether there is a specific policy on computerised testing or not, the legal and ethical restrictions on the use of psychological tests remain.

However, South African professionals should take cognisance of the responsibilities for test users listed in the ITC's guidelines (ITC, 2005). Using computerised and internet-delivered testing requires a higher level of technological sophistication, a greater awareness of security issues and a responsible concern for the welfare of the respondent. Furthermore, our local regulations require that a psychology professional take personal responsibility for assessment work. This is difficult to do with unsupervised testing, where the test user cannot even be certain that the equipment on which the test will be completed will be adequate for testing purposes. Computers should not be used to mass-produce assessments. We must never lose sight of the fact that we work with individuals who have constitutionally protected rights.

References

Agnew, M. (2003). *Manual for the GeneSys Integrated Assessment System Version 3*. Pulloxhill: Psytech International.

Aprolab (2010). *About Dr Taylor*. Retrieved June 20, 2010, from http://www.aprolab.co.za/content/abouttaylor.html.

Axiom Software (no date). *Professional Personality Profiling for Everyone*. Retrieved December 3, 2010, from www.axiomsoftware.com.

Brosnan, M. J. (1998). *The Psychological Impact of Information Technology.* New York, NY: Routledge.

Bugbee, A. C. & Bernt, F. M. (1990). Testing by computer: Findings in six years of use 1982–1988. *Journal of Research on Computing in Education, 23(1),* 87–100.

Cognadev (2010). *Cognadev*. Retrieved June 20, 2010, from http://www.cognadev.com/.

Department of Health (1977). *Regulation R1863 of Act No. 56 of 1974.* Pretoria: Department of Health.

Department of Health (2006). *Regulation R717 of Act No. 56 of 1974.* Pretoria: Department of Health.

HPCSA (Health Professions Council of South Africa) (2006). *Form 257: South African Guidelines on Computer-based and Internet-based Testing.* Pretoria: Health Professions Council of South Africa.

ITC (International Test Commission) (2005). *International Guidelines on Computer-Based and Internet-Delivered Testing.* Retrieved September 30, 2010, from http://www.intestcom.org/Downloads/ITC%20Guidelines%20on%20Computer%20-%20version%202005%20approved.pdf.

JvR Group (2010). *Psychological Test Providers in Africa.* Retrieved June 20, 2010, from http://www.jvrafrica.co.za/.

Legg, S. M. & Buhr, D. C. (1992). Computerised adaptive testing with different groups. *Educational Measurement: Issues and Practice,* Summer, 23–27.

M&M Initiatives (2010). *LPCat: Computerised Adaptive Testing.* Retrieved June 20, 2010, from http://www.mminitiatives.com/mnm_products.htm.

Moe, K. C. & Johnson, M. F. (1988). Participants reaction to computerized testing. *Journal of Educational Computing Research, 4(1),* 79–86.

Neethling Brain Instruments (2010). *NBI Profiles.* Retrieved June 20, 2010, from http://www.nbiprofile.com/index.htm.

Owen, K. (1989a). *Test and Item Bias: The Suitability of the Junior Aptitude Tests as a Common Test Battery for White, Indian and Black Pupils in Standard 7.* Pretoria: Human Sciences Research Council.

Owen, K. (1989b). The suitability of Raven's Progressive Matrices for various groups in South Africa. *Personality and Individual Differences, 13(2),* 149–159.

Plato Learning (2010). *Our History.* Retrieved June 20, 2010, from http://www.plato.com/About-Us/Our-Company/History.aspx.

Professional Board for Psychology (2006). *Training and Examination Guidelines for Psychometrists.* Pretoria: Human Sciences Research Council.

Psytech International Limited (2010). *iSupervise.* Retrieved June 20, 2010, from http://www.psytech.com/newsite5/software-GeneSysiSupervise.php.

Psytech South Africa. (2010). *Access to Psytech SA Tests.* Retrieved June 20, 2010, from http://www.psytech.co.za.

Schuhfried Gmbh (2010). *Vienna Test System.* Retrieved June 20, 2010, from http://www.schuhfried.at/en/products/vienna-test-system-vts.html.

SHL Group (no date). *SHL Verify.* Retrieved December 6, 2010, from http://www.shl.com/WhatWeDo/AbilityScreeningAndTesting/Pages/Verify.aspx.

SHL South Africa (no date). *General Information.* Retrieved December 6, 2010, from http://www.training.shl.co.za/asp/Conf.asp.

Sutton, R. (1991). Equity and computers in the schools: A decade of research. *Review of Educational Research, 61(4),* 475–503.

Taylor, J. M. & Radford, E. J. (1986). Psychometric testing as an unfair labour practice. *South African Journal of Psychology, 16*, 79–96.

Taylor, T. R. (1987). *Test Bias: The Roles and Responsibilities of Test Users and Test Publishers*. Pretoria: Human Sciences Research Council.

Taylor, T. R. & Boeyens, J. C. A. (1991). The comparability of the scores of blacks and whites on the South African Personality Questionnaire: An exploratory study. *South African Journal of Psychology, 21*, 1–10.

Technology Access Foundation (2010). *Overview of TAF*. Retrieved June 18, 2010, from http://www.techaccess.org/index.html.

Thomas International (2010). *Welcome to Thomas International*. Retrieved June 20, 2010, from http://www.thomas.co.za/.

Tredoux, N. (1985). *The Development and Programming of a Computerised Situation Simulation for Managers*. Johannesburg: National Institute of Personnel Research.

30 The ImPACT neurocognitive screening test: a survey of South African research including current and projected applications

A. B. Shuttleworth-Edwards, V. J. Whitefield-Alexander and S. E. Radloff

In recent decades, the development of computerised neurocognitive screening has revolutionised medical management in the sports concussion arena by making possible preseason (baseline) testing of large numbers of athletes, and repeat follow-up testing of the concussed athlete, to monitor recovery and facilitate safe return-to-play decisions (Moser et al., 2007). The aim of this chapter is to introduce the most widely employed instrument of this genre, the ImPACT (Immediate Postconcussion Assessment and Cognitive Testing) test (Iverson, Lovell & Collins, 2002), and to review the available South African normative research data in respect of the instrument to date.[1] While the test has potential for wide application beyond the sports concussion arena (as discussed in the concluding section of this chapter), its development within the sports injury context calls for background detail in this regard.[2]

Mild traumatic brain injury (concussion) in sport

Mild traumatic brain injury (MTBI), typically referred to as 'concussion' in the sports arena, is a common feature amongst both amateur and professional sports alike (Cassidy, Carroll, Peloso, Borg & Von Holst, 2004). While once considered to be a 'routine risk' associated with participation in the game, the impact of these injuries has gained significant international interest and concern amongst sports and health professionals in the past three decades (Barth et al., 1989; Collins, Lovell & McKeag, 1999; Shuttleworth-Edwards, Border, Reid & Radloff, 2004), and is currently considered by the Centers for Disease Control and Prevention (CDC, 1997) to be of epidemic proportions. The incidence of the concussive injury varies widely depending on the sport, such that in one comparative high school study US football accounted for 63 per cent of all cases, wrestling for 10.5 per cent, girls' soccer for 6.2 per cent, boys' soccer for 5.7 per cent, girls' basketball for 5.2 per cent, boys' basketball for 4.2 per cent, softball for 2.1 per cent, baseball for 1.2 per cent, field hockey for 1.1 per cent and volleyball for 0.5 per cent (Powell & Barber-Foss, 1999).

Given the wide participation in the sport of rugby union in South Africa, of particular relevance is research documenting a higher rate of concussion for rugby union rather than for rugby league, American football and soccer (Cassidy et al., 2004).[3] Generally there is also a greater risk of injury in rugby union. In a survey of three South African schools' top teams, an incidence of 2.3 concussions per rugby-playing schoolboy has been recorded, compared with an average incidence of 0.4 concussions for an equivalent group of field hockey players (Shuttleworth-Edwards, Border et al., 2004). Importantly, another South African incidence study in respect of rugby union (Shuttleworth-Edwards, Noakes et al., 2008), revealed that tighter control of medical management of the concussive injury was associated with a higher concussion incidence – that is, less under-reporting of the injury – due to increased awareness about the nature and potential seriousness of this injury amongst the coaches and athletes themselves. In this study the average incidence per rugby-playing season over a five-year period (2002–2006) was shown to range massively from 4 per cent to 14 per cent at school level and 3 per cent to 23 per cent at adult level.

In light of the clearly documented prevalence of MTBI (concussion) in the sports arena, there has been growing concern about the extent of cognitive, emotional and behavioural changes that are known to occur in association with this injury (Shuttleworth-Edwards & Whitefield, 2007). More immediate acute sequelae typically resolve within three months post-injury, and effects which persist for longer than this are viewed as relatively intractable (that is, chronic) (Reitan & Wolfson, 1999). Sequelae typically include dysfunction in memory, learning and processing speed, as demonstrated on psychometric testing (Erlanger, Kutner, Barth & Barnes, 1999; Hinton-Bayre, Geffen & Friiss, 2004; Lezak, Howieson & Loring, 2004; Tromp & Mulder, 1991), as well as a cluster of commonly self-reported physical, emotional and behavioural sequelae, including headache, dizziness, blurred vision, anxiety, depression, sleep disturbance, noise and light sensitivity, fatigue, poor concentration, impulsivity, argumentativeness and irritability (Lezak et al., 2004; Reitan & Wolfson, 1999). Such effects will be pronounced in the acute phase of recovery, gradually petering out or reaching a plateau of chronic disability in certain areas. A substantial proportion of around 10–30 per cent of individuals that sustain even a single MTBI do sustain chronic impairment, particularly those with prior vulnerability such as cognitive or psychiatric disability (Reitan & Wolfson, 1999; Ruff, 2005).

With increasing attention being paid to the phenomenon of *cumulative* MTBI within the contact sports arena, there has been a gathering weight of research that points to permanent neurocognitive deficits demonstrated on objective testing, or symptomatic dysfunction based on self-reports, in players of these sports, including soccer (Witol & Webbe, 2003), Australian rules football (Cremona-Meteyard & Geffen, 1994), American football (Iverson, Gaetz, Lovell & Collins, 2004), and rugby union (Shuttleworth-Edwards, Border et al., 2004; Shuttleworth-Edwards & Radloff, 2008; Shuttleworth-Edwards, Smith & Radloff, 2008), with problems being more pronounced in professional and older players who have longer and/or more intensive exposure to the sport (Shuttleworth-Edwards, Border et al., 2004; Baroff, 1998). The crucial management issue associated with the sports concussive injury is that there are known risks of allowing concussed athletes to return to play before they are fully recovered from the injury (Aubry et al., 2002; Shuttleworth-Edwards, 2009). Risks of premature return to play include: (i) the possibility of rapid herniation and sudden death (Second Impact Syndrome) following a second, even mild, impact to the vulnerable brain; and/or (ii) increased risk of permanent intellectual decline (Cantu, 1998; Hovda, Le & Lifshitz, 1995; McCrory & Berkovic, 1998). It is in relation to this post-injury monitoring of recovery from the injury that neuropsychological assessment has been identified as a critical element.

Neuropsychological assessment in the sports context

Neuropsychological assessment is widely acknowledged as being more sensitive to the subtle neurocognitive effects of MTBI than any other diagnostic tool (Anderson, 1996; Rees, 2003). However, classically employed paper-and-pencil tests that tap the typically affected domains of attention, concentration, memory and processing speed (for example, the Digit Symbol Substitution Test, the Digit Symbol Incidental Recall, the Trail Making Test, the Digit Span Test and memory tests from the Wechsler Memory Scales) are also sensitive to the effects of practice as a result of repeat testing, with the greatest effects likely to occur between the first and second test administrations (Lezak et al., 2004; Strauss, Sherman & Spreen, 2006). This is a problem for clinicians evaluating recovery from MTBI in athletes where serial testing over short time intervals is necessary. Moreover, such commonly employed paper-and-pencil tests require individual administration and scoring, usually by a registered practitioner, and this is too labour-intensive and costly for baseline and follow-up testing of large numbers of athletes.

Accordingly, computer-based neuropsychological test batteries were developed specifically within the sports context, in order to address difficulties encountered with paper-and-pencil measures (Schnirring, 2001; Shuttleworth-Edwards & Border, 2002). Computer-based neuropsychological tests allow for the randomisation of test stimuli, thereby minimising practice effects (Lovell & Collins, 2002). In addition, in comparison with paper-and-pencil tests, computerised tests provide a more accurate measurement of processes such as reaction time and processing speed in milliseconds, thereby increasing the reliability of the testing process; they allow for the evaluation of a large number of athletes with minimal labour required; the data received can be easily stored and accessed at a later date; and lastly, such tests allow for the rapid production of automatically scored test data in a computer-generated clinical report (Lovell & Collins, 2002). Consequently, the use of computerised neurocognitive assessment batteries within the sports arena has gained ratification at a series of international symposiums held on concussion management over the past decade, and the view has been endorsed that neuropsychological evaluation should play an integral part in the overall management and treatment of athletes who have sustained concussions in sport (Aubry et al., 2002; McCrory et al., 2005; McCrory et al., 2009). The preferred mode for this evaluation is via computerised testing under the interpretive guidance of the clinical neuropsychologist (Echemendia, Herring & Bailes, 2009).

Currently, there are a number of computer-based neuropsychological tests available specific to the sports management context, including Cogsport (CogState Ltd, Melbourne), Headminder or Concussion Resolution Index (Headminder Inc., New York), ANAM (Automated Neuropsychological Assessment Metric) (developed by the US Department of Defense) and ImPACT (ImPACT Inc., Pittsburgh, PA). With the exception of Cogsport, which is based on the test stimulus of a pack of playing cards, these programs incorporate test constructs that were modelled on traditional neuropsychological tests and designed to measure the cognitive domains sensitive to the effects of MTBI (Podell, 2004). ImPACT is the most widely used of these programs worldwide, and compared with the above-listed programs offers the most comprehensive range of functional domains and symptoms to be checked. Moreover, the ImPACT test is the only one of these programs to date that has gained registration with the Health Professions Council of South Africa (HPCSA), and since its registration in 2002 has provided the basis for extensive clinical practice and research output within the South African arena. Commensurate with the HPCSA regulations on the use of computerised testing (HPCSA, 2006), the ImPACT test, while requiring the services of a registered psychologist for its interpretation, can be administered by a trained technician, thereby ensuring the suitability of this test for large-scale national application.

The ImPACT program

The ImPACT program was developed in a research context in order to evaluate cognitive outcome following concussion (Iverson et al., 2002; Collins et al., 1999). It was designed to assess multiple aspects of neuropsychological functioning, including attention span, sustained and selective attention, reaction time, and both verbal and visual dimensions of memory. The test has been refined over the years to incorporate a number of versions, including ImPACT-2.0 and ImPACT-3.0. The developers are working on making two versions available that will take the place of all prior versions, simply called ImPACT Desktop Version (developed between 2000 and 2007) and ImPACT Online (developed from 2007 to 2012). The test can be administered in numerous languages including English, Afrikaans, Spanish, French, Italian, Swedish, Czech, German, Japanese and Portuguese. The test is mouse-driven and can be loaded onto a standard desktop computer, or can be accessed online. An automatically generated report reflects the percentile ranking of each composite score on a testee's neurocognitive profile, calculated on the basis of age-adjusted US norms.

ImPACT-2.0 and ImPACT-3.0 have been used for the studies conducted in South Africa thus far, depending on which version was available for use at the time. Versions 2.0 and 3.0 consist of (i) a brief questionnaire to elicit demographic, medical and scholastic details; (ii) a symptom questionnaire; and (iii) a neurocognitive test battery. The ImPACT symptom scale consists of 22 symptoms commonly experienced after concussion that have to be rated as absent, partially present or definitely present on a 6-point Likert scale (Lovell et al., 2006) (see Table 30.1). The neurocognitive screening aspect is made up of six test modules that assess aspects of cognitive functioning relating to attention, memory, reaction time and processing speed, the results of which are combined to produce four basic composite scores in the domains of Verbal Memory, Visual Memory, Visual Motor Speed and Reaction Time, and a fifth composite score delineated as Impulse Control that serves as a validity indicator (Iverson, Lovell & Collins, 2003; Schatz, Pardini, Lovell & Collins, 2006) (see Table 30.2). The ability areas called upon for each of the six test modules are further delineated in Table 30.3.

Table 30.1 Delineation of the ImPACT postconcussion 6-point Likert scale

Symptom	None	Mild		Moderate		Severe	
Headache	0	1	2	3	4	5	6
Nausea	0	1	2	3	4	5	6
Vomiting	0	1	2	3	4	5	6
Balance problems	0	1	2	3	4	5	6
Dizziness	0	1	2	3	4	5	6
Fatigue	0	1	2	3	4	5	6
Trouble falling asleep	0	1	2	3	4	5	6
Sleeping more than usual	0	1	2	3	4	5	6
Sleeping less than usual	0	1	2	3	4	5	6
Drowsiness	0	1	2	3	4	5	6
Sensitivity to light	0	1	2	3	4	5	6
Sensitivity to noise	0	1	2	3	4	5	6
Irritability	0	1	2	3	4	5	6
Sadness	0	1	2	3	4	5	6
Nervousness	0	1	2	3	4	5	6
Feeling more emotional	0	1	2	3	4	5	6
Numbness or tingling	0	1	2	3	4	5	6
Feeling slowed down	0	1	2	3	4	5	6
Feeling mentally 'foggy'	0	1	2	3	4	5	6
Difficulty concentrating	0	1	2	3	4	5	6
Difficulty remembering	0	1	2	3	4	5	6
Visual problems	0	1	2	3	4	5	6

Source: Adapted from Lovell et al. (2006).

Table 30.2 Delineation of the ImPACT neurocognitive composite and contributing scores

Composite scores	Contributing scores
Verbal Memory	• Word Memory (learning and delayed) • Symbol Match (memory score)
Visual Memory	• Design Memory (learning and delayed) • X's and O's (percentage correct)
Reaction Time	• X's and O's (average counted correct reaction time) • Symbol Match (average weighted reaction time for correct responses) • Colour Match (average reaction time for correct responses)
Visual Motor Speed	• X's and O's (average correct distracters) • Symbol Match (average correct responses) • Three Letters (number of correct numbers correctly counted)
Impulse Control*	• X's and O's (number of incorrect distracters) • Colour Match (number of errors)

Source: Adapted from Iverson et al. (2002).

Note: *The Impulse Control composite score serves to measure profile validity, with a score > 20 implicating poor effort (Schatz et al., 2006).

Table 30.3 Ability areas tapped by the ImPACT test modules

Test module	Ability areas
Word Memory	Immediate and delayed memory for words
Design Memory	Immediate and delayed memory for designs
X's and O's	Attention, concentration, working memory and reaction time
Symbol Match	Visual processing speed, learning and memory
Colour Match	Focused attention, response inhibition, reaction time
Three Letters	Attention, concentration, working memory, visual-motor speed

Source: Adapted from Iverson et al. (2002).

Reliability and validity of the ImPACT test

The ImPACT test consists of a near-infinite number of random forms, thereby minimising practice effects, and has shown good test-retest reliability (Maroon, Field, Lovell, Collins & Post, 2002). In respect of the Memory composite, it has been demonstrated that controls did not increase with multiple testing, while concussed athletes performed more poorly on the Verbal Memory test at 36 hours, 4 days and 7 days post-injury compared to their baseline scores (Lovell et al., 2003). In a study on high school athletes, ImPACT was administered four times, two to eight days apart (Iverson et al., 2003). Test-retest correlation coefficients for the Memory composite ranged from 0.66 to 0.85, for the Processing Speed composite from 0.75 to 0.88, and for the

Reaction Time composite from 0.62 to 0.66 across the various test sessions. The Reaction Time composite was highly consistent across all testing intervals, while the Memory and Processing Speed composites revealed weaker correlations between the first and second test occasions, compared with the second and third, and third and fourth, occasions. Therefore, while there was some improvement after the first test interval, there was little practice effect shown after subsequent administrations.

In a study investigating the diagnostic utility of ImPACT and the Postconcussion Symptom Scale (Schatz et al., 2006), it was demonstrated that the combined sensitivity of ImPACT and the symptom score (that is, the probability that a test result will be positive when a concussion is present) was 81.9 per cent, and the specificity (that is, the probability that a test result will be negative when a concussion is not present) was 89.4 per cent. The Schatz et al. study followed on a series of earlier studies attesting to the efficacy of the ImPACT Memory and Reaction Time composites that supported the presence of concussive injury in general, including the mildest Grade 1 concussion (Lovell, Collins, Iverson, Johnston & Bradley, 2004; Lovell et al., 2003). Construct convergent and divergent validity was demonstrated via a factor analysis revealing a two-factor solution of Processing Speed and Memory, with the Symbol Digit Modalities Test of processing speed correlating more highly with the Visual Motor Speed and Reaction Time composites than the two memory composites (Iverson, Lovell & Collins, 2005).

Overall, therefore, the ImPACT test reports excellent test-retest reliability, minimal practice effects and good construct validity when examined in relation to the commonly employed neuropsychological tests. The diagnostic sensitivity and specificity of the test in respect of MTBI is excellent.

South African research using the ImPACT test

Under the coordination of the first author of this chapter, and in collaboration with the developers of the ImPACT program at the University of Pittsburgh Medical Center Sports Concussion Program, a series of National Research Foundation-funded postgraduate research studies using the ImPACT test has been in progress in South Africa since 2002, with a view to investigating the chronic neuropsychological effects of participation in the contact sport of rugby union. Studies targeting demographically equivalent comparative groups of contact and noncontact sports players were initiated in the Western Cape, Eastern Cape and KwaZulu-Natal at high school, university, club and provincial levels, some of which are still ongoing. In addition, there has been growing use of the test at the school and professional levels on a commercial basis in order to facilitate concussion management. The first set of noncontact sport normative indications arising out of these research studies, specifically in respect of Grade 12 male, predominantly white English-speaking high school athletes, has been isolated for presentation in this chapter (Whitefield, 2006).

Research study: South African normative data for noncontact sport high school athletes

The sample for this research consisted of all final-year, sports-playing Grade 12 high school boys from an English-medium school in the Western Cape Province, who were targeted over a two-year period for participation in the study, which was designed to compare contact with noncontact sports players. The objective was to investigate the effect of long-term participation in a contact sport, and to derive normative data in respect of this cohort of predominantly white South African schoolboys in attendance at an educationally advantaged English-medium school. The initial pool comprised 297 boys, and following exclusions a total of 189 athletes made up the final sample. Exclusion criteria included being not actively involved in any sport; having a history of substance abuse, learning disorder, Attention Deficit Disorder, any grades repeated, neurological or psychiatric disorder, moderate or severe traumatic brain injury; being fatigued or poorly motivated; having an overly low Wechsler Adult Intelligence Scale–III (WAIS-III) Vocabulary scaled score (< 8), or an abnormally raised score on the Impulse Control composite (> 20).

The sample was further divided between a contact sports group (n = 115) made up of individuals participating in rugby, soccer and Jeet Kune Do, and a noncontact group for the purposes of comparative nonclinical normative data (n = 74), made up of individuals participating in field hockey (n = 29), basketball (n = 11), water polo (n = 10), athletics (n = 5), tennis (n = 3), squash (n = 3), swimming (n = 3), cycling (n = 3), cricket (n = 2), rowing (n = 2), golf (n = 2) and gymnastics (n = 1). Demographic features of the noncontact norming sample were an age range of 16 to 18 years (mean = 17.08; SD = 0.33) and an above-average Vocabulary scaled score (mean = 12.26; SD = 1.90). A history of mild traumatic brain injury was not used as an exclusion criterion in this study, as it was anticipated that this feature would serve to differentiate the contact and noncontact sports groups on neuropsychological testing. While the contact sports players reported a history of on average 1.28 concussions, the noncontact sports players reported on average only 0.27 concussions, implying that minimal if any individuals in the latter group had sustained more than one concussion ($p = 0.001$).

Written consent to conduct the research at the school and within school hours was obtained from the Western Cape Department of Education as well as from the school headmaster. All Grade 12 parents were sent letters informing them of the nature and purpose of the research, and were given the option of withdrawing their children from the study by signing an attached waiver form. Written consent was received from all participants prior to testing. Testing took place between February and April and was conducted by two postgraduate psychology students trained in the administration of the ImPACT test; standardised test instructions were applied. The ImPACT program had been loaded by the school technician, and participants were tested in groups of approximately 25 boys in the school computer laboratory, without any noise or distractions, and with an overall testing time of approximately 20 to 30 minutes.

Prior to the commencement of ImPACT testing, the WAIS-III Vocabulary subtest (Wechsler, 1997) was administered to establish the equivalence of the contact and noncontact groups in the study, in respect of intellectual potential. While this test is administered orally for individual assessments, in order to facilitate group assessment participants were instructed to write their definitions in booklets which were provided, and no heed was taken of the discontinuation rule. Although the administration deviated from the standard procedure, it provided a parameter for excluding abnormally low-functioning individuals from the sample, and served to suggest that the cohort was of at least average to above-average intellectual potential (see data cited above), an observation that is commensurate with the relatively advantaged educational background of the cohort under investigation. The ImPACT Impulse Control composite scores were used as validity indicators for exclusion purposes only, whereas the composite scores for the other four composites (Verbal Memory, Visual Memory, Visual Motor Speed and Reaction Time) were subjected to group statistical analysis, including the calculation of means and standard deviations. These were then descriptively compared with the available age-equivalent data from the ImPACT -2.0 US norming sample (Iverson et al., 2002).

The results are presented in Table 30.4, and reveal that the South African ImPACT mean scores for predominantly white English-speaking noncontact sports players with advantaged education are broadly equivalent to the age-equivalent US data, with most scores falling well within the US normative ranges. Reaction Time falls just above the US normative bracket in the direction of being marginally, but not clinically significantly, slower by .02 of a second.

Table 30.4 Preseason noncontact group cognitive mean scores for South African high school male athletes in comparison with age-equivalent US average normative ranges on the ImPACT test

	South African mean scores	US normative ranges
	N = 74	N = 158
Verbal Memory	85.41	80–92
Visual Memory	77.77	71–88
Visual Motor Speed	37.79	33.7–42.5
Reaction Time	0.60	0.58–0.50

Source: Data for US normative ranges derived from Iverson et al. (2002).

In respect of the ImPACT symptom scale (see Table 30.5), the findings reveal that the average total symptom score reported by a predominantly white English-speaking cohort of South African male athletes was 12.5, compared with a normal range of only 1 to 6 for US male athletes.

Accordingly, it appears that South African high school male athletes of this demographic description have a tendency to report substantially more postconcussive symptoms on average than the US high school male athlete, with a mean score that rates as 'unusual', bordering on 'high', according to the US classification.

Table 30.5 Preseason noncontact group total symptom mean score for South African high school male athletes in comparison with age-equivalent US normative ranges on the ImPACT test

SA symptom means	USA symptom ranges (classification)
N = 74	N = 588
	0 (Low–Normal)
	1–6 (Normal)
12.50	7–13 (Unusual)
	14–21 (High)
	22+ (Very High)

Source: Data for US symptom ranges derived from Iverson et al. (2002).

The normative data derived for the ImPACT test in respect of this South African predominantly white male high school population of noncontact sports athletes reveals a neurocognitive profile that is highly equivalent to the age-equivalent US normative data on this test. This finding reflects the fact that the sample is drawn from South African learners within a relatively advantaged English-medium educational setting, and consequently they do not reveal any disadvantaged ability when completing the ImPACT neurocognitive test in comparison to the average US athlete similarly enjoying Westernised first-world high school standards. The finding is commensurate with prior South African cross-cultural studies across a spectrum of traditional paper-and-pencil cognitive tests (including the WAIS-III and Wechsler Intelligence Scale for Children–IV (WISC-IV), and other miscellaneous neurocognitive tests), that consistently demonstrate equivalence of cognitive test performance with the US standardisations for South African white and black testees being educated in formerly white South African English-medium high school and university settings (Shuttleworth-Edwards, Gaylard & Radloff, chapter 2, this volume; Shuttleworth-Edwards, Kemp, Rust, Muirhead, Hartman & Radloff, 2004; Shuttleworth-Edwards, Van der Merwe, Van Tonder & Radloff, chapter 3, this volume; Shuttleworth-Jordan, 1996). However, there was unusually high symptom reporting for the South African sample compared with the US normative data, implicating cross-cultural variations in symptom reporting between these two groups that warrants more in-depth evaluation beyond the scope of the available data, as to why this should be the case.

Importantly, the outcome on the present research was specifically in respect of a *noncontact* sports cohort of Grade 12 high school boys in the age range 16–18. However, it replicates the outcome of a previously published normative comparison conducted by the present authors in respect of *contact* sports players tested for commercial purposes at preseason (Shuttleworth-Edwards, Whitefield-Alexander, Radloff, Taylor & Lovell, 2009). In this study, the relative normality of the scores for contact sports players was presumed in that testing at *preseason* usually occurs following a three- to four-month break from playing the sport, thereby precluding the confounding effect of any cognitive fall-off due to cumulative head and body impacts sustained during a rugby/football season. In this previously published study the ImPACT composite test scores and total symptom scores for South African rugby players (that is, players of rugby union) were compared with those of US football players in three different age groups (11–13 years, 14–16 years, 17–21 years) (see Table 30.6), and revealed remarkably equivalent neurocognitive scores across all the composites between the comparison groups at each age stage, with small effect sizes of no clinical relevance. However, for the total symptom score there was a consistent tendency for the South African contact sport players to report substantially more symptoms than their US age-equivalent peers, with medium effect sizes implicating clinically relevant differences.

Table 30.6 Means of ImPACT neurocognitive composite scores for South African rugby and US football players across three age groups

Neurocognitive measures	SA mean score	USA mean score
11–13 years	**(n = 301)**	**(n = 775)**
Verbal Memory composite	80.20	82.10
Visual Memory composite	69.50	71.90
Visual Motor composite	31.30	30.80
Reaction Time composite	0.63	0.66
Impulse Control composite	8.40	8.40
Total Symptom composite	8.10	3.70
14–16 years	**(n = 997)**	**(n = 4081)**
Verbal Memory composite	82.00	81.80
Visual Memory composite	73.30	70.80
Visual Motor composite	33.90	34.90
Reaction Time composite	0.60	0.60
Impulse Control composite	8.10	7.70
Total Symptom composite	8.90	6.00
17–21 years	**(n = 319)**	**(n = 4784)**
Verbal Memory composite	84.10	83.50
Visual Memory composite	76.00	72.90
Visual Motor composite	38.10	38.40
Reaction Time composite	0.57	0.58
Impulse Control composite	6.90	6.00
Total Symptom composite	10.80	5.30

Source: Adapted from Shuttleworth-Edwards et al. (2009).

The overall implication of both these comparative normative studies is that the ImPACT test can be used appropriately in South Africa on educationally advantaged individuals who are proficient in English in the age range 11 to 21 years, making use of the automatically generated age-related percentile scores that appear on the report printout for neurocognitive screening. However, when evaluating a symptom profile across the same age spectrum, a degree of greater leniency should be allowed for a South African testee's baseline symptom score compared with the US norms. The fact that the tendency for enhanced symptom reporting amongst the South African schoolboys occurs for both contact and noncontact sports groups, and across *all* the adolescent and young adult age groups, does suggest that there is a cultural underpinning to this variation. In other words, it would appear that the effect cannot be attributed to factors such as age-specific stressors (for example, the stress of being in a specific grade) or the deleterious neurological consequences of participation in rugby rather than American football.

Importantly, all the data presented in this chapter are with reference to groups of predominantly white English first-language athletes from relatively advantaged educational backgrounds. Therefore, it cannot be assumed that there will be equivalence of normative data on the ImPACT neurocognitive test profile for South African testees who are from educationally disadvantaged backgrounds – for example, those educated within the former Department of Education and Training township coloured and black schools – and/or testees whose first language is not English. Prior South African cross-cultural research referred to above (Shuttleworth-Edwards, Gaylard et al., chapter 2, this volume; Shuttleworth-Edwards, Kemp et al., 2004; Shuttleworth-Edwards, Van der Merwe et al., chapter 3, this volume; Shuttleworth-Jordan, 1996) has revealed a significant lowering of cognitive test performance in both the verbal and nonverbal areas in respect of such testees, and until more specific research is available on the ImPACT test on these populations, some similar lowering should be anticipated. In the sports arena, the attainment of a preseason baseline test profile is particularly crucial for individuals who differ from the norm group, in that their post-injury scores can be compared with their own pre-injury test profiles, and this goes some way towards circumventing the problem of lack of appropriate norms.

Concluding comments and future directions

The past four decades have seen the dramatic development of modern clinical neuropsychology into a discipline that has gained substantial recognition within the medical and legal fraternities (Lezak et al., 2004; Walsh, 1991). In hospital settings, departments of neurology and neurosurgery routinely call upon the assessment services of the clinical neuropsychologist to facilitate their diagnostic and rehabilitation decisions. For disability claims in medico-legal settings, the clinical neuropsychologist is a core member of the team of expert witnesses employed for the evaluation of disability following brain injury. Until recently, the tools employed by the neuropsychologist were a spectrum of paper-and-pencil tests typically including a test of general intellectual functioning such as one of the Wechsler scales, and a collection of additional tests to evaluate more specific functional modalities such as verbal tasks, speeded and unspeeded visuoperceptual skills, visual and verbal memory, and executive functions (Lezak et al., 2004; Strauss et al., 2006). The problem is that such evaluations are labour-intensive and costly, in that the battery normally takes two to three hours to administer, and several more hours to score and interpret. Consequently, there has been a limit on the ability to utilise such evaluations on a mass basis, and this in turn has been restrictive in considering new and wider applications of neuropsychological evaluation.

However, this limitation has changed dramatically within the past decade with the advent of the computerised neurocognitive screening instrument, exemplified in the present chapter by the ImPACT test. As is clear from the description of this test presented in this chapter, it consists of a number of neurocognitive tasks that are known to be particularly sensitive to the generalised effects of diffuse brain impairment in association with concussive brain injury. Yet, in contrast to the traditional paper-and-pencil battery, the test can be administered by trained technicians on large groups of testees, and the results are immediately automatically scored and saved online, such that the overall process per test takes a maximum of 20 to 30 minutes. Accuracy on speeded tasks is particularly facilitated in this process compared with traditional paper-and-pencil test options, and there is a much reduced problem with practice effects due to the availability of multiple randomised versions of the tasks. Consequently, whereas this was formerly not a pragmatic option, neuropsychological evaluation (including preseason testing and the follow-up of the concussed athlete) is being viewed within the sports medicine arena as a cornerstone of the modern approach to concussion management (Aubry et al., 2002; McCrory et al., 2009; Moser et al., 2007).

While the sports milieu has been the setting for the development of bulk employment of neurocognitive screening via a test such as ImPACT, the instrument is gaining recognition as having the potential for wider application. There is a spectrum of neuropathology in addition to concussion that may present in relatively early stages with decline in the areas of attention, concentration, processing speed, and short-term and delayed memory due to the non-specific effects of diffuse brain pathology. Such pathology includes Mild Cognitive Impairment (MCI) (a preclinical dementia that has more pronounced effects than normal cognitive aging), Alzheimer's disease, HIV/AIDS dementia, alcohol dementia, dementias in association with other toxic substances, dementias due to metabolic and endocrine disturbance, and so on (Lezak et al., 2004; Lishman, 1999). In addition, psychiatric disturbance such as depression, post-traumatic stress disorder and anxiety disorders may affect these same functional modes deleteriously.

Notably, the ImPACT test has revealed sensitivity to neurocognitive decline in association with HIV/AIDS dementia (Shuttleworth-Edwards & Whitefield-Alexander, 2010) and depression (Iverson, 2006). While subtle, such cognitive decline may have clinically relevant everyday occupational consequences, and once identified on the basis of screening using a test such as ImPACT, the observation can be followed up with more comprehensive neuropsychological evaluation to evaluate the implications in an individual case, and to supply specific recommendations. Within the aviation context, the possibility of baseline screening of all pilots, cabin crew and ground-control personnel is being considered, followed by routine retesting as part of the regular medical examination on an annual or biannual basis (Shuttleworth-Edwards & Whitefield-Alexander, 2010). The objective would be for early detection of cognitive fall-off in association with incipient neurological or psychiatric disorder in the interests of aviation safety. Further, ImPACT is being widely employed in the US military to monitor the consequences of combat trauma to the brain and psychiatrically (Lovell, Collins, Pardini, Parodi & Yates, 2005). Another avenue for consideration is the implementation of baseline screening for individuals in settings where there is risk of hypoxia and/or exposure to toxic substances (for example, deep-sea divers or employees in an asbestos factory), with routine follow-up to ensure that they are not suffering any associated negative consequences (Shuttleworth-Edwards & Whitefield-Alexander, 2011).

This chapter has described the ImPACT test, a frequently employed neurocognitive screening instrument used within the sports concussion arena. South African specific normative data have been presented, and comparative indications with US normative data described. It has been indicated that there is a need for additional normative data on South Africans whose first language is not English and who come from relatively disadvantaged educational backgrounds. Although developed within the sports context to screen for concussion, thereby promoting the facility for mass testing to facilitate medical management of the athlete, the sensitive screening capacity of this time- and cost-effective instrument promises much wider application for the identification of diffuse brain damage effects in association with a wide spectrum of commonly presenting neuropathological conditions. The ability to conduct large-scale neuropsychological screening for the identification of brain damage effects (for example, in sport, the military, aviation, and hypoxic or toxic work environments) constitutes a giant leap forward specifically for the discipline of clinical neuropsychology, as well for the psychological assessment forum generally within psychology.

Notes

1 Acknowledgements are due to the South African National Research Foundation and the Rhodes University Joint Research Council for funding of the ImPACT normative research studies, and to the collaborating researchers and developers of the ImPACT program at the University of Pittsburgh Medical Center Sports Concussion Program, Pittsburgh, USA.

2 Declaration of interest: The first and second authors of this chapter are involved in the commercial use of ImPACT within South Africa and the UK.

3 Rugby union is one of a cluster of rugby football games which originated from soccer, the oldest and most widely played of all the football games (Micheli & Riseborough, 1974). In 1823 a schoolboy at Rugby School in England, whilst playing soccer, picked up the ball and ran with it to put it across the goal line. Over a period of 30 years this approach took on and developed into the completely separate game of rugby football, which later splintered and developed into several modes: rugby union; rugby league;

American football; and Australian rules football. Rugby union is now an extremely popular and fast-growing spectator sport worldwide, and is played at school, university and professional levels in countries such as England, Wales, Scotland, the USA, Canada, Argentina, France, Japan, Australia, New Zealand, Zimbabwe and South Africa.

References

Anderson, S. J. (1996). Sports-related head injuries: A neuropsychological perspective. *Sports Medicine*, September, 23–27.

Aubry, M., Cantu, R., Dvorak, J., Graf-Baumann, T., Johnston, K. M., Kelly, J. et al. (2002). Summary and agreement statement of the 1st International Symposium on Concussion in Sport, Vienna, 2001. *Clinical Journal of Sport Medicine, 12,* 6–11.

Baroff, G. S. (1998). Is heading a soccer ball injurious to brain function? *Journal of Head Trauma Rehabilitation, 13,* 45–52.

Barth, J. T., Alves, W. M., Ryan, T. V., Macciocchi, S. N., Rimel, R. W., Jane, J. A. et al. (1989). Mild head injury in sports: Neuropsychological sequelae and recovery of function. In H. S. Levin, H. Eisenberg & A. Benton (Eds), *Mild Head Injury* (pp. 257–275). Oxford: Oxford University Press.

Cantu, R. (1998). Second-impact syndrome. *Clinics in Sports Medicine, 17,* 37–43.

Cassidy, J. D., Carroll, L. J., Peloso, P. M., Borg, J. & Von Holst, H. (2004). Incidence, risk factors and prevention of mild traumatic brain injury: Results of the WHO collaborating centre task force on mild traumatic brain injury. *Journal of Rehabilitation Medicine, Suppl. 43,* 28–60.

CDC (Centers for Disease Control and Prevention) (1997). Sports-related recurrent brain injuries – United States. *Morbidity Mortality Weekly Report, 46,* 224–227.

Collins, M. W., Lovell, M. R. & McKeag, D. (1999). Current issues in managing sports-related concussion. *Journal of the American Medical Association, 282,* 193–198.

Cremona-Meteyard, S. L. & Geffen, G. M. (1994). Persistent visuospatial attention deficits following mild head injury in Australian rules football players. *Neuropsychologist, 32,* 649–662.

Echemendia, R., Herring, S. & Bailes, J. (2009). Who should conduct and interpret the neuropsychological assessment in sports-related concussion? *British Journal of Sports Medicine, 43,* i32–i35.

Erlanger, D. M., Kutner, K. C., Barth, J. T. & Barnes, R. (1999). Neuropsychology of sports-related head injury: Dementia pugilistica to post concussions syndrome. *The Clinical Neuropsychologist, 13,* 193–209.

Hinton-Bayre, A. D., Geffen, G. & Friiss, P. (2004). Presentation and mechanisms of concussion in professional rugby league football. *Journal of Science Medicine and Sport, 7,* 275–289.

Hovda, D. A., Le, H. M. & Lifshitz, J. (1995). Long-term changes in metabolic rates for glucose following mild, moderate and severe concussive head injuries in adult rats. *Neurosurgery, A,* 375–376.

HPCSA (Health Professions Council of South Africa: Professional Board for Psychology) (2006). *South African Guidelines on Computerised Testing.* Report No. Form 257. Pretoria: Health Professions Council of South Africa.

Iverson, G. (2006). Sensitivity of computerized neuropsychological screening in depressed university students. *The Clinical Neuropsychologist, 20,* 695–701.

Iverson, G. L., Gaetz, M., Lovell, M. R. & Collins, M. W. (2004). Cumulative effects of concussion in amateur athletes. *Brain Injury, 18,* 433–443.

Iverson, G. L., Lovell, M. R. & Collins, M. W. (2002). *Immediate Postconcussion Assessment and Cognitive Testing (ImPACT) Normative Data Version 2.0.* Pittsburgh, PA: ImPACT Applications Inc.

Iverson, G. L., Lovell, M. R. & Collins, M. W. (2003). Interpreting change on ImPACT following sport concussion. *Clinical Neuropsychology 17(4),* 460–467.

Iverson, G. L., Lovell, M. R. & Collins, M. W. (2005). Validity of ImPACT for measuring processing speed following sports-related concussion. *Journal of Clinical and Experimental Neuropsychology, 27,* 683–689.

Lezak, M. D., Howieson, D. B. & Loring, D. W. (2004). *Neuropsychological Assessment* (4th edition). Oxford: Oxford University Press.

Lishman, W. (1999). *Organic Psychiatry: The Psychological Consequences of Cerebral Disorder* (3rd edition). Oxford: Blackwell Science.

Lovell, M. R. & Collins, M. W. (2002). New developments in the evaluation of sports-related concussion. *Current Sports Medicine Reports, 1,* 287–292.

Lovell, M. R., Collins, M. W., Iverson, G. L., Field, M., Maroon, J. C., Cantu, R. et al. (2003). Recovery from mild concussion in high school athletes. *Journal of Neurosurgery, 98,* 296–301.

Lovell, M. R., Collins, M. W., Iverson, G. L., Johnston, K. M. & Bradley, J. P. (2004). Grade 1 or 'ding' concussions in high school athletes. *American Journal of Sports Medicine, 32(1),* 47–54.

Lovell, M. R., Collins, M., Pardini, J. E., Parodi, A. & Yates, A. (2005). Management of cerebral concussion in military personnel: Lessons learned from sports medicine. *Operative Techniques in Sports Medicine, 13,* 212–221.

Lovell, M., Iverson, G., Collins, M., Podell, K., Johnston, K., Pardini, D. et al. (2006). Measurement of symptoms following sports-related concussion: Reliability and normative data for the Post-Concussion Symptom Scale. *Applied Neuropsychology, 13,* 166–175.

Maroon, J. C., Field, M., Lovell, M. R., Collins, M. & Post, J. (2002). The evaluation of athletes with cerebral concussion. *Clinical Neurosurgery, 49,* 319–332.

McCrory, P. & Berkovic, S. F. (1998). Second impact syndrome. *Neurology, 50,* 677–683.

McCrory, P., Johnston, K., Meeuwisse, W., Aubry, M., Cantu, R., Dvorak, J. et al. (2005). Summary and agreement statement of the 2nd International Conference on Concussion in Sport, Prague 2004. *Clinical Journal of Sport Medicine, 15,* 48–55.

McCrory, P., Meeuwisse, W., Johnston, K., Dvorak, J., Aubry, M., Molloy, R. et al. (2009). Consensus statement on concussion in sport: The 3rd International Conference on Concussion in Sport held in Zurich, November 2008. *British Journal of Sports Medicine, 43,* i76–i84.

Micheli, L. J. & Riseborough, E. M. (1974). The incidence of injuries in rugby football. *Journal of Sports Medicine, 2,* 93–97.

Moser, R. S., Iverson, G. L., Echemendia, R. J., Lovell, M. R., Schatz, P., Webbe, F. M. et al. (2007). NAN position paper. Neuropsychological evaluation in the diagnosis and management of sports concussion. *Archives of Clinical Neuropsychology, 22,* 909–916.

Podell, K. (2004). Computerized assessment of sports-related brain injury. In M. Lovell, R. Echemendia, J. Barth & M. Collins (Eds), *Traumatic Brain Injury in Sports: An International Neuropsychological Perspective* (pp. 375–393). Lisse: Swets & Zeitlinger.

Powell, J. W. & Barber-Foss, K. D. (1999). Traumatic brain injury in high school athletes. *Journal of the American Medical Association, 282,* 958–963.

Rees, P. M. (2003). Contemporary issues in mild traumatic brain injury. *Archives of Physical Medicine Rehabilitation, 84,* 1885–1894.

Reitan, R. M. & Wolfson, D. (1999). The two faces of mild head injury. *Archives of Clinical Neuropsychology, 14,* 191–202.

Ruff, R. (2005). Two decades of advances in understanding of mild traumatic brain injury. *Journal of Head Trauma Rehabilitation, 20,* 5–18.

Schatz, P., Pardini, J., Lovell, M. & Collins, M. (2006). Sensitivity and specificity of the ImPACT test battery for concussion in athletes. *Archives of Clinical Neuropsychology, 21,* 91–99.

Schnirring, L. (2001). How effective is computerized concussion management? *The Physician and Sports Medicine, 29,* 11–16.

Shuttleworth-Edwards, A. B. (2009). Convolutions of the 'silent concussion': A neuropsychologist's response to the dark ages of rule-based return-to-play decisions. *Archives of Neurology, 66,* 420–421.

Shuttleworth-Edwards, A. B. & Border, M. A. (2002). Computer-based screening in concussion management: Use versus abuse. *British Journal of Sports Medicine, 36,* 473.

Shuttleworth-Edwards, A. B., Border, M., Reid, I. & Radloff, S. (2004). South African Rugby Union. In M. R. Lovell, R. E. Echemendia, J. T. Barth & M. W. Collins (Eds), *Traumatic Brain Injury in Sports: An International Neuropsychological Perspective* (pp. 149–168). Lisse: Swets & Zeitlinger.

Shuttleworth-Edwards, A. B., Kemp, R., Rust, A., Muirhead, J., Hartman, N. & Radloff, S. (2004). Cross-cultural effects on IQ test performance: A review and preliminary normative indications on WAIS-III test performance. *Journal of Clinical and Experimental Neuropsychology, 26,* 903–920.

Shuttleworth-Edwards, A. B., Noakes, T. D., Radloff, S. E., Whitefield, V. J., Roberts, C. O., Clark, S. J. et al. (2008). The comparative incidence of reported concussions for follow-up management in South African Rugby Union. *Clinical Journal of Sport Medicine, 18,* 403–409.

Shuttleworth-Edwards, A. B. & Radloff, S. E. (2008). Compromised visuomotor processing speed in players of Rugby Union from school through to the adult national level. *Archives of Clinical Neuropsychology, 23,* 511–520.

Shuttleworth-Edwards, A. B., Smith, I. & Radloff, S. E. (2008). Neurocognitive vulnerability amongst university rugby players versus noncontact sport controls. *Journal of Clinical and Experimental Neuropsychology, 30,* 870–884.

Shuttleworth-Edwards, A. B. & Whitefield, V. J. (2007). Ethically we can no longer sit on the fence: A neuropsychological perspective on the cerebrally hazardous contact sports. *South African Journal of Sports Medicine, 19,* 32–38.

Shuttleworth-Edwards, A. B. & Whitefield-Alexander, V. J. (2010). The implementation of routine neurocognitive screening to improve airline safety: An overdue aid to medical evaluation. Invited address in a workshop on Psychological Assessment of Aircrew at the Biennial Conference of the South African Society for Aerospace & Environmental Medicine. Pretoria, September 9–12.

Shuttleworth-Edwards, A. B. & Whitefield-Alexander, V. J. (2011). The utility of computerized neurocognitive screening using the ImPACT programme within the diving context. Invited presentation at the 17th International Congress of Hyperbaric Medicine. Cape Town, March 16–19.

Shuttleworth-Edwards, A. B., Whitefield-Alexander, V. J., Radloff, S. E., Taylor, A. M. & Lovell, M. R. (2009). Computerized neuropsychological profiles of South African versus United States athletes: A basis for commentary on cross-cultural norming issues in the sports concussion arena. *The Physician and Sports Medicine, 37,* 45–51.

Shuttleworth-Jordan, A. B. (1996). On not reinventing the wheel: A clinical perspective on cultural aspects of test usage in South Africa. *South African Journal of Psychology, 26(2)*, 96–102.

Strauss, E., Sherman, E. M. S. & Spreen, O. (2006). *A Compendium of Neuropsychological Tests* (3rd edition). Oxford: Oxford University Press.

Tromp, E. & Mulder, T. (1991). Slowness of information processing after traumatic head injury. *Journal of Clinical and Experimental Neuropsychology, 13*, 821–830.

Walsh, K. (1991). *Understanding Brain Damage: A Primer of Neuropsychological Evaluation* (2nd edition). Melbourne: Churchill Livingstone.

Wechsler, D. (1997). *The Wechsler Adult Intelligence Scale – Third Edition (WAIS-III)*. San Antonio, TX: Psychological Corporation.

Whitefield, V. J. (2006). 'Glory is temporary, brain injury is forever.' A neuropsychological study on the cumulative effects of sports-related concussive brain injury amongst Grade 12 school boy athletes. PhD dissertation, Rhodes University, Grahamstown.

Witol, A. D. & Webbe, F. M. (2003). Soccer heading frequency predicts neuropsychological deficits. *Archives in Clinical Neuropsychology, 18*, 397–417.

31 A family consultation model of child assessment

Z. Amod

Innovative assessment procedures, which take into account contextual factors such as language, culture, education, socio-economic status and recent educational policy developments, are needed in South Africa. In the democratic South Africa, Education White Paper 6 (Department of Education, 2001) calls for assessment practices that are less expert-driven, non-deficit-focused and linked to curriculum support. The Initial Assessment Consultation (IAC) approach, which is the focus of this chapter, encompasses and attempts to address these needs. This shared problem-solving approach to child assessment has at its core a focus on collaboration with parents and caregivers, as well as with significant others such as teachers, with the purpose of facilitating learning and the empowerment of clients. The approach is based on a sound philosophical and theoretical foundation and is a departure from the belief that assessment and intervention are discrete clinical procedures.

The IAC approach to child assessment, which represents a paradigm shift in assessment practice, was initially developed by Adelman and Taylor (1979) at the Fernald Institute at the University of California to address prevailing criticisms of conventional assessment procedures. For more than two decades, the IAC family participation and consultation model of assessment has been adapted and implemented at the University of the Witwatersrand. The key principles of the IAC approach are applied by many local professionals and training institutions that work within the assessment, remedial and educational fields. Research has supported the usefulness of this holistic and egalitarian form of assessment (Amod, 2003; Amod, Skuy, Sonderup & Fridjhon, 2000; Levin, 2003; Manala, 2001; Skuy, Westaway & Hickson, 1986; Warburton, 2008), which mirrors the more democratic environment of post-apartheid South Africa, with its endorsement of human rights, its sensitivity towards cross-cultural differences and its changing educational policies on assessment practice.

Background to the IAC approach

The IAC model provides an optimal and broad framework for assessment practice. Adelman and Taylor (1983; 1993; 2010) reject the reductionist view of behavioural, emotional and learning problems as reflecting internal deficits and pathology within the individual. They caution against the risk of misdiagnosis and bias towards labelling. As an alternative, they propose an interactional framework within which socio-emotional issues and barriers to learning can be understood. These issues are conceptualised along a continuum that encompasses internal and extrinsic variables, or a combination of both. The ecosystemic model is particularly useful in that it reflects a holistic, culturally and environmentally based view of learning and mental health issues. The IAC model encompasses Bronfenbrenner's (1979) ecological model, which posits that external interacting systems (such as family and school, and their reciprocal interaction) influence children's developmental trajectory.

Basic premises of the IAC approach

The IAC assessment model was developed in reaction to the criticisms and limitations of prevailing assessment practices. It contests the assumptions of the medical model and exemplifies best-practice principles in assessment, which are founded on a postmodernist approach that examines a plurality of possible causes. The model transcends the biological reductionist criticism levelled against the medical model in that it examines the reciprocal relationships between personal and environmental variables (Adelman & Taylor, 1979; Skuy et al., 1986). Because of its transactional character, the IAC approach offers a broader scope of inquiry and understanding by allowing an investigation into interpersonal, intrapersonal and environmental variables.

Table 31.1 A comparison of the traditional testing approach and the IAC model of assessment

Traditional testing	IAC
Person-centred.	Dynamic interaction between person and environmental variables.
Pathology/internal deficit model.	Holistic; intrapersonal, societal, cultural and environmentally based conceptualisation of mental health.
Usually reliance on product-related, 'static' testing (IQ scores).	Broad conceptualisation of assessment. Incorporates diagnostic teaching or counselling and process-based and interactive assessment procedures.
Often premature, person-focused assessment.	Ecosystemic assessment.
Problem with culture fairness.	Assessment is contextualised.
Psychologist as expert – offers 'expert' prescriptions.	Joint problem-solving with active parent and family participation and engagement. Psychologist as collaborative consultant.
Often once-off testing process.	Assessment seen as an ongoing process.
Criticism regarding inadequate link between assessment and intervention.	Facilitates link between assessment and intervention, which are seen as being inextricably linked.

Table 31.1 provides a comparison between the IAC approach and traditional psychometric assessment procedures. The latter tend to be person-centred, mainly focusing on internal deficits of the learner. They are also expert-driven and have been criticised for not making an adequate link between assessment and intervention. The IAC model of assessment attempts to address some of the limitations of conventional testing.

A key assumption underpinning the IAC approach is that assessment is a joint problem-solving approach involving the consultant, the family and/or significant others and the child. Through this experience, clients and consultants together pave the way to reach an understanding of client concerns so as to make appropriate intervention decisions. A step-by-step procedure, which is discussed later in this chapter, serves as a catalyst for change. The IAC's shared problem-solving paradigm assumes client motivation and capability. There is an assumption that the client wants to alter a 'discomforting status quo' and has 'some degree of relevant skills to do so' (Adelman & Taylor, 1979, p.58). Client control, consent, commitment and competence are all vital to the outcome of the IAC process.

The IAC approach presents a departure from the belief that assessment and intervention are discrete clinical procedures. Adelman and Taylor (1983; 2010) maintain that in practice, assessment is an integral part of the treatment plan; it is the first intervention which highlights the existence and definition of a problem. It is this aspect of the intervention process which leads to decision-making relating to problems. This approach draws from the fields of both mental health and education, as well as from interactional epistemology.

The problem-solving approach inherent in the IAC family conferences allows the family to own the situation and take charge, instead of relying on an 'expert' to solve the problem. The latter position has dominated past intervention strategies, because society has cast psychologists in the role of unquestionable 'experts' (Skuy et al., 1986). The IAC approach demystifies this conception by recasting the entire assessment method in terms of a more equitable problem-solving approach (Skuy et al., 1986). Change, according to the model, must come from within the family rather than from the outside.

Adelman and Taylor (1983) have questioned the utility of gathering and analysing the large amount of test data generated by conventional testing procedures, especially where there are concerns related to methodological, conceptual and ethical factors. To justify the inclusion of an assessment procedure, it must provide certainty about the interpretations and judgements made from the information provided (Adelman & Taylor, 1983). Current over-reliance on test findings alone frequently results in unreliable and invalid data being used in decision-making and support delivery (Snyder & Lopez, 2005). The movement away from product-related test results (for example, IQ scores) is particularly relevant in the South African context, where most practitioners, like their overseas counterparts, acknowledge that the process of assessment is far broader than psychometric testing. Within the IAC approach, psychometric testing is just one of the various methods of eliciting data. Other important sources include, in various combinations, diagnostic teaching and/or counselling, perceptions of the child and significant others, observational reports, informal teacher assessments, school reports and other relevant data such as medical and paramedical reports.

Central ideas related to the intervention theory

The structure of the IAC is based on several theoretical and pragmatic approaches to assessment and intervention, which are described below.

The family system

The involvement of psychologists with families in the assessment process has received considerable attention (Carnahan & Simeonsson, 1992; Davis & Gettinger, 1995; Gaughan, 1995; Ho & Gonzales, 2002; Mowder, Smith, Moy & Pedro, 1995). In keeping with ecosystemic theory, the IAC model stresses the importance of family participation and the participation of significant others in the child's life, in both the assessment and intervention planning phases. Not only is the child assessed in relation to his or her unique context, but the formulation of relevant interventions must also take the child's family and wider systems into account. The participation of the family in assessment provides the assessor with a wider range of information, in that the assessor has access to the family's perceptions, is made more aware of the values and needs of the family, and is also able to observe the family interactions. The experiences and perceptions of the family, as well as observations of family interactions, can serve to validate or invalidate formal test findings.

Freundl, Compas, Nelson, Adelman and Taylor (1982) studied three patterns of family participation: parents interviewed first, children interviewed first, and family interviewed as a unit. These were evaluated in terms of the impact of assessment information, client satisfaction and follow-through on decisions. Their findings suggested that assessment of the family as a unit was highly effective, and no less effective than the other patterns assessed. They hypothesised, however, that full family participation may have further psychological and long-term practical benefits, such as feelings of competence and self-determination for the child. Freundl et al. (1982) suggested, furthermore, that family involvement in decision-making that stresses open communication may, if successful, encourage the family to engage in such communication outside of the assessment setting.

Optimal accommodative match and the notion of a valid contract

Two central ideas that constitute the cornerstones of the IAC assessment approach are the establishment of (i) an optimal accommodative match and (ii) a valid contract.

The optimal accommodative match refers to the requirement that the process and content not be too disparate from clients' current way of understanding their world. Decisions made in the IAC process must be based on the mutual understanding between the consultant and the client. This concept is helpful in the South African situation. The pursuit of an accommodative match legitimises clients' understanding of their problems (based on their socio-cultural background, for instance). It is also particularly important in the South African context that the alternatives for intervention generated from assessment take into consideration the limited resources of many parents, schools and communities. For example, it may not be practical to recommend that the child attend a programme of language enrichment; rather, the incorporation of activities that can be done within the contexts of home and school may be more viable.

The idea of a valid contract involves the need to elicit informed consent and mutual active commitment from all parties in terms of intervention objectives and procedures. Research supports the importance of people being involved in decision-making which affects them (Adelman & Taylor, 1979; Amod et al., 2000). The active involvement of clients in the IAC procedure facilitates self-determination and 'ownership' with regard to the intervention and decision-making process. The notion of a valid contract balances the scales between the assessor and the client. According to Kriegler and Skuy (1996), the IAC does not, as was past practice, perpetuate an authoritarian dichotomy between 'expert' and client.

Family participation empowers the family, especially the child. Client participation mediates a sense of competence to the child, which can then become a source of motivation. With active participation of the clients, interventions can be seen not only as a means of solving problems, but also as a way of affording the opportunity to mediate problem-solving skills (Adelman & Taylor, 1979).

The IAC procedure: application of the shared problem-solving process

Although most professional assessment and consultation activities can be conceptualised as problem-solving, the process may not be shared (Adelman & Taylor, 2010). The essence of the shared assessment process, as applied in the IAC, is that clients work together with the consultant to gather and interpret the assessment data and to determine alternatives for intervention. This process not only takes into account the importance of client consent and empowerment, but is the core value of the IAC approach to assessment and it characterises a shift away from the traditional medical model. The traditional structure of service provision tended to replicate the pattern of power deprivation that many clients felt in other significant areas of their lives (Saleeby, 1997). The benefits of client empowerment are that it helps people to take charge and control of their lives, learn new ways to think about their situation and adopt new behaviours that give them more satisfactory and rewarding outcomes (Hancock, 1997).

Approaches similar to that of the IAC are applied within a few other settings in South Africa (Warburton, 2008). The IAC procedure, as expounded by Adelman and Taylor (1979; 1983; 2010) and adapted for use at the University of the Witwatersrand, consists of the following steps:

1. An initial screening, usually via the telephone.
2. Completion of a questionnaire by parents and/or significant others regarding individual perceptions of concerns, background information, previous interventions, how they think their concerns could be addressed, and so forth.

3. Gathering of records and reports from other professionals and agencies, as determined by the client.
4. Analysis of the questionnaire, reports and records by the consultant to determine the need to expand upon or corroborate information.
5. The holding of a group conference with relevant parties (IAC session I). Generally the child, parents and possibly the siblings and/or significant others are invited to this session (depending on parental preference).
6. Testing, if necessary. Assessment through a brief period of instruction or counselling may be indicated instead, or in some instances a multidisciplinary team assessment may be necessary. There is liaison with the school, with the consent of the family.
7. A second group conference is held with the child and his or her parents or family members (IAC session II). The purpose of this feedback session is to expand on the understanding of the concerns (after gathering further information), and to generate alternatives and decisions to address the identified concerns.
8. A few weeks later, a follow-up is conducted via the telephone or a conference is held with the family to evaluate progress with regard to alternatives decided upon in the IAC sessions and to assess satisfaction with the service. Further assessment sessions and a subsequent conference may be held if necessary, to review and possibly revise the original decisions.

The family conferences are conducted in a fairly structured way. The areas of discussion are documented under certain headings, and summaries are written up on a large chart or sheet of paper for all participants to peruse. This provides clients with access to all available information. Common and divergent perspectives on the problem are highlighted, and areas of success as well as perceived solutions are discussed.

In the initial family interview, agreement is sought regarding the goals of the assessment. The child's strengths and interests are then elicited. This contributes to a holistic understanding of the child and is in line with the focus on asset-based assessment procedures (Bouwer, 2005). Family members are in the unique position of having an intimate understanding of their child's strengths and interests, temperament and what motivates the child. Concerns regarding the child and an understanding of these concerns are discussed, after which alternatives are generated and examined, as possible solutions to the difficulties and concerns identified. Evaluating the advantages and disadvantages of each alternative with the participants further clarifies each person's idea of a best solution. In this way participants make decisions based on their own understanding, through facilitation by the consultant, rather than relying too much on expert advice.

Depending upon the decisions taken in the initial IAC session, information is gathered during the ensuing week(s) from a number of sources which could include informal and formal assessment procedures, observation, available reports, liaison with the school and/or diagnostic teaching or counselling. Once the understanding of the concerns has been thus broadened, a follow-up consultation is held where further decisions regarding intervention are made jointly by the participants. Such intervention may target changes in the environment or aspects thereof, and/or may be directed at the child him- or herself. The telephonic follow-up or case conference to discuss and evaluate the assessment outcome and decisions made reflects the view of assessment as an ongoing process.

The framework of the IAC structure, which uses a chart to record the family conference discussions, aids the process of problem resolution. Such a framework makes concrete abstract formulations in such a way that a clearer picture of the problem is drawn and the different perceptions of the participants are recorded. The experience of actively working through each column of the chart allows for enactment of phases of problem resolution on the 'stage' of the IAC room. Through this problem-solving process the consultant is also provided with valuable insights into family structure and interaction, and the family is given the opportunity of expressing its communication channels, blocks, areas of conflict, and capacity or reasons for failure to resolve conflict.

Uses and practical application of the IAC approach in the South African context

A number of psychology training institutions in South Africa use an approach to assessment based on the broad principles embodied in the IAC model of assessment. Postgraduate students at the University of the Witwatersrand undertake practical work using the IAC approach with children, adolescents and their families. A number of these graduates have adapted principles and procedures compatible with the IAC in their practices (Warburton, 2008).

Psychological assessment needs to be grounded in a workable model as a framework for practice. The IAC approach has been found to have particular relevance to the South African context, as it has several innovative features incorporated into the assessment procedure. The conceptual shift represented by the IAC approach, from an individual pathology orientation to an interactional and family empowerment focus, circumvents many of the criticisms of traditional assessment procedures. The basic principles of active participation, self-determination, joint decision-making, consumer orientation and a holistic and systemic framework are in keeping with the values of transparency and democracy advocated in the South African Constitution.

In utilising an approach such as the IAC model, assessment is viewed in its broadest sense, drawing upon multiple sources of data other than formal testing procedures. Where tests are used, these need to be justified by clear rationales, which encourages reflective and ethical psychological practice; and unnecessary testing is eliminated. Other alternatives that can be used in the IAC assessment process include prescribed periods of assessment through instruction or teaching, and assessment through counselling. The former alternative could include, for instance, the introduction of a reading programme, and pre- and post-intervention measures could be obtained of the child's functioning. This form of dynamic assessment of the child's learning potential is described in chapter 9 of this volume. As regards assessment through counselling, an example would be the use of play-based assessment as described by Linder (1993).

Limitations of the IAC approach

Adelman and Taylor (1979) mention certain limitations of the IAC approach, stating that some clients tend to rely excessively on professionals for diagnoses and prescriptions and would prefer to have definite answers given to them. They also mention that children may be reluctant to voice and share their perceptions in front of their family members. Certain reservations have also been expressed about the ability of younger children and those with severe problems to participate in a meaningful way in the IAC process. The IAC framework needs to be used and applied flexibly, to meet the diverse needs of children and their families or caregivers.

Another limitation of the IAC approach could be that important and possibly confrontational issues may be overlooked. In terms of the psychodynamic approach, it might be argued that defences, denial and repressed memories may prevent clients from presenting the whole truth. It is therefore argued that, in applying the IAC process, the consultant needs to be psychotherapeutically well skilled.

Research on the IAC approach

Studies conducted on the IAC approach by Adelman and Taylor (1979) and those conducted in South Africa (Amod, 2003; Amod et al., 2000; Dangor, 1983; Manala, 2001; Mugnaioni, 2008; Skuy et al., 1986) have looked at client satisfaction with services rendered. The perceptions of consultants using this approach to assessment have also been surveyed (Dangor, 1983; Levin, 2003; Mugnaioni, 2008; Warburton, 2008). These exploratory quantitative descriptive studies, which span a period of about three decades, utilised structured questionnaires and rating scales for the collection of data. While the sample sizes used in these studies have generally been small, which may affect the validity of the findings, they have supported the usefulness of the IAC approach to assessment as perceived by clients and consultants. Client satisfaction with professional services is an obvious aspect of the quality of service delivery and a relevant outcome measure (Human & Teglasi, 1993; Rey, Plapp & Simpson, 1998). Furthermore, as noted by Rey et al. (1998), learning about facets that alter parental satisfaction may facilitate the design of services that are more effective and acceptable to consumers.

Initial research carried out by Adelman and Taylor (1979) indicated client satisfaction with the IAC procedure: 24.4 per cent were satisfied, and 65.9 per cent were very satisfied with the procedure. They also found that 72.8 per cent of clients had followed through on decisions made in the IAC, while a further 18.7 per cent had either begun the process or had chosen alternatives not mentioned in the IAC. Adelman and Taylor (1979) concluded that their preliminary findings suggested that the IAC approach was a viable alternative to other existing assessment practices, and that it was effective in generating decisions about the nature of psychoeducational services needed. The fact that 90.3 per cent of clients were satisfied with the programme, and that 91.5 per cent had either acted on decisions made or were implementing other alternatives, suggested that family participation in a problem-solving paradigm provides a valuable framework for assessment.

There is a general lack of research on models of assessment, not only in South Africa but also elsewhere in the world. Amongst the pilot studies that have been conducted at the University of the Witwatersrand, Dangor (1983) assessed the effectiveness of the IAC by means of family perceptions, as well as the perceptions of student consultants. The sample in this study included 40 families who constituted 90 per cent of the clients seen within a 6-month period, as well as 20 student assessors. The findings indicated a high degree of client family satisfaction with the IAC model, favouring the continued use of the IAC. Client families endorsed the joint decision-making process between the consultants and themselves as being highly positive, and regarded decisions emanating from the IAC as being very worthwhile. Students found the structure of the IAC helpful, and they viewed the emphasis on the child's strengths positively. According to Dangor (1983), there was no discrepancy between family and students' perceptions of the IAC. Dangor noted that the degree of respondent motivation to complete the questionnaires was an extraneous variable in the study which was difficult to control. Families needed reminders before returning the questionnaires. She suggested that further studies needed to be conducted using objective change criteria, to gauge the effectiveness of the IAC model.

Findings by Dangor (1983) and those yielded previously in the USA were supported by a further study by Skuy et al. (1986). Participants in the latter study were 84 client families, who constituted 93 per cent of the 90 clients attended to over a period of 8 months. The findings of this study demonstrated positive attitudes to the IAC procedure as measured by (i) clients' satisfaction with the process; (ii) their perceived ability to participate in the process; and (iii) the efficacy of the shared problem-solving approach in ensuring a link between assessment and intervention. A further finding was that 93 per cent of the sample had implemented the decisions taken in the parent feedback interview of the IAC process.

Skuy et al. (1986) found positive correlations between decision-making, active participation in assessment, and attitudes towards the consultants and the services provided by them. They concluded that decision-making arising from the assessment and active participation in the assessment were associated with positive attitudes towards consultants and the services which they offered. Significant positive correlations were also reported between improvement in six problem-area variables, which included the presenting problem, school, behaviour, motivation, emotional functioning and family relationships. A limitation of the Skuy et al. (1986) study was the lack of a control group which would have afforded the opportunity to compare the IAC with other models of assessment. Also, there do not appear to be any comparable studies to suggest that decisions are more frequently implemented using the IAC framework than when other assessment approaches are used.

Concerns related to the use of a Eurocentric model of assessment in South Africa, such as the IAC approach, prompted the study by Amod et al. (2000). This study indicated that the IAC was an effective assessment approach across racial and cultural groups within the client population seen at the University of the Witwatersrand. Fifty client families out of those seen over a period of two years were surveyed. The questionnaire, which was constructed in this study to measure client feedback and perceived improvement in problem areas, was based on that used previously by Skuy et al. (1986). In addition to the original questionnaire, questions were added relating to cross-cultural issues. The replication of the questionnaire and the use of the same dimensions allowed for a qualitative comparison to be made between the results obtained and the findings of the Skuy et al. (1986) study.

The results of the Amod et al. (2000) study corroborated the positive findings of Skuy et al. (1986). Clients were highly satisfied with the IAC process and their involvement in it, as well as with the efficiency and efficacy of the shared problem-solving process in ensuring a link between assessment and intervention. Ninety-four per cent of the clients in this study implemented decisions taken in the IAC, while a similar number of clients (93 per cent) did so in the Skuy et al. study. The findings further suggested that race and culture were not a significant factor in relation to attitudes towards the IAC. There were two exceptions to this. Firstly, a significantly larger number of black respondents indicated that they would have wished for greater decision-making on the part of the consultant, as compared with their white, coloured and Indian counterparts. This could be related to the fact that people who were most disempowered by the apartheid system may not have been used to a participative style, and hence expected professionals to take responsibility for decision-making.

Secondly, the fact that Indian and African extended families participated in the assessment to a significantly greater extent than white and coloured families ties in with the cultural differences among the groups in this regard (Amod et al., 2000). Among the African and Indian families in South Africa, emphasis is placed on the role of grandparents and the extended family in the lives of parents and children.

A limitation of the Amod et al. (2000) study was the inability to control for extraneous variables which could have contributed to perceived client changes, such as school and teacher changes, increased motivation, and change in family dynamics. Furthermore, while the study focused on attitudes towards the IAC process and the implementation of decisions, there were no further reports of clients' long-term adherence, or objective measures of improved functioning in problem areas.

Given the lack of comparative studies involving the IAC, Manala (2001) conducted a survey of parents' views on two approaches to assessment. One approach was the IAC and the other was a psychodynamic-social model used at a community internship site. The latter approach to assessment starts with an initial intake interview which is attended by the parents only, and has a psychodynamic focus. The psychosocial history of the child and family is recorded. This intake interview is discussed at a case conference, and suggestions for further interventions are evaluated by the therapeutic team. Interventions may include parent counselling, play therapy, emotional assessment and/or psychoeducational assessment. Testing is not always advocated. Manala (2001) found that there was no significant difference in the respondents' perceptions, and both approaches to assessment were rated as being highly satisfying. She proposed an integrated assessment model which incorporates cognitive and psychodynamic insights and involves the entire family in the assessment.

The IAC formed part of a broader study conducted by Amod (2003), in which a problem-solving psychoeducational assessment model was designed and implemented in a school district consisting mainly of schools of lower socio-economic status. In this mixed-methods action research study using a control group, 12 district support team members (including psychologists and learning support specialists) and 47 school-based support team members were trained on the IAC. Levin (2003), an intern psychologist, facilitated the training of the district support team. The IAC trainees implemented this approach within 10 schools which included 54 learners and their parents. A range of measures were utilised in this study, such as pre- and post-intervention questionnaires, pupil screening scales, school adjustment scales and family grids, as well as focus group interviews. The results reflected positive attitudes and a strong concordance in the perceptions of the respondents (IAC consultants, parents, learners and teachers), in relation to the IAC procedure. The majority of the perceptions were highly positive about the active participation of parents and families in the assessment process. This was the first study of the IAC that was conducted out of the 'clinical' university setting and extended to schools and the community. The successful application of the IAC tool within a school district attests to its flexibility and utility within different settings.

A case study using the IAC approach to assessment and an ecosystemic intervention programme consisting of learning support, play therapy and parent counselling was conducted by Mugnaioni (2008). Qualitative methods of data collection were used, and thematic content analysis was employed to analyse the data. Mugnaioni concluded that an ecosystemic approach to assessment and intervention was a viable process in understanding and supporting an underachieving, anxious child. She did, however, state that more research was needed to add validity to the findings of her study. Constraints in applying an ecosystemic approach to assessment and intervention were also noted, since successful implementation of this approach required time, expertise and the necessary financial and structural support.

In a recent, non-experimental exploratory pilot study, Warburton (2008) investigated past student consultants' (N = 40) perceptions of the effectiveness of the IAC as a framework for the assessment process, and their use of this approach at internship sites or other places of work. A self-designed questionnaire, which was pilot-tested on a representative sample, was administered in this study. Thematic content analysis was used to analyse the data. The results of the study suggested that the IAC is perceived as an effective approach to assessment, as it helps to contextualise the client and is a collaborative and interactive process (100 per cent of the respondents indicated this). Respondents viewed the IAC process as conducive to involving all stakeholders, such as the child, the family or other caregivers and the teacher, in the assessment and intervention planning process. The majority of the sample (92 per cent) expressed satisfaction with the IAC model's ecosystemic and holistic approach, which they regarded as practical and flexible, while 72 per cent saw the value of the IAC as being its client- and family-centred focus. Warburton (2008) found that many of the principles of the IAC continued to be adopted by past students at their internship sites or places of work.

A limitation of the Warburton (2008) study was the low return rate of the questionnaires, which resulted in a small sample size. Further, since the majority of the respondents had less than five years of work experience, they may not have had an extensive background experience against which to critically compare and evaluate the IAC model in relation to other approaches to assessment.

Conclusion

The IAC model, with its sound philosophical, theoretical and ethical foundations, is well suited to meeting the needs of psychological assessment practice and intervention in South Africa. Studies conducted thus far, although limited to the context of the University of the Witwatersrand, have shown that the IAC is an effective assessment approach across cultural groups. The holistic and joint child and family participatory emphasis of the IAC complements the government's emphasis on addressing barriers to learning and development. Furthermore, the IAC process is congruent with the principles of best practice in the field of assessment, which move beyond a conventional testing approach.

References

Adelman, H. S. & Taylor, L. (1979). Initial assessment and related consultation. *Learning Disability Quarterly, 2*, 52–64.

Adelman, H. S. & Taylor, L. (1983). *Learning Disabilities in Perspective.* Glenview, IL: Scott, Foresman.

Adelman, H. S. & Taylor, L. (1993). *Learning Problems and Learning Disabilities: Moving Forward.* Pacific Grove, CA: Brooks/Cole.

Adelman, H. S. & Taylor, L. (2010). *Mental Health in Schools: Engaging Learners, Presenting Problems and Improving Schools.* Thousand Oaks, CA: Corwin.

Amod, Z. (2003). A problem-solving psychoeducational assessment model for implementation by educators in South African schools. Unpublished PhD dissertation. University of the Witwatersrand, Johannesburg.

Amod, Z., Skuy, M., Sonderup, L. & Fridjhon, P. (2000). Effectiveness of the Initial Assessment and Consultation process (IAC) with different cultural groups in South Africa. *International Journal of Special Education, 15(1)*, 1–11.

Bouwer, C. (2005). Identification and assessment of barriers to learning. In E. Landsberg, D. Kruger & N. Nel (Eds), *Addressing Barriers to Learning: A South African Perspective* (pp. 45–60). Pretoria: Van Schaik.

Bronfenbrenner, U. (1979). *The Ecology of Human Development: Experiments by Design and Nature.* Cambridge, MA: Harvard University Press.

Carnahan, S. L. & Simeonsson, R. J. (1992). Family involvement in child assessment. *International Journal of Cognitive Education and Mediated Learning, 2(3)*, 224–232.

Dangor, Z. M. (1983). Assessment services at a university education clinic. Unpublished Master's research report. University of the Witwatersrand, Johannesburg.

Davis, S. K. & Gettinger, M. (1995). Family-focused assessment for identifying family resources and concerns: Parent preferences, assessment information and evaluation across three methods. *Journal of School Psychology, 33(2)*, 99–121.

Department of Education (2001). *Education White Paper 6 Special Needs Education: Building an Inclusive Education and Training System*. Pretoria: Department of Education.

Freundl, P. C., Compas, B. E., Nelson, P., Adelman, H. S. & Taylor, L. (1982). Learning and behaviour problems. *Journal of Clinical Child Psychology, 11(3)*, 238–242.

Gaughan, E. (1995). Family assessment in psychoeducational evaluation: Case studies with the Family Adaptibility and Classroom Evaluation Scales. *Journal of School Psychology, 33(1)*, 7–28.

Hancock, M. R. (1997). *Principles of Social Work Practice: A Generic Practice Approach*. London: Hawarth Press.

Ho, B. S. & Gonzales, R. (2002). An applied research study of family-centered practices in an ethnically diverse elementary school. *The California School Psychologist, 6*, 27–38.

Human, M. T. & Teglasi, H. (1993). Parents' satisfaction and compliance with recommendations following psychoeducational assessment of children. *Journal of School Psychology, 31*, 449–467.

Kriegler, S. M. & Skuy, M. (1996). Perspectives on psychological assessment in South African schools. In P. Engelbrecht, S. M. Kriegler & M. I. Booysen (Eds), *Perspectives on Learning Difficulties: International Concerns and South African Realities* (pp. 109–122). Pretoria: Van Schaik.

Levin, T. T. (2003). Learning support through shared problem-solving: A model of psychoeducational assessment and intervention for District Support Teams. Unpublished Master's research report. University of the Witwatersrand, Johannesburg.

Linder, D. W. (1993). *Transdisciplinary Play-Based Assessment: A Functional Approach to Working with Young Children*. London: Brooks.

Manala, J. T. (2001). Parents' perceptions of assessment practices at two Johannesburg clinics. Unpublished Master's research report. University of the Witwatersrand, Johannesburg.

Mowder, B. A., Smith, H. Y., Moy, L. & Pedro, M. (1995). Parent role characteristics: Parent views and their implications for school psychologists. *Psychology in the Schools, 32*, 27–37.

Mugnaioni, M. V. (2008). Assessing and supporting an underachieving anxious child: Using a constructivist ecosystemic approach in a South African university training context. Unpublished Master's research report. University of the Witwatersrand, Johannesburg.

Rey, J. M., Plapp., J. M. & Simpson, P. L. (1998). Parental satisfaction and outcome: A four-year study in a child and adolescent mental health service. *Australian and New Zealand Journal of Psychiatry, 33(1)*, 22–29.

Saleeby, D. (1997). *The Strengths Perspective in Social Work Practice*. New York, NY: Addison-Wesley Longman.

Skuy, M., Westaway, M. & Hickson, J. (1986). Cross-cultural applications of an innovative educational assessment process. *Journal of Personality and Social Psychology, 1(3)*, 411–421.

Snyder, C. R. & Lopez, S. J. (2005). *Handbook of Positive Psychology*. New York, NY: Oxford University Press.

Warburton, B. (2008). The perceptions of student consultants towards the Initial Assessment and Consultation (IAC) model of assessment. Unpublished Master's research report. University of the Witwatersrand, Johannesburg.

32 Qualitative career assessment in South Africa

M. Watson and M. McMahon

The history of career assessment spans more than a century, with its origins in the early 1900s. It is a history that is recursively related to the development of career theory and practice. Thus the philosophy of career assessment reflects and informs the career psychology discipline of the times. The predominant approach to career practice through most of the last century was a directive, matching approach resulting from a focus on quantitative career assessment. There is also a long history to qualitative career assessment, but it is a history that has been subsumed by the dominant story of quantitative career assessment (McMahon, 2008; McMahon & Patton, 2006). The first part of this chapter provides an overview of quantitative career assessment and then introduces qualitative career assessment. The second part of the chapter focuses on a qualitative career assessment instrument that has been developed in South Africa, the My System of Career Influences (MSCI) reflection process, beginning with an introduction to its theoretical foundation, the Systems Theory Framework (STF) of career development.

Quantitative career testing

De Bruin and De Bruin (2006) make an important distinction between the words 'testing' and 'assessment'. Psychological testing means just that – the administration, scoring and collating of tests, which in career counselling could involve abilities, interests, values and personality traits. Assessment, on the other hand, is a broader, more holistic concept which is inclusive of but not limited to psychological testing. Assessment reflects a process of giving meaning to information (psychometric or otherwise); it promotes greater career and self-exploration in a client. This section describes testing in career counselling, while the next section examines the role of assessment in career counselling.

Much of the history of career psychology has reflected on the dominant role of testing. There is general agreement that the dominant role of career testing evident internationally is similarly reflected at a national level. Lamprecht (2002, p.121), for instance, states that career counselling in South Africa has 'over the last 50 years been dominated by the practice of standardised, psychometric tests'. Lamprecht argues that the trait-factor approach on which some of the more popular careers tests are founded still remains the career counselling approach of most South African practitioners.

Historically, a trait-factor approach to career counselling (as well as its updated person–environment fit approach) reflects a logical-positivist world view which values objective data and measurement that allows the career counsellor to predict career choice (McMahon & Patton, 2006). Career testing encourages the gathering and interpretation of psychometric information at a point in time, thus limiting the possibility of a process approach to career counselling which would more actively involve the client.

While any psychometric test has the potential to be utilised in a qualitative way, as discussed later in this chapter, there is a range of career tests available in South Africa that provide scores and are predominantly used in a limited, quantitative manner by many career counsellors. These tests reflect diverse theoretical backgrounds. By far the most popular questionnaire is the Self-Directed Search (SDS) (Holland, 1985), which provides interest scores that enable a matching process between an individual's interest profile and a corresponding work environment. This questionnaire is directly based on the original trait-factor approach to career counselling and its more recent derivative, person–environment fit. It has been adapted for use in South Africa (Bisschoff, 1993). Research on the use of the SDS in South Africa has been mixed. Nel (2006) provides a comprehensive description of such research and concludes that the SDS still maintains its preferred psychometric status in South Africa. More recently Watson, Foxcroft and Allen (2007) found that the SDS codes of working field guides did not match the codes ascribed to them in a South African dictionary of occupations.

Several career tests are based on Super's (1990) career developmental approach. Three of these tests have been specifically adapted for use in South Africa: the Career Development Questionnaire (CDQ) (Langley, 1990); the Life Roles Inventory (LRI) (Langley, 1992); and the Values Scale (VS) (Langley, Du Toit & Herbst, 1992). The CDQ provides scores on self-information, decision-making skills, the gathering of career information, the integration of self- and career information, and career planning that reflect an individual's state of readiness to make a career decision. Low scores would indicate the need for remediation of those aspects of career development. The LRI positions the role of work within other life roles and provides an assessment of an individual's relative participation in, commitment to and value expectations of five life roles. As such, the LRI provides a more holistic perspective on the role of work in an individual's life. The VS provides scores on 22 values that could relate to the work role, and provides individuals with the opportunity to rank the importance of such roles in relation to the meaning they would seek from the work role.

Other popular career tests are the Jung Personality Questionnaire (Du Toit, 1987), which has been standardised for use in South Africa, and the Myers-Briggs Type Indicator (Myers & McCaulley, 1985). Both are personality questionnaires which encourage greater self-understanding in clients. They also allow for a matching process in which the client's personality trait scores are compared with the scores of individuals working in the occupations in which the client has expressed interest.

Clearly, the popularity of these quantitative tests has been much evident over several decades in South Africa. Whether these tests have served us well would depend on how they have been incorporated into the career assessment process. De Bruin and De Bruin (2006) warn us not to hold stereotypical perceptions of standardised career tests in South Africa but, equally, such tests offer the great temptation of being utilised in stereotypical and limited ways. As De Bruin and De Bruin note, '[i]t is the uses to which they are put, and the manner in which this is done, that can be good or bad' (p.130). Unfortunately a restricted, cost-effective (in terms of time and client expectations) use of most of these measures has led to consistent criticism of quantitative career tests in South Africa.

Lamprecht (2002) points to several concerns that have been raised about quantitative career assessment. There is the criticism that such tests portray a limited, less holistic view of the client's life, reducing clients' lives to scores concerning the working role only. Lamprecht argues that quantitative testing creates work identities for clients and little more. Related to this criticism is the increasing concern that contextual factors are insufficiently considered during quantitative career assessment, that clients are reduced to 'psychometric selves' (Lamprecht, 2002, p.124) and that the interpretation of quantitative scores is decontextualised. Another concern is that quantitative scores may lead to information overload in that a major part of the career counselling process is spent processing psychometric information, which may limit the potential for other activities to happen.

Qualitative career assessment

In recent decades there has been a movement in career psychology towards theories and practices informed by a constructivist world view, which places emphasis on individuals identifying their life themes and constructing their own career stories (see, for example, Amundson's (2009) active engagement, Cochran's (1997) narrative career counselling, Peavy's (1998) SocioDynamic approach, Pryor and Bright's (2011) chaos theory, and Savickas et al.'s (2009) life designing). This movement shifts the focus of career assessment from interpreting scores to reflecting on individuals' stories (McMahon & Patton, 2002; Savickas, 1993). In essence, clients play a more active role in the career counselling process through interpreting their career assessment within the parameters of their life contexts, as well as through the resultant career stories that they tell. When considering the increasingly unpredictable and complex world of work in which individuals may make several career decisions and transitions, encouraging active participation by career clients is critical to encouraging them to take greater responsibility for their decisions and to learn processes and strategies that they may apply to subsequent decisions. McMahon and Patton (2006) suggest that career counselling is under pressure to be more interpretive, and for its assessment approaches to accommodate constant change both in society and in the workplace. Qualitative career assessment allows the career counselling process to reflect these macro-systemic challenges and, at the same time, to engage in what Blustein (2001, p.176) has termed 'experience-near connections to clients'.

Qualitative career assessment is in itself a process, one that is more informal, less standardised and less reliant on scores than other assessment processes. It promotes self- and career exploration (De Bruin & De Bruin, 2006) and it encourages the client to explore the influence of not only intrapersonal factors but also external, systemic influences on personal career development, such as family, peer group, cultural context and societal-environmental barriers. The goal in qualitative career assessment is thus less on an end-process decision outcome and more on an exploration process and contextualisation that will lead to an effective career decision. With its emphasis on process, qualitative career assessment encourages a collaborative career counselling relationship between the career counsellor and the client. Thus clients assume a role of active agent in the career choice process, as compared to the more passive client role presented by traditional career testing, which enables them to experience and learn processes and approaches which they can apply to subsequent decisions.

The promotion of qualitative career assessment raises several philosophical issues about career assessment. One such issue is whether career assessment should be psychological or psychosocial in nature. Most career assessment in South Africa could be considered as psychological in its approach. However, Watson, Duarte and Glavin (2005) argue that career assessment should be psychosocial, that it should focus on assessing the relationship between individuals and the broader contextual factors that may influence their career development. A further issue is that of validation, with most career measures in South Africa validated in terms of the applicability of international measures in a variety of cultural contexts. Thus the focus has been on the construct, concurrent and predictive validation of quantitative career measures, rather than on the use of qualitative career assessment that explores career development within the cultural context in which an individual may be embedded (Watson et al., 2005). With qualitative career assessment, the issue of validity is, rather, defined by the appropriateness of the career assessment introduced into the career counselling process. Given that clients will be active partners in this qualitative career assessment, the issue of validity becomes mutually defined.

Common to most qualitative career assessment processes is their flexibility and usefulness with clients from diverse backgrounds (De Bruin & De Bruin, 2006). In addition, qualitative career assessment encourages a collaborative relationship between the client and the career counsellor, who jointly undertake and interpret the career assessment process. This process is continuous in nature, rather than a point-in-time intervention like quantitative career testing.

There are recognised limitations to qualitative career assessment, such as the fact that it can be time-consuming and labour-intensive. This form of assessment has also been criticised for its questionable validity and reliability. The issue of validity and reliability, however, needs to be understood in terms of the differing world views of quantitative and qualitative career testing and assessment. The cost-effectiveness of qualitative career assessment may need to be understood in relation to the shorter- and longer-term goals of the career assessment process. In the context of South Africa, cost-effectiveness is particularly pertinent in terms of both time and money. In addition, the public perception of the career counselling process is generally that it will be of a short and structured duration, leading often to resistance on the part of both the career counsellor and the client to adopt a more exploratory approach. On the other hand, if the goal of career counselling is genuine exploration that will empower the client for the future, qualitative career assessment can nurture and stimulate such an exploratory process.

A wide variety of qualitative career assessment processes are available to career counsellors. Several of the more popular of these approaches will now be described. The first of these is *card sorts*, which is often used in qualitative career assessment and is possibly the best-known approach. Here clients have to sort out a pack of cards (relating to interests, values, aptitudes and personality traits) in terms of how important or not the cards are to their lives. This sorting may also be undertaken by significant others in the client's life. Most card sets are grounded in theories of classification and in this regard, therefore, may not be truly qualitative. An example of a constructivist card sort is the Intelligent Career Card Sort® (Parker, 2006), which uses three sets of cards focusing on self-awareness, each set reflecting a way of knowing: knowing-how, knowing-why and knowing-whom.

Reflecting its constructivist underpinnings, qualitative career assessment places great emphasis on story and narrative. A narrative approach may involve the writing of essays by clients about their lives. Essay-writing exercises may be unstructured or structured, and the career counsellor and the client will jointly analyse the essay for significant life themes. Stories may also be elicited through *unstructured interviews* and *life stories* (see, for example, Hartung, 2007), and Fritz and Beekman (2007) describe a process of *reflective journal writing* which could focus on a career or life transition.

Collages are frequently used in qualitative career assessment as they can provide clients with insight into their values, interests and personality traits. This qualitative assessment involves cutting out pictures from old magazines in order to illustrate themes, whether those as broad as how clients see themselves (for example, a collage titled 'my strengths') or more specifically structured themes such as what clients' projected future could be. Fritz and Beekman (2007) suggest that a collage could also focus on themes such as 'this is not me' or 'this is what I am good at'. Instead of pictures, clients can also be encouraged to choose personal artefacts that would help tell their story (Fritz & Beekman, 2007).

The use of *metaphor* in qualitative career assessment involves the choice of word images that reflect on clients in relation to their career developmental concerns. Lamprecht (2002) refers to this form of assessment as flights of the imagination. For a fuller description of the use of metaphor, the reader is referred to the extant literature (for example, McMahon, 2008). There are also qualitative assessment processes that allow clients to discover themes and patterns from different chapters of their lives – for example, the *genogram* and *timelines*.

Some qualitative career assessment approaches have been developed from specific career theory frameworks such as Peavy's (1998) life-space map and Amundson's (2009) pattern identification exercise. In the South African context, Maree, Bester, Lubbe and Beck (2001) argued a decade ago about the limitations and irrelevance of quantitative career assessment, and Maree (2009) has more recently argued for the greater relevance of qualitative career assessment. The present chapter considers the development, application and research in South Africa of one such qualitative career assessment process, the MSCI (McMahon, Patton & Watson, 2005a; 2005b). The MSCI operationalises the STF of career development (McMahon & Patton, 1995; Patton & McMahon, 1999; 2006) and a brief description of this theoretical framework is provided in the following section of the chapter. Thereafter, the MSCI will be described and then an overview of research related to the MSCI will be presented.

The STF of career development

Part of a more recent movement in career theory that reflects a constructivist perspective of career development, the STF (McMahon & Patton, 1995; Patton

Figure 32.1 The Systems Theory Framework of career development

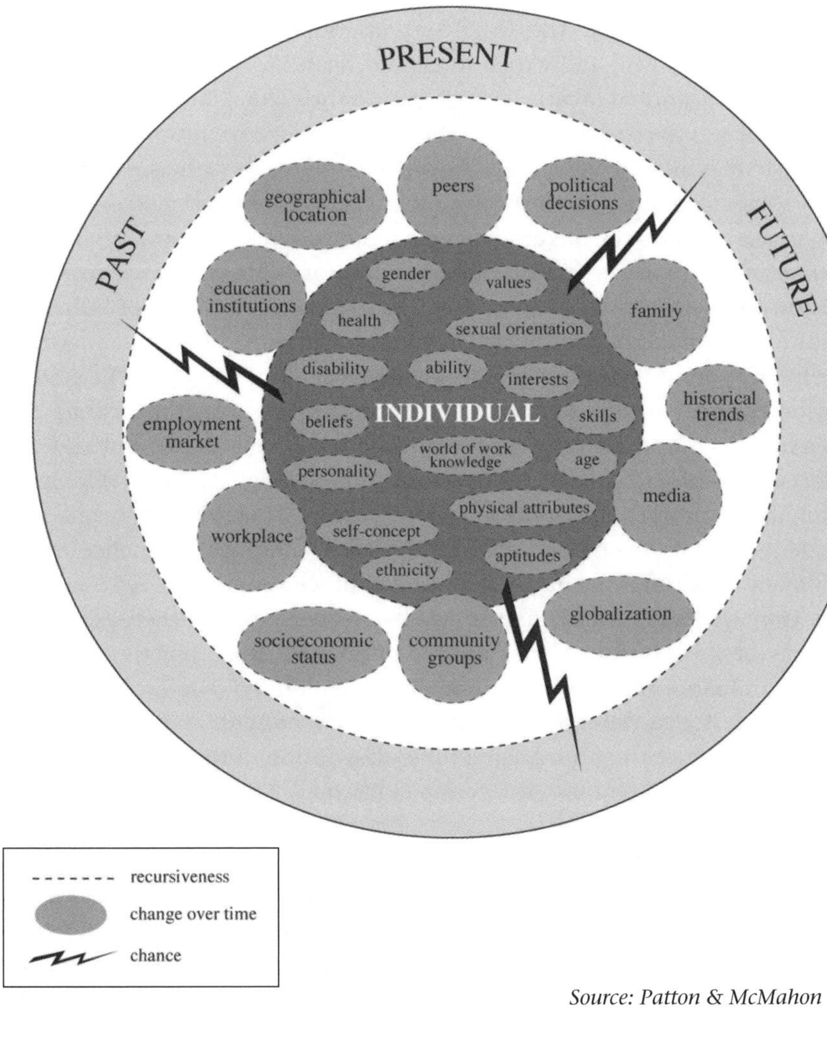

Source: Patton & McMahon (1999).

& McMahon, 1999; 2006) provides a meta-theoretical framework which conceptualises individual career development within a broader system of contextual influences. Within its holistic framework, the STF conceptualises career development in terms of both content and process influences which can impact on an individual's career development. The STF locates the individual at the heart of a complex and dynamic system of interconnecting influences on career development. The content influences depict the complexity of career development, and the process influences depict its dynamic nature. The STF is portrayed in Figure 32.1.

The central circle in the diagram represents the individual system, within which are a range of intrapersonal influences such as gender, interests, age, abilities, personality factors and an individual's sexual orientation. Of particular importance in the South African context is the STF's consideration of the individual in context, rather than the individual in isolation. Thus the individual system is sited within larger contextual systems – that is, the social system and the environmental-societal system. Culture is not included as a specific influence, because it is regarded as a personal construct by individuals which is recursively connected to their context. The social system comprises the more immediate context within which the individual lives, and relates to social influences such as the family, educational institutions, peers and the media. Encompassing both the individual and the social systems is the macro context of the environmental-societal system, which includes macro-systemic influences such as geographical location, socio-economic circumstances, political decisions and globalisation.

The process influences of recursiveness, change over time and chance are illustrative of the dynamic nature of career development, as is evident in the interaction that can occur within and between the three systems of influence. The multidirectional and nonlinear interaction between influences, in which change in one part of the system results in change in another part of the system, demonstrates the concept of recursiveness (that is, interaction within and between influences). Recursiveness is represented in Figure 32.1 by dotted lines. The process influence of chance suggests that an individual's career development does not always proceed along predetermined paths. Thus, chance events such as accidents, illness or natural disasters may significantly influence career development. Superimposed on all content and process influences is the context of time. Time changes both the nature and the degree of influence. For example, family may be an influence across the life of an individual, but the nature of the family influence may be quite different in childhood, adolescence and as an older adult. Across time, the past influences the present, and together, past and present influence the future. For a fuller description of the STF, the reader is referred to the extant literature (for example, Patton & McMahon, 2006; Patton, McMahon & Watson, 2006).

The STF has been criticised for not offering in-depth accounts of the influences. However, as a meta-theoretical framework and not a theory, that is not the intention of the STF, as detailed accounts of some influences are found in the extant literature (for example, Holland (1985) provides a detailed account of interests). A strength of the STF is that it includes influences that may be pervasive in the career development of individuals but that have received little or no attention in the extant literature. Such influences may be incorporated into the stories of clients engaged in practical applications of the STF, such as the MSCI.

The MSCI

The MSCI (McMahon et al., 2005a; 2005b) is a qualitative career assessment instrument developed from the STF. It provides individuals with the opportunity to reflect on their systems of influence in a step-by-step process. As a consequence of such reflection, individuals are able to create their own career stories (McMahon, Patton & Watson, 2004) and gain a better understanding of the uniqueness, wholeness and interconnectedness of the influences on their career development. To date, an adolescent version (McMahon et al., 2005a; 2005b) has been published and a subsequent adult version has been developed (McMahon, Watson & Patton, in press a; in press b).

The MSCI (both the adolescent and adult versions) is a booklet of 12 pages, each of which contains brief information, a set of instructions, illustrative examples and the space for reflections to be recorded. The first section of the booklet guides individuals through a process of reflection on their present career situation in terms of their occupational aspirations, work experience, life roles, previous decision-making they may have made, and the support networks available to them. In the second section of the booklet, individuals are able to diagrammatically identify and prioritise their career influences, by thinking in turn about who they are (that is, the individual system of the STF), about the people around them (that is, the social system of the STF), about society and the environment (that is, the environmental-societal system of the STF), and about their past, present and future (that is, the context of time in the STF system).

Once individuals have completed a sequential exploration of their different systems of influence, they are provided with an opportunity to summarise their reflections of their identified influences on a page titled 'representing my system of career influences'. The subsequent step is to present these reflections diagrammatically on a chart titled 'my system of career influences' which is, in essence, a personalised STF. The penultimate page of the booklet, titled 'reflecting on my system of career influences', provides individuals with the opportunity to reflect on the insights they may have gained through the whole guided process, resulting in their completing their action plan on the subsequent page. For a fuller description of the MSCI, the reader is referred to the extant literature (for example, McMahon et al., 2005a; 2005b). The MSCI is subject to the same criticisms directed more generally at qualitative career assessment that have been outlined earlier in this chapter. In particular, the MSCI does not generate 'answers' in the form of occupational titles or work environments that more predictive quantitative assessment may do. However, this is not its purpose; rather, its aim is to contextualise and present in story form individuals' career decisions. A particular strength of the MSCI is that it may be used individually or in group settings such as classrooms and corporate career development programmes.

Researching the MSCI

Because quantitative and qualitative assessment are based on different premises, the parameters for validating the psychometric properties of quantitative career measures cannot be applied to qualitative career assessment measures. Thus a first step in the development of the MSCI was to develop rigorous guidelines for the development and evaluation of qualitative career assessment (McMahon, Patton & Watson, 2003).

Development of the MSCI (Adolescent Version)

The adolescent version of the MSCI was developed over four years and involved a three-stage cross-national trialling process (McMahon et al., 2004; 2005a; 2005b; McMahon, Watson & Patton, 2005). Each subsequent stage involved refinement of the layout, the language and the instructions. Importantly, a trial with English-speaking South African adolescents from socio-economically disadvantaged backgrounds and between the ages of 13 and 17 years indicated the need for an introductory process to familiarise the adolescents with systems thinking. Consequently a set of case studies was included in the *Facilitators' Manual*, to enhance the MSCI learning process. Positive feedback was received on the *Facilitators' Manual* and also on the supplementary career development learning activities provided in the manual, including the activity to introduce adolescents to systemic thinking. In summary, the three-year trialling of the MSCI suggested that adolescents can create their own meaningful stories through a reflective, qualitative career assessment process. It represents a meaningful learning experience that is 'theoretically grounded, client oriented, holistic, sequential' (McMahon et al., 2005a, p.40). In a further development, the MSCI has now been translated into the Chinese, Dutch, French and Icelandic languages.

Development of the MSCI (Adult Version)

A consequence of the trialling of the MSCI (Adolescent Version) was feedback calling for an adult version of the MSCI. Trials of a modified MSCI for adults (McMahon et al., in press a; in press b) were conducted internationally in Australia, South Africa and Great Britain, with feedback being provided both by facilitators as well as by adult participants in the three countries. Trials included males and females from trade, managerial and professional backgrounds, and from urban and rural locations and settings such as a large public sector organisation and small–medium enterprises. The results were overwhelmingly positive, with most participants indicating that the MSCI (Adult Version) was helpful to them and would be helpful to their friends. In terms of the South African trialling, participants indicated that the MSCI assessment process had increased their awareness of the diversity and critical importance of systemic influences in their lives, and provided them with the opportunity to 'put things into perspective'. It challenged participants to confront and act on perspectives that they had gained. Facilitators' feedback was positive. The South African facilitator commented on the usefulness of both the case studies in the *Guide* and the broader theoretical sections that conceptualised the nature of qualitative career assessment.

Research and application of the MSCI

The usefulness of the MSCI as a qualitative career assessment tool has been demonstrated in several South African research projects to date (McMahon & Watson, 2006). For instance, McMahon, Watson, Foxcroft and Dullabh (2008) report on the career development of South African adolescents residing in a children's home for a minimum of three years. This study examined the usefulness of the STF and the MSCI in understanding how contextual factors may impact on adolescent career development. The results indicated that the adolescents identified with all influences within the three systems of the STF and that parental influence was important in their career development. Other results indicated that working overseas was identified as an important influence.

The MSCI has also been researched in terms of both individual and group intervention. For instance, the MSCI has proved useful in enhancing the career development of middle-class South African high school students (Kuit, 2005). Kuit used the MSCI in a collaborative group approach in order to help adolescents elaborate their career narrative and find meaning in their personal career development. Similarly, in a case study approach, McMahon and Watson (2008) described the use of the MSCI in individual career counselling with a Grade 12 high school student which demonstrated how the client could take a more active role in the career counselling process, and how career decisions can be considered, re-evaluated and reprioritised more holistically within the broader context of an individual's system of influences.

In a further case study, Watson and McMahon (2009) described the case of a 33-year-old English-speaking black South African higher education student with whom they made use of the MSCI (Adult Version). The case study illustrated how career counsellors can assist tertiary students to reflect on intrapersonal strengths and macro-systemic barriers and, in doing that, link their life stories to their career choices. This particular study was responding to persistent calls for the development of more qualitative career counselling models and assessment processes that would reflect the realities of counselling in a developing world context (Maree & Molepo, 2006; Watson, 2006).

Collett's (2011) research on black South African adolescents and their parents of middle-class socio-economic status demonstrates an increasing acculturation in the adolescents' perceptions of the systemic influences on their career development. The significance of Collett's research focus cannot be overstated, as career psychology has been criticised internationally and within South Africa for its predominant focus on white middle-class samples (Watson, 2010).

The studies reported in this section of the chapter demonstrate qualitative research that attempts to meet the proposed goals for career psychology set out at the start of the previous decade (Savickas, 2001). Firstly, this body of research attempts to better interrelate research with practice, and to provide alternative methods of research through the use of the STF and the MSCI. Secondly, this research has focused on more disadvantaged populations through the use of an assessment process that can be regarded as locally as well as internationally grounded. The authors of this chapter are aware that the chapter emphasises a minority qualitative perspective within a book that is predominantly quantitative in its content focus. It is to this issue that we turn in concluding the chapter.

Conclusion

There are several issues to consider in relation to the role of qualitative and quantitative career assessment. Lamprecht (2002) sees the two forms of testing and assessment as largely incompatible. Even when he suggests that they could be combined, he urges that the psychometric information should 'not be regarded as the main sources of information' (p.126). The position of the present chapter's authors is that this is not an either/or situation, that we need to explore possibilities for the coexistence of quantitative and qualitative career assessment. As De Bruin and De Bruin (2006, p.130) have argued, 'a comprehensive and collaborative approach to career assessment where both standardised psychological tests and qualitative career assessment procedures have a role to play, depending on the needs of the client' is what is called for. Nevertheless, the present authors would argue further that quantitative career assessment needs to be qualitatively understood, that any assessment without contextualisation runs the risk of being limited in its interpretation. This is particularly the case when career assessment is undertaken in a developing world context with a diversity of cultural groups.

A second issue to consider is that the use of qualitative career assessment is not new. As indicated at the start of this chapter, it has a long but neglected history. Part of this neglect reflects the development of career psychology in more stable, measurable times. In a sense, increasing globalisation and the consequent changing nature of work calls for career practitioners to revisit the need for more qualitative career assessment. Thus, Blustein, Kenna, Murphy, DeVoy and DeWine (2005, p.352) point out that qualitative career assessment is moving 'from the margins into the center of contemporary inquiry'. While this may be true, there has been a lack of contextually relevant qualitative career assessment processes that are grounded in the local contexts in which they can be used. This chapter has explored the potential of qualitative career assessment to accommodate the less tangible and therefore less measurable variables that may influence individual career development.

This brings us to our final point: that this chapter has described to the reader an example of a qualitative approach to career assessment, the MSCI, which is sensitive to variables such as culture, socio-economic background, barriers to career development and other contextual influences that have been less focused on in quantitative career assessment. In addition, given the limitations discussed earlier, the MSCI's capacity to be used in group and education settings suggests that it is a cost-effective approach to qualitative career assessment in South Africa. Such an approach would seem to be exceptionally relevant in the present context within which most South Africans live.

References

Amundson, N. E. (2009). *Active Engagement* (3rd edition). Richmond, British Columbia: Ergon Communications.

Bisschoff, R. (1993). *Self-Directed Search Questionnaire (SDS).* Pretoria: Human Sciences Research Council.

Blustein, D. L. (2001). Extending the reach of vocational psychology: Toward an inclusive and integrative psychology of working. *Journal of Vocational Behavior, 59,* 171–182.

Blustein, D. L., Kenna, A. C., Murphy, K. A., DeVoy, J. E. & DeWine, D. B. (2005). Qualitative research in career development: Exploring the center and margins of discourse about careers and working. *Journal of Career Assessment, 13,* 351–370.

Cochran, L. (1997). *Career Counseling: A Narrative Approach.* Thousand Oaks, CA: Sage.

Collett, G. (2011). Systemic influences on black South African adolescents' career development: Adolescent and parental perspectives. Unpublished Master's dissertation. Nelson Mandela Metropolitan University, Port Elizabeth.

De Bruin, K. & De Bruin, G. P. (2006). Career assessment. In G. B. Stead & M. B. Watson (Eds), *Career Psychology in the South African Context* (2nd edition, pp. 129–136). Pretoria: Van Schaik.

Du Toit, L. B. H. (1987). *Manual for the Jung Personality Questionnaire.* Pretoria: Human Sciences Research Council.

Fritz, E. & Beekman, L. (2007). Engaging clients actively in telling stories and actualising dreams. In K. Maree (Ed.), *Shaping the Story: A Guide to Facilitating Narrative Career Counselling* (pp. 163–175). Pretoria: Van Schaik.

Hartung, P. J. (2007). Career construction: Principles and practice. In K. Maree (Ed.), *Shaping the Story: A Guide to Facilitating Narrative Career Counselling* (pp. 103–120). Pretoria: Van Schaik.

Holland, J. L. (1985). *Professional Manual for the Self-Directed Search* (revised edition). Odessa, FL: Psychological Assessment Resources.

Kuit, W. (2005). The career development of South African Grade 11 adolescents: A career systems and discursive perspective. Unpublished Master's dissertation. Nelson Mandela Metropolitan University, Port Elizabeth.

Lamprecht, J. C. (2002). Career assessment skills. In K. Maree & L. Ebersöhn (Eds), *Lifeskills and Career Counselling* (pp. 119–127). Johannesburg: Heinemann.

Langley, R. (1990). *The Career Development Questionnaire (CDQ): Manual.* Pretoria: Human Sciences Research Council.

Langley, R. (1992). *The Life Roles Inventory (LRI): Manual.* Pretoria: Human Sciences Research Council.

Langley, R., Du Toit, R. & Herbst, D. L. (1992). *Manual for the Values Scale.* Pretoria: Human Sciences Research Council.

Maree, J. G. (2009). Career counseling in the 21st century: South African institutions of higher education at the crossroads. *South African Journal of Higher Education, 23(2),* 436–458.

Maree, J. G., Bester, S. E., Lubbe, C. & Beck, C. (2001). Post-modern career counselling to a gifted black youth: A case study. *Gifted Education International, 15(3),* 324–338.

Maree, K. & Molepo, M. (2006). The use of narratives in cross-cultural career counselling. In M. McMahon & W. Patton (Eds), *Career Counselling: Constructivist Approaches* (pp. 69–81). London: Routledge.

McMahon, M. (2008). Qualitative career assessment: A higher profile in the 21st century? In J. Athanasou & R. van Esbroeck (Eds), *International Handbook of Career Guidance* (pp. 587–601). New York, NY: Springer Verlag.

McMahon, M. & Patton, W. (1995). Development of a systems theory of career development. *Australian Journal of Career Development, 4(2),* 15–20.

McMahon, M. & Patton, W. (2002). Using qualitative assessment in career counselling. *International Journal for Vocational and Educational Guidance, 51,* 51–66.

McMahon, M. & Patton, W. (2006). Qualitative career assessment. In M. McMahon & W. Patton (Eds), *Career Counselling: Constructivist Approaches* (pp. 163–175). London: Routledge.

McMahon, M., Patton, W. & Watson, M. (2003). Developing qualitative career assessment processes. *The Career Development Quarterly, 51,* 194–202.

McMahon, M., Patton, W. & Watson, M. (2004). Creating career stories through reflection: An application of the Systems Theory Framework of career development. *Australian Journal of Career Development, 13(3),* 13–16.

McMahon, M., Patton, W. & Watson, M. (2005a). *The My System of Career Influences (MSCI): Facilitators' Manual.* Camberwell, Melbourne: ACER Press.

McMahon, M., Patton, W. & Watson, M. (2005b). *The My System of Career Influences (MSCI): Reflecting on My Career Decisions.* Camberwell, Melbourne: ACER Press.

McMahon, M. & Watson, M. (2006). Career research in a postmodern era. *Australian Journal of Career Development, 15(2),* 26–31.

McMahon, M. & Watson, M. (2008). Systemic influences on career development: Assisting clients to tell their career stories. *The Career Development Quarterly, 56,* 280–288.

McMahon, M., Watson, M., Foxcroft, C. & Dullabh, A. (2008). South African adolescents' career development through the lens of the Systems Theory Framework: An exploratory study. *Journal of Psychology in Africa, 18(4),* 531–538.

McMahon, M., Watson, M. & Patton, W. (2005). Qualitative career assessment: Developing the My System of Career Influences Reflection Activity. *Journal of Career Assessment, 13,* 476–490.

McMahon, M., Watson, M. B. & Patton, W. (in press a). *My System of Career Influences (MSCI) (Adult Version): Work Booklet.* Brisbane: Australian Academic Press.

McMahon, M., Watson, M. B. & Patton, W. (in press b). *My System of Career Influences (MSCI) (Adult Version): Facilitators' Guide.* Brisbane: Australian Academic Press.

Myers, I. B. & McCaulley, M. H. (1985). *Manual: A Guide to the Development and Use of the Myers-Briggs Type Indicator.* Palo Alto, CA: Consulting Psychologists Press.

Nel, Z. J. (2006). The career choice theory of John Holland. In G. B. Stead & M. B. Watson (Eds), *Career Psychology in the South African Context* (2nd edition, pp. 35–50). Pretoria: Van Schaik.

Parker, P. (2006). Card sorts: Constructivist assessment tools. In M. McMahon & W. Patton (Eds), *Career Counselling: Constructivist Approaches* (pp. 176–186). London: Routledge.

Patton, W. & McMahon, M. (1999). *Career Development and Systems Theory: A New Relationship.* Pacific Grove, CA: Brooks/Cole.

Patton, W. & McMahon, M. (2006). *Career Development and Systems Theory: Connecting Theory and Practice* (2nd edition). Rotterdam: Sense Publishers.

Patton, M., McMahon, M. & Watson, M. (2006). Career development and systems theory: Enhancing our understanding of career. In G. B. Stead & M. B. Watson (Eds), *Career Psychology in the South African Context* (2nd edition, pp. 65–78). Pretoria: Van Schaik.

Peavy, R. V. (1998). *SocioDynamic Counselling: A Constructivist Perspective.* Victoria, British Columbia: Trafford.

Pryor, R. & Bright, J. (2011). *The Chaos Theory of Careers: A New Perspective on Working in the Twenty-first Century.* New York, NY: Routledge.

Savickas, M. L. (1993). Career counseling in the postmodern era. *Journal of Cognitive Psychotherapy: An International Quarterly, 7,* 205–215.

Savickas, M. L. (2001). The next decade in vocational psychology: Mission and objectives. *Journal of Vocational Behavior, 59,* 284–290.

Savickas, M. L., Nota, L., Rossier, J., Dauwalder, J-P., Duarte, M. E., Guichard, J. et al. (2009). Life designing: A paradigm for career construction in the 21st century. *Journal of Vocational Behavior, 75,* 239–250.

Super, D. E. (1990). A life-span, life-space approach to career development. In D. Brown & L. Brooks (Eds), *Career Choice and Development: Applying Contemporary Theories to Practice* (2nd edition, pp. 197–261). San Francisco, CA: Jossey-Bass.

Watson, M. B. (2006). Career counselling theory, culture and constructivism. In M. McMahon & W. Patton (Eds), *Career Counselling: Constructivist Approaches* (pp. 45–56). London: Routledge.

Watson, M. (2010). Career psychology in South Africa: Addressing and redressing social justice. *Australian Journal of Career Development, 19,* 24–29.

Watson, M., Duarte, M. E. & Glavin, K. (2005). Cross-cultural perspectives on career assessment. *The Career Development Quarterly, 54,* 29–35.

Watson, M. B., Foxcroft, C. D. & Allen, L. J. (2007). Tracking Holland interest codes: The case of South African field guides. *Australian Journal of Career Development, 16(2),* 51–59.

Watson, M. & McMahon, M. (2009). Career counselling in South African higher education: Moving forward systemically and qualitatively. *South African Journal of Higher Education, 23(3),* 470–481.

33 Psychological assessment and workplace transformation in South Africa: a review of the research literature

K. Milner, F. Donald and A. Thatcher

This chapter is set against the backdrop of a post-apartheid South African society that requires radical transformation of its institutions and organisations in order to attain the ideals of a just and equitable social order. The need for the transformation of South African organisations has been recognised at all levels of the South African economy. At a national, policy-making level the need for transformation has been acknowledged in various forms of legislation and policy – notably legislation and policy relating to black economic empowerment (BEE) and employment equity. At an organisational level there has also been a growing appreciation of the need for transformation, partly in response to the broader legislative environment but also in response to the increasing diversity of the South African workplace, the challenges of globalisation, and the need to redress past inequities.

Depending on how they are used, psychological assessment instruments can play a role either in organisational transformation or in maintaining the status quo.[1] Psychometric tests and other forms of assessment take on a gatekeeping role when used in an organisational context, and therefore can be a key determinant of access to both employment opportunities as well as career mobility. To quote Sehlapelo and Terre Blanche (1996, p.49):

> Given South African Psychology's intimate relationship with psychometrics and the continued prevalence of psychometric testing in modern day South Africa, it should obviously be an important site of transformation. The fact is that if psychological tests are used on a large scale to determine who gains access to economic and educational opportunities, and if psychology as a profession is truly interested in empowerment, the reform of testing practices should be one of its priorities. However, testing practices, i.e. the day-to-day use of tests as opposed to technical issues of test construction and validation tends to receive inadequate research attention.

Other authors, including Claassen (1997), Foxcroft (1997) and Nzimande (1995), have made similar claims. Criticisms of assessment instruments (particularly psychometric tests) in use in South African organisations include the fact that many psychometric tests are not standardised for use on a South African population and are thus inherently culturally biased (Bedell, Van Eeden & Van

Staden, 1999; Wallis & Birt, 2003). Critical reviews of assessment tools and practices in South Africa have thus contributed to a body of knowledge that positions assessment as a contested terrain.

In summary, the imperatives for workplace transformation mentioned earlier, the potential inherent in psychological assessment for acting as either a tool for, or an obstacle to, this transformation, and the controversies surrounding the history and current use of psychological assessment in South African organisations (Foxcroft & Roodt, 2008; Magwaza, 1995; Moerdyk, 2009; Sehlapelo & Terre Blanche, 1996; Stead, 2002), point to the need for ongoing evaluation of the work being done in relation to psychological assessment at work. Our aim in this chapter is to evaluate the South African research attention that has been devoted to psychological assessment over the past ten years, and assess the extent to which this research specifically addresses concerns regarding assessment and organisational transformation. In doing so, we draw on organisational justice theory in order to position our analysis within a sound theoretical framework.

An organisational justice framework

> Organisational justice – members' sense of the moral propriety of how they are treated – is the 'glue' that allows people to work together effectively. Justice defines the very essence of individuals' relationship to employers.
>
> (Cropanzano, Bowen & Gilliland, 2007, p.34)

The reason for choosing organisational justice as a framework for organising our evaluation of research on assessment in organisations is straightforward. If psychological assessment is to have any credibility as a decision-making tool in the South African workplace it must, first and foremost, show that it is fair. Within the context of transformation, however, the issue of fairness is not always straightforward. What fairness is, and how it is perceived, is the key concern of the organisational justice literature. Greenberg (1990, p.400) specifically states that the organisational justice literature has 'grown around attempts to describe and explain the role of fairness as a consideration in the workplace'. Fairness, as viewed from an organisational justice perspective, is not a unitary construct (see the section on dimensions of organisational justice below). Its value for the purpose of this chapter lies in acknowledging that fairness can take on different guises in different contexts. For example, standardising tests for a South African population for different norm groups within that population may meet the criteria for procedural justice, in that standardisation addresses cross-cultural bias. However, it will not necessarily advance the transformation agenda of redressing past injustice and creating a more equitable post-apartheid society, which may need to be viewed in relation to distributive justice.

An organisational justice perspective on assessment, and particularly research into assessment, thus allows us to broaden the lens through which we view psychological assessment. It enables a move away from what De Wolff

(1993) terms the 'prediction paradigm', which treats assessment primarily as a psychometric exercise concerned with the test's factor structure, and statistical reliability and validity (Cropanzano & Wright, 2003), towards a more holistic evaluation of the entire assessment process.[2]

Dimensions of organisational justice

In a meta-analysis of 25 years of organisational justice research, Colquitt, Conlon, Wesson, Porter and Ng (2001) established that distributive justice, procedural justice and interpersonal justice have a unique contribution to make to understanding individuals' perceptions of fairness. A brief explanation of these dimensions is provided below.

Distributive justice

Based on the work of Adams (1965) on equity in social exchange as a prime motivator of human behaviour, distributive justice deals with 'the distribution of the conditions and goals which affect individual (psychological, social and economic) wellbeing' (Deutsch, 1975, p.137). Essentially, distributive justice is concerned with the way in which a particular outcome is viewed by the recipient of that outcome (Cropanzano & Greenberg, 1997). There appear to be 'three allocation rules that can lead to distributive justice ... : equality (to each the same), equity (to each in accordance with contributions) and need (to each in accordance with the most urgency)' (Cropanzano et al., 2007, p.37).

Procedural justice

Procedural justice is concerned with 'the justice of the formal allocation processes' (Cropanzano et al., 2007, p.36). It refers to the way in which outcomes are allocated but not to the outcomes themselves. Leventhal (1980) is credited with identifying six criteria for determining whether a process is fair: consistency, bias-free, accuracy, correctability, opportunity for representation of all stakeholders, and ethicality.

Interactional justice

Interactional justice refers to the 'importance of the quality of the interpersonal treatment people receive when procedures are implemented' (Colquitt et al., 2001, p.426). The current understanding of interactional justice divides it into two types: interpersonal justice – being treated with dignity and respect; and informational justice – provision of explanations as to how and why decisions were made.

The way in which we utilise these three components of organisational justice in analysing South African research on psychological assessment is discussed in the following section, and the procedure for delineating the scope of our investigation, in terms of identifying relevant research articles, is presented. Thereafter, the way in which this research is categorised in relation to the above three dimension of organisational justice is described.

Procedure used for the literature search and analysis

The literature search aimed to identify empirical research and position papers that have been published since 2000 and which either use South African data or refer to assessment in South Africa. The date 2000 was chosen as this limited the search to research data that could be clearly identified as being from post-apartheid years, and specifically since the enactment of the Employment Equity Act (No. 55 of 1998), while simultaneously focusing on relatively up-to-date articles. Initially the search focused on South African academic journals which were likely to contain information on assessment in organisations. These included the *South African Journal of Industrial Psychology* (SAJIP), the *South African Journal of Psychology* (SAJP), the *South African Journal of Human Resource Management* (SAJHRM), *Psychology in Society* (PINS), the *Journal of Psychology in Africa* (JPA) and the *South African Journal of Business Management* (SAJBM). From all these journals, the SAJIP yielded the most articles (N = 46) and the SAJHRM, JPA, PINS and SAJBM contained the least relevant studies (N = 0 in each case).

Next, databases were searched; these included Ebsco Host, Proquest, PsycINFO, Science Direct and Wiley InterScience. Google Scholar and Yippy were also searched to ensure that coverage had been sufficiently broad. These databases were chosen because, between them, they cover many thousands of academic, peer-reviewed and research-based journals. Many of these journals are listed in Thomson Reuters (formerly ISI) Web of Knowledge, indicating their standing in the academic world of research. Further, research based on South African data need not be restricted to South African journals, but may be published in international journals. Lastly, references in relevant articles were followed up. It is acknowledged that there is a great deal of valuable information in organisations, and test publishers' data banks. However, it was decided to exclude these sources and rather to focus on research that had been peer-reviewed and was publicly available. This is not intended to devalue the importance of unpublished research.

The search terms used were initially broad, and were then narrowed to improve the nature of the hits and to approach the issue from different angles using more selective search terms. All searching was done in English. A number of search strategies were implemented, using different combinations of root words and subsequently additional words to streamline or direct the outcome of the search. Searches included searching for individual words, words in combination, and specific phrases. Boolean search techniques were also used with 'and'/'or'/'not' combinations. Terms used included 'fairness', 'bias', 'psychometric', 'assessment', 'test', 'staffing', 'selection' and 'South Africa'. In addition, the names of specific psychometric tests used in South African industry were also considered in place of 'psychometric' or 'assessment'. Studies that did not specifically investigate assessment within the broad context of organisations were not included in our analysis (for example, studies investigating psychometric instruments that are commonly used in organisational settings, but that only used a student sample and did not make explicit reference to applicability in organisational settings, were not included in our analysis).

Articles were analysed in the following manner. Firstly, they were divided into two key categories – those containing empirical primary data versus those that provided commentary or were conceptual or theoretical in nature. Next, the types of assessments covered by the articles were noted. The third step was to identify the types of justice included in the data in empirical articles, or discussed in theoretical articles. It is important to note that merely mentioning issues related to legal compliance, bias and fairness in the literature review of empirical articles was not seen as being a sufficient indicator of research into these issues. Rather, the aim of the study and its data needed to examine justice, bias and/or fairness directly.

The framework used for categorising justice issues in assessment was based on Gilliland (1993) and De Jong and Visser (2000a).

Research which tackled issues of standardisation, job-relatedness, predictive validity, face validity, the opportunity to perform, and adherence to standardised and consistent administration methods was considered to address procedural justice. Standardisation could refer either to the assessment instrument itself (for example, ensuring that the items were relevant for the South African context), the assessment scores (for example, the establishment of appropriate norm groups) or the delivery of the assessment (for example, administered in a consistent manner). Since all these issues deal with either the development or the administration of the assessments they are procedural in nature. Thus, reliability, validity, standardisation and differential item functioning were categorised as procedural justice. In addition, issues related to language usage and translation and to availability of test administrators were included in this category.

The authors cited above include interpersonal treatment information received in procedural justice. However, to maintain consistency with the types of justice established by Colquitt et al. (2001), these were categorised as interactional justice in the current study. Interactional justice included the interpersonal effectiveness of the test administrator and the propriety of questions. Informational justice included communication and openness about the assessment process and feedback.

Research focusing explicitly on equity, equality and special needs (for example, employment equity and transformation) is considered to address distributive justice, in line with Gilliland (1993) and De Jong and Visser (2000a).

Based on the foregoing discussion, we interrogate this literature through three questions:

1. What types of assessments have been scrutinised in the literature? In other words, are we still narrowly focused on psychological testing or are we starting to address a broader conceptualisation of psychological assessment?
2. What is the paradigmatic nature of the theory and research on organisational assessment in South Africa? Does it conform to De Wolff's (1993) prediction paradigm or does it address broader societal and contextual issues?
3. What, if any, aspects of organisational justice are being evaluated with regard to psychological assessment in the South African workplace? From a transformational standpoint, issues of distributive justice are of key concern here.

The texts on which our interrogation focuses are listed in Table 33.1.

Table 33.1 Literature assessed in the review

Author/s	Date	Empirical/ theoretical	Types of assessment	Types of justice addressed
Abrahams	2001	Theoretical	Psychometric testing in general	Distributive: Emphasises the need to transform society from a historical and socio-political perspective
Abrahams	2002	Empirical	Sixteen Personality Factor Questionnaire (16PF)	Procedural: Study of bias
Barnard & Schaap	2005	Empirical	Technical Test Battery	Procedural: Concurrent validity and legal compliance
Coetzee & Schaap	2005	Empirical	Multifactor Emotional Intelligence Scale, Multifactor Leadership Scale	Procedural: Relationship between emotional intelligence and leadership
De Beer	2004	Empirical	Learning Potential Computerised Adaptive Test (LPCAT)	Procedural: Study of bias
De Beer	2005	Empirical	LPCAT	Procedural: Study of bias
De Beer	2006	Empirical	LPCAT	Procedural: Study of bias
De Bruin	2000	Empirical	Comrey Personality Questionnaire, 16PF	Procedural: Factor structure of tests
De Bruin, De Bruin, Dercksen & Cilliers-Hartslief	2005	Empirical	Raven's Progressive Matrices, Five Factor–Nonverbal Personality Questionnaire	Procedural: Predictive validity
De Jong & Visser	2000b	Empirical	Interviews, curriculum vitae, work sample tests, biographical information blank, written ability/ psychometric tests, personal references, personality tests, honesty tests, personal contacts, graphology	Procedural: Job-relatedness, predictive validity, face validity, opportunity to perform, consistent administration, propriety of questions, extent of use, employers' rights Distributive: Equity Informational: Explanations provided
De Kock & Schlechter	2009	Empirical	Raven's Advanced Progressive Matrices, Blox Test	Procedural: Predictive validity

continued →

Author/s	Date	Empirical/ theoretical	Types of assessment	Types of justice addressed
De Lange, Fourie & Van Vuuren	2003	Empirical	360-degree questionnaire, assessment centre	Procedural: Psychometric properties and usefulness
Du Toit & De Bruin	2002	Empirical	Holland's typology	Procedural: Structural validity
Foxcroft	2004	Theoretical	Psychometric testing in general	Procedural: Issues in the development of multicultural tests
Henning, Theron & Spangenberg	2004	Empirical	Predictive Index	Procedural: Internal structure
Heuchert, Parker, Stumpf & Myburgh	2000	Empirical	Revised NEO Personality Inventory (NEO-PI-R)	Procedural: Factor structure
Huysamen	2004	Theoretical	Psychometric testing in general	Procedural: Bias and differential item functioning
Huysamen	2006	Theoretical	Psychometric testing in general	Procedural: Reliability estimates
Jonker & Vosloo	2008	Empirical	Schutte Emotional Intelligence Scale	Procedural: Psychometric properties
Joubert & Kriek	2009	Empirical	Occupational Personality Questionnaire 32 Version i (OPQ32i)	Procedural: Psychometric properties
La Grange & Roodt	2001	Empirical	Customer Contact Styles Questionnaire Version 5.2 (CCSQ5.2), Verbal Evaluation Test, Customer Contact Competency Inventory (CCCI)	Procedural: Predictive validity
Laher	2008	Theoretical	NEO-PI-R	Procedural: Psychometric properties and differential scores
Lopes, Roodt & Mauer	2001	Empirical	APIL-B	Procedural: Predictive validity
Meiring, Van de Vijver & Rothmann	2006	Empirical	Fifteen Factor Questionnaire Plus (15FQ+)	Procedural: Study of bias

Author/s	Date	Empirical/ theoretical	Types of assessment	Types of justice addressed
Meiring, Van de Vijver, Rothmann & Barrick	2005	Empirical	Cognitive and personality test: 15FQ+, 16PF, South African Personality Questionnaire (SAPQ), NEO	Procedural: Need for legal compliance, study of bias
Muller & Schepers	2003	Empirical	SpEEx, Raven's Advanced Progressive Matrices	Procedural: Predictive validity using multicultural sample
Murphy & Maree	2009	Theoretical	Dynamic testing in general	Procedural: Psychometric properties and differential scores
Nel & De Villiers	2004	Empirical	Emotional Competency Inventory	Procedural: Predictive validity
Nicholls, Viviers & Visser	2009	Empirical	CCSQ7.2, CCCI, Personnel Test Battery	Procedural: Predictive validity
Nzama, De Beer & Visser	2008	Empirical	15FQ+, Cognitive Process Profile (CPP), structured interview	Procedural: Need for legal compliance, predictive validity
Paterson & Uys	2005	Empirical	Psychometric tests in general	Procedural: Development of tests; availability of appropriate tests; standards for use; cross-cultural applicability; competence of testers; legal compliance; changing world of work Distributive: Focus on impact of responsible selection on the selection and development of previously disadvantaged individuals; relationship between scientific bias and fairness perceptions
Pelser, Bergh & Visser	2005	Empirical	TRAM 1 Learning Potential, Vienna Test System	Procedural: Concurrent validity
Potgieter & Van der Merwe	2002	Theoretical	Competency-based assessments	Procedural: Guidelines for developing competency-based assessments

continued →

Author/s	Date	Empirical/ theoretical	Types of assessment	Types of justice addressed
Prinsloo & Ebersöhn	2002	Theoretical	16PF	Procedural: Construct validity and bias
Rothmann & Cilliers	2007	Theoretical	Mainly psychometric personality tests and 15FQ+	Procedural: Need for legal compliance; cross-cultural appropriateness Distributive: Changes in the workplace mentioned, but not with view to transformation or assessing people for future organisation
Schaap	2001	Empirical	PIB / SpEEx	Procedural: Bias and differential item functioning
Schaap & Basson	2003	Empirical	PIB / SpEEX Motivation Index	Procedural: Bias and construct equivalence
Schaap & Vermeulen	2008	Empirical	PIB / SpEEx	Procedural: Studies construct equivalence and bias; discusses language and translation issues
Schepers	2002	Empirical	Computerised information-processing test	Procedural: Develops and evaluates tests with intercorrelations and factor analyses
Schroder	2004	Theoretical	In-basket	Procedural: Use of in-baskets only versus range of assessment techniques
Spangenberg & Theron	2003	Empirical	In-basket	Procedural: Validity of an in-basket
Spangenberg & Theron	2004	Theoretical	In-basket	Procedural: Ethics of use of in-basket in leadership development
Stead	2002	Theoretical	Psychometric tests in general	Procedural: Need for legal compliance; more research on bias and other psychometric properties; shortage of skilled test developers needed to develop or adapt tests; language issues Distributive: Acknowledges need to redress past

Author/s	Date	Empirical/ theoretical	Types of assessment	Types of justice addressed
Stuart & Paquet	2001	Empirical	Bar-On Emotional Quotient Inventory (Bar-On EQ-i), Multifactor Leadership Questionnaire	Procedural: Examines relationship between the two questionnaires
Sugreen & Schepers	2006	Empirical	SpEEx, Multifactor Leadership Questionnaire	Procedural: Focus on psychometric properties and usefulness
Theron	2007	Theoretical	Psychometric tests in general	Procedural: Need for legal compliance Distributive: Recognises that tests regulate access to resources; refers to Mandela's call for transformation; recognises that merely eliminating bias will not eradicate adverse impact; considers fairness models
Theron	2009	Theoretical	Psychometric tests in general	Distributive: Examines adverse impact ratios
Theron & Roodt	2000	Empirical	360-degree marketing competency assessment	Procedural: Focus is on mental models and not bias or justice
Theron & Roodt	2001	Empirical	360-degree project management competency assessment	Procedural: Inter-rater reliability
Van der Merwe	2002	Empirical	Psychometric tests in general, group interaction exercise, in-basket, interviews, presentations	Procedural: Organisation's test policy, need for legal compliance; competence of testers; cross-cultural bias; psychometric properties; overall selection process
Van de Vijver & Rothmann	2004	Theoretical	Psychometric tests, interviews	Procedural: Need for legal compliance; psychometric properties; multicultural issues; tester competence; administration conditions
Van Eeden & Mantsha	2007	Empirical	16PF	Procedural: Translation into Tshivenda

continued →

Author/s	Date	Empirical/ theoretical	Types of assessment	Types of justice addressed
Viljoen, Schepers & Van Zyl	2001	Empirical	Learning Style Preference Questionnaire	Procedural: Examines effects of gender, educational qualifications and functional disciplines, but not race. Focus is not on justice but on development and evaluation of scale
Visser & Du Toit	2004	Empirical	Occupational Personality Questionnaire (OPQ)	Procedural: Factor structure of OPQ
Visser & Viviers	2010	Empirical	OPQ32N	Procedural: Psychometric properties to achieve legal compliance
Vorster & Roodt	2003	Empirical	360-degree supervisory competency questionnaire	Procedural: Focus on psychometric properties but not on bias or justice. Includes differences between language groups
Wallis	2004	Theoretical	Psychometric tests in general	Procedural: Ethics of use of in-basket in leadership development
Wallis & Birt	2003	Empirical	16PF	Procedural: Multicultural understanding of language in test items

Based on the above evaluation we are able to start proposing some answers to the questions we posed earlier. These are addressed question by question in the following section.

Analysis of the literature reviewed

1. What types of assessments have been scrutinised in the literature? Are we still narrowly focused on psychological testing or are we starting to address a broader conceptualisation of psychological assessment?

It is evident from Table 33.1 that the majority of research attention remains focused on a fairly narrow range of assessments, primarily individual psychometric tests. There is some evidence of research, for example in the work of Visser and Matthews (2005), De Lange, Fourie and Van Vuuren (2003) and Spangenberg and Theron (2004), which addresses a broader range of assessment techniques, including interviews, in-basket techniques, biographical blanks and competency-based assessments. Over and above this, Van der Merwe (2002) is one of the few authors who address broader assessment concerns, specifically the issue of how assessment is actually practised within organisations in South Africa. This is a small, qualitative study but it gives some insight into which tests are used in industry and for what purpose.

Finally, we must acknowledge that there are social context elements beyond organisational assessment practices that will also impact on the assessment climate in organisations, and that will influence transformation efforts. For example, Martin and Durrheim (2006) found that the attitudes, perceptions, stereotypes and discourses of the owners of recruitment agencies (especially racial stereotypes and discourses) negatively influenced organisational transformation. Recruitment agencies are important (but not the only) gatekeepers of access to employment opportunities, and therefore the stereotypes and discourses evident in Martin and Durrheim's (2006) findings would impact on procedural and distributive justice in relation to transformation in assessment practices (that is, they may determine which people arrive at an organisation as applicants to be assessed). Their article is not, however, included in Table 33.1 as it does not address assessment.

2. What is the paradigmatic nature of the theory and research on organisational assessment in South Africa? Does it conform to De Wolff's (1993) prediction paradigm or does it address broader societal and contextual issues?

However, there are two issues that emerge from standardisation. Firstly, norm groups must be representative of the people being assessed. In the South African context norm groups are often simplified in terms of race, gender and/or educational level. While this simplification is necessary, it does hide the complexities inherent in terms such as 'race' and 'gender'. This simplification means that there is little engagement with definitions of race (or gender or educational level) and instead these categories are tied to the historical descriptors that may not always be productive in relation to transformative efforts. Of course, it is unsurprising that these categories proliferate in the published articles as these are the categories used in South African legislation, notably the Employment Equity Act.

Secondly, standardisation cannot replace validity. It is quite possible that if 'groups' have different norm scores they may also have differential (predictive) validity curves. The vast majority of the research we surveyed, if not all of it, is firmly located within the prediction paradigm. It is important to note, however, that unlike the situation in other countries, the proliferation of reliability and validity studies is not merely a psychometric exercise but is, to some extent, a response to the criticisms levelled against the testing industry in South Africa – in particular, the charge that psychometric tests have in the past been used, at worst, in support of a racist agenda of white supremacy and, at best, in a manner that tended to ignore systematic biases in favour of whites. This is evident in the large number of studies which cite legal compliance with employment equity legislation as the raison d'être for the research. In this regard South African academic engagement with assessment is some way ahead of other countries in addressing the socio-political context in which testing is taking place, albeit in relation to a research agenda that remains within a fairly narrow prediction paradigm.

Bedell et al. (1999, p.5) warn that an emphasis on the psychometric properties (they are primarily interested in test bias) 'precludes a focus on making the testing context more human and democratic'. The pitfalls of a narrow, prediction approach to psychological assessment are explored in terms of the argument that, in its very design, psychological testing draws on a historical perspective. Psychological assessments are designed to assess what once 'was' in the organisation and not what 'can be'. In Theron's (2009, p.184) words, expressed in psychometric language, 'selection decisions should be based on expected criterion performance, estimated without systematic group-related prediction error from the predictor'. He notes that under-represented groups may therefore be unfairly disadvantaged by such prediction paradigms. In the South African context, psychological assessments are legally required by the Employment Equity Act to be valid, reliable, fairly applied, and not biased against any employee or group of employees. In the published South African literature and in the work of the Psychometrics Committee of the Professional Board for Psychology, the emphasis has been on producing psychological tests (and, to a lesser extent, psychological assessments such as competency-based interviews and behavioural assessments) that are valid and reliable, and by implication tests that are therefore more culturally fair. However, reliability and validity in these contexts only refer to information that has been gathered in the past (Theron, 2009).

The two most important validity measures for psychological assessment are criterion-related validity and predictive validity. In order to establish the effectiveness of a psychological test using criterion-related validity, one must use a criterion measure that is already available in the organisation (for example, common criterion measures are organisational level, performance ratings or existing psychological assessment measures). Similarly with predictive validity, the psychological assessment is of necessity compared with some predictive measure that is already in existence in the organisation (such as success in the organisation, organisational mobility, career progression, and so on). Predictive validity, in this sense, is not a true prediction of a future state but a prediction of whether a person will be as 'successful' in the organisation as others have been in the past. This assumes that the parameters for success remain unchanged. For example, if the predictive measure is career progression, then the reasons for promotion in the organisation must remain the same before and after transformation for the predictive measure to be valid (and it should be noted, in terms of this argument, that if a certain population group was favoured for promotion during a transformation process but not before, then promotion cannot be a considered as a valid predictive measure).

In essence then, criterion measures and predictive measures of these types only ensure that psychological assessment can determine the extent to which an individual is likely to succeed in a position based on past yardsticks for effectiveness. Unfortunately this is not particularly useful for transforming an organisation (since the assessment only tells the test administrator what was a good criterion or a good predictor for the existing organisation or the past organisation, but not for a new, transformed organisation). For transformation (and to identify a 'true' predictor), the psychological assessment needs to tell the test administrator whether a person will meet the needs of an organisation that is not yet in existence. Psychological assessments that have been shown to be reliable and valid (even for different groups of test-takers) are therefore in danger of maintaining the status quo in an organisation (that is, allowing the organisation to 'defensibly' use psychological assessments to recruit the same types of people). As Theron (2009, p.183) argues, 'valid selection procedures used in a fair and nondiscriminatory manner that optimises utility very often result in adverse impact against members of protected groups'. In other words, Theron (2009) argues that even assessments that are valid and reliable in determining success in the organisation based on success in the past may only perpetuate unjust organisational practices, even if assessment is applied in a fair manner.

This argument is not intended to undermine the importance of valid and reliable assessments, the fair and consistent administration of assessments, the use of appropriate norm groups, and assessments that are relevant for the organisation's needs and the test-takers' attributes. What we are saying, though, is that these aspects provide necessary but not sufficient conditions to enable the transformation of our country's organisations. When assessments are not developed specifically for the South African population, standardisation is a useful starting point. Standardisation primarily involves establishing relevant norm groups that enable people administering the assessments to make fair judgements between norm groups. Of course, it is also possible to perform post-transformation validation studies to determine whether the psychological assessments were indeed effective in enabling transformation. Examples of research that has begun to engage with the issue of psychological assessment and transformation and its complexities are Theron's (2007; 2009) papers addressing adverse impact in the South African context. Theron (2009) advocates a more nuanced approach to understanding diversity and suggests paying more attention to understanding job competency potential rather than existing skill/attribute sets.

In summary, South African research is predominantly undertaken within the prediction paradigm, but this is perhaps largely due to the need to ensure compliance with the Employment Equity Act. We support the need for culturally fair, valid and reliable tests in South Africa, but the academic community needs to be wary of the proliferation of validity and reliability studies that are essentially little more than psychometric exercises. These are important for industry but tend to be atheoretical in nature and therefore do not always advance disciplinary knowledge in particularly meaningful ways.

3. What, if any, aspects of organisational justice are being evaluated with regard to psychological assessment in the South African workplace? From a transformational standpoint, issues of distributive justice are of key concern here.

Given that we have already found that the majority of, though not all, research in South Africa focuses fairly narrowly on psychometric testing, and tends to fall within De Wolff's (1993) prediction paradigm, it is unsurprising when looking at the research through an organisational justice lens that procedural justice tends to be the dominant justice dimension that is addressed in the published research literature. There is some literature which addresses interactional justice, in the sense that practitioners are exhorted to ensure that interactional justice precepts are adhered to in all selection-type processes and procedures, including assessment (see, for example, De Jong & Visser, 2000b; Paterson & Uys, 2005; Visser & De Jong, 2001). However, there is very little research evidence pertaining to interactional justice and assessment in South Africa. Given the distinct mistrust that seems to exist amongst 'recipients' of assessments in South African industry (Sehlapelo & Terre Blanche, 1996; Stead, 2002), it would seem that this could be a fruitful area for future research. For example, language equivalence in the assessment instruments themselves has been looked at (see, for example, Abrahams, 2002; Foxcroft, 2004; Jonker & Vosloo, 2008; Joseph & Van Lille, 2008; Meiring, Van de Vijver & Rothmann, 2006; Schaap & Basson, 2003; Schaap & Vermeulen, 2008; Van Eeden & Mantsha, 2007; Visser & Matthews, 2005), but what about language differences in test administration? Are the subtle and not-so-subtle nuances of race and racial dynamics in South Africa shaping the way in which assessment 'recipients' are treated and how they experience their assessment encounters? Is the process of assessment, as practised in organisations, transparent enough to meet the requirements of interactional justice?

There is virtually no research in South Africa addressing distributive justice concerns. This is in line with international research trends, where distributive justice is regarded as a lesser concern in selection (Cropanzano et al., 2007) and, by implication, in assessment. However, we propose that within the context of transformation the issue of distributive justice is paramount. As Stone-Romero and Stone (2005, p.458) argue:

> There is considerable evidence that members of out-groups have long experienced lower levels of positively valent outcomes than members

of in-groups. Regrettably, the outcomes experienced by out-group members are often unrelated or weakly related to their potential or actual contributions (inputs). Thus, they have been treated unfairly vis à vis the equity norm.

Certainly, the history and legacy of apartheid in South Africa have violated the equity norm in organisations for generations. Research that focuses on procedural justice – that is, on ensuring that there is no bias, adverse impact or unfairness in current assessment tools or practices – does not sufficiently address the key issues of *redress* that are central to debates about the transformation of South African institutions and organisations, and also the transformation of psychology itself as a discipline in South Africa.

Conclusion

The aim of this chapter has been to view South African assessment research through an organisational justice lens, in order to evaluate the contribution of assessment research to transformation in South African organisations. The chapter has argued that relatively significant progress has been made in responding to the challenge posed by legislation and the powerful critiques of psychometric research and practices in South Africa. This progress is reflected in the focus and growth in research on procedural justice in assessment. However, the literature review has found that interactional justice has been addressed to a far more limited extent, and distributive justice has been virtually ignored. This has important implications for the credibility of assessment in relation to transformation in South Africa. Assessment still seems to be approached from within a narrow predictive paradigm, with an emphasis on psychometric testing and the psychometric properties associated therewith. There is a sense that this results in a somewhat mechanical approach, where the emphasis is on meeting the legal requirements rather than engaging fully with the transformation imperatives of the country. Assessment is still in danger of being associated with a powerful elite pursuing a managerialist agenda. We propose that a way of addressing this is to encourage more research on the following issues:

- the ways in which assessment is practised in organisations and the decision-making processes associated with these assessments;
- the perceptions and experiences of the recipients of assessment practices in organisations;
- creative ways of addressing criterion measures that facilitate transformation (this may be occurring in organisations but being treated as an internal organisational matter, rather than as an issue of academic concern); and
- addressing the roles of the stakeholders in different types of research and encouraging a broader and more critical approach to assessment in South Africa, especially in the light of current debates on race and racial categories in post-apartheid South Africa.

Notes

1 In this chapter, 'transformation' refers specifically to attempting redress for previously disadvantaged groups and not to organisational transformation in a more general sense (for example, structural or technological change).

2 For the purposes of this chapter, the assessment process and its component parts are defined as follows:

A psychometric test is a 'sample of behaviour gathered under standardized conditions with clearly defined rules for scoring the sample, with a view to describing current behaviour or to predicting future behaviour' (Moerdyk, 2009, p.270).

Psychological assessment 'is the larger social process by which a test is administered, interpreted, and used to render a decision. Testing is only one aspect of assessment, although it is an important one' (Cropanzano & Wright, 2003, p.9).

This broader view of psychological assessment also incorporates assessments other than tests, including interviews, work samples and assessment centres, as well as the procedures of selecting, administering, giving feedback and decision-making involving these assessments.

References

Abrahams, F. (2001). The use and abuse of psychological testing in industry: An overview. In C. R. Stones (Ed.), *Socio-Political and Psychological Perspectives on South Africa* (pp. 197–214). New York, NY: Nova.

Abrahams, F. (2002). The (un)fair usage of the 16PF (SA92) in South Africa: A response to C. H. Prinsloo & I. Ebersöhn. *South African Journal of Psychology, 32(3)*, 58–61.

Adams, J. S. (1965). Inequity in social exchange. In L. Berkowitz (Ed.), *Advances in Experimental Social Psychology* (pp. 267–299). New York, NY: Academic Press.

Barnard, M. & Schaap, P. (2005). The concurrent validity of the Technical Test Battery as an indicator of work performance in a telecommunications company. *South African Journal of Industrial Psychology, 31(2)*, 71–77.

Bedell, B., Van Eeden, R. & Van Staden, F. (1999). Culture as a moderator variable in psychological test performance: Issues and trends in South Africa. *Journal of Industrial Psychology, 25(3)*, 1–7.

Claassen, N. C. W. (1997). Cultural differences, politics and test bias in South Africa. *European Review of Applied Psychology, 47(4)*, 297–307.

Coetzee, C. & Schaap, P. (2005). The relationship between leadership behaviour, outcomes of leadership and emotional intelligence. *South African Journal of Industrial Psychology, 31(3)*, 31–38.

Colquitt, J. A., Conlon, D. E., Wesson, M. J., Porter, C. O. L. H. & Ng, K. Y. (2001). Justice at the millennium: A meta-analytic review of 25 years of organizational research. *Journal of Applied Psychology, 86(3)*, 425–445.

Cropanzano, R., Bowen, D. E. & Gilliland, S. W. (2007). The management of organizational justice. *Academy of Management Perspectives, 21(4)*, 34–48.

Cropanzano, R. & Greenberg, J. (1997). Progress in organizational justice: Tunnelling through the maze. In C. L. Cooper & I. T. Robertson (Eds), *International Review of Industrial and Organizational Psychology* Volume 12 (pp. 317–372). Chichester: Wiley.

Cropanzano, R. & Wright, T. A. (2003). Procedural justice and organizational staffing: A tale of two paradigms. *Human Resource Management Review, 13(1)*, 7–39.

De Beer, M. (2004). Use of differential item functioning (DIF) analysis for bias analysis in test construction. *South African Journal of Industrial Psychology, 30(4)*, 52–57.

De Beer, M. (2005). Development of the Learning Potential Computerised Adaptive Test (LPCAT). *South African Journal of Psychology, 35(4)*, 717–747.

De Beer, M. (2006). Dynamic testing: Practical solutions to some concerns. *South African Journal of Industrial Psychology, 32(4)*, 8–14.

De Bruin, G. (2000). An inter-battery analysis of the Comrey Personality Scales and the 16 Personality Factor Questionnaire. *South African Journal of Industrial Psychology, 26(3)*, 4–7.

De Bruin, K., De Bruin, G. P., Dercksen, S. & Cilliers-Hartslief, M. (2005). Predictive validity of general intelligence and Big Five measures for adult basic education and training outcomes. *South African Journal of Psychology, 35(1)*, 46–57.

De Jong, A. & Visser, D. (2000a). Black and white employees' fairness perceptions of personnel selection techniques. *South African Journal of Psychology, 30(4)*, 17–24.

De Jong, A. & Visser, D. (2000b). Organisational justice rules as determinants of black and white employees' fairness perceptions of personnel selection techniques. *South African Journal of Industrial Psychology, 26(1)*, 29–38.

De Kock, F. & Schlechter, A. (2009). Fluid intelligence and spatial reasoning as predictors of pilot training performance in the South African Air Force (SAAF). *South African Journal of Industrial Psychology, 35(1)*, 31–38.

De Lange, M., Fourie, L. & Van Vuuren, L. J. (2003). Reliability of competency-based, multidimensional, multiple-rater performance ratings. *South African Journal of Industrial Psychology, 29(2)*, 39–48.

Deutsch, M. (1975). Equity, equality, and need: What determines which value will be used as the basis of distributive justice? *Journal of Social Issues, 31(3)*, 137–149.

De Wolff, C. J. (1993). The prediction paradigm. In H. Schuler, J. Farr & M. Smith (Eds), *Personnel Selection and Assessment: Individual and Organizational Perspectives* (pp. 253–261). Hillsdale, NJ: Lawrence Erlbaum.

Du Toit, R. & De Bruin, G. P. (2002). The structural validity of Holland's R-I-A-S-E-C model of vocational personality types for young black South African men and women. *Journal of Career Assessment, 10(1)*, 62–77.

Foxcroft, C. D. (1997). Psychological testing in South Africa: Perspectives regarding ethical and fair practices. *European Journal of Psychological Assessment, 13(3)*, 229–235.

Foxcroft, C. D. (2004). Planning a psychological test in the multicultural South African context. *South African Journal of Industrial Psychology, 30(4)*, 8–15.

Foxcroft, C. D. & Roodt, G. (2008). *An Introduction to Psychological Assessment in the South African Context* (3rd edition). Cape Town: Oxford University Press.

Gilliland, S. W. (1993). The perceived fairness of selection systems: An organizational justice perspective. *Academy of Management Review, 18(4)*, 694–734.

Greenberg, J. (1990). Organizational justice: Yesterday, today, and tomorrow. *Journal of Management, 16(2)*, 399–432.

Henning, R., Theron, C. C. & Spangenberg, H. H. (2004). An investigation into the internal structure of the unit performance construct as measured by the Performance Index (PI). *South African Journal of Industrial Psychology, 30(2)*, 26–36.

Heuchert, J. W. P., Parker, W. D., Stumpf, H. & Myburgh, C. P. H. (2000). The Five-Factor Model of personality in South African college students. *American Behavioral Scientist, 44(1)*, 112–125.

Huysamen, G. K. (2004). Statistical and extra-statistical considerations in differential item functioning analyses. *South African Journal of Industrial Psychology, 30(4)*, 44–57.

Huysamen, G. K. (2006). Recent proposals to estimate transient error within the classical test theory tradition. *South African Journal of Industrial Psychology, 32(4)*, 41–47.

Jonker, S. S. & Vosloo, C. (2008). The psychometric properties of the Schutte Emotional Intelligence Scale. *South African Journal of Industrial Psychology, 34(2)*, 21–30.

Joseph, L. & Van Lille, B. (2008). Investigating subscale differences among race and language groups on the Occupational Personality Profile. *South African Journal of Psychology, 38(3)*, 501–514.

Joubert, T. & Kriek, H. J. (2009). Psychometric comparison of paper-and-pencil and online personality assessments in a selection setting. *South African Journal of Industrial Psychology, 35(1)*, 78–88.

La Grange, L. & Roodt, G. (2001). Personality and cognitive ability as predictors of the job performance of insurance sales people. *South African Journal of Industrial Psychology, 27(3)*, 35–43.

Laher, S. (2008). Structural equivalence and the NEO-PI-R: Implications for the applicability of the Five Factor Model of personality in an African context. *South African Journal of Industrial Psychology, 34(1)*, 76–80.

Leventhal, G. S. (1980). What should be done with equity theory? New approaches to the study of fairness in social relationships. In K. J. Gergen, M. S. Greenberg & R. H. Willis (Eds), *Social Exchange: Advances in Theory and Research* (pp. 27–55). New York, NY: Plenum.

Lopes, A., Roodt, G. & Mauer, R. (2001). The predictive validity of the APIL-B in a financial institution. *South African Journal of Industrial Psychology, 27(1)*, 61–69.

Magwaza, S. (1995). Humanising and democratizing assessments. *People Dynamics, 13*, 12–15.

Martin, G. & Durrheim, K. (2006). Racial recruitment in post-apartheid South Africa: Dilemmas of private recruitment agencies. *Psychology in Society, 33*, 1–15.

Meiring, D., Van de Vijver, F. J. R. & Rothmann, S. (2006). Bias in an adapted version of the 15FQ+ in South Africa. *South African Journal of Psychology, 36(2)*, 340–356.

Meiring, D., Van de Vijver, F. J. R., Rothmann, S. & Barrick, M. R. (2005). Construct, method, and item bias of cognitive and personality tests in South Africa. *South African Journal of Industrial Psychology, 31(1)*, 1–8.

Moerdyk, A. (2009). *The Principles and Practice of Psychological Assessment*. Pretoria: Van Schaik.

Muller, J. & Schepers, J. (2003). The predictive validity of the selection battery used for junior leader training within the South African National Defence Force. *South African Journal of Industrial Psychology, 29(3)*, 87–98.

Murphy, R. & Maree, D. J. F. (2009). Revisiting core issues in dynamic assessment. *South African Journal of Psychology, 39(4)*, 420–431.

Nel, H. & De Villiers, W. S. (2004). The relationship between emotional intelligence and job performance in a call centre environment. *South African Journal of Industrial Psychology, 30(3)*, 75–81.

Nicholls, M., Viviers, A. M. & Visser, D. (2009). Validation of a test battery for the selection of call centre operators in a communications company. *South African Journal of Psychology, 39(1)*, 19–31.

Nzama, L., De Beer, M. & Visser, D. (2008). Predicting work performance through selection interview ratings and psychological assessment. *South African Journal of Industrial Psychology, 34(3),* 39–47.

Nzimande, B. (1995). To test or not to test? Unpublished paper presented at the Congress of Psychometrics for Psychologists and Personnel Practitioners, Pretoria, June 5.

Paterson, H. & Uys, K. (2005). Critical issues in psychological test use in the South African workplace. *South African Journal of Industrial Psychology, 31(3),* 12–22.

Pelser, M., Bergh, Z. C. & Visser, D. (2005). The concurrent validity of learning potential and psychomotor ability measures for the selection of haul truck operators in an open-pit mine. *South African Journal of Industrial Psychology, 31(2),* 58–70.

Potgieter, T. E. & Van der Merwe, R. P. (2002). Assessments in the workplace: A competency-based approach. *South African Journal of Industrial Psychology, 28(1),* 60–66.

Prinsloo, C. H. & Ebersöhn, I. (2002). Fair usage of personality assessment in South Africa: A response to Abrahams and Mauer with special reference to issues of research methodology. *South African Journal of Psychology, 32(3),* 48–57.

Rothmann, S. & Cilliers, F. V. N. (2007). Present challenges and some critical issues for research in industrial/organisational psychology in South Africa. *South African Journal of Industrial Psychology, 33(1),* 8–17.

Schaap, P. (2001). Determining differential item functioning and its effect on the test scores of selected PIB indexes, using item response theory techniques. *South African Journal of Industrial Psychology, 27(2),* 32–38.

Schaap, P. & Basson, J. S. (2003). The construct equivalence of the PIB/SpEEx motivation index for applicants from diverse cultural backgrounds. *South African Journal of Industrial Psychology, 29(2),* 49–59.

Schaap, P. & Vermeulen, T. (2008). The construct equivalence and item bias of the PIB/SpEEx conceptualisation-ability test for members of five language groups in South Africa. *South African Journal of Industrial Psychology, 43(3),* 29–38.

Schepers, J. M. (2002). Construction of a computerised information-processing test battery. *South African Journal of Industrial Psychology, 28(2),* 55–66.

Schroder, H. M. (2004). The fallacy of using in-basket based measures for the validation of leadership dimensions. *South African Journal of Industrial Psychology, 30(2),* 106.

Sehlapelo, M. & Terre Blanche, M. (1996). Psychometric testing in South Africa: Views from above and below. *Psychology in Society, 21,* 49–59.

Spangenberg, H. H. & Theron, C. C. (2003). Validation of the high performance leadership competencies as measured by an assessment centre in-basket. *South African Journal of Industrial Psychology, 29(2),* 29–38.

Spangenberg, H. H. & Theron, C. C. (2004). Rejoinder to articles by Harold M. Schroder: The fallacy of using in-basket based measures for the validation of leadership dimensions. *South African Journal of Industrial Psychology, 30(2),* 107–108.

Stead, G. B. (2002). The transformation of psychology in a post-apartheid South Africa: An overview. *International Journal of Group Tensions, 31(1),* 79–102.

Stone-Romero, E. F. & Stone, D. L. (2005). How do organizational justice concepts relate to discrimination and prejudice? In J. Greenberg & J. A. Colquitt (Eds), *Handbook of Organizational Justice* (pp. 439–462). Mahwah, NJ: Lawrence Erlbaum Associates.

Stuart, A. & Paquet, A. (2001). Emotional intelligence as a determinant of leadership potential. *South African Journal of Industrial Psychology, 27(3),* 30–34.

Sugreen, G. & Schepers, P. (2006). The association of the selected SpEEx-battery indices with the constructs of the Multifactor Leadership Questionnaire. *South African Journal of Industrial Psychology, 32(1)*, 42–51.

Theron, C. (2007). Confessions, scapegoats and flying pigs: Psychometric testing and the law. *South African Journal of Industrial Psychology, 33(1)*, 102–117.

Theron, C. (2009). The diversity-validity dilemma: In search of minimum adverse impact and maximum utility. *South African Journal of Industrial Psychology, 35(1)*, 183–195.

Theron, D. & Roodt, G. (2000). Mental models as moderating variable in 360-degree competency assessments. *South African Journal of Industrial Psychology, 26(7)*, 14–19.

Theron, D. & Roodt, G. (2001). An evaluation of the 360° project management competency assessment questionnaire. *South African Journal of Industrial Psychology, 2(2)*, 51–56.

Van der Merwe, R. (2002). Psychometric testing and human resource management. *South African Journal of Industrial Psychology, 28(2)*, 77–86.

Van de Vijver, F. J. R. & Rothmann, S. (2004). Assessment in multicultural groups: The South African case. *South African Journal of Industrial Psychology, 30(4)*, 1–7.

Van Eeden, R. & Mantsha, T. R. (2007). Theoretical and methodological considerations in the translation of the 16PF5 into an African language. *South African Journal of Psychology, 37(1)*, 62–81.

Viljoen, M. J., Schepers, J. M. & Van Zyl, K. (2001). The construction and evaluation of a normative learning style preference questionnaire. *South African Journal of Industrial Psychology, 27(3)*, 51–60.

Visser, D. & De Jong, A. (2001). Comparing fairness perceptions of personnel selection techniques of American, French and South African job applicants. *Journal of Industrial Psychology, 27(2)*, 62–68.

Visser, D. & Du Toit, J. M. (2004). Using the Occupational Personality Questionnaire (OPQ) for measuring broad traits. *South African Journal of Industrial Psychology, 30(4)*, 65–77.

Visser, D. & Matthews, J. D. L. (2005). The power of non-verbal communication: Predicting job performance by means of thin slices of non-verbal behaviour. *South African Journal of Psychology, 35(2)*, 362–383.

Visser, D. & Viviers, R. (2010). Construct equivalence of the OPQ32N for black and white people in South Africa. *South African Journal of Industrial Psychology, 36(1)*, 1–11.

Vorster, A. & Roodt, G. (2003). A psychometric approach to supervisory competency assessment. *South African Journal of Industrial Psychology, 29(3)*, 38–44.

Wallis, T. (2004). Psychological tests do not measure what they claim to measure: A re-evaluation of the concept of construct validity. *South African Journal of Psychology, 34(1)*, 101–112.

Wallis, T. & Birt, M. (2003). A comparison of native and non-native English-speaking groups' understanding of the vocabulary contained within the 16PF (SA92). *South African Journal of Psychology, 33(3)*, 182–190.

34 Assessment of prior learning: a South African perspective

R. Osman

Assessment in all its dimensions is a contested idea. Part of the contestation rests on the potential for assessment practices to exclude individuals, be it from work, from university and from schooling or, of course, from life opportunities. This contestation is sharpened when assessment of individuals on the basis of race is used to exclude individuals and indeed whole communities from equal opportunities to access work, university, school or any other context which has the potential to enhance a person's livelihood. In South Africa, a country which is strongly racialised, and one in which race was used as a factor to exclude the majority from access to basic opportunities, assessment and rethinking assessment take on a profound role – a role that must ensure the equalisation of opportunities between people, rather than the continued differentiation of opportunities offered to people, based on race. This will require careful shifts in how we think about assessment and how we practise it. We need to develop a view about what a just and equal society means for all of us, individually and collectively, and we need to rigorously explore the implications this has for assessment. Whatever the position that we take on this matter, it is clear that the implications for assessment in all its dimensions ought to be not only significant, but also society-changing in the most positive of ways.

This chapter argues that a greater understanding of alternative and even complementary approaches to psychometric testing and assessment would make an important contribution to conceptualising and implementing assessment practices that are fair as well as transparent, and that have an equalising effect in a divided society such as ours. However, there is a need to identify and even to develop such alternative and complementary approaches to psychometric testing in such a manner that assessors can engage with them effectively. With this need in mind, this chapter will explore a practical form of assessment that could potentially complement and perhaps even enhance psychometric testing in the South African context. It will proffer the portfolio of learning as an effective way to assess the prior learning of adults in higher education. By focusing on the assessment of prior knowledge, irrespective of where such knowledge originates, the chapter offers insights into the transformative potential of the portfolio for individual learning and development.

Recognition of Prior Learning: the South African context

The Recognition of Prior Learning (RPL) approach foregrounds ideas about open and fair processes of access and assessment. It is also a process through which an individual can make a claim to knowledge that she or he has which is up for assessment and evaluation. The aim of this assessment, undertaken by an assessor, is to validate such knowledge either for entry into an existing academic programme in a university or for obtaining a credit within such a programme. RPL can also be used to accredit an assessee's learning in terms of what they know and can do in a particular domain or field of expertise. This form of accreditation or recognition does not depend on any prerequisites, such as a previous qualification. What it does is provide access to learning, and encourages adults to seek opportunities for further learning and education. Ralphs (2012) reminds us that RPL was introduced in South Africa to address the transformation imperatives after 1994, by attempting to provide access to learning for those who had been excluded due to apartheid, and to encourage lifelong learning by creating opportunities for learning obtained from other sites, such as work and recreation, to be accredited. Finally, RPL was introduced as part of the National Qualifications Framework (NQF) so that the learning which was acquired informally could interface seamlessly with other forms of learning in the framework, ensuring that all people would find their place in the framework and not only those who had a formal qualification. This strong social justice agenda, coupled with a developmental agenda of providing new learning routes and pathways for those who had been excluded by apartheid, is what characterised the introduction of RPL in South Africa.

Overall, the uptake of RPL in South African higher education has been uneven. To date, national guidelines for the implementation of RPL are vague, and there is a dearth of research on existing RPL programmes and very little on the experiences of people who have participated in such programmes – that is, assessors and recipients. No comparative studies of RPL practices across academic and occupational settings are available, and most studies focus on RPL as an assessment device, examining the procedures rather than the methods of RPL interventions (Ralphs, 2007).

Ralphs (2007) points out that the uptake is in small projects in the fields of adult education, teacher education, nursing education, and management and leadership, based in higher education institutions. Where the uptake is bigger, it is usually in sectors that have to comply with newly established legal and professional standards, such as the financial and constructions sectors.

In addition to the practical challenges associated with RPL, the assessment of prior learning raises many questions in the realm of assessment. For example, what assessment methods can be used which allow for assessing the specificity of prior knowledge and, at the same time, for standardisation? Do we understand the complexity of assessing RPL in different contexts, and are the contexts comparable? The practice of assessment, psychometric or otherwise, raises questions of what knowledge can be assessed. Whose knowledge is valid? How should it be validated and against what criteria? What are the costs to assessors as they come into direct conflict with normative values, beliefs and assumptions about assessment prevalent in higher education institutions?

While this chapter may not fully answer all of these questions, it makes visible critical issues about RPL and its assessment dimensions – issues overlooked and sometimes ignored in debates about testing and assessment. It makes clear that in the final analysis all forms of assessment, whether these are psychometric or alternative forms, are underpinned by a particular theory of knowledge and learning, and of the value of such knowledge and learning. How we get our assessees to talk about this learning, and how we choose to assess or recognise this learning, is a complex and far from neutral process. Michelson, Mandell et al. (2004, p.23) remind us that 'such decisions reflect the stated or unstated ideological frameworks that mould our understanding of the social, cultural, economic, and historical contexts within which we and our students live'.

Portfolios as a complementary tool to assessment

Portfolios of learning are usually opportunities for assessees to express the knowledge, understandings and skills that they have gained from experiential activities, be it in the workplace, recreationally or through the activities of life and living. Through a process of reflecting on this learning, an assessee is able to compile a portfolio of learning, which is then assessed or evaluated for its fit with relevant learning outcomes in an institution, a degree programme or a course. The degree of fit will determine whether the assessee can claim a credit for such learning and avoid having to redo or repeat what is already known from experience. This process of reflecting on one's learning and then representing it in a way that matches the learning outcomes of a programme or course sometimes enables the assessee to develop a deeper understanding of his or her own knowledge. Unlike psychometric testing, which can be completed in a short period of time and interpreted relatively easily, reflecting on one's learning in a portfolio of activities is time-intensive, in that the assessee/RPL applicant is expected to receive feedback on their representation of the knowledge. This process of formative feedback is ongoing while the portfolio of experience is being developed. Coupled with this formative feedback is the need for an assessee-friendly environment in which such feedback and assessment occur. Such feedback and assessment also require sustained guidance, mentoring and support from the assessor.

This emphasis on reflection draws on the work of Kolb (1984), who posited an experiential learning cycle as the basis of adult learning. He suggested that adult learners engage in a process that takes them from a concrete experience to reflection, to drawing inferences and making generalisations on the basis of experience, and then testing these inferences by engaging in a new experience. Challis (1993, p.40) points out that 'it is important to remember here that past experiences are being recalled in order to identify not the events themselves, but the learning that can be identified as having arisen from that experience'.

Similarly, Whitaker (1989, p.11) states unequivocally that 'experience is good for many things, but ... credit should be awarded ... only for *learning* and not for experience' (emphasis in original).

Assessment techniques used in the portfolio method include interviews, reflective writing tasks, portfolios of learning and portfolio development courses, with portfolios of learning and portfolio development courses playing a significant role. Typically, such portfolios require assessees to reflect on prior experience by analysing learning moments and events that were significant to them. This usually culminates in a reflective essay in which assessees move beyond description of experience to analysis of learning that has emerged from such experience (Castle & Attwood, 2001). Assessees then assemble evidence that supports such claims of learning from experience, which includes certificates of formal learning and project work done by the assessee as well as testimonials from the workplace. An alternative to the reflective essay would be a task that requires assessees to reflect on their prior learning and represent this learning in a way that would be comparable to competencies set for the courses in which access or credit is being sought. The emphasis, in the portfolio approach to assessment results, is on an enhanced sense of individual well-being, respect for experience and individual empowerment through education. In South Africa, this form of assessment is in sharp contrast to the types of assessments that were used under apartheid, which were designed and implemented to undermine learners' sense of self-worth.

Michelson (1997; 1998) cautions that the reflective, autobiographical modes are not appropriate for all assessees. Similarly, Usher (1989) reminds us that the emphasis on articulating learning with outcomes and competencies is reminiscent of behaviourist approaches to assessment. In South Africa, Volbrecht (2009) also cautions that the effectiveness of the portfolio process depends on reflection, and this requires the assessee to use information from informal learning settings clearly and accurately. This is not always possible, as sometimes experience has to be extracted from the distant past and information about such learning is not readily available. Cretchley and Castle (2001, p.489) also point out that this assessment process through portfolios can be 'unwieldy' and require 'high-level language skills'. Again, this is potentially exclusionary if the portfolio process is conducted in a language that is different to the one that the assessor speaks. In some ways this language difference or the need for high-level language skills could alienate the assessee from his or her experience (Osman, 2004; Trowler, 1996). This echoes the repeated difficulties mentioned elsewhere in this volume regarding language proficiency and assessment. In spite of this critique, the portfolio approach is attractive because it provides an opportunity for adult learners to make what they have learnt from experience visible and measurable. This approach to assessment also gives assessees an enhanced understanding of themselves as knowledge makers and knowledge seekers. The potential for achieving self-empowerment and self-knowledge is worthwhile in itself. Volbrecht (2009) rightly asserts that RPL should be about learning and about assessment. In some ways this holds true for all forms of assessment – there is a need for a learning dimension to assessment, or what

Boud (2000, p.151) calls 'sustainable assessment'. Boud argues that assessment practices in higher education 'tend not to equip students well for the processes of effective learning in a learning society ... sustainable assessment encompasses the abilities required to undertake those activities that necessarily accompany learning throughout life in formal and informal settings' (p.151).

Is an RPL assessment through the portfolio valid?

Andersson (2006, p.40) offers an interesting position on the question of the validity of RPL assessments – be they formative assessments (like the portfolio discussed in this chapter) or summative assessments (like multiple-choice questions): 'To make claims of validity you have to know what you intend to assess.' Depending on what is being assessed, Andersson, drawing on the work of Kvale (1996), offers four types of validity: predictive, pragmatic, content and communicative validity. He argues that if the function of RPL through the portfolio is the development of the individual and his or her learning, then pragmatic validity is high because it is related to the formative function of RPL. By way of contrast, the predictive validity of RPL assessment through the portfolio may be low, as it will be difficult to tell how the assessee will do in the programme or course to which she or he has gained access after having completed the portfolio. Despite evidence of statistical validity in psychometric tests, this is generally based on the assumption that all individuals tested come from the same backgrounds, an assumption that cannot be made in South Africa.

Final thoughts

This chapter has foregrounded a number of questions relating to RPL and ways of thinking about acquired knowledge and its assessment. Portfolios as a complementary tool for assessment, particularly in occupational and aptitude testing, are an innovation that will require a variety of shifts. They require an institutional culture that is responsive to subjective orientations to assessment, an orientation not commonly found in South African universities. Using portfolios to assess students calls for assessors who understand psychometric testing and alternative forms of testing such as portfolios, who can cross the boundary between these approaches and then assist in a viable collaboration between different forms of assessment. Portfolios of assessment cannot replace psychometric assessment, as they are focusing on slightly different objectives, but they may complement psychometric assessment and assessment for learning. Messick (1989) reminds us that assessments construct societies, and have consequences for societies. The task before us is to deconstruct and undo the negative effects of and attitudes towards assessment in our society, and to be vigilant about the effects of assessment on society, since, 'all acts of assessment involve more than is apparent and we must judge them accordingly' (Boud, 2000, p.166). RPL gives assessees an opportunity to exercise a measure of control over assessment, and is transparent and fair. It does not discriminate between assessees (as psychometric tests do), and instead discriminates between different levels of learning from experience. While no single approach to portfolios as a means of assessment can be deemed most appropriate, they should be seen as an alternative form of assessing adult students' prior knowledge – an idea and practice of assessment that is open to change and possibilities. They also hold promise for affirming adult students entering higher education, as they learn about themselves and feel confident as learners and as human beings. In South Africa, where educational assessment under apartheid was synonymous with undermining adults' sense of themselves as human beings and as learners, individual and collective assessment through portfolios could be one of the thrusts for equity in education. More importantly, entrenched educational inequalities in South Africa compel teachers in higher education to explore alternatives to the logic and practice of assessment, as is evidenced by the chapters in this volume. The challenge is to engage in such an exploration with integrity, and to work responsibly with claims about assessment being objective and fair.

References

Andersson, P. (2006). Different faces and functions of RPL: An assessment perspective. In P. Andersson & J. Harris (Eds), *Re-theorising the Recognition of Prior Learning* (pp. 31–50). Leicester: National Institute of Adult Continuing Education.

Boud, D. (2000). Sustainable assessment: Rethinking assessment for the learning society. *Studies in Continuing Education, 22(2)*, 151–167.

Castle, J. & Attwood, G. (2001). Recognition of prior learning (RPL) for access or credit? Problematic issues in a university adult education department in South Africa. *Studies in the Education of Adults, 33(1)*, 60–72.

Challis, M. (1993). *Introducing APEL*. London: Routledge.

Cretchley, G. & Castle, J. (2001). OBE, RPL and adult education: Good bedfellows in higher education in South Africa? *International Journal of Lifelong Education, 26(6)*, 487–501.

Kolb, D. A. (1984). *Experiential Learning*. New York, NY: Prentice-Hall.

Kvale, S. (1996). Evaluation as construction of knowledge. In P. Hayhoe & J. Pan (Eds), *East–West Dialogue in Knowledge and Higher Education* (pp. 117–140). New York, NY: M. E. Sharp.

Messick, S. (1989). Validity. In R. L. Linn (Ed.), *Educational Measurement* (3rd edition, pp. 13–104). New York, NY: Macmillan.

Michelson, E. (1997). The politics of memory: The recognition of experiential learning. In S. Walters (Ed.), *Globalization, Adult Education and Training: Impacts and Issues* (pp. 141–153). London: Zed Books.

Michelson, E. (1998). *Expanding the Logic of Portfolio-assisted Assessment: Lessons from South Africa*. New York, NY: National Centre on Adult Education.

Michelson, E., Mandell, A. & Contributors (2004). *Portfolio Development and the Assessment of Prior Learning* (2nd edition). Sterling, VA: Stylus.

Osman, R. (2004). Making the invisible visible: Portfolios and prior knowledge in higher education. *South African Journal of Higher Education, 18(3)*, 305–315.

Ralphs, A. (2007). Specialised pedagogy: A comparative study of RPL practices within the changing landscape of the NQF in South Africa: Conceptual maps and navigation tools. Paper presented at the 5th International Research Work and Learning Conference. Cape Town, December 3–5.

Ralphs, A. (2012). Exploring RPL: Assessment device and/or specialised pedagogical practice. *Journal of Education 53*, 75–96.

Trowler, P. (1996). Angels in marble? Accrediting prior experiential learning in higher education. *Studies in Higher Education, 21(1)*, 17–30.

Usher, R. (1989). Qualification, paradigms and experiential learning in higher education. In O. Fulton (Ed.), *Access and Institutional Change* (pp. 64–81). Milton Keynes: Society for Research into Higher Education & Open University Press.

Volbrecht, T. (2009). New courses for Trojan horses: Rethinking RPL in a South African teacher education curriculum. *Studies in Continuing Education, 31(1)*, 13–27.

Whitaker, U. (1989). *Assessing Learning: Standards, Principles and Procedures*. Philadelphia, PA: Council for Adult Experiential Learning.

35 Large-scale assessment studies in South Africa: trends in reporting results to schools

A. Kanjee

The significant increase in the use of large-scale assessment studies (LSAS) for education reform (Benveniste, 2002; Kellaghan & Greaney, 2001; UNESCO, 2000) can be attributed to a number of causes, including the focus on learning outcomes as an indicator for education quality, the emphasis on the results agenda as advocated by the international donor community (Lockheed, 2011), and the impact of globalisation on education in general and assessment in particular (Carnoy, 2000; Jansen, 2001). The focus on measuring learning outcomes as an indicator of education quality was advocated at the 1990 Education For All (EFA) world conference in Jomtien (UNESCO, 2000), and reinforced at the 2000 EFA world conference in Dakar (Kellaghan & Greaney, 2003). The emphasis on cognitive outcomes is best understood when viewed in the context of the following argument presented in the EFA Global Monitoring Report (UNESCO, 2004, p.43):

> ... there is good evidence to suggest that the quality of education – as measured by test scores – has an influence upon the speed with which societies can become richer and the extent to which individuals can improve their own productivity and incomes. We also know that years of education and acquisition of cognitive skills – particularly the core skills of literacy and numeracy – have economic and social pay-offs ... Education systems that are more effective in establishing cognitive skills to an advanced level and distributing them broadly through the population will bring stronger social and economic benefits than less effective systems.

While LSAS have the potential to significantly impact on what is taught and how it is taught (Abu-Alhija, 2007; Black & Wiliam, 2007), there has been limited focus on the impact of these studies on the learning and teaching process (Kellaghan & Greaney, 2003; Pellegrino, Chudowsky & Glaser, 2001; UNESCO, 2000). It is also widely recognised that the number of countries conducting LSAS is likely to increase in the future (Forster, 2002). Given the significant financial and human resource investments required for conducting LSAS, there is an urgent need to ensure that these studies yield greater value for money – that is, an increase in learning outcomes. However, there is limited information pertaining to the cost benefit of these studies (Kellaghan & Greaney, 2001).

That LSAS can play a useful role in the learning and teaching process is beyond question (Schiefelbein & Schiefelbein, 2003). What is critical, however, is how information obtained from large-scale assessments is utilised to impact on education reform in general, and improving learning outcomes in particular. This chapter reviews how LSAS have been applied in the South African context and determines whether, and how, these studies have reported information that can be used in improving learning outcomes.

The chapter begins with a definition of LSAS, highlighting their different applications in addressing the information needs of teachers and policy makers. Next, trends in the use of LSAS, with some examples of different formats for analysis and reporting information, are noted. The chapter concludes by highlighting some of the challenges in the effective use of LSAS in South Africa.

Definition and uses of large-scale assessment

The primary use of assessment is to obtain relevant information to support learning, to monitor the functioning of learners or education systems, to hold institutions accountable and to certify or select learners (Black & Wiliam, 2007; Kellaghan & Greaney, 2003). A useful criterion for distinguishing the purpose of assessment is whether the assessments are planned and applied by (i) the teacher in the classroom or (ii) relevant authorities outside the classroom – that is, at the school, district, province, national, regional or international level. Classroom assessments are primarily used to support learning, are used on a daily basis by teachers and learners, and comprise a range of methods that include practical work, group work, oral presentations and tests. In addition, end-of-year examinations are also conducted by teachers to certify learner competence to proceed to the next grade level. Assessments that are planned and conducted from outside the classroom are used to (i) certify learner competence (for example, national examinations); (ii) monitor and evaluate the functioning of an education system or intervention project (for example, national or district assessment studies conducted to identify areas in need of intervention); (iii) hold teachers, schools or districts accountable (for example, by attaching sanctions or rewards based on results); or (iv) support learning (for example, by providing feedback to teachers for use in addressing common errors made by learners).

In this chapter, a large-scale assessment is defined as any assessment conducted from outside the classroom for the purpose of certification, monitoring and evaluation, accountability and supporting learning.

Review of recent research on assessment

Recent research findings on the use of assessment, at both the systems and classroom levels, have resulted in a significant shift in how assessments are used in the education sector (Abu-Alhija, 2007, Black & Wiliam, 1998; Brown & Hattie, 2003; Harlen, 2005). These findings have provided a richer and deeper understanding of the different functions and uses of assessment, the tensions arising when different functions are conflated, and how to effectively use assessments to support teachers in enhancing learning within the classroom.

Black and Wiliam (2007) distinguish between three practical functions of assessment: evaluative, summative and formative. Evaluative assessments are used to evaluate institutions and curricula, and serve the purpose of accountability; summative assessments are used to certify achievement or potential – that is, provide evidence pertaining to what learners have been or will be able to do; and formative assessment provides feedback to learners about how to go about improving their performance – that is, evidence about learning based on the here and now. All three functions are applicable to LSAS (Shavelson, Black, Wiliam & Coffey, 2003), while only the summative and formative functions are applicable to classroom assessments (Black & Wiliam, 2007; Harlen, 2005).

Pertaining to the use of assessment in practice, a number of studies have demonstrated the tensions created when the same assessments are required to serve multiple purposes (Abu-Alhija, 2007; Harlen, 2005; Shavelson et al., 2003). Black and Wiliam (2007, p.8) note that

> while the formative and summative functions of assessment may not be completely incompatible, there are clearly tensions between the two, because they serve different needs. Where the formative function is paramount, the requirement is for evidence that provides a dependable guide to instructional action, so the inferences are very much in the 'here and now'. Where the summative function is paramount, the requirement is for evidence that supports inferences about what the student has been, is, or might be able to do ...

While Harlen (2005) also argues for maintaining the distinction between formative and summative functions, he further notes that the assessment system should be planned and implemented to enable evidence of students' ongoing learning to be used for both purposes.

Addressing the challenges in effectively using large-scale assessments in New Zealand, Brown and Hattie (2003) propose eight principles for developing a national assessment system to support teachers in enhancing learning. The principles assert that 'national' assessment should

- mirror important rich ideas;
- make rich ideas rather than items dominant;
- have low-stakes consequences;
- use more than tests to communicate standards;
- ensure that 'national' compatibility information is available;
- ensure that teachers value it as part of teaching;
- assess what is taught; and
- provide meaningful feedback to all participants.

These principles have been applied in the successful implementation of the Assessment Tools for Teaching and Learning programme in New Zealand (Brown & Hattie, 2003).

Assessment in South Africa

Besides public examinations that have been a feature of the South African education landscape for several decades, the number of other LSAS that have been conducted since the mid-1990s has also increased significantly (Kanjee, 2006). These studies have been conducted at different levels of the system – national, provincial and district – by education departments, research agencies, non-governmental organisations as well as universities (Department of Education, 2003; 2004; Kanjee, 2006). In addition, significant resources have been invested in implementing these studies. However, limited information is available on the impact of LSAS on learning and teaching practices in South African schools, in particular on how information from these studies has been used to support teachers in improving learning in the classroom. In this section, a number of these studies are reviewed to identify, in each case, the purpose of the study and the target audience, and to provide examples of results reported (focusing specifically on mathematics) that could be of use to teachers in the classroom. First, a brief review is presented of the role of assessment under the apartheid regime to provide a context for understanding the changes that have taken place since then and the challenges that need to be addressed.

Two main points emerge from an analysis of the history of assessment practices in South Africa. First, assessment practices were closely linked to the oppressive apartheid policies of the state, and second, current assessment practices within the education sector emerged and developed from within the psychological sector in South Africa. From the very beginning, (intelligence) testing in South Africa has been used by the state to produce theories of intellectual differences between races (Appel, 1989; Bulhan, 1980; Mathonsi, 1988; Nzimande, 1995; Swartz, 1992; Whittaker, 1990). With regard to his research on the 'Educability of the South African Native', Fick (1929, cited in Whittaker, 1990, p.56) concluded that 'the inferiority of the Native (African) in educability as shown by the measurement of their actual achievement in education, limits considerably the proportion of Natives who can benefit by education of the ordinary type beyond the rudimentary level'.

Although conducted in the context of psychology, and not specifically for educational purposes, the findings of these (certainly at that stage) prominent and influential academics laid the foundation for the way in which educational assessment was to be conducted in South Africa in later years. This is demonstrated by both Mathonsi (1988) and Nzimande (1995), who argue that tests were intentionally misused to deprive blacks of access to resources and opportunity, and that the intellectual development of blacks was stifled in a conscious and systematic manner to meet the needs of the white minority for a cheap source of labour. This took the form of an elaborate system of tests and examinations by means of which control of and entry into the economy was regulated (Swartz, 1992). It is thus no surprise that the emphasis in education was geared towards rote learning, and was examination-orientated. The development of critical thought and active student participation in the learning-teaching process was actively discouraged; rather, students were viewed as mere passive recipients of information (Kallaway, 1984).

The primary purpose of assessment was for classification – for example, into different grade levels – and for selection for promotion purposes. The use of assessment for monitoring, evaluation, diagnosis of learner problems or early identification of learning difficulties was certainly not a common phenomenon, especially in black schools (Malaka, 1995). Malaka attributes this, at the classroom level, to the lack of emphasis on assessment in teacher training programmes, the poor qualifications of teachers in general and in the area of assessment in particular, and the limited time spent on assessing learners. At the provincial or national level, reasons for the lack of an adequate assessment system can clearly be linked to the government's apartheid policies and, to some extent, to the lack of technical expertise (Kanjee, 1998). This situation, however, proved beneficial to the apartheid state as any system that allowed for critical evaluation of the education system or development of relevant intervention strategies would have been perceived as a threat to state hegemony. The fact that the development of any technical expertise in the area of assessment was not actively promoted, and that most of the available expertise was located in the state-controlled, or at the very least state-aligned (and -funded) organisations, attests to this fact (Cloete, Muller & Orkin, 1986).

Recently, however, assessment has taken centre stage in many debates, research projects, conferences and policy documents, where the critical and relevant issues are beginning to be addressed (Department of Education, 1998; 2007; Kanjee, 1998; 2006; Lubisi & Murphy, 2002; Taylor & Vinjevold, 1999). For example, the Curriculum 2005 review committee argued for the need for 'a coherent policy document on assessment aligned with the curriculum and containing clear guidelines and procedures, and greater attention to assessment in teacher preparation for the new curriculum' (Department of Education, 2000, p.19). In addition, the national assessment policy passed in December 1998 for the General Education and Training band, Grades R–9 and Adult Basic Education and Training, was recently revised with a greater emphasis being placed on the formative use of assessment information in the classroom (Department of Education, 2007). Kanjee (2006) provides an overview of the increasing use of national assessment studies in South Africa since the mid-1990s. It is within this context that the value and use of LSAS in South Africa should be viewed.

LSAS in South Africa

A review of LSAS conducted in South Africa over the past decade reveals a range of different purposes for these studies. Table 35.1 summarises the primary purposes, target audiences, grade levels and content areas targeted, and time periods during which these studies were conducted.

Table 35.1 Summary of LSAS conducted in South Africa since 1996

Name	Purpose	Primary audience	Organisation	Content	Date
Grade 9 Longitudinal Study	To 'establish a benchmark instrument that could be used to monitor changes in learner achievement over time' (Govender, 1998, p.3)	Researchers	HSRC	Grade 9: English, Maths, Science	1996
Monitoring Learning Achievement project	To 'provide up to date information for decision makers at national and sub-national level …' (Chinapah et al., 2000, p.4)	Policy makers	Department of Education & UNESCO/UNICEF	Grade 4: Literacy, Life Skills, Numeracy	1999
District-Wide Reading Improvement Program	To (i) determine the level of reading attainment of Grade 3 learners in the Gauteng Department of Education District S1 (Benoni/Brakpan); (ii) track the reading attainment gap between historically advantaged and disadvantaged schools; (iii) obtain information to guide intervention programmes for improving the reading ability of Foundation Phase learners in the district; and (iv) serve as a baseline for evaluation of current and future intervention programmes (Gauteng Department of Education, 2000)	District officials	Gauteng Dept. of Education, District S1	Grade 3: English Reading and Writing	1999
Evaluation of the Quality Learning Programme	To 'determine the impact of the intervention programs on the performance of districts, schools, teachers and learners' (Kanjee & Prinsloo, 2005, p.2)	Funders, programme managers	HSRC	Grades 9 and 11: English, Maths	2000, 2002, 2004
Grade 3 Systemic Evaluation	To '(a) serve as a baseline for future systemic evaluation studies, and (b) make appropriate recommendations regarding national education policy implementation' (Department of Education, 2003, p.7)	Policy makers	Department of Education	Grade 3: Literacy, Life Skills, Numeracy	2001, 2007

Name	Purpose	Primary audience	Organisation	Content	Date
Assessment Modelling Initiative	To 'pilot a District Assessment System comprising: development of Assessment Resource Banks (ARBs) for assisting educators improve learning, and conducting uniform assessments to determine changes in performance of Grade 3 learners' (Claassen, Makgamatha & Kanjee, 2003, p.1)	Teachers, district officials, programme managers, funders	HSRC	Grades R– 6: Maths/Numeracy, Literacy/English Grade 3: Literacy, Numeracy	2001–2003 2000, 2001, 2002
Monitoring Trends in Education Quality	To '(a) demonstrate best practices regarding the implementation of national assessment (systemic evaluation) studies in South Africa, with specific focus on methods and procedures for data analysis, reporting and use; (b) identify standards of performance and apply appropriate methods of establishing and reporting on these standards; (c) measure changes in Grade 9 learner performance from 1996 to 2002; (d) identify and develop relevant indicators to accurately represent the context of learning and teaching across the range of schools; (e) identify factors that affect learner performance; and (f) establish a national baseline for Grade 9 to monitor the impact of the new curriculum' (Kanjee & Povey, 2006, p.3)	Policy makers, researchers	HSRC	Grade 9: English, Maths, Science	2002, 2010
Grade 6 Systemic Evaluation	To 'benchmark performance and track the progress made towards the achievement of the transformational goals of access, redress, equity and quality' (Department of Education, 2004, p.6)	Policy makers	Department of Education	Grade 6: English, Maths, Science	2004
Teacher Guides	To '(i) share information on what learners were able and not able to do in the Mathematics task, (ii) provide examples of questions used in the systemic evaluation as well as typical answers that learners gave, (iii) provide some "Tips for teaching" to address similar problems among learners' (Department of Education, 2005, p.2)	Teachers	Department of Education	Grade 6: English, Maths, Science	2005

continued →

Name	Purpose	Primary audience	Organisation	Content	Date
Integrated Education Programme Evaluation	To '(i) evaluate progress made towards achieving the overall project goal of improving student performance in participating schools, and (ii) determine the extent to which the IEP intervention has made an impact on the teaching and learning in IEP schools' (JET, 2008, p.3)	Funders, programme managers	JET Education Services	Grade 3: Literacy, Numeracy Grade 6: Maths, Science	2004, 2005, 2006
Primary Mathematics Research Project	To 'make available to policy makers and other participants in the education system, an accurate, empirical and national picture of what was happening to primary-level mathematics ...' (Schollar, 2004, p.8)	Policy makers, researcher	E Schollar & Associates	Grades 5 & 7: Numeracy/Maths	2004
Assessment of Language and Mathematics Skills	'(i) to measure achievement in mathematics and language of WCED learners, (ii) to benchmark WCED learners' achievement against student achievement in other countries, (iii) to prioritise learners with potential and inform the WCED's trajectory of developing and supporting effective learning and teaching processes' (Heugh, Diedricks, Prinsloo & Herbst, 2007, p.4)	Policy makers, school principals, learners	Western Cape Education Department (WCED)	Grade 8: Maths, English	2006
SACMEQ	To (i) equip educational planners in member countries with the technical skills needed for effectively monitoring and evaluating schooling and the quality of education, and (ii) engage in collaborative research which address priority policy concerns regarding enhancing the quality of education and achieving EFA goals (Moloi & Strauss, 2005)	Policy makers	Department of Education / UNESCO	Grade 6: English, Maths	2001, 2007

Name	Purpose	Primary audience	Organisation	Content	Date
Trends in International Mathematics and Science Study (TIMSS)	To allow the comparison of performance with other countries and to contribute to improved policy and practice (Reddy, 2006a)	Policy makers, researchers	HSRC / International Association for the Evaluation of Educational Achievement	Grade 8: Maths, Science	1995, 1999, 2003
Progress in International Reading Literacy Study (PIRLS)	The Progress in International Reading Literacy Study was conducted to compare learners' levels of literacy in Grade 4 across a sample of participating countries (approximately 40) (Howie et al., 2009)	Policy makers, researchers	University of Pretoria / IEA	Grade 4	2006
Common Tasks of Assessments	Assessment of Grade 9 learners in Maths, Science and English. Assessment intended to introduce an end-of-compulsory-schooling exit certificate (General Education and Training Certificate). However, this idea was dropped in 2011 in favour of a Grade 9 ANA	Learners, parents, teachers	Provincial and National Departments of Education	Grade 9 Languages and Mathematics	Piloted in 2002. Applied by provinces from 2003 to 2008
Annual National Assessments (ANA)	'At the individual learner level, the ANA results will provide teachers with empirical evidence on what the learner can and/or cannot do at a particular stage or grade and do so at the beginning of the school year. At systemic level, ANA provides reliable data for policy decisions related to provision and support required at various levels of the system. The ANA will make it easier for district offices to determine where support is most urgently needed and by allowing principals, teachers and parents to plan in a more informed manner how to improve performance' (Department of Basic Education, 2010)	Learners, parents, teachers, education officials	Department of Basic Education	Grades 1–6 From 2012: Grade 9	Piloted from 2008; first administered in 2011

A review of the listed studies reveals a number of trends. First, only one of the studies, Assessment Modelling Initiative, focused specifically on providing information to teachers to address the formative functions of assessment, while the primary purposes for the rest of the studies listed were to provide information to policy makers, to evaluate specific intervention programmes, and to obtain baseline information. Recently, the Annual National Assessments (ANA) (Department of Basic Education, 2011) were introduced to provide information to teachers and parents. However, no strategies or systems are in place for the effective dissemination and reporting of assessment information. Second, the most common form of reporting learner performance was based on mean percentage scores, usually reported at national, provincial or district level. Information was also aggregated by gender, language (home language versus language of learning and teaching) and geographical location (urban versus rural). Information was generally presented using both tables and graphs, and reported by learning area (for example, Mathematics) as well as the subdomains assessed (for example, by learning outcomes or by content areas like numeracy or geometry). Third, the provision of relevant examples, taken from responses to test questions, to demonstrate specific response patterns of learners, was a feature of many studies. Fourth, in at least one of the studies reviewed, the following innovations (at least in the South African context) were noted: (i) assessment of teacher content knowledge; (ii) use of advanced data analysis techniques – that is, path analysis and multilevel modelling – to identify impact on learner performance and to determine factors affecting learner performance respectively; (iii) use of matrix sampling designs to obtain comprehensive and in-depth coverage of the curriculum outcomes and assessment standards; and (iv) use of item response theory to equate scores from tests administered at different points in time. Two examples relating to these trends, derived from the studies reviewed, are discussed next.

The Grade 6 Systemic Evaluation

Figure 35.1 Mathematics achievement levels by province

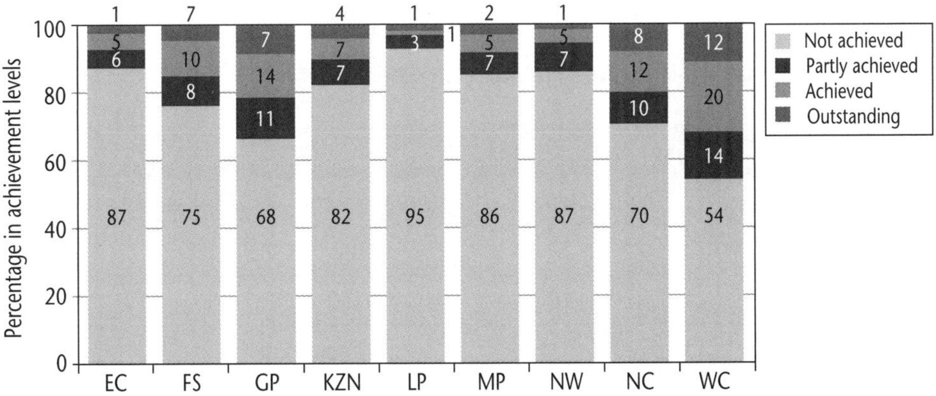

Source: Department of Education (2004, p.82).

The Grade 6 Systemic Evaluation study was conducted by the Department of Education to determine the context within which learning and teaching were taking place and the levels of learner performance across the nine provinces (Department of Education, 2004). Scores for each learning area were reported according to the four achievement levels outlined in the national curriculum, to demonstrate the performance levels at which learners were functioning (see Figure 35.1). At the national level, 81 per cent of learners were functioning at the 'Not Achieved' level in Mathematics, while a small percentage of learners, 12 per cent, were found to be functioning at or above the required Grade 6 level, that is 'Achieved' and 'Outstanding' combined.

The innovation of the Grade 6 study was the reporting of results to teachers. Specifically, Teacher Guides were developed from items administered during the Systemic Evaluation study to provide 'tips' for teachers to use in the classroom to improve learning. The Guides were developed for each of the three learning areas assessed – English, Mathematics and Science – and comprised examples of learner performance on different sections of the learning area, examples of item tasks presented to learners (Figure 35.2), information describing the items (Figure 35.3), average national scores obtained by learners (Figure 35.4), and examples and explanations of learner responses (Figure 35.5).

Figure 35.2 Example of an item

2.1 Understanding number operations

Assessment of understanding number operations includes assessing the ability to do basic calculations and perform simple operations that involve addition, subtraction, multiplication and division, and using these operations to solve given problems.

Example 1: Problem solving using basic operations

In this question learners were required to calculate the cost of items and to write correct answers in the spaces provided on the order form.

Complete the following order form for your school:

ORDER FORM			
Description	No. of items	Price per item	Cost in Rand
Whistle	5	R25	
Soccer Ball	10	R300	
		Total cost	

Source: Department of Education (2005, p.9).

Figure 35.3 Information describing the item

Characteristics of Example 1

Learning outcome:	LO 1: Numbers, operations and relationships
Assessment standard:	Solves problems in context including contexts that may be used in building awareness of other learning areas, as well as human rights, social, economic and environmental issues such as: • financial (including buying and selling, profit and loss, and simple budgets)
Question type:	Short answer
Grade level:	Grade 5
Difficulty level:	Medium
Cognitive category:	Solving routine problems
Correct answer(s):	A = R125 B = R3 000 C TOTAL COST = R3 125
Mark allocation:	3 marks
Scoring guide/key:	3 marks for three correct answers 2 marks for two correct answers 1 mark for one correct answer 0 marks for incorrect answer or no response

Source: Department of Education (2005, p.10).

Figure 35.4 Average scores obtained by learners

Example 1: Results

	% of learners per option
One answer correct	24
Two answers correct	7
Three answers correct	8
Incorrect	46
No response	15
Total	**100**

Most learners did not do well in this question. A few (8%) got all three required answers correct and showed a clear understanding of the problem by ***multiplying*** the cost of one item by the number of items in each case and then ***adding*** to get the total cost for all the items.

Source: Department of Education (2005, p.10).

Figure 35.5 Examples and explanations of learner responses

Example 1: Learner responses

Correct response

ORDER FORM			
Description	No. of items	Price per item	Cost in Rand
Whistle	5	R25	125
Soccer Ball	10	R300	3000
		Total cost	3125

✓

Incorrect response

ORDER FORM			
Description	No. of items	Price per item	Cost in Rand
Whistle	5	R25	R30
Soccer Ball	10	R300	R4000
		Total cost	R70000

✗

In this example, the incorrect responses revealed a number of problem areas:

- In the first row of the order form the learner clearly added the "No. of items (5)" to the "Price per item (R25)" and obtained R30 as the answer.
- In the second row it looks as if both addition and multiplication were used, suggesting a lack of certainty as to which operation was required. When probably adding 10 to R300 a further problem area was displayed, viz. a lack of knowledge of place value, resulting in 'tens' being added to 'hundreds'.
- Lack of knowledge of *place value* was again shown when the learner tried to add the two sub-answers (R30 and R4 000) in the last column of the order form. Here it is uncertain whether the learner tried to multiply as well, probably by 10.

The following possibilities need to be considered and specific steps taken to address them if found to be true:

- Lack of familiarity with tabulated information (e.g. an order form)
- Lack of understanding of place value which then leads to incorrect operations (e.g. in addition and, most likely, in subtraction as well)
- Using 'techniques' without understanding the full process involved in a given operation (e.g. the tendency to add a zero to the answer when multiplying or even adding).

Source: Department of Education (2005, p.11).

The Southern African Consortium for Monitoring Education Quality

The Southern African Consortium for Monitoring Education Quality (SACMEQ) conducts regional assessment surveys within the 15 southern African countries to equip educational planners in member countries with the technical skills needed for effectively monitoring and evaluating schooling and the quality of education, and to engage in collaborative research which addresses priority policy concerns focused on enhancing the quality of education. Since 1995, three regional surveys have been conducted. In the most recent survey, conducted in 2007, a new dimension was added: knowledge about HIV/AIDS. Specifically, learners and teachers were assessed in the following five dimensions: definitions and terminology, transmission mechanisms, avoidance behaviours, diagnosis and treatment, and myths and misconceptions (SACMEQ, 2010).

The instrument for this assessment was based on the assumption that knowledge about HIV/AIDS was a necessary, but not sufficient, requirement to ensure that young people would adopt behaviours that would protect and promote their own health and the health of others, and that ignorance about HIV/AIDS could never provide a sound foundation for wise behaviour. The scores on the HIV-AIDS Knowledge Test (and their standard errors of sampling) have been summarised in Table 35.2 for Grade 6 pupils and their teachers. As noted in Table 35.2, results indicate low levels of knowledge among learners and relatively high levels among teachers. However, an unexplained issue that requires further research relates to the reasons why teachers have not transferred, or were unable to transfer, more knowledge about HIV/AIDS to their learners.

Table 35.2 Performance of Grade 6 pupils and teachers on the SACMEQ HIV/AIDS knowledge test

School system	Pupils						Teachers					
	Transformed score		Reached minimal level		Reached desirable level		Transformed score		Reached minimal level		Reached desirable level	
	Mean	SE	%	SE	%	SE	Mean	SE	%	SE	%	SE
Mauritius	453	5	17	2	2	1	698	6	98	1	63	3
Lesotho	465	4	19	1	5	1	751	8	99	1	82	3
Zimbabwe	477	5	30	2	4	1	785	7	99	0	93	2
Seychelles	488	2	25	1	3	0	789	3	99	0	95	0
Zambia	488	4	35	2	4	1	744	7	98	1	86	2
Uganda	489	4	33	2	4	1	708	9	98	1	72	3
Botswana	499	4	32	2	7	1	782	6	100	0	93	2
SACMEQ	500	4	36	2	7	1	746	7	99	1	82	2
Zanzibar	501	3	38	1	4	0	657	5	94	1	45	3
Namibia	502	3	36	2	6	1	764	6	100	1	87	2
South Africa	503	4	35	2	8	1	781	6	100	0	93	2
Mozambique	507	6	40	2	8	2	741	7	99	1	81	3
Kenya	509	4	39	2	7	1	793	8	100	0	95	2
Malawi	512	5	43	2	9	1	714	9	99	1	72	4
Swaziland	531	3	52	2	4	1	759	7	100	0	89	2
Tanzania	576	4	70	2	24	1	724	7	99	1	82	3

Source: SACMEQ (2010, p.2).

Challenges in the implementation of LSAS in South Africa

A number of challenges, at the systems and classroom levels, need to be addressed for the successful implementation of LSAS to take place, and thereby to enhance learning in the classroom. These are discussed below.

Policies and guidelines

The development and implementation of appropriate policies is critical for ensuring the effective use of assessment information to improve the learning of all children within the education sector. The latest national assessment policy (Department of Education, 2007) calls for enhancing the use of assessment to improve learning within the classroom. Action Plan 2014 (Department of Basic Education, 2010) also specifies that reports must be provided to parents pertaining to their children's levels of performance as well as their strengths and weaknesses, with the expectation that parents will assist their children or pressurise schools to address their children's needs. However, in both documents, there is no clear strategy on how this will be achieved, and how information should be reported and disseminated to parents and teachers, nor any strategy on what support will be provided to assist parents and teachers in implementing the policy.

A possible solution is to implement a national reporting framework that provides clear guidelines and tools for parents and teachers, as well as district and provincial officials, on how to analyse, interpret and apply assessment information for improving learning. Specifically, information must be reported against clear performance standards and performance level descriptors, so as to provide information on what learners know and can do and to highlight specific strengths and weaknesses of learners that need to be addressed.

Capacity and skills of teachers and education officials

The development of relevant capacity and skills of teachers and education officials to effectively use assessment information for improving learning is a major challenge facing education systems all over the world. South Africa is no different. Key reasons for this include the limited training provided during pre-service teacher training programmes and limited in-service professional development support. In addition, the high administrative burden associated with implementing effective assessments is also a mitigating factor.

A key solution to this challenge lies in the introduction and/or expansion of specific assessment-related courses into the programmes provided to trainee teachers. In addition, the application of relevant assessment methods and techniques should also serve as a key criterion against which trainee teachers are evaluated. Similar programmes should also be provided as in-service professional development and support by the national and provincial departments of education. An area for additional research pertains to current assessment practices – specifically, the ways in which teachers and education officials obtain assessment information and how they use this information for improving learning.

Systems, structure and resources

The structure, organisation and available resources, both human and financial, of an assessment system largely determine access to and effective use of assessment information. Within the education sector in South Africa, there are significant variations at the national, provincial and district levels regarding how assessment systems are implemented. Specifically, provinces differ in terms of where responsibility for assessment is located (that is, in a curriculum unit, an examinations unit or a specific assessment unit), allocation of staff and funding, as well as in their strategies for collecting, analysing, reporting and disseminating assessment information.

Effective solutions to these problems are complex and difficult to implement. However, any solution must (i) account for the different contexts within which district and provincial education officials operate, as well as the context within which teaching and learning occurs; (ii) ensure that the critical role of assessment in improving learning is both understood and actively promoted; (iii) ensure that senior officials prioritise the use of assessment for improving learning, and that this is reflected in the allocation of resources; and (iv) ensure that appropriate structures and processes are established to enhance the flow and use of assessment information at all levels of the education system.

Conclusion

The effective use of assessment information can have a significant positive impact on improving learning in South African schools. In particular, LSAS have the potential to contribute to the information needs of teachers and education officials in order to provide both cognitive and noncognitive information, which can then be used to develop and implement relevant interventions for improving learning and teaching. To date, there has been limited focus of LSAS on supporting the formative functions of assessment. Given the significant investments in these studies over the past decade, and their potential to address the learning needs of all children, there is an urgent need to ensure that LSAS in South Africa are more effectively applied. However, for this to succeed, a number of key practical challenges need to be addressed, as identified earlier in this chapter.

Given the steady improvement of expertise and experience within the country, as well as the available resources and continued applications of LSAS in the future, ensuring that the potentially significant impact of LSAS on formative functions of assessment is realised in South African schools seems to be largely dependent on political will, and on effective collaboration between the key education role players. It should, however, be noted that in the quest to improve learning in South African schools, assessment is but one, albeit critical, element, and is thus only a means to an end.

References

Abu-Alhija, F. N. (2007). Large-scale testing: Benefits and pitfalls. *Studies in Educational Evaluation, 33*, 50–68.

Appel, S. W. (1989). 'Outstanding individuals do not arise from ancestrally poor stock': Racial science and the education of black South Africans. *Journal of Negro Education, 58*, 554–557.

Benveniste, L. (2002). The political structuration of assessment: Negotiating state power and legitimacy. *Comparative Education Review, 46*, 89–118.

Black, P. & Wiliam, D. (1998). Inside the black box: Raising standards through classroom assessment. *Phi Delta Kappa, October*, 139–148.

Black, P. & Wiliam, D. (2007). Large-scale assessment systems: Design principles drawn from international comparisons. *Measurement, 5(1)*, 1–53.

Brown, G. T. & Hattie, J. A. (2003). *A National Teacher-Managed, Curriculum-Based Assessment System: Assessment Tools for Teaching and Learning (asTTle)*. Technical Report Number 41. University of Auckland, Auckland.

Bulhan, A. B. (1980). Psychological research in Africa: Genesis and function. *Race and Class, 23*, 25–41.

Bulhan, H. A. (1993). Imperialism in studies of the psyche: A critique of African psychological research. In L. J. Nicholas (Ed.), *Psychology and Oppression: Critiques and Proposals* (pp. 1–34). Johannesburg: Skotaville.

Carnoy, M. (2000). *Globalisation and education reform: What planners need to know*. Paris: IIEP–UNESCO.

Chinapah, V., H'ddigui, M., Kanjee, A., Falayojo, W., Fomba, C. O., Hamissou, O., Rafalimanana, A. & Byamugisha, A. (2000). *With Africa for Africa: Towards Quality Education for All*. Pretoria: Human Sciences Research Council.

Claassen, N. C. W., Makgamatha, M. & Kanjee, A. (2003). *Grade 3 Summative Assessment Results*. Report submitted to the Research Triangle Institute for the District Development Support Programme. Pretoria: Human Sciences Research Council.

Cloete, N., Muller, J. & Orkin, M. (1986). How we learned to stop worrying and love the HSRC. *Psychology and Society*, 6, 29–46.

Department of Basic Education (2010). National Education Policy Act: Action plan to 2014: Towards the realisation of schooling 2025: Draft. Pretoria: Department of Basic Education.

Department of Basic Education (2011). *Report on the 2011 Annual National Assessments*. Pretoria: Department of Basic Education.

Department of Education (1998). Assessment policy in the General Education and Training band: Grades R to 9 and ABET. Pretoria: Department of Education.

Department of Education (2000). *A South African Curriculum for the Twenty-first Century: Report of the Review Committee on Curriculum 2005*. Pretoria: Department of Education.

Department of Education (2003). *National Report on Systemic Evaluation: Mainstream Education – Foundation Phase*. Pretoria: Department of Education.

Department of Education (2004). *Grade 6 Systemic Evaluation Report*. Pretoria: Department of Education.

Department of Education (2005). *Grade 6 Systemic Evaluation Teacher Guide*. Pretoria: Department of Education.

Department of Education (2007). *National Policy on Assessment and Qualifications for Schools in the General and Further Education and Training Band*. Pretoria: Department of Education.

Forster, M. (2002). *National Monitoring of Learning Achievement in Developing Countries.* UNICEF Education Section Working Paper. New York, NY: UNICEF.

Gauteng Department of Education (2000). *Technical Report: Instrument Design and Administration of the Grade 3 District-Wide Reading Assessment.* Benoni, Gauteng: District S1, Gauteng Department of Education.

Govender, L. (1998). *The 1996 South African Longitudinal Survey of Scholastic Achievement.* Pretoria: Human Sciences Research Council.

Harlen, W. (2005). Teachers' summative practices and assessment for learning – tensions and synergies. *Curriculum Journal, 16(2),* 207–223.

Heugh, K., Diedricks, G. A. M., Prinsloo, C. H. & Herbst, D. L. (2007). *Assessment of Language and Mathematics Skills of Grade 8 Learners in the Western Cape in 2006.* Pretoria: Human Sciences Research Council.

Howie, S. J., Venter, E. J., Van Staden, S., Zimmerman, L., Long, C., Scherman, V. & Archer, E. (2009). *South African Children's Reading Achievement: Summary Report on PIRLS 2006.* Pretoria: Centre for Evaluation and Assessment.

Jansen, J. (2001). School autonomy and evaluation: On the politics of performance in South Africa. *Prospectus, 31(1),* 553–562.

JET Education Services (2008). *Integrated Education Program (IEP) Report: Final Measurement of IEP Learner Performance in Grades 3 and 6.* Report commissioned by RTI International under contract to USAID. Johannesburg: JET Education Services.

Kallaway, P. (1984). An introduction to the study of education for blacks in South Africa. In P. Kallaway (Ed.), *Apartheid and Education* (pp. 1–44). Johannesburg: Ravan Press.

Kanjee, A. (1998). Educational transformation and assessment research in South Africa: The role of the Human Sciences Research Council. Paper presented at the annual conference of the International Association for Educational Assessment. Barbados, May 11–15.

Kanjee, A. (2006). Improving learner achievement in schools: Application of national assessments in South Africa. In S. Buhlungu, J. Daniel, R. Southall & J. Lutchman (Eds), *State of the Nation: South Africa 2007* (pp. 470–499). Cape Town: HSRC Press.

Kanjee, A. & Povey, J. (2006). Monitoring trends in education quality: Technical report. Unpublished report. Pretoria: Human Sciences Research Council.

Kanjee, A. & Prinsloo, C. (2005). *Improving Learning in South African Schools: The Quality Learning Project Summative Evaluation.* Report commissioned by the JET Education Trust. Pretoria: Human Sciences Research Council.

Kellaghan, T. & Greaney, V. (2001). *Using Assessment to Improve the Quality of Education.* Paris: UNESCO.

Kellaghan, T. & Greaney, V. (2003). Monitoring performance: Assessment and examinations in Africa. Paper presented at the Association for the Development of Education in Africa (ADEA) Biennial Meeting. Grand Baie, Mauritius, December 3–6.

Lockheed, M. (2011). Policies, performance and panaceas: What international assessments are good for (and not good for) in developing countries. Paper presented at the Annual Meeting of the Comparative and International Education Society. Montreal, Canada, May 1–5.

Lubisi, R. C. & Murphy, R. J. L. (2002). Assessment in South African schools. *Assessment in Education, 9(2),* 256–268.

Malaka, L. M. (1995). Assessment skills of teachers: A study of South African teachers. Unpublished PhD dissertation. University of Massachusetts, Amherst.

Mathonsi, E. N. (1988). *Black Matriculation Results: A Mechanism of Social Control.* Johannesburg: Skotaville.

Moloi, M. & Strauss, J. (2005). *The SACMEQ II Project in South Africa: A Study of the Conditions of Schooling and the Quality of Education.* Harare: SACMEQ.

Nzimande, B. (1995). To test or not to test? Paper presented at the Congress of Psychometrics for Psychologists and Personnel Practitioners. Council for Scientific and Industrial Research, Pretoria, June 13–14.

Pellegrino, J. W., Chudowsky, N. & Glaser, R. (2001). *Knowing What Students Know: The Science and Design of Educational Assessment.* Washington, DC: National Academy Press.

Reddy, V. (2006a). *Mathematics and Science Achievement in South African Schools in TIMSS 2003.* Cape Town: HSRC Press.

Reddy, V. (Ed.) (2006b). *Marking Matric: Overview and challenges.* Cape Town: HSRC Press.

SACMEQ (Southern African Consortium for Monitoring Education Quality) (2010). How successful are HIV-AIDS prevention education programmes? *SACMEQ Policy Issues Series 3.* Paris: UNESCO.

Schiefelbein, E. & Schiefelbein, P. (2003). From screening to improving quality: The case of Latin America. *Assessment in Education, 10(2),* 141–154.

Schollar, E. (2004). *The Primary Mathematics Research Project: An Empirical Investigation into the Outcomes of Mathematics Education in South African Primary Schools.* Report prepared for the Shuttleworth Foundation. Johannesburg: Eric Schollar & Associates.

Shavelson, R. J., Black, P. J., Wiliam, D. & Coffey, J. E. (2003). On aligning formative and summative assessment. Paper presented at the National Research Council Workshop on Assessment in Support of Instruction and Learning: Bridging the Gap Between Large-scale and Classroom Assessment. Washington DC, January 23–24.

Swartz, D. (1992). Issues in the reform of the system of certification South Africa. In E. Unterhalter, H. Wolpe & T. Botha (Eds), *Education in a Future South Africa: Policy Issues and Transformation.* Trenton, NJ: Africa World Press.

Taylor, N. & Vinjevold, P. (1999). *Getting Learning Right: Report on the President's Education Initiative Research Project.* Johannesburg: Joint Education Trust.

Umalusi (2006). Draft criteria for evaluation, accreditation and monitoring of examination bodies. Pretoria: Umalusi.

UNESCO (2000). *EFA 2000 Assessment Surveys: Monitoring Learning Achievement.* Paris: UNESCO.

UNESCO (2004). *EFA Global Monitoring Report 2005. Education for All: The Quality Imperative.* Paris: UNESCO.

Whittaker, S. B. (1990). A critical historical perspective on psychology in Azania/South Africa. Paper presented at the Psychology and Apartheid Conference. University of the Western Cape, Bellville, March 29–31.

36 Current and future trends in psychological assessment in South Africa: challenges and opportunities

S. Laher and K. Cockcroft

In the last 20 years, with the advent of a new democratic political dispensation, the field of psychological assessment in South Africa has developed in many ways. Most notable have been the influx of international tests and the Employment Equity Act (No. 55 of 1998). This Act was specifically promulgated to recognise that as a result of apartheid and other discriminatory laws and practices, there are disparities in employment, occupation and income in the labour market which have created such pronounced disadvantages for certain categories of people that they cannot be addressed by simply repealing discriminatory laws. Hence, the Employment Equity Act proposes a number of actions, the most prominent being that of affirmative action, to address the broader inequalities that exist in the workplace in South Africa. The Act also states that all psychological instruments used on South Africans should be reliable, valid, unbiased and fair for all groups in the country. This is a novel approach to legislation, since internationally the governance of psychological testing generally falls under the auspices of the psychological registration bodies. The promulgation of this legislation has led to increased 'conscientisation' of researchers, practitioners and the public. As a consequence, validation studies of the types discussed by Milner, Donald and Thatcher in chapter 33 of this volume have been undertaken. A number of private companies and institutions have also started using only those tests that are supported by a solid body of empirical research. However, a number of challenges remain. Rather than viewing each as an insurmountable obstacle, we attempt in this chapter to present them as challenges to be overcome, each giving rise to a unique set of opportunities.

Policy implications of the Employment Equity Act

Although the majority of practitioners are using tests ethically and responsibly, there is no active control mechanism to manage this effectively. The Health Professions Council of South Africa (HPCSA) has a Psychometrics Committee under the Professional Board for Psychology. The Psychometrics Committee has a mandate to evaluate tests to determine whether they are reliable, valid and fair before registering them for use in the country. However, there is currently no legislation indicating that only HPCSA-registered tests may be used. This has been proposed in the most recent amendments to the Employment Equity Act, but the contentious nature of this proposal, and objection from the Association of Test Publishers amongst others, have led to the promulgation of the amendments being postponed. These disagreements have delayed progress in psychological assessment development and practice in South Africa.

Arising from this are several more challenges and associated opportunities, particularly if the amendments to the Employment Equity Act are eventually promulgated. These amendments propose that only psychologists and psychometrists be permitted to utilise psychological tests and assessments. They also propose that only registered psychometric instruments may be used in the country, thus intensifying the stringency of the legislation on psychological testing in South Africa. This is potentially advantageous in that, if regulated and managed correctly, it will ensure that psychological assessment is practised ethically and appropriately, allowing no opportunity to repeat the abuses of the past. There will be an increased opportunity to promote and instil the development of an 'ethical consciousness', as was identified by Coetzee in chapter 28. While in principle this proposal is seductive, practically it raises a host of additional challenges. Primary among these are that the body responsible for registering psychological tests is currently not managing this task. In order to manage the influx of tests to be registered should the Employment Equity Act amendments be promulgated, the Psychometrics Committee of the HPCSA's Professional Board for Psychology will have to be expanded. It will have to consider the creation of an extended group of people willing to review tests, as proposed by Foxcroft (2004), with regard to developing suitable tests for the multicultural South African context. However, obtaining funding for this purpose will be a considerable challenge.

The need for skilled personnel

In addition to the abovementioned concern, a further concern is that there is a limited number of individuals with the requisite specialist measurement skills and knowledge of assessment in South Africa. Foxcroft (2004) points out that there has been limited transfer of test development skills to a new generation of researchers, since postgraduate psychology programmes tend to focus on developing psychology practitioners, and states that 'it remains unfortunate that at this critical moment, when psychological test development stands at the threshold of a new era in which new tests should be developed from a multicultural rather than a monocultural perspective, there is a critical shortage of experienced test developers in South Africa' (p.8). Despite the importance of psychological assessment both locally and globally, it is marginalised in South African academic curricula. South Africa has registration categories for psychologists specialising in clinical, counselling, educational and industrial psychology, and most recently in forensic and neuropsychology, but a specialisation in psychometrics falls into the category of a psychometrist or a psychological counsellor – a level that is academically lower than that of a psychologist. The HPCSA and academic institutions need to consider the introduction of a specialist area devoted to psychological assessment that ranks equal in stature to registration as a psychologist, with its own scope of practice.

The need for a specialisation in psychological assessment would also address the potential increase in demand for these skills, should the amendments to the Employment Equity Act be promulgated. If only psychologists and psychometrists are authorised to use psychological tests, as proposed in the amendments, this is likely to place a heightened demand on a small pool of practitioners. This opportunity is countered by the fact that there will in all likelihood not be sufficient numbers of qualified practitioners to meet the demand.

This raises both a challenge and an opportunity for psychology departments across the country. Students are increasingly realising the potential for pursuing careers in psychological assessment. As such, the demand for psychometric programmes is increasing. However, using Gauteng as an example, there are only three training institutions in this province which offer this option. Two of them require the students to locate and organise their own internship sites, and one of them organises the internship site but charges a premium fee. There is little standardisation across the programmes, although all conform to the Guidelines for Psychometrists document provided by the HPCSA (2010). It is recommended that academic institutions take cognisance of these developments and develop and strengthen psychometric programmes.

The current Employment Equity Act requires that psychological tests be scientifically reliable, valid and fair, and that imported, etic tests be explored for utility in South Africa only if they can be appropriately adapted and translated. It also requires that more local, emic instruments be developed. The Human Sciences Research Council (HSRC) had a unit devoted to test development and adaptation which was dissolved following the governmental transformation in 1994, and all test material was subsequently sold to local test publishers. Research from this unit of the HSRC, unless published in academic journals, is not easily accessible. The current test publishers conduct some research on the ex-HSRC and other instruments that they market, but this is minimal and not widely available. Most test publishers tend to focus only on their marketable instruments, the majority of which are etic in nature, as is evidenced in some of the chapters in this book. Thus, the challenge is to meet the increasing demand for practitioners with test development and adaptation skills, and the opportunity arising from this is clear – the creation of a new academic specialisation to develop these scarce skills in the country.

Aside from the role of academic institutions in providing training, a possibility is that the government consider setting up a body similar to that of the HSRC unit – that is, one that receives partial funding from government and partial funding from private donors and corporate businesses. One of the reasons for suggesting that government contribute only partially to funding such an initiative stems from the history associated with psychological assessment. Comprehensive government control of the use and distribution of tests might repeat the problems experienced under the previous dispensation, where a relatively small number of instruments received official sanctioning and support. According to Heuchert (personal communication, March 9, 2012), in the past 'this led to groupthink, an insular approach and premature foreclosing on the very complex issue of trying to evaluate and assess the human psyche in all its intricacies'. This needs to be avoided in future planning for the field of psychological assessment in South Africa.

Practical constraints

This proposal may be idealistic, given the lack of resources in South Africa, both human and financial. Consequently, there may not be funds available to finance assessment projects, which battle for a priority position against the background of HIV/AIDS, poverty, crime and corruption. Funding for psychological assessment (and other psychological services) is also a problem on a practical level, since the majority of the population relies on public health care. In these settings there are very few adequate environments for testing; test material is often old, incomplete and/or unavailable; and there is a very limited or nonexistent budget to purchase and upgrade test materials. Hence, practitioners in these situations are faced with the ethical dilemma of committing copyright infringements by using photocopied materials or denying individuals much-needed services. This challenge can be translated into an opportunity for government to improve service delivery in these settings, firstly by identifying and acknowledging this as a concern, and then by allocating a budget to cover the costs of such materials. Assessment practitioners and researchers also need to consider developing local or emic tests in order to address the challenge of the exorbitant fees charged for purchasing etic instruments.

Etic versus emic tests

The use of imported instruments (an etic approach), adapted versions of imported instruments (a pseudo-etic approach) or locally developed instruments (emic instruments) is highly debated. Many argue that the use of etic instruments is both necessary and justified since most companies that use assessment instruments are multinational. As such, South Africa needs to be represented globally on an equal footing with other countries. In contrast, many clinicians argue that for various reasons, most notably those of culture and language, more emic instruments are necessary. Anderson (2001, p.33), for example, makes a strong argument for the collection of local neuropsychological normative data by pointing out that 'the injudicious use of imported normative data could result in an unacceptably high diagnostic rate of neuropsychological impairment in otherwise healthy South Africans'. In 1996, Shuttleworth-Jordan argued for adaptation and standardisation of well-researched international tests, rather than 'reinventing the wheel' by developing completely new tests.

This issue is best illustrated in the area of personality testing. The Five-Factor Model (FFM) of personality and the Revised NEO Personality Inventory (NEO-

PI-R) are currently regarded as the 'gold standard' in personality assessment against which all other objective tests are compared (see Laher, chapter 18, this volume). Laher's chapter provides evidence for the utility, albeit limited, of the NEO-PI-R in South Africa. The NEO-PI-R has not been adapted or standardised for the South African context and therefore represents an etic test. More recent findings support the utility of the instrument but are limited to student samples. Taylor and De Bruin (chapter 16, this volume) have developed the Basic Traits Inventory (BTI) for use in South Africa. As indicated in their chapter, the BTI was constructed based on the FFM. Thus, it represents more of a pseudo-etic approach than an emic one.

More recently, work has been under way on a truly emic personality instrument, the South African Personality Inventory (SAPI) (Laher, 2010; Meiring, 2006). The project aims at developing a single, unified personality inventory for South Africa that incorporates both universal (etic) and unique (emic) personality factors found across the diversity of cultures in this country. The first stage of this project explored indigenous perceptions of personality, primarily through the work of Nel (2008). He explored personality structure in each of the 11 language groups in South Africa. Structured interviews were conducted in the native languages of 1 308 South Africans to gather information about personality-descriptive terms. This resulted in 50 000 personality-descriptive terms, which were reduced to 190 personality dimensions via the use of cluster analysis. The 190 dimensions were further clustered and finally resulted in 9 clusters – namely, Extraversion, Soft-heartedness, Conscientiousness, Emotional Stability, Intellect, Openness, Integrity, Relationship Harmony and Facilitating, with the first 6 labels being more closely related to the FFM and the last 3 being more indigenous personality constructs (Nel, 2008). The quantitative phase of this project is currently under way and involves administering 2 500 items to 4 language groupings in South Africa. Results have not yet been published for this (Meiring, 2010). As is evident from this example, the process of test development is lengthy and complicated, and while emic instruments are useful, they come with their own challenges. Aside from the practical problems associated with test development – that is, lack of skilled personnel and funding – there is also the challenge that if South Africa is to establish and maintain its position internationally in the discipline, we need to employ and adapt etic instruments.

Quite often test developers argue forcibly for the universal applicability of their instruments. South Africa, with its multilingual and culturally diverse population, provides a perfect environment for such claims to be empirically tested. The issue of cultural diversity encompasses current understandings of both culture as well as acculturation, and this leads to another set of challenges and opportunities.

Defining culture

Internationally and locally, the cross-cultural applicability of psychological instruments is often pronounced on, but the term 'culture' is seldom defined. In many international studies 'culture' refers to either nationality or ethnicity, while locally 'culture' is often a euphemism for race. Consequently, 'culture' in South African research and practice is often represented by the racial categories black, coloured, white and Indian, or language groupings based on ethnicity such as isiZulu, Sesotho, Tshivenda, and so on. It can be argued that this type of classification represents a perpetuation of the apartheid classification systems. However, this way of grouping individuals is endorsed by the Employment Equity Act.

In order to 'promote the constitutional right of equality and the exercise of true democracy; eliminate unfair discrimination in employment; ensure the implementation of employment equity to redress the effects of discrimination; [and] achieve a diverse workforce broadly representative of the South African people' amongst other things (Preamble to the Employment Equity Act), the Act proposes affirmative action in Chapter 3. According to Section 15(1), '[a]ffirmative action measures are measures designed to ensure that suitably qualified people from designated groups have equal employment opportunities and are equitably represented in all occupational categories and levels in the workforce of a designated employer'. Designated groups are defined in the Act as 'black people, women and people with disabilities', where '"black people" is a generic term which means Africans, Coloureds and Indians' (Chapter 1, Definitions). This suggests that psychometric studies should be considering differences across gender and racial groupings.

The issue is complex, as there is no doubt that culture affects behaviour and the psychological constructs being measured (Bedell, Van Eeden & Van Staden, 1999), and the extent of cultural diversity in South Africa makes the development of tests that are valid, unbiased and fair for all groups in the country extremely difficult. It is necessary for individuals working in this field to actively engage in this debate, since it is becoming increasingly evident that race groupings are no longer valid indicators for differences amongst South Africans. The concept of culture is also more complex than merely being reduced to race, language and/or ethnicity. Many have argued that issues of acculturation are becoming more salient in the South African context. This argument is addressed in the next section.

Acculturation

Some practitioners in the field of psychological assessment argue that 'degree of acculturation' should be considered a key variable in contemporary research and practice in this field. For example, McCrae, Costa and Martin (2005) suggest that in a number of studies ancestry and culture are confounded, thus increasing the necessity for studies on acculturation. This is particularly the case in the African and South African contexts, where 'politically liberated Africans are now challenged by the opportunities and risks of modern technology and, above all, by the fast pace of worldwide transformation and change' (Okeke, Draguns, Sheku & Allen, 1999, p.240). Acculturation has been defined as 'those phenomena which result in individuals having different cultures coming into continuous first-hand contact with subsequent changes in the original cultural patterns of either or both groups' (Redfield, Linton & Herskovits, 1936 quoted in Van de Vijver & Phalet, 2004, p.216). The difficulty in terms of psychological assessment is that different groups in South Africa are in various stages of acculturation (Shuttleworth-Jordan, 1996).

The general perception tends to be that in South Africa, African individuals are acculturated into the white, Western, usually individualist, culture. However, since 1994, it has become increasingly evident from daily interactions that acculturation is occurring in both directions. White South Africans are absorbing aspects of African culture possibly as much as African people are absorbing aspects of Western culture. Most of us have experience of this, with a clear example being the recent FIFA World Cup event where, for the first time, South Africans were presented as a cohesive nation and not as separate race groups. The varying levels of acculturation present a challenge to research and practice in psychological assessment, while simultaneously providing unique opportunities for South Africa to contribute meaningfully to the international arena. Many scales have recently been developed to measure acculturation. A constructive suggestion would be for these scales to be explored. The opportunity exists for either the creation or the adaptation of an acculturation scale that can routinely be employed in research to better understand the acculturation construct and its role in the South African context. Looking beyond the traditional variables of language, race and ethnic group, it might be interesting to explore the stage of identity development that the individual is at. This could be used to provide a context for the interpretation of other test data. The qualitative approach to career assessment, as described by Watson and McMahon (see chapter 32, this volume), is indicative of assessment within this tradition.

The economic divide

'Acculturation' may also be a more academic or socially acceptable way of describing the broader and more pervasive economic divide that exists in South Africa. Although South Africa is now part of a digitised, globalised society, it remains a very unequal society, with the majority of the population still not having access to basic resources, opportunities, employment and education. This divided access is frequently described in the literature and is said to pervade all aspects of South African life, from politics and economics through to education (see Devey, Skinner & Valodia, 2006; Skinner & Valodia, 2006). In the psychological literature, reference in this regard is often made to urban versus rural samples (Foxcroft, 2002; Foxcroft & Davies, 2008). Whilst we acknowledge that the urban–rural distinction is important, and has made and will continue to make important contributions to our understanding of the challenges facing psychological assessment in South Africa, we do believe that the divide is much deeper than geographical location.

South Africa has a 'second economy', which parallels the 'first economy' and functions independently of formal market and banking systems (Mbeki, 2003; The Presidency, 2007). Furthermore, the 'first economy' operates in such a way that it often undermines the growth of the 'second economy', leaving little space for class mobility and equality. Thus, those individuals trapped within this second economy have very little class mobility and, as argued by Philip and Hassen (2008), are unable to escape the cycle of poverty and inequality that entraps them. South Africa has the world's highest Gini coefficient, which, according to Leibrandt, Woolard, Finn and Argent (2010), increased from .66 to .70 in the period from 1993 to 2008. Although it is still the African population that suffers most from this lack of opportunity, there is a growing middle and upper class among this group. Van der Berg, Burger and Louw (2010) and Seekings and Natrass (2006) argue that the increase in the Gini coefficient is primarily a result of the growing class divide, particularly amongst the indigenous African population in South Africa. There is no denying that a vast divide exists between those who do and those who do not have access to resources (Leibrandt et al., 2010). It is recommended that future research in psychological assessment take socio-economic indicators (which encompass quality of education) into account, as these are better representations of the divisions present in South Africa than race, ethnicity and/or language.

The quality of education

Linked in part to socio-economic status, as well as to the debate on the utility of race as an indicator, is quality of education. Equal access to education and opportunity are proposed for all, and there has been a segment of the population across the various race and language groups that has been the recipient of these opportunities. In this context, the use of race and language variables is regarded as no longer valid. In this regard, Shuttleworth-Edwards, Van der Merwe, Van Tonder and Radloff (chapter 3, this volume) suggest that quality of education is a more discriminating variable than race when considering performance on intelligence tests. By quality of education, Shuttleworth-Edwards et al. are referring to the distinction between relatively advantaged education within the historically white private and/or former Model C educational institutions (Private/Model C schooling), and relatively disadvantaged education within the black and coloured township educational institutions (Township schooling). Their research has revealed considerable lowering of Wechsler Intelligence Scale for Children (Fourth Edition) (WISC-IV) IQ test scores (of 20 to 30 IQ points) in association with relatively disadvantaged education, when compared to the British standardised norms. This is particularly salient in light of recent proposed government policies on both school readiness and vocational counselling. Some provincial departments of education have imposed an informal moratorium on school readiness testing within their schools. School readiness assessment is a highly contentious issue in South Africa, as discussed by Amod and Heafield in chapter 6 of this volume. With the historical misuse of assessment measures, which perpetuated exclusionary practices and an inequitable education system, still vivid in South African society's collective memory, school readiness assessment is understandably still viewed with suspicion. In addition, some of the psychological tools used to assess readiness either do not have local norms or these are outdated (Foxcroft, Paterson, Le Roux & Herbst, 2004). Some attempts are made to address this; for example, Theron (chapter 5, this volume) demonstrates how one such test, the Junior South African Individual Scales (JSAIS), can be interpreted in a multicultural (and crime-ridden) context. She urges practitioners not to limit the JSAIS to a measure of intelligence, but to use it to comment qualitatively on children's level of resilience and readiness for formal learning.

Unfortunately, such useful information only takes us part of the way towards addressing the challenge of school readiness assessment, as the negative perception of such assessment persists. Further, socio-economic divisions that persist in South Africa exacerbate developmental and emotional differences between children. The purpose of school readiness assessment, as indicated by Amod and Heafield (chapter 6), is not only to determine readiness for formal school entry, but also to identify preschool children who could benefit from additional stimulation programmes, learning support or retention in order to develop and consolidate skills which are absent. By denying children this opportunity we thwart their prospects for learning and achievement in a Western education system.

Language and literacy

South Africa has 11 official languages and the Language-in-Education Policy (Department of Education, 1997) promotes multilingualism in our schools through use of more than one language of learning and teaching, and/or by offering additional languages as fully fledged subjects, and/or by applying special immersion or language maintenance programmes, or through other means approved by the head of the provincial education department. In addition, many employers require that future employees be fluent in another South African language as well as English in order to be able to better assist clients. These are all reasonable suggestions, given that the majority of South Africans (91.8 per cent of the population) speak English as their second language (Statistics South Africa, 2001).

Research has consistently demonstrated how taking a test in a language that is not one's first language can impact on test results (see Abrahams, 2002; Foxcroft, 2004; Franklin-Ross, 2009; Heuchert, Parker, Stumpf & Myburgh, 2000; Horn, 2000; Meiring, Van de Vijver & Rothmann, 2006; Nel, 2008; Taylor, 2000; 2004; Van de Vijver & Rothmann, 2004; Van Eeden & Mantsha, 2007; Vogt & Laher, 2009). Nell (1994) has argued that language is the most important variable that influences test performance. If an individual takes a test in a language in which she or he is not proficient, it is exceedingly difficult to determine whether poor performance is a result of language difficulties or difficulty in terms of the construct being measured. Thus, it is salient that home language issues also be examined as a challenge to psychological assessment in South Africa.

Another commonly held assumption is that home language is representative of an individual's language proficiency. This is flawed since, as with culture, an individual's home language indicates nothing about his or her proficiency in English, which is usually what questions about home language are intended to uncover. Medium of instruction at school is probably a better indicator than home language of an individual's language proficiency in English.

Discussions of language and assessment raise further challenges. According to Project Literacy (2010), a non-governmental organisation that delivers adult basic education and training in South Africa, there are 4.7 million South Africans who have not attended school and are completely illiterate. There are a further 4.9 million adult South Africans who are functionally illiterate – that is, they left school before Grade 7. The majority of existing psychological assessment procedures require some degree of literacy. Both the challenge and the opportunity inherent in this would be the development of assessment methods to service this group. Since this problem is not unique to South Africa, solutions in this regard have the potential to be of international relevance.

Test translation

A further, related challenge is that of using test material in English and administering it to individuals whose proficiency in English may be limited. Notwithstanding the dynamic interplay between language, culture and thought, on a practical level translation of test materials presents a myriad of challenges, foregrounded by the fact that South Africa has 11 official languages. The difficulty is compounded by the fact that some indigenous South African languages do not have equivalent words or idiomatic expressions to those used in English (Horn, 2000). For example, 'green' and 'blue' are expressed by the same word in isiXhosa, while Afrikaans has no words for 'sexy' or 'weird'; there are no single words in isiXhosa for 'manipulation', 'morality', 'intentions', 'roller-coaster', or 'jittery', and only one word in this language for the English terms 'vision', 'dream', 'fantasy' and 'imagination' (Horn, 2000). In this context, translation difficulties are aggravated when working with clinical instruments such as the Beck Depression Inventory or the Millon Clinical Multiaxial Inventory – III, which require the translation of clinical terms. When no translated instruments are available, practitioners often rely on the services of an interpreter. In a clinical setting, this is most likely to be a nurse, an intern or a student, while in schools this is usually undertaken by teachers and/or cleaning staff, usually on an ad hoc basis. The limitations and dangers inherent in this practice are self-evident. Again, this points to the need to train more skilled individuals, both in psychological assessment and in allied professions such as interpretation.

Response bias

An aspect that is linked to both culture and language, and that is currently receiving much research interest in the field of psychological assessment, is response bias. In personality psychology, for example, it is quite common to find response biases operational in non-Western cultures. Taylor and De Bruin (see chapter 16, this volume) have considered this with regard to the BTI. Other researchers have argued that any personality differences observed between cultures may not necessarily be true differences, but may occur due to differences in response styles and response biases in African samples (see Piedmont, Bain, McCrae & Costa, 2002). Allik and McCrae (2004) argue that acquiescent response biases, as well as a tendency to avoid extreme responses, are more prominent in collectivistic cultures. Hamamura, Heine and Paulhus (2008) also argue that extreme response styles are more characteristic in those of European heritage, while moderate response styles are more characteristic in those of East Asian heritage. They also cite literature which suggests that North Americans of European heritage have higher levels of extreme responding as compared to African-Americans and Latino Americans. They conclude that this may be due to a tendency towards dialectical thinking (a tolerance of contradictory beliefs) that is more prominent in East Asian cultures, and/or to social desirability.

These findings are in contradiction to the findings of Bernardi (2006), who reports that social desirability response bias decreases as a country's level of individualism increases. Furthermore women, according to Bernardi, are more likely to exhibit social desirability response bias. Bernardi's study was conducted with samples from 12 countries – namely, Australia, Canada, China, Colombia, Ecuador, Hong Kong, Ireland, Japan, Nepal, South Africa, Spain and the USA. Bernardi does not provide the demographic breakdown of each of the samples. Rather, he divides them up into cultural areas defined as More Developed Latin, Less Developed Latin, More Developed Asian, Asian Colonial, and Anglo. He includes South Africa in the Anglo group along with Australia, Canada, Ireland and the USA. Without the demographic breakdown it is difficult to decide whether this was appropriate or not, but in Bernardi's study South Africa was clustered closer to the individualism dimension, and given the arguments presented in this book and in this chapter specifically, this may have been erroneous. Either way, this highlights the need for more research on response biases, whether they be extreme or acquiescent responding or social desirability responding.

Qualitative approaches

To address issues such as varying levels of literacy and test-wiseness, psychological assessment is moving away from the more traditional testing approach to more of an assessment focus. Hence, practitioners are consistently encouraged to use a battery of tests, to take an appropriate history and to explore collateral information before making decisions and recommendations (Foxcroft, 2004). In an organisational setting, testing forms only one part of the selection procedure. Interviews, in-basket tasks, role plays and group activity are frequently employed in addition to traditional testing (Moerdyk, 2009). Watson and McMahon (chapter 32, this volume) provide a comprehensive description of the manner in which qualitative information and techniques can be used effectively in career assessment. The reader is also referred to Maree (2007) and

Stead and Watson (2006) for further information on narrative approaches to career counselling. Osman (chapter 34, this volume) issues the challenge to assessment practitioners to equalise opportunities between people rather than differentiating opportunities based on race. Recognition of Prior Learning (RPL) provides an opportunity for individuals to present their gained life experiences to be meaningfully considered in occupational and aptitude assessment situations.

In addition, given the educational disparities in South Africa, learning potential approaches hold promise in identifying those who have the potential for development and who could benefit from further training (Amod & Seabi, chapter 9, this volume; De Beer, chapter 10, this volume). Proponents of this approach hold that intellectual ability is not static but can be modified. The development of the appropriate cognitive processes to function optimally in the world is dependent upon the individual's opportunity to benefit from appropriate mediation experiences (Feuerstein, 1980). The nature and extent of the mediation would provide an indication of the learning potential of the testee, and provide guidance for further educational intervention. This approach could be used in conjunction with Howard Gardner's (1993) theory of multiple intelligences. He suggests that it is far more fruitful to describe cognitive ability in terms of a profile of relative strengths and weaknesses, rather than focusing on a single general intelligence score. Unfortunately, no standardised and normed test of multiple intelligences exists yet. Those that can be found on the internet are based to varying degrees on Gardner's ideas, and have not been psychometrically validated.

Development of indigenous knowledge systems

None of the challenges presented here are new. Many have already been taken up as opportunities. Etic instruments have been developed. Pseudo-etic efforts are continuously undertaken with adaptations of intelligence, personality, interest and aptitude instruments. Emic approaches are also undertaken. Some of these, such as the Jung Personality Questionnaire and Self-Directed Search, represent work undertaken before 1994 by the HSRC. The work on the Sixteen Personality Factor Questionnaire (16PF) began with the HSRC, but is now being continued by local test distributors. Instruments such as the BTI and recent developments with the SAPI represent more recent emic approaches which hold promise. Work has been done to explore the possibilities of assessing intelligence and aptitude dynamically (see, in this volume, Amod & Seabi, chapter 9; De Beer, chapter 10; Taylor, chapter 11), thus addressing some of the challenges posed by language and education, although factors related to socio-economic status remain. In the area of career assessment there has also been substantial progress, with the use of qualitative, lifestyle narratives (see Watson & McMahon, chapter 32, this volume). However, none of these have yet addressed an important challenge – namely, the general acceptance of and subscription to Western, Eurocentric theoretical models and paradigms.

Earlier in the chapter we alluded to the FFM and the NEO-PI-R being the gold standard against which all personality instruments are evaluated. However, the FFM has been found to be lacking, particularly when used in Asian and African cultures (see Cheung, Cheung, Howard & Lim, 2006; Cheung, Leung, Fan, Song, Zhang & Zhang, 1996; Laher, 2008; 2011; Laungani, 1999; McCrae, Terracciano et al., 2005a; 2005b; Nel, 2008; Okeke et al., 1999; Pervin, 1999; Rossier, Dahourou & McCrae, 2005; Van Eeden & Mantsha, 2007). This finding prompted Cheung and colleagues to conduct research with the Chinese lexicon, resulting in the development of the Chinese Personality Assessment Inventory (CPAI) (Cheung et al., 1996) and subsequently the Cross-Cultural Personality Assessment Inventory – 2 (CPAI-2) (Cheung, 2004; Cheung, Cheung, Zhang, Leung, Leong & Yeh, 2008).

The BTI is a personality inventory developed in the South African context in accordance with the FFM (Taylor, 2004; Taylor & De Bruin, 2006). It measures the five factors of Neuroticism, Extraversion, Openness to Experience, Agreeableness and Conscientiousness, but unlike the NEO-PI-R, the BTI has five facets within each factor. The nomenclature and flavour of some of the facets are similar to those of the NEO-PI-R, but others have a slightly different focus. For example, Extraversion in the BTI consists of Gregariousness, Positive Affectivity, Ascendance, Excitement-Seeking and Liveliness (Taylor, 2004; Taylor & De Bruin, 2006). Although not as clear as the SAPI example given earlier, this nonetheless draws attention to the differences in the construct meanings and operationalisations across cultures.

Another locally developed instrument, the SAPI, reveals some new facets, as well as slightly different facets, to express traditional domains (Laher, 2010; Meiring, 2006; Nel, 2008). For example, the scale of Relationship Harmony is seen as one of the dimensions indigenous to South Africans and consists of the subscales of Approachability, Conflict-Seeking, Interpersonal Relatedness (also a factor on the CPAI-2) and Meddlesome. These scales, particularly those of Interpersonal Relatedness and Meddlesome, are not covered by the FFM. Extraversion is a universal scale, but in the South African context using the SAPI, it has subscales of Dominance, Expressiveness, Positive Emotionality and Sociability (Nel, 2008). Thus, Extraversion is different in a South African sample to that typically described by the FFM, with Dominance being included here, whereas Assertiveness is included in the Neuroticism factor in the NEO-PI-R. Expressiveness is defined as the inclination to share one's feelings or problems with others, and can be seen as a combination of Warmth (E) and Feelings (O) on the NEO-PI-R. Positive Emotionality can be seen as a combination of the Extraversion Positive Emotions facet, as well as the Extraversion facet of Gregariousness. However, the facets of Excitement-Seeking and Activity do not appear in the SAPI operationalisation of Extraversion, indicating the different flavour of some of the domains in other cultures.

It is evident from the research and arguments presented above that the opportunity exists within the psychological assessment research community to develop emic theoretical approaches to accompany emic instruments. South Africa provides a unique context for the development of indigenous knowledge within the field of psychological assessment. Such knowledge needs to be incorporated into theory and introduced into international mainstream research. Dialogue and discussion around this topic have been largely neglected, and must be invited if South African research in this field is to develop to maturity.

South Africa's global position

Often we argue that South African psychology, much like psychology in most other developing countries, operates on the periphery of international psychology, with the USA and Europe being at the centre. This argument is no longer sufficient. South Africa has both the talent and the context to become a more dominant player in the field. The proposal that South Africa provide international leadership in psychological assessment is based on several reasons. The first, as already stated, is the practical one that multinational companies would advocate. However, there are other reasons of greater value. South Africa is a developing nation that has proven that it has the capacity to be progressive in a number of fields. Our Constitution, a peaceful transition to democracy, the Truth and Reconciliation hearings, the work on HIV/AIDS, and attempts to eliminate racism are amongst a few areas in which South Africa leads. By virtue of the country's history, as well as its cultural diversity, South Africa provides an excellent environment for research on both etic and emic instruments.

Conclusion

The compilation of chapters in this book was intended to address some of the challenges raised here. Test development and use have been occurring in a 'haphazard, uncoordinated manner' (Foxcroft, 1997, p.234) and the purpose of this text has been to collate these data. A further aim was to force practitioners to evaluate the utility of South African and international tests that are commonly used. Most practitioners have embraced a multi-method assessment approach, in which practitioners are aware that test results are only one part of the larger process. As Claassen (1997, p.306) states, '[n]ever can a test score be interpreted without taking note of and understanding the context in which the score was obtained'. However, as is evident from the chapters in the book and the arguments presented in this chapter, we need to go further. Psychological assessment has come of age in South Africa, and the active pool of researchers and practitioners involved in the writing and reviewing of aspects of this book is evidence enough of the diverse talent present in our country to meet these challenges constructively.

References

Abrahams, F. (2002). The (un)fair usage of the 16PF (SA92) in South Africa: A response to C. H. Prinsloo and I. Ebersöhn. *South African Journal of Psychology, 32(3)*, 58–61.

Allik, J. & McCrae, R. R. (2004). Toward a geography of personality traits: Patterns of profiles across 36 cultures. *Journal of Cross-Cultural Psychology, 35*, 13–28.

Anderson, S. J. (2001). On the importance of collecting local neuropsychological normative data. *South African Journal of Psychology, 31*, 29–34.

Bedell, B., Van Eeden, R. & Van Staden, F. (1999). Culture as a moderator variable in psychological test performance: Issues and trends in South Africa. *South African Journal of Industrial Psychology, 25(3)*, 1–7.

Bernardi, R. A. (2006). Associations between Hofstede's cultural constructs and social desirability response bias. *Journal of Business Ethics, 65*, 45–53.

Cheung, F. M. (2004). Use of Western and indigenously developed personality tests in Asia. *Applied Psychology: An International Review, 53*, 173–191.

Cheung, S. F., Cheung, F. M., Howard, R. & Lim, Y-H. (2006). Personality across the ethnic divide in Singapore: Are 'Chinese traits' uniquely Chinese? *Personality and Individual Differences, 41*, 467–477.

Cheung, F. M., Cheung, S., Zhang, J., Leung, K., Leong, F. & Yeh, K. H. (2008). Relevance of Openness as a personality dimension in Chinese culture: Aspects of its cultural relevance. *Journal of Cross-Cultural Psychology, 39*, 81–108.

Cheung, F. M., Leung, K., Fan, R. M., Song, W. Z., Zhang, J. X. & Zhang, J-P. (1996). Development of the Chinese Personality Assessment Inventory (CPAI). *Journal of Cross-Cultural Psychology, 27*, 181–199.

Claassen, N. C. W. (1997). Cultural differences, politics and test bias in South Africa. *European Review of Applied Psychology, 47(4)*, 297–307.

Department of Education (1997). *Language-in-Education Policy*. Retrieved July 20, 2011, from http://www.education.gov.za/LinkClick.aspx?fileticket=XpJ7gz4rPT0%3D&tabid=390&mid=1125.

Devey, R., Skinner, C. & Valodia, I. (2006). The state of the informal economy. In S. Buhlungu, J. Daniel, R. Southall & J. Lutchman (Eds), *The State of the Nation (2005–2006)*. Cape Town: HSRC Press.

Feuerstein, R. (1980). *Instrumental Enrichment: An Intervention Programme for Cognitive Development*. Baltimore, MD: University Park Press.

Foxcroft, C. D. (1997). Psychological testing in South Africa: Perspectives regarding ethical and fair practices. *European Journal of Psychological Assessment, 13(3)*, 229–235.

Foxcroft, C. D. (2002). Ethical issues related to psychological testing in Africa: What I have learned (so far). In W. J. Lonner, D. L. Dinnel, S. A. Hayes & D. N. Sattler (Eds), *Online Readings in Psychology and Culture* (Unit 5, Chapter 4). Retrieved May 16, 2010, from http://orpc.iaccp.org/index.php?view=article&catid=23%3Achapter&id=45%3Afoxcroft&format=pdf&option=com_content.

Foxcroft, C. D. (2004). Planning a psychological test in the multicultural South African context. *South African Journal of Industrial Psychology, 30(4)*, 8–15.

Foxcroft, C. D. & Davies, C. (2008). Historical perspectives on psychometric testing in South Africa. In C. van Ommen & D. Painter (Eds), *Interiors: A History of Psychology in South Africa* (pp. 152–182). Pretoria: Unisa Press.

Foxcroft, C., Paterson, H., Le Roux, N. & Herbst, D. (2004). *Psychological Assessment in South Africa: A Needs Analysis. The Test Use Patterns and Needs of Psychological Assessment Practitioners*. Pretoria: Human Sciences Research Council.

Franklin-Ross, D. (2009). Exploring language bias in the NEO-PI-R. Unpublished Master's dissertation. University of the Witwatersrand, Johannesburg.

Gardner, H. (1993). *Multiple Intelligences: The Theory in Practice*. New York, NY: Basic Books.

Hamamura, T., Heine, S. J. & Paulhus, D. L. (2008). Cultural differences in response styles: The role of dialectical thinking. *Personality and Individual Differences, 44*, 932–942.

Heuchert, J. W. P., Parker, W. D., Stumpf, H. & Myburgh, C. P. H. (2000). The Five-Factor Model of personality in South African college students. *American Behavioral Scientist, 44*, 112–125.

Horn, B. S. (2000). A Xhosa translation of the revised Neo Personality Inventory: A pilot study. Unpublished Master's dissertation. University of Port Elizabeth, Port Elizabeth.

HPCSA (Health Professions Council of South Africa) (2010). *The Professional Board for Psychology: Training and Examination Guidelines for Psychometrists*. Retrieved June 15, 2012, from http://www.hpcsa.co.za/downloads/psycho_policy/form_94.pdf.

Laher, S. (2008). Structural equivalence and the NEO-PI-R: Implications for the applicability of the Five Factor Model of personality in an African context. *South African Journal of Industrial Psychology, 34(1)*, 76–80.

Laher, S. (2010). Personality theory and assessment research in South Africa: A review. Paper presented at the 16th South African Psychology Congress. International Convention Centre, Durban, August 3–6.

Laher, S. (2011). The applicability of the NEO-PI-R and the CPAI-2 in South Africa. Unpublished PhD dissertation. University of the Witwatersrand, Johannesburg.

Laungani, P. (1999). Cultural influences on identity and behaviour: India and Britain. In Y. T. Lee, C. R. McCauley & J. G. Draguns (Eds), *Personality and Person Perception across Cultures* (pp. 191–212). Mahwah, NJ: Lawrence Erlbaum Associates.

Leibrandt, M., Woolard, I., Finn, A. & Argent, J. (2010). *Trends in South African Income Distribution and Poverty since the Fall of Apartheid*. OECD Social, Employment and Migration Working Papers, No. 101. Paris: Organisation for Economic Cooperation and Development.

Maree, K. (2007). *Shaping the Story: A Guide to Facilitating Narrative Counselling*. Pretoria: Van Schaik.

Mbeki, T. (2003). The second economy, what it is and what is needed to meet the growth and development challenges it presents. Address of the President to the National Council of Provinces (NCOP). Retrieved December 7, 2009, from http://www.info.gov.za/speeches/2003/03111115461004.htm.

McCrae, R. R., Costa, P. T., Jr & Martin, T. A. (2005). The NEO-PI-3: A more readable revised NEO Personality Inventory. *Journal of Personality Assessment, 84*, 261–270.

McCrae, R. R., Terracciano, A. & 79 members of the Personality Profiles of Cultures Project. (2005a). Universal features of personality traits from the observer's perspective: Data from 50 cultures. *Journal of Personality and Social Psychology, 88*, 547–561.

McCrae, R. R., Terracciano, A. & 78 members of the Personality Profiles of Cultures Project. (2005b). Personality profiles of cultures: Aggregate personality traits. *Journal of Personality and Social Psychology, 89*, 407–425.

Meiring, D. (2006). *South African Personality Inventory Project*. Retrieved October 11, 2007, from http://www.meiringd.co.za/sapi.htm.

Meiring, D. (2010). The SAPI in South Africa. Paper presented at the Annual Congress of the Society for Industrial/Organisational Psychology in South Africa. The Forum Campus, Bryanston, Johannesburg, July 29–30.

Meiring, D., Van de Vijver, F. J. R. & Rothmann, S. R. (2006). Bias in an adapted version of the 15FQ+ questionnaire in South Africa. *South African Journal of Psychology, 36(2)*, 340–356.

Moerdyk, A. (2009). *The Principles and Practice of Psychological Assessment*. Pretoria: Van Schaik.

Nel, J. A. (2008). Uncovering personality dimensions in eleven different language groups in South Africa: An exploratory study. Unpublished PhD dissertation. University of the North-West, Potchefstroom.

Nell, V. (1994). Interpretation and misinterpretation of the South African Wechsler-Bellevue Adult Intelligence Scale: A history and a prospectus. *South African Journal of Psychology, 24(2), 100–109.*

Okeke, B. I., Draguns, J. G., Sheku, B. & Allen, W. (1999). Culture, self and personality in Africa. In Y. T. Lee, C. R. McCauley & J. G. Draguns (Eds), *Personality and Person Perception across Cultures* (pp. 139–162). Mahwah, NJ: Lawrence Erlbaum Associates.

Pervin, L. A. (1999). The cross-cultural challenge to personality. In Y. T. Lee, C. R. McCauley & J. G. Draguns (Eds), *Personality and Person Perception across Cultures* (pp. 23–44). Mahwah, NJ: Lawrence Erlbaum Associates.

Philip, K. & Hassen, E. (2008). *The Review of the Second Economy Programmes: An Overview for the Presidency's 15-Year Review.* Pretoria: Trade and Industrial Policy Secretariat.

Piedmont, R. L., Bain, E., McCrae, R. R. & Costa, P. T., Jr (2002). The applicability of the Five-Factor Model in a sub-Saharan culture: The NEO-PI-R in Shona. In R. R. McCrae & J. Allik (Eds), *The Five-Factor Model of Personality across Cultures* (pp. 155–174). New York, NY: Kluwer Academic.

The Presidency (2007). *Towards a Fifteen-Year Review.* Pretoria: Government Communication and Information Service.

Project Literacy (2010). *Project Literacy: Leaders in Adult Learning.* Retrieved July 3, 2010, from http://www.projectliteracy.org.za/.

Rossier, J., Dahourou, D. & McCrae, R. R. (2005). Structural and mean level analyses of the Five-Factor Model and locus of control: Further evidence from Africa. *Journal of Cross-Cultural Psychology, 36,* 227–246.

Seekings, J. & Nattrass, N. (2006). *Class, Race, and Inequality in South Africa.* Pietermaritzburg: University of KwaZulu-Natal Press.

Shuttleworth-Jordan, A. B. (1996). On not re-inventing the wheel: A clinical perspective on culturally relevant test usage in South Africa. *South African Journal of Psychology, 26(2),* 96–102.

Skinner, C. & Valodia, I. (2006). Two economies: Mistaken idea. *South African Labour Bulletin, 30,* 57–60.

Statistics South Africa (2001). *Census 2001.* Retrieved May 21, 2010, from http://www.statsa.gov.za/publications/populationstats.asp.

Stead, G. B. & Watson, M. B. (2006). *Career Psychology in the South African Context* (2nd edition). Pretoria: Van Schaik.

Taylor, I. A. (2000). The construct comparability of the NEO-PI-R questionnaire for black and white employees. Unpublished PhD dissertation. University of the Free State, Bloemfontein.

Taylor, N. (2004). The construction of a South African five-factor personality questionnaire. Unpublished Master's dissertation. Rand Afrikaans University, Johannesburg.

Taylor, N. & De Bruin, G. P. (2006). *Basic Traits Inventory: Technical Manual.* Johannesburg: Jopie van Rooyen & Partners.

Van der Berg, S., Burger, R. & Louw, M. (2010). Post-apartheid South Africa: Poverty and distribution. In M. Nissanke & E. Thorbecke (Eds), *Trends in an Era of Globalization: The Poor under Globalization in Africa, Asia, and Latin America.* Oxford: Oxford University Press.

Van de Vijver, F. J. R. & Phalet, K. (2004). Assessment in multicultural groups: The role of acculturation. *Applied Psychology: An International Review, 53,* 215–236.

Van de Vijver, F. & Rothmann, S. (2004). Assessment in multicultural groups: The South African case. *South African Journal of Industrial Psychology, 30,* 1–7.

Van Eeden, R. & Mantsha, T. (2007). Theoretical and methodological considerations in the translation of the 16PF5 into an African language. *South African Journal of Psychology, 37(1),* 62–81.

Vogt, L. & Laher, S. (2009). The relationship between individualism/collectivism and the Five Factor Model of personality: An exploratory study. *Psychology in Society, 37,* 39–54.

Contributors

Sumaya Laher (PhD) is an associate professor in the Department of Psychology, University of the Witwatersrand. Her research interests are in the fields of psychological assessment, particularly personality theory and assessment, cross-cultural issues in relation to mental health and illness and the interface between religion and psychology.

Kate Cockcroft (PhD) is an associate professor in the Department of Psychology at the University of the Witwatersrand. She conducts research in the field of developmental cognitive psychology, particularly intelligence, memory and language, as well as cognitive assessment in the South African context.

Zaytoon Amod (PhD) is a senior lecturer in the Department of Psychology at the University of the Witwatersrand. Her research interests include psycho-educational assessment within the South African context, the promotion of preventative mental health programmes and holistic methods of assisting individuals to achieve their cognitive and socio-emotional potential.

Katherine Bain (PhD) currently works as a clinical psychologist and lecturer at the University of the Witwatersrand. Her research interests are currently focused in the area of attachment, the interface between attachment and culture, and parent-infant psychotherapy.

Fatima Bhabha is an associate and head of both the Psychometric Advisory Services and Bureau Departments at Jopie van Rooyen & Partners (JvR). She is a certified trainer on the Myers-Briggs Type Indicator (MBTI) Certification Programme in sub-Saharan Africa.

Marita Brink (PhD) is a clinical psychologist in private practice. She supervises the work of qualified psychologists and facilitates workshops for professionals and students at the University of Johannesburg and North-West University. She has been doing Rorschach training on a basic and an advanced level since 1974.

Nicoleen Coetzee (PhD) is a lecturer in the Department of Psychology at the University of Pretoria. Her research interests include the development and standardisation of psychological instruments, particularly instruments that could be used when conducting trans-disciplinary research in the South African context.

Marié de Beer (PhD) is a professor in the Department of Industrial and Organisational Psychology at the University of South Africa. She has been involved in psychological test development and validation research for more than 20 years. She developed the Learning Potential Computerised Adaptive Test (LPCAT), which measures learning potential.

Gideon de Bruin (D.Litt. et Phil, Psychology) is a professor and head of the Department of Industrial Psychology and People Management at the University of Johannesburg. His research focuses on cross-cultural psychological assessment, with a particular emphasis on personality, career development and work-related stress.

Diana de Sousa is currently completing her PhD in the area of learning disabilities. Her research interests include literacy skills in primary school learners, language acquisition, reading, spelling, and remediation of learning difficulties in young monolingual and bilingual children.

Fiona Donald (PhD) is a senior lecturer in the Department of Psychology at the University of the Witwatersrand. She has extensive experience in researching and implementing assessment in organisations in southern Africa.

David Edwards (PhD) is a professor in the Department of Psychology at Rhodes University where he conducts and supervises case study research on psychotherapy. He runs a clinical practice, as well as a professional training programme in schematherapy, designed for challenging cases that do not respond to short-term interventions.

Emma-Kate Gaylard practises as a clinical psychologist in Johannesburg, focusing on child assessment and psychotherapy. She runs a company called Child Matters that arranges professional development workshops focusing on emotional and learning disorders in childhood and adolescence.

Renate Gericke is a clinical psychologist and lecturer at the University of the Witwatersrand. Her research interests include the mother–child attachment relationship, epistemological convergences and divergences between attachment theory and psychoanalytic theory and developmental presentations of pathology in children.

Kirston Greenop (PhD) is a research psychologist who specialises in the areas of cognitive psychology, neuropsychology and research methods. She currently works in the private sector, researching strategic socio-economic issues of relevance to business.

Deidre Heafield is a registered educational psychologist working in private practice. Her interests include cognitive and developmental assessment, as well as therapeutic work with children with a range of learning disabilities.

Lorna Jacklin (PhD) is an adjunct professor of paediatrics in the Faculty of Health Sciences, University of the Witwatersrand, and principal consultant paediatrician at the Charlotte Maxeke Johannesburg Academic Hospital. A certified neurodevelopmental specialist with a wide range of interests including autism and child abuse, she is also a registered trainer in the use of the Griffiths scales of mental development.

Tina Joubert is a registered industrial psychologist and senior research consultant with SHL South Africa. She is involved in research in the field of personality as well as cognitive assessment in the South African context. Her latest area of interest lies in the cross-cultural transportability of bio-data measures in the South African context.

Anil Kanjee (PhD) is a research professor and coordinator of the postgraduate programme in the Department of Educational Studies, Tshwane University of Technology. His research focuses on assessment for learning approaches in schools and universities, reporting and using assessment results, item response theory and data analysis, and the application of ICTs for teacher professional development.

Kathy Knott is a director at Jopie van Rooyen & Partners (JvR). She is a counselling psychologist and a certified trainer on a number of tools, specifically the Myers-Briggs Type Indicator (MBTI) Certification Programme, in sub-Saharan Africa. She manages the South African range of assessments at JvR.

Marilyn Lucas (PhD) is a professor and holds the Chair of Neuropsychology/Cognitive Neuropsychology at the University of the Witwatersrand. She is particularly interested in the clinical practice of neuropsychology, including assessment and rehabilitation.

Mary McMahon (PhD) is a senior lecturer in the School of Education at the University of Queensland. She researches and publishes in a range of career development methods and is particularly interested in developing practical applications of systemic and narrative approaches for use by adolescents, parents and practitioners.

Karen Milner (PhD) is an associate professor in Industrial/Organisational Psychology at the University of the Witwatersrand. Her research focuses on workplace health promotion.

Yvonne Oosthuizen is a psychometrist who has worked for Jopie van Rooyen & Partners (JvR) for the past five years. Currently she heads up the Human Resources Department at the JvR Group.

Ruksana Osman (PhD) is a full professor and head of the School of Education, and convener of the UNESCO Chair in Teacher Education for Diversity and Development at the University of the Witwatersrand. Her research has focused on equity and access to learning in higher education. Within this broad framework, she has researched the assessment and recognition of prior learning in teacher education and higher education.

Rabia Patel is a lecturer in the Department of Psychology at Rhodes University. Her research interests include developmental and mental health issues related to children, adolescents and adults living with HIV. She is also involved in employee wellness issues.

Cas Prinsloo (D Litt et Phil, Psychology) is a chief research specialist with the Human Sciences Research Council. He studies language and literacy acquisition and development among primary school learners from the perspectives of psycholinguistics and cognitive neuropsychology. He was involved in adapting and standardising versions of the Sixteen Personality Factor Questionnaire for South African use.

Sarah Radloff (PhD) is a professor in the Department of Statistics at Rhodes University. Her fields of specialisation are applied statistics, multivariate data analysis, generalised linear models, and econometrics.

Jessica Rice is currently completing a Masters degree in Neuropsychology. Her research interests are in the field of traumatic brain injury, emotion-based decision-making, manganism toxicity, cross-language transfer of spelling strategies, phonological awareness in learning to spell, as well as simultaneous and sequential cognitive processing in monolingual and bilingual children.

Joseph Seabi is a registered educational psychologist and a lecturer in the Department of Psychology at the University of the Witwatersrand. His research focusses on dynamic assessment, childhood psychopathology, career counselling, academic under-preparedness of first year students, and environmental health psychology.

Ann Shuttleworth-Edwards is professor emerita and full professor on a research contract in association with the Psychology Department at Rhodes University. Her research interests include brain dysfunction in association with participation in contact sports, and the collection of normative data for commonly employed cognitive tests.

Nicola Taylor (PhD) is an associate and the head of the Research Department at Jopie van Rooyen & Partners (JvR). Her research focus is on cross-cultural psychological assessment, particularly within the fields of personality and cognitive ability assessment, test construction, and the validation of psychometric assessments in the South African context.

Terence Taylor (D Litt et Phil) is the owner of Aprolab. The company creates and markets psychometric instruments and training programmes. He has been involved in test construction and cognitive research throughout his career and over the past two decades has focused on the assessment of learning potential and the development of critical thinking capabilities.

Andrew Thatcher (PhD) is a professor and Chair of Industrial/Organisational Psychology at the University of the Witwatersrand. He conducts research in the field of technology use and technology adoption focusing on technology adoption in under-resourced areas and the adoption and use of 'green' technologies.

Linda Theron (DEd) is a professor in the School of Education Sciences at North-West University. She is a qualitative researcher and her research and publishing are committed to understanding why and how some South African youth resile. She is the principal South African investigator in the five country 'Pathways to Resilience' study, led by Michael Ungar.

Nanette Tredoux is the director of Psytech, South Africa. She is also a board member on the Professional Board for Psychology at the HPCSA. Her research interests are in psychological assessment and she has written on various tests, issues of ethics in assessment and computerised assessment.

Adele van der Merwe is a counselling psychologist who completed cross-cultural research on the WISC-IV as part of her Masters degree at Rhodes University. She conducts both psychotherapy and assessment in her private practice.

Rene van Eeden (PhD) is an associate professor in the Department of Psychology at the University of South Africa. She has been involved in the development and cross-cultural validation of cognitive and personality measures for use in the South African context. Her publications include work on personality assessment in an organisational context, as well as on leadership and organisational dynamics.

Phia van Tonder is a clinical psychologist who completed cross-cultural research on the WISC-IV as part of her Masters degree at Rhodes University in Grahamstown, South Africa. She is currently working at the Forensic Unit for the Eastern Cape Department of Health.

Nadene Venter is a registered industrial psychologist and the managing director at SHL South Africa. She is a regular contributor at both scientific and professional events on various topics including talent acquisition and development, innovations in assessment, and strategic talent management and serves on the Executive for the Society for Industrial & Organisational Psychology in South Africa (SIOPSA).

Mark Watson is a professor in the Psychology Department of the Nelson Mandela Metropolitan University. He specialises, researches and practises in career, school and adolescent psychology and has published extensively in international journals. He has also contributed chapters to international career texts, and is on the editorial advisory board of several international career journals.

Victoria Whitefield-Alexander (PhD) is a counselling and research psychologist affiliated to the Crescent Clinic in Kenilworth, Cape Town. As clinician and researcher, she works closely in association with the Rhodes University National Sports Concussion Initiative (NSCI) and is co-director of ImPACT Applications South Africa.

Charles Young (DCounsPsych) is a senior lecturer and academic coordinator of the Professional Programmes in Clinical and Counselling Psychology at Rhodes University. His research interests include issues of student mental health and well-being and the application of cognitive psychotherapies in South African contexts.

Index

B

C

M

N